COGNITIVE APPROACHES TO OBSESSIONS AND COMPULSIONS
THEORY, ASSESSMENT, AND TREATMENT

COGNITIVE APPROACHES TO OBSESSIONS AND COMPULSIONS
THEORY, ASSESSMENT, AND TREATMENT

EDITED BY

RANDY O. FROST
Department of Psychology, Smith College, Northampton, MA, USA

GAIL STEKETEE
School of Social Work, Boston University, Boston, MA, USA

2002

Pergamon
An Imprint of Elsevier Science

Amsterdam – Boston – London – New York – Oxford – Paris
San Diego – San Francisco – Singapore – Sydney – Tokyo

ELSEVIER SCIENCE Ltd
The Boulevard, Langford Lane
Kidlington, Oxford OX5 1GB, UK

First edition 2002

Library of Congress Cataloging in Publication Data
A catalog record from the Library of Congress has been applied for.

British Library Cataloguing in Publication Data
A catalogue record from the British Library has been applied for.

ISBN 0-08-043410-X

♾ The paper used in this publication meets the requirements of ANSI/NISO Z39.48-1992 (Permanence of Paper).
Printed in The Netherlands.

Contents

Section E: Therapy Effects on Cognition

Appendices

Contributors

Nader Amir

Department of Psychology, University of Georgia, Athens, Georgia, USA

Martin M. Antony

Anxiety Treatment and Research Centre, St. Joseph's Healthcare, Hamilton, Ontario, Canada

Martine Bouvard

Unité de Traitment de l'Anxiété, Hôpital Neurologique et Neuro-Chirurgical, Lyon, France

John E. Calamari

Finch University of Health Services/The Chicago Medical School, North Chicago, Illinois, USA

Cheryl N. Carmin

Department of Psychiatry, University of Illinois-Chicago, Chicago, Illinois, USA

David A. Clark

Department of Psychology, University of New Brunswick, Fredericton, New Brunswick, Canada

Davide Coradeschi

Department of General Psychology, University of Padova, Padova, Italy

Teresa M. Deer

Finch University of Health Services/The Chicago Medical School, North Chicago, Illinois, USA

Stella Dorz

Department of General Psychology, University of Padova, Padova, Italy

Paul M. G. Emmelkamp

Department of Clinical Psychology, University of Amsterdam, Amsterdam, The Netherlands

Elizabeth Forrester

Department of Psychology, Institute of Psychiatry, De Crespigny Park, Denmark Hill, London, UK

Randy O. Frost

Department of Psychology, Smith College, Northampton, Massachusetts, USA

Beth S. Gershuny

OCD Clinic, Massachusetts General Hospital-East, Charleston, Massachusetts, USA

Amy S. Janeck   Department of Psychology, University of British Columbia, Vancouver, British Columbia, Canada

Michael J. Kozak   Center for Scientific Review, National Institute of Mental Health, Bethesda, Maryland, USA

Michael Kyrios   Department of Psychology, University of Melbourne, Victoria, Australia

John S. March   Departments of Psychiatry and Psychology: Social and Health Sciences, Duke University Medical Center, Durham, North Carolina, USA

Dean McKay   Department of Psychology, Fordham University, New York, USA

Peter D. McLean   University of British Columbia Hospital and University of British Columbia, Vancouver, British Columbia, Canada

Fugen Neziroglu   Bio-Behavioral Institute, Great Neck, New York, USA

Caterina Novara   Department of General Psychology, University of Padova, Padova, Italy

Sophie Oh   Department of Psychology, University of Melbourne, Victoria, Australia

Gilbert Pinard   Department of Psychiatry, McGill University, Montreal, Quebec, Canada

C. Alec Pollard   Saint Louis Behavioral Medicine Institute, Louis, Missouri, USA

Christine Purdon   Department of Psychology, University of Waterloo, Waterloo, Ontario, Canada

Josée Rhéaume   Hotel-Dieu de Levis Hospital, Levis, Quebec, Canada

John H. Riskind   Department of Psychology, George Mason University, Fairfax, Virginia, USA

Paul Salkovskis   Department of Psychology, Institute of Psychiatry, De Crespigny Park, Denmark Hill, London, UK

Ezio Sanavio   Department of General Psychology, University of Padova, Padova, Italy

Roz Shafran   Department of Psychiatry, Oxford University, Warneford Hospital, Oxford, UK

Kenneth J. Sher   Department of Psychology, University of Missouri-Columbia, Columbia, Missouri, USA

Claudio Sica   Department of General Psychology, University of Padova, Padova, Italy

Gregoris Simos   Community Mental Health Center and Department of Psychiatry, Aristotelian University of Thessaloniki, Thessaloniki, Greece

Ingrid Söchting   Department of Psychiatry, Richmond Hospital, Richmond, British Columbia, Canada

Debbie Sookman   Department of Psychology, McGill University Health Centre (RVH), Montreal, Quebec, Canada

Gail Steketee   School of Social Work, Boston University, Boston, Massachusetts, USA

Kevin P. Stevens   Bio-Behavioral Institute, Great Neck, New York, USA

Steven Taylor   Department of Psychiatry, University of British Columbia, Vancouver, British Columbia, Canada

Dana S. Thordarson   Department of Psychiatry, University of British Columbia, Vancouver, British Columbia, Canada

Anton J.L.M. van Balkom   Department of Psychiatry and Institute for Research in Extramural Medicine, Vrije Universiteit, Amsterdam, The Netherlands

Patricia van Oppen   Department of Psychiatry and Institute for Research in Extramural Medicine, Vrije Universiteit, Amsterdam, The Netherlands

Ricks Warren   Pacific University, Portland, Oregon, USA

Maureen L. Whittal   Anxiety Disorder Unit, University of British Columbia Hospital and University of British Columbia, Vancouver, British Columbia, Canada

Pamela S. Wiegartz	Department of Psychiatry, University of Illinois-Chicago, Chicago, Illinois, USA
Sabine Wilhelm	OCD Clinic, Massachusetts General Hospital-East, Charleston, Massachusetts, USA
Nathan L. Williams	Department of Psychology, George Mason University, Fairfax, Virginia, USA
Kimberly Wilson	OCD Clinic, Massachusetts General Hospital-East, Charleston, Massachusetts, USA
Jose A. Yaryura-Tobias	Bio-Behavioral Institute, Great Neck, New York, USA

Preface

Formed in 1996, the Obsessive Compulsive Cognitions Working Group (OCCWG) is an active international consortium of clinical researchers who are dedicated to the study of cognitive aspects of obsessive compulsive disorder (OCD). This group grew out of strong collegial interests in understanding and accurately assessing cognitive aspects of OCD. Now with more than 40 members from nine countries, the OCCWG has been very successful in generating methods for assessing cognitive interpretations and beliefs associated with OCD and testing these in large samples of participants.

This book represents a concerted effort on the part of OCCWG members and their collaborators. Chapters in this volume articulate cognitive theoretical models, assessment of cognitions and cognitive aspects of treatments for OCD and related disorders. These chapters represent the most recent theoretical understanding and research findings about cognition and OCD.

The first chapter by Dr. Steven Taylor sets the stage for this volume by providing some background on the interest in cognitive theory regarding obsessive compulsive disorder (OCD), and history about the development of the research group that is responsible for all of the chapters in this book. A final chapter includes our own musings about the research findings in this book and where we believe more research is needed and might lead us. In between are 23 chapters divided into five sections covering the following topics: domains of beliefs in OCD, measurement of cognition, cognitive aspects of disorders related to OCD, cognitive aspects of special populations with OCD, and cognitive aspects of therapy. Each chapter was written by experts and reviewed carefully by section editors who are also members of the OCCWG. Commentaries by senior researchers in these areas follow each section of the book. We believe the result is a remarkably comprehensive picture of cognitive aspects of OCD as they are understood at the present time.

Research is moving rapidly in this field, and we expect to find that a considerable amount of important new knowledge will be produced on cognition and OCD in the coming years. Each chapter offers new questions and ideas and strategies for pursuing them. We will be very satisfied if this volume helps shape new directions in research on cognitive aspects of OCD.

We would like to thank the members of the Obsessive Compulsive Cognitions Working Group for their tireless devotion to the study of cognition in obsessive compulsive disorder and for their work on writing and editing the chapters in this volume. We also thank the many OCD patients who have contributed to the research enterprise of the Working Group in research laboratories throughout the world. Finally, we would like to thank Ashley Bowers for her help in proofreading and pulling together the final stages of this volume.

Gail Steketee
Randy Frost

Chapter 1

Cognition in Obsessive Compulsive Disorder: An Overview

Steven Taylor

Introduction

Obsessive compulsive disorder (OCD) is among the most common anxiety disorders, with a lifetime prevalence of approximately 2.3 percent (Weissman *et al.*, 1994). It often begins in adolescence or early adulthood, usually with a gradual onset (American Psychiatric Association [APA], 2000). The disorder tends to be chronic if untreated, with symptoms waxing and waning in severity, often in response to stressful life events (Rasmussen & Eisen, 1992). OCD is characterized by clinically significant obsessions, compulsions, or both. Obsessions are intrusive and distressing thoughts, images, or impulses. Common examples of obsessions include intrusive thoughts of being contaminated, recurrent doubts that one has not turned off the stove, and disturbing thoughts of harming loved ones. Compulsions are repetitive, intentional behaviors that the person feels compelled to perform, often with a desire to resist. Compulsions are typically intended to avert some feared event or to reduce distress. They may be performed in response to an obsession, such as repetitive hand-washing in response to obsessions about contamination. Alternatively, compulsions may be performed in accordance to certain rules, such as checking three times that the stove is switched off before leaving the house. Compulsions can be overt (e.g., cleaning) or covert (e.g., thinking a "good" thought to undo or replace a "bad" thought). Compulsions are excessive or not rationally connected to what they are intended to prevent.

OCD is commonly comorbid with other disorders, such as other anxiety disorders, mood disorders, eating disorders, and substance use disorders (APA, 2000). The degree of insight associated with OCD varies within and between individuals (Kozak & Foa, 1994). Insight refers to the degree that sufferers recognize that their obsessions and compulsions are unreasonable and due to a psychiatric disorder. Insight varies along a continuum, ranging from good to extremely poor insight. In their calmer moments, OCD sufferers with good insight are able to recognize, for example, that their concerns with contamination are excessive, or that repeated checking of door locks is unnecessary. OCD sufferers with extremely poor insight believe their obsessions and compulsions are entirely reasonable and appropriate. In terms of DSM-IV, the latter people would be diagnosed as having OCD comorbid with either Delusional Disorder or Psychotic Disorder Not Otherwise Specified

(APA, 2000). An OCD sufferer's insight may change over time, and so comorbid diagnoses may change accordingly.

Obsessions and compulsions, of insufficient severity to meet DSM-IV criteria for OCD, are common in the general population (Frost & Gross, 1993; Frost, Sher, & Geen, 1986; Frost & Shows, 1993; Rachman & de Silva, 1978; Salkovskis & Harrison, 1984). Compared to clinical obsessions, those found in the general population — so-called *normal obsessions* — tend to be less frequent, shorter in duration, and associated with less distress (Rachman & de Silva, 1978; Salkovskis & Harrison, 1984). Normal and clinical obsessions and compulsions share common themes such as violence, contamination, and doubt (Rachman & de Silva, 1978; Salkovskis & Harrison, 1984). Normal and clinical compulsions also have common themes (e.g., repetitive checking of locks and switches). These similarities suggest that the study of normal obsessions and compulsions may shed light on the mechanisms of OCD.

With regard to the treatment of OCD, serotonergic pharmacotherapies (e.g., clomipramine, fluvoxamine) and behavior therapy (exposure plus response prevention) are both effective in reducing OC symptoms (van Balkom *et al.*, 1994) and both normalize activity in brain structures implicated in OCD such as the right caudate nucleus (Baxter *et al.*, 1992). Exposure and response prevention involves exposing patients to distressing but harmless stimuli (e.g., touching a "contaminated" object such as a trash can), and then helping patients prevent themselves from engaging in compulsions (e.g., refraining from hand-washing; for details see Steketee, 1993). Exposure and response prevention and pharmacotherapies are equally effective, although there is ample room for improving both interventions. Some patients are unable or unwilling to complete these therapies, while other patients show limited improvement despite adequate adherence. Still others display treatment gains in the short term, only to relapse later on. Combining behavioral and pharmacological treatments has produced disappointing results, with most studies finding combined treatments to be no better than behavior therapy alone (O'Connor, Todorov, Robillard, Borgeat, & Brault, 1999; Hohagen *et al.*, 1998; Kobak, Greist, Jefferson, Katzelnick, & Henk, 1998; van Balkom & van Dyck, 1998; van Balkom *et al.*, 1994, 1998).

Advances in understanding the causes of OCD may lead to improved treatments. The repetitiveness and fixedness of obsessions and compulsions suggests that cognitive factors play an important role (Rachman & Hodgson, 1980). The remainder of this introductory chapter will present an overview of theoretical approaches to OCD, with an emphasis on cognitive approaches and their implications for treatment. This is followed by a review of the remaining sections in this volume, which extend in various ways the analysis of cognition in OCD.

Theoretical Approaches

There are many psychological and biological theories of OCD. Most theories offer only sketches of putative mechanisms without providing details of psychopathological processes (see Jakes, 1996, for a detailed critique). Few theories have been subject to extensive empirical evaluation. Some theories account for only a subset of OC phenomena, while others fail to account for the widespread occurrence of OC-like phenomena in the general population (e.g., normal obsessions). Among the most prominent theoretical approaches are conditioning models and cognitive models.

Conditioning Models

Conditioning models (e.g., Rachman & Hodgson, 1980; Teasdale, 1974) are based on the notion that fears are acquired by classical conditioning and maintained by operant conditioning. The latter consists of learned avoidance or escape responses. A person with washing compulsions, for example, may have a conditioned fear of contamination. Avoidance and escape from "contaminated" stimuli (e.g., public washrooms) persists because they result in the absence or reduction of distress. Avoidance and escape prevents the fear from being extinguished, thereby maintaining OCD. Conditioning models proved valuable because they led to treatment involving exposure and response prevention, one of the most effective interventions for OCD.

Despite their strengths, conditioning models have several important limitations. Although they account for compulsions, they do not adequately explain the causes of obsessions, and fail to explain why compulsions are so persistent and repetitive (Gray, 1982). Conditioning models also fail to account for the fact that people with OCD display a broad range of insight into the reasonableness of their obsessions and compulsions, and any given person's insight can fluctuate over time and circumstance.

Cognitive Approaches

Several cognitive models have been proposed. They fall into two broad classes: those proposing that OCD is due to some dysfunction in cognitive processing, and those postulating specific dysfunctional beliefs as causes of obsessions and compulsions.

Dysfunctions in General Cognitive Processes. Several studies have found that people with OCD, compared to people without the disorder, often have poorer performance on neuropsychological measures such as tests of executive functioning (planning, reasoning, set shifting) and memory (e.g., Alarcón, Libb, & Boll, 1994; Mataix-Cols *et al.*, 1999; Purcell, Maruff, Kyrios, & Pantelis, 1998; Savage *et al.*, 2000; Schmidke, Schorb, Winkelmann, & Hohagen, 1998). Such deficits are not found in all patients, and even when present they tend to be mild. Nevertheless, the findings led some theorists to suggest that OCD arises from aberrations in general information processing systems (e.g., Pitman, 1987; Reed, 1985), possibly due to dysregulated neural circuitry (e.g., Otto, 1990). The deficits are general in the sense that they affect all information that is processed, including information related to the person's obsessional concerns (e.g., contamination stimuli) and affectively neutral information.

Reed's (1985) cognitive–structural model is an example of this class of models. Reed proposed that OCD arises from the failure to spontaneously structure one's experiences (and memories), which leads to a compensatory over-structuring. Thus, people with OCD are said to have difficulty categorizing their experiences, which leads to doubting, indecision, rumination, and particular compulsions such as checking rituals. There are several important limitations to this model. Among the most important is that it lacks motivation (Jakes, 1996). Why should it matter to a person if he or she is unable to spontaneously structure his or her experiences? Why should this provoke distress and compulsive rituals?

More generally, there are four major problems with the dysfunctional processing models. First, it is not clear whether the poor performance on neuropsychological tests is a cause or consequence of OCD. Second, the models do not account for the heterogeneity of OCD symptoms; why does one person develop checking compulsions while another develops hoarding rituals? Third, the models do not account for the fact that mild neuropsychological deficits have been found in many disorders, including panic disorder, social phobia, posttraumatic stress disorder, and bulimia nervosa (e.g., Alarcón *et al.*, 1994; Beckham, Crawford, & Feldman, 1998; Jones, Duncan, Brouwers, & Mirksy, 1991; Lucas, Telch, & Bigler, 1991; Vasterling, Brailey, Constans, & Sutker, 1998). Fourth, exposure and response prevention is an effective treatment for OCD, but this would not be predicted from these models. If dysfunctional processing plays any causal role in OCD, it is most likely to be a nonspecific vulnerability factor that is neither a necessary nor sufficient cause of obsessions and compulsions.

Cognitive Specificity and Dysfunctional Beliefs. Among the most promising contemporary models of OCD are those based on Beck's (1976) cognitive specificity hypothesis, which proposes that different types of psychopathology arise from different types of dysfunctional beliefs. Unipolar mood disorders, for example, are said to be associated with beliefs about loss, failure, and self-denigration (e.g., "I am a failure"). Various personality disorders are said to be characterized by distinct dysfunctional beliefs; e.g., dependent personality disorder is associated with beliefs like "I can function only if I have access to someone competent" (Beck, Freeman, & Associates, 1990). Social phobia is thought to be associated with beliefs about rejection or ridicule by others (Beck & Emery, 1985; e.g., "It's devastating to be criticized"). Panic disorder is said to be associated with beliefs about impending death, insanity, or loss of control (Beck, 1988; Clark, 1986; e.g., "My heart will stop if it beats too fast").

Several theorists have proposed that obsessions and compulsions arise from specific sorts of dysfunctional beliefs. Among the most sophisticated of these models is Salkovskis' cognitive–behavioral approach (e.g., Salkovskis, 1985, 1989, 1996). This and similar models form the theoretical foundation for much of the work described in this volume. Salkovskis' theory begins with the well-established finding that intrusions (i.e., thoughts, images, and impulses that intrude into consciousness) are experienced by most people. An important task for any theory is to explain why almost everyone experiences cognitive intrusions (at least at some point in their lives), yet only some people experience intrusions in the form of clinical obsessions (i.e., intrusions that are unwanted, distressing, and difficult to remove from consciousness).

Salkovskis argued that cognitive intrusions — whether wanted or unwanted — reflect the person's current concerns arising from an "idea generator" in the brain. The concerns are automatically triggered by internal or external reminders of those concerns. For example, intrusive thoughts of harming others may be triggered by encountering potentially dangerous objects (e.g., sharp kitchen knives). Salkovskis proposed that intrusions develop into obsessions only when intrusions are appraised as posing a threat for which the individual is personally responsible. To illustrate, consider the intrusive image of stabbing one's child. Most people experiencing such an intrusion would regard it as a meaningless cognitive event, with no harm-related implications ("mental flotsam"). Such an intrusion can develop into a clinical obsession if the person appraises it as having serious consequences for which he or she is personally responsible. That would happen if the person made an appraisal such as the following: "Having thoughts about stabbing my child means that I really want to hurt her — that means I'm a dangerous person who must take extra precautions to make sure I don't lose control." Such appraisals evoke distress and motivate the person to try to suppress or remove the unwanted intrusion (e.g., by replacing it with a "good" thought), and to attempt to prevent any harmful events associated with the intrusion (e.g., by removing all sharp objects from the house).

Compulsions (neutralizing behaviors) are conceptualized as efforts to remove intrusions and to prevent any perceived harmful consequences. Salkovskis advanced two main reasons why compulsions become persistent and excessive: (a) they are reinforced by immediate distress reduction and by temporary removal of the unwanted thought (negative reinforcement); and (b) they prevent the person from learning that their appraisals are unrealistic (e.g., the person fails to learn that unwanted harm-related thoughts do not lead to acts of harm). Compulsions influence the frequency of intrusions; compulsive rituals can become reminders of intrusions and thereby trigger reoccurrence of the latter. For example, compulsive hand-washing can remind the person that he or she may become contaminated. Attempts at distracting oneself from unwanted intrusions paradoxically increase the frequency of intrusions, possibly because the distracters become reminders (retrieval cues) of the intrusions. Compulsions can strengthen one's perceived responsibility. That is, the absence of the feared consequence after performing the compulsion reinforces the belief that the person is responsible for removing the threat.

Other factors also may influence the occurrence of intrusive thoughts. Mood-dependent recall is thought to influence the occurrence (accessibility) of intrusions and harm-related appraisals. Anxious mood is thought to increase the likelihood that intrusions will be triggered, whereas depressed or dysphoric mood is thought to increase the likelihood of harm-related appraisals.

To summarize, when a person appraises intrusions as posing a threat for which he or she is personally responsible, the person becomes distressed and attempts to remove the intrusions and prevent their perceived consequences. This increases the frequency of intrusions. Thus, intrusions become persistent and distressing. In other words, they escalate into clinical obsessions. Other factors, such as mood state-dependent recall also contribute to the occurrence of obsessions. Compulsions maintain the intrusions, and prevent the person from evaluating the accuracy of his or her appraisals.

Why do some people, but not others, make harm- and responsibility-related appraisals of their intrusive thoughts? Life experiences shape the basic assumptions we hold about ourselves and the world (Beck, 1976). Salkovskis (1985) proposed that assumptions about blame, responsibility, or control play an important role in OCD, as illustrated by beliefs such as "Having a bad thought about an action is the same as performing the action," and "Failing to prevent harm is the same as having caused the harm in the first place." These assumptions can be acquired from a strict moral or religious upbringing, or from other experiences that teach the person codes of conduct and responsibility (Salkovskis, Shafran, Rachman, & Freeston, 1999).

Strong beliefs in personal responsibility can occur in the general population (as a vulnerability factor for OCD), although people with OCD are expected to have the strongest of these beliefs. Other types of dysfunctional beliefs also may be important in OCD, including beliefs about the importance of one's thoughts, the importance of controlling thoughts, and perfectionism (Freeston, Rhéaume, & Ladouceur, 1996). Thus, contemporary cognitive–behavioral theories propose that particular types of dysfunctional beliefs play an important role in the etiology and maintenance of OCD, with responsibility beliefs being among the most important. Strength of these beliefs presumably influences the person's insight into his or her OCD. As research progresses we may be able to eventually discover the content-specific information processing biases (e.g., selective attention to contamination-related stimuli) associated with particular dysfunctional beliefs, and also identify the biological correlates of the cognitive mechanisms specified in Salkovskis' and related models (e.g., the neuroanatomic correlates of the idea generator).

These models have led to a promising new cognitive–behavioral therapy. As in traditional behavior therapy for OCD, it involves exposure and response prevention exercises. However, the exercises are framed as behavioral experiments to test appraisals and beliefs. To illustrate, consider a patient who has recurrent images of terrorist hijackings, and a compulsion to repeatedly telephone airports to warn them. This patient is found to hold a belief such as "Thinking about terrorist hijackings will make them actually occur." To challenge this belief, the patient and therapist can devise a test that pits this belief against a more realistic belief (e.g., "My thoughts have no influence on the occurrence of hijackings"). A behavioral experiment might involve deliberately bringing on thoughts of a hijacking and then evaluating the consequences. Methods derived from Beck's cognitive therapy (e.g., Beck & Emery, 1985) are also used to challenge OCD-related beliefs and appraisals.

Obsessive Compulsive Cognitions Working Group

The Obsessive Compulsive Cognitions Working Group (OCCWG) is an international group of investigators sharing a common interest in understanding the role of cognitive factors in OCD. Extending the work of Salkovskis and others, the group began by developing a consensus regarding the most important beliefs (and associated appraisals) in OCD (OCCWG, 1997). Responsibility beliefs and other belief domains were identified, as summarized in Table 1.1. Self-report inventories were developed to assess these domains, which can be used in research into the nature and treatment of OCD (OCCWG, 2001).

Eventually these scales may be used to assess patients' cognitive profiles in order to guide the optimal selection of interventions (Taylor, 1999). Consider, for example, the profiles for two hypothetical OCD patients in Figure 1.1. Patient A tends to overestimate threat, is intolerant of uncertainty, and has inflated responsibility. In other words, this patient is characterized by especially strong beliefs about the necessity of detecting and preventing harm from external sources. This patient suffers from compulsive checking

Table 1.1: Consensus from the Obsessive Compulsive Cognitions Working Group (1997): Important OCD-related Beliefs.

Belief domains	Definitions and examples
Over-importance of thoughts	Belief that the occurrence of a thought, image, or impulse implies something very important. Included in this domain are beliefs that reflect thought–action fusion. That is, beliefs that the mere presence of a "bad" thought can produce a "bad" outcome. Examples: "Having a bad thought is the same as doing a bad deed;" "Having violent thoughts means I will lose control and become violent."
Importance of controlling one's thoughts	Overvaluation of the importance of exerting complete control over intrusive thoughts, images, and impulses, and the belief that this is both possible and desirable. Examples: "I should be able to gain complete control of my mind if I exercise enough will power;" "I would be a better person if I gained control over my thoughts."
Perfectionism	Belief that: (1) there is a perfect solution to every problem; (2) that doing something perfectly is possible and necessary; and (3) that even minor mistakes have serious consequences. Examples: "It is important to keep working at something until its done just right;" "For me, failing partly is as bad as failing completely."
Inflated responsibility	Belief that one is especially powerful in producing and preventing personally important negative outcomes. These outcomes are perceived as essential to prevent. They may be actual, that is, having consequences in the real world, and/or at a moral level. Such beliefs may pertain to responsibility for doing something to prevent or undo harm, and responsibility for errors of omission and commission. Examples: "I often think I am responsible for things that go wrong;" "If I don't act when I foresee danger, I am to blame for any bad consequences."
Overestimation of threat	Beliefs indicating an exaggerated estimation of the probability or severity of harm. Examples: "I believe the world is a dangerous place"; "Small problems always seem to turn into big ones in my life."
Intolerance for uncertainty	This domain encompasses three types of beliefs: (1) beliefs about the necessity for being certain; (2) beliefs that one has a poor capacity to cope with unpredictable change; and (3) beliefs about the difficulty of adequate functioning in inherently ambiguous situations. Examples: "It is possible to be absolutely certain about the things I do if I try hard enough;" "I cannot tolerate uncertainty."

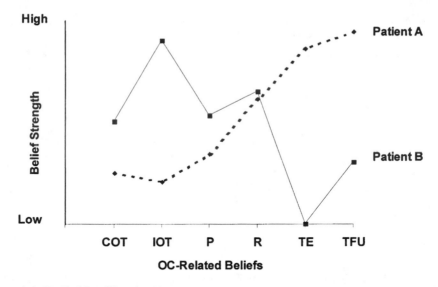

Figure 1.1: Belief Profiles for Two Hypothetical OCD Patients.
(COT = beliefs about the importance of controlling one's thoughts, IOT = overimportance of thoughts, P = perfectionism, R = inflated responsibility, TE = overestimation of threat, TFU = intolerance for uncertainty). Reprinted from S. Taylor (1999), 'Treatment of obsessive compulstive disorder: Progress, prospects, and problems.' *Cognitive and Behavioral Practice*, 6, 342–344. Reprinted with permission of the Association for Advancement of Behavior Therapy.

(e.g., checking the stove, electrical appliances, and door locks). Cognitive approaches to OCD suggest that these symptoms can be treated by restructuring the patient's beliefs about threat, uncertainty, and responsibility. Patient B presents with a different pattern of beliefs. This patient has especially strong beliefs in the over-importance of thoughts, and in the excessive need to control thoughts. The patient also is perfectionistic and has an inflated sense of personal responsibility. Patient B has harm-related obsessions. Cognitive–behavioral therapy for this patient would target beliefs about intrusive thoughts and responsibility as a means of treating the obsessions.

Overview of this Volume

The remainder of this volume describes the current state of progress of the OCCWG. The chapters are divided into several sections. Chapters in the first section contain detailed descriptions of the six cognitive domains and how they relate to one another, along with discussions of how these domains are related to OCD symptoms and other clinical problems. The second section focuses in more detail on the measurement of cognition in OCD. The section opens with a description of the development of the instruments to measure the six domains: the Obsessive Beliefs Questionnaire (OBQ) and the Interpretation of Intrusions Inventory (III) and a brief review of data on the reliability and validity of the current versions of these instruments. The remaining chapters broaden the focus to consider non-questionnaire methods of assessing OCD-related cognition, such as information-processing paradigms. The relationship between the domains and cognitive processing is discussed, and the nature of insight in OCD is considered.

The third section consists of chapters examining the role of cognition in OCD-spectrum and related disorders. The notion of spectrum disorders is a fuzzy concept, based primarily on the phenomenological similarity between OC symptoms and the symptoms of other disorders. For instance, in body dysmorphic disorder, obsessive fears focused on imagined physical defects bear many similarities to obsessive fears in OCD. Spectrum and related disorders are of interest because they may arise from mechanisms similar to those involved in OCD. Understanding the nature and treatment of the spectrum and related disorders therefore may shed light on the etiology and treatment OCD, and vice versa. The chapters in this section review body dysmorphic disorder, eating disorders, mood disorders, and psychotic disorders. The relationship between OCD and these disorders is described, including phenomenological and cognitive similarities and differences.

The fourth section examines the role of OCD cognitions and cognitive processes in various populations, including children, the elderly, subclinical OCD, and severe OCD. OCD cognitions across different cultures are also examined. The chapters describe the cognitive features in each population, including those features that distinguish one population from another. Assessment and treatment issues for each population are also discussed.

The final section focuses on the effects that therapies have on OCD symptoms and cognitions. If OCD is due, at least in part, to dysfunctional beliefs, then treatments that produce enduring reductions in OCD should produce corresponding cognitive changes. The chapters examine the cognitive and symptomatic effects of various therapies, including behavioral and cognitive–behavioral therapies, and pharmacotherapies. Related issues are also addressed, such as the effects of beliefs on treatment adherence.

The summary chapter draws the findings and conclusions of the various chapters together to consider future directions for theory, research, and treatment. Important issues include whether focusing on belief domains will actually lead to better understanding and treatment of OCD. Questions regarding the interrelation and origins of these domains are also considered. To facilitate future research, the OBQ and III are presented in appendices, along with their scoring keys.

Over the past few decades, great strides have been made in furthering our understanding of the nature and treatment of OCD. Much remains to be learned. The chapters in this volume highlight our contributions to understanding the role of cognition in this common and debilitating disorder. Although the chapters are authored by specific individuals, many of the ideas and conclusions are the result of discussions among the OCCWG members. It is notable that such a large group of experts, each with their own views and opinions, were able to work together in such a stimulating, productive fashion. This was made possible by the consummate coordination of the OCCWG chairs, Randy Frost and Gail Steketee.

References

Alarcón, R. D., Libb, J. W., & Boll, T. J. (1994). Neuropsychological testing in obsessive–compulsive disorder: a clinical review. *Journal of Neuropsychiatry and Clinical Neurosciences*, *6*, 217–228.

American Psychiatric Association. (2000). *Diagnostic and statistical manual of mental disorders* (4th ed., text revision). Washington, DC: Author.

van Balkom, A. J. L. M., & van Dyck, R. (1998). Combination treatments for obsessive–compulsive disorder. In R. P. Swinson, M. M. Antony, S. Rachman, & M. A. Richter (eds), *Obsessive–compulsive disorder: theory, research, and treatment* (pp. 349–366). New York: Guilford.

van Balkom, A., van Oppen, P., Vermeulen, A., van Dyck, R., Nauta, M., & Vorst, H. (1994). A meta-analysis on the treatment of obsessive compulsive disorder: a comparison of antidepressants, behavior, and cognitive therapy. *Clinical Psychology Review*, *14*, 359–381.

van Balkom, A. J. L. M., de Hann, E., van Oppen, P., Spinhoven, P., Hoogduin, K. A. L., & van Dyck, R. (1998). Cognitive and behavioral therapies alone versus in combination with fluvoxamine in the treatment of obsessive compulsive disorder. *Journal of Nervous and Mental Disease*, *186*, 492–499.

Baxter, L. R., Schwartz, J. M., Bergman, K. S., Szuba, M. P., Guze, B. H., Mazziotta, J. C., Alazraki, A., Selin, C. E., Ferng, H.-K., Munford, P., & Phelps, M. E. (1992). Caudate glucose metabolic rate changes with both drug and behavior therapy for obsessive–compulsive disorder. *Archives of General Psychiatry*, *49*, 681–689.

Beck, A. T. (1976). *Cognitive therapy and the emotional disorders*. New York: International Universities Press.

Beck, A. T. (1988). Cognitive approaches to panic disorder: theory and therapy. In S. Rachman & J. D. Maser (eds). *Panic: psychological perspectives* (pp. 91–109). Hillsdale, NJ: Erlbaum.

Beck, A. T., & Emery, G. (1985). *Anxiety disorders and phobias: a cognitive perspective*. New York: Basic Books.

Beck, A. T., Freeman, A., & Associates. (1990). *Cognitive therapy of personality disorders*. New York: Guilford.

Beckham, J. C., Crawford, A. L., & Feldman, M. E. (1998). Trail Making Test performance in Vietnam combat veterans with and without posttraumatic stress disorder. *Journal of Traumatic Stress*, *11*, 811–819.

Clark, D. M. (1986). A cognitive approach to panic. *Behaviour Research and Therapy*, *24*, 461–470.

Freeston, M. H., Rhéaume, J., & Ladouceur, R. (1996). Correcting faulty appraisals of obsessional thoughts. *Behaviour Research and Therapy*, *34*, 433–446.

Frost, R. O., & Gross, R. C. (1993). The hoarding of possessions. *Behaviour Research and Therapy*, *31*, 367–381.

Frost, R. O., Sher, K. J., & Geen, T. (1986). Psychopathology and personality characteristics of nonclinical compulsive checkers. *Behaviour Research and Therapy*, *24*, 133–143.

Frost, R. O., & Shows, D. L. (1993). The nature and measurement of compulsive indecisiveness. *Behaviour Research and Therapy*, *31*, 683–692.

Gray, J. A. (1982). *The neuropsychology of anxiety*. London: Oxford University Press.

Hohagen, F., Winkelmann, G., Raeuchle, H. R., Hand, I., Koenig, A., Muenchau, N., Hiss, H., Kabisch, C. G., Kaeppler, C., Schramm, P., Rey, E., Aldenhoff, J., & Berger, M. (1998). Combination of behaviour therapy with fluvoxamine in comparison with behaviour therapy and placebo: results of a multicentre study. *British Journal of Psychiatry*, *173* (Suppl. 35), 71–78.

Jakes, I. (1996). *Theoretical approaches to obsessive–compulsive disorder*. Cambridge: Cambridge University Press.

Jones, B. P., Duncan, V. V., Brouwers, P., & Mirsky, A. F. (1991). Cognition in eating disorders. *Journal of Clinical and Experimental Neuropsychology*, *13*, 711–728.

Kobak, K. A., Greist, J. H., Jefferson, J. W., Katzelnick, D. J., & Henk, H. J. (1998). Behavioral versus pharmacological treatments of obsessive compulsive disorder: a meta-analysis. *Psychopharmacology*, *136*, 205–216.

Kozak, M. J., & Foa, E. B. (1994). Obsessions, overvalued ideas, and delusions in obsessive–compulsive disorder. *Behaviour Research and Therapy*, *32*, 343–353.

Lucas, J. A., Telch, M. J., & Bigler, E. D. (1991). Memory functioning in panic disorder: a neuropsychological perspective. *Journal of Anxiety Disorders*, *5*, 1–20.

Mataix-Cols, D., Junque, C., Sanchez-Turet, M., Vallejo, J., Verger, K., & Barrios, M. (1999). Neuropsychological functioning in a subclinical obsessive–compulsive sample. *Biological Psychiatry*, *45*, 898–904.

Obsessive Compulsive Cognitions Working Group. (1997). Cognitive assessment of obsessive–compulsive disorder. *Behaviour Research and Therapy*, *35*, 667–681.

Obsessive Compulsive Cognitions Working Group. (2001). Development and initial validation of the Obsessive Beliefs Questionnaire and the Interpretation of Intrusions Inventory. *Behaviour Research and Therapy*, *39*, 987–1006.

O'Connor, K., Todorov, C., Robillard, S., Borgeat, F., & Brault, M. (1999). Cognitive behaviour therapy and medication in the treatment of obsessive compulsive disorder: a controlled study. *Canadian Journal of Psychiatry*, *44*, 64–71.

Otto, M. W. (1990). Neuropsychological approaches to obsessive–compulsive disorder. In M. A. Jenike, L. Baer, & W. E. Minichiello (eds), *Obsessive–compulsive disorders: theory and management* (pp. 132–148). Chicago: Year Book Medical.

Pitman, R. A. (1987). A cybernetic model of obsessive–compulsive pathology. *Comprehensive Psychiatry*, *28*, 334–343.

Purcell, R., Maruff, P., Kyrios, M., & Pantelis, C. (1998). Neuropsychological deficits in obsessive–compulsive disorder: a comparison with unipolar depression, panic disorder, and normal controls. *Archives of General Psychiatry*, *55*, 415–423.

Rachman, S., & Hodgson, R. J. (1980). *Obsessions and compulsions*. Englewood Cliffs, NJ: Prentice Hall.

Rachman, S., & de Silva, P. (1978). Abnormal and normal obsessions. *Behaviour Research and Therapy*, *16*, 233–248.

Rasmussen, S. A., & Eisen, J. L. (1992). The epidemiology and clinical features of obsessive compulsive disorder. *Psychiatric Clinics of North America*, *15*, 743–758.

Reed, G. F. (1985). *Obsessional experience and compulsive behaviour: a cognitive structural approach*. New York: Academic.

Salkovskis, P. M. (1985). Obsessional–compulsive problems: a cognitive–behavioural analysis. *Behaviour Research and Therapy*, *25*, 571–583.

Salkovskis, P. M. (1989). Cognitive–behavioural factors and the persistence of intrusive thoughts in obsessional problems. *Behaviour Research and Therapy*, *27*, 677–682.

Salkovskis, P. M. (1996). Cognitive–behavioral approaches to the understanding of obsessional problems. In R. M. Rapee (ed.), *Current controversies in the anxiety disorders* (pp. 103–134). New York: Guilford.

Salkovskis, P. M., & Harrison, J. (1984). Abnormal and normal obsessions: a replication. *Behaviour Research and Therapy*, *22*, 549–552.

Salkovskis, P. M., Shafran, R., Rachman, S., & Freeston, M. H. (1999). Multiple pathways to inflated responsibility in obsessional problems: possible origins and implications for therapy and research. *Behaviour Research and Therapy*, *37*, 1055–1072.

Savage, C. R., Deckersbach, T., Wilhelm, S., Rauch, S. L., Baer, L., Reid, T., & Jenike, M. A. (2000). Strategic processing and episodic memory impairment in obsessive compulsive disorder. *Neuropsychology*, *14*, 141–151.

Schmidtke, K., Schorb, A., Winkelmann, G., & Hohagen, F. (1998). Cognitive frontal lobe dysfunction in obsessive–compulsive disorder. *Biological Psychiatry*, *43*, 666–673.

Steketee, G. S. (1993). *Treatment of obsessive compulsive disorder*. New York: Guilford.

Taylor, S. (1999) Introduction to the special series. Treatment of obsessive–compulsive disorder: progress, prospects, and problems. *Cognitive and Behavioral Practice*, *6*, 342–345.

Teasdale, J. D. (1974). Learning models of obsessional–compulsive disorder. In H. R. Beech (ed.), *Obsessional states* (pp. 197–229). London: Methuen.

Vasterling, J. J., Brailey, K., Constans, J. I., & Sutker, P. B. (1998). Attention and memory dysfunction in posttraumatic stress disorder. *Neuropsychology*, *12*, 125–133.

Weissman, M. M., Bland, R. C., Canino, G. J., Greenwald, S., Hwu, H.-G., Lee, C. K., Newman, S. C., Oakley-Browne, M. A., Rubino-Stipec, M., Wickramaratne, P. J., Wittchen, H.-U., & Yeh, E.-K. (1994). The cross national epidemiology of obsessive compulsive disorder. *Journal of Clinical Psychiatry*, *55* (Suppl. 3), 5–10.

Section A

Domains of Beliefs in Obsessive Disorder: An Overview

Chapter 2

Importance of Thoughts

Dana S. Thordarson and Roz Shafran

Definition and History of Importance of Thoughts Concept

The importance of thoughts domain of cognition in obsessive compulsive disorder (OCD) comprises beliefs and interpretations involving excessive importance attached to negative intrusive thoughts (*Obsessive Compulsive Cognitions Working Group* [OCCWG], *1997*). More specifically, importance of thoughts refers to general beliefs and specific interpretations in one of three themes:

a) Negative intrusive thoughts indicate something significant about oneself (e.g., that one is terrible, weird, abnormal).
b) Having negative intrusive thoughts increases the risk of bad things happening (e.g., having the thoughts means they are likely to come true, having impulses means one is likely to act on them).
c) Negative intrusive thoughts must be important merely because they have occurred.

    The importance of thoughts domain comprises interpretations and beliefs that have also been described as moral thought–action fusion (thoughts are morally equivalent to actions), likelihood thought–action fusion (having bad thoughts can increase the risk of bad things happening), and magical thinking (similar to likelihood thought–action fusion, that thoughts alone can cause bad things to happen).

History of the Concept of Importance of Thoughts

Careful clinical observations have long documented the exaggerated importance that patients with OCD appear to place on their intrusive thoughts. For example, a patient described by Conolly (1830) was considered to be unable to distinguish her "fancies" from facts, and Maudsley (1895) wrote that such a patient ". . . is constrained to think of doing an indecent act and is in fright lest he should someday do it" (p. 184). In the early part of the 20th Century, Bleuler (1934/1916) observed that "the patients also fear that they might destroy their beloved ones through a thought ('omnipotence of thought')" (p. 561).
    The excessive importance placed on thoughts by obsessional patients has also been

noted in passing during the course of studies that predated cognitive theories of OCD. Rachman (1971) stated that, "obsessional ruminations are likely to produce increases in responsiveness (sensitization) because of their special significance" (p. 231). In addition, in his paper describing the satiation method for the modification of obsessions (prolonged exposure to obsessions), Rachman (1976) wrote ". . . our satiation patients are told that most people experience unwanted, unacceptable intrusive thoughts but that they rarely attach significance to these useless ideas and therefore can dismiss them easily. The patients are encouraged to regard their obsessions as alien and useless . . ." (p. 438). This hypothesis, that people with OCD tend to attach excessive importance to their intrusive thoughts, and that they should be encouraged to see them as unimportant, continues to hold currency almost 25 years later.

Cognitive Theory

Despite these early observations, it was only with the publication of Salkovskis' seminal paper proposing a cognitive–behavioral theory of obsessive compulsive disorder that the interpretation of intrusive thoughts was brought to the forefront of cognitive theory and treatment (Salkovskis, 1985). Salkovskis (1985, 1989, 1996) proposed that, in OCD, normal intrusive thoughts are appraised as indicating possible responsibility for harm or its prevention, and that the interpretation of the thought in terms of responsibility leads to distress and compulsive behavior. Specific assumptions which were suggested to interact with the intrusion to result in an appraisal of responsibility include "Having a thought about an action is like performing the action" (p. 579).

Other Descriptions of Importance of Thoughts and Related Constructs

Another way in which thoughts are given exaggerated importance was described and termed "the psychological fusion of thoughts and actions" (Rachman, 1993). In this paper, which considered the relationship between responsibility, guilt and obsessions, Rachman suggested that thought–action fusion (TAF) may be a common factor that serves to inflate the importance of intrusive thoughts. Soon afterwards, Tallis (1994) published two case examples of people with TAF and examined the origins of their beliefs. The first patient had, at the age of six, prayed that her grandfather would die, and he died of a heart attack the next day. The second patient, who had been sexually abused by her father, had prayed that her father would go away or be taken away and, within a week, he was killed in an accident. Tallis suggested that these unfortunate coincidences may have resulted in the development of the patients' TAF and led to the subsequent development of OCD.

Later work developed the concept of TAF further and divided it into two components: moral TAF and likelihood TAF (Rachman, Thordarson, Shafran, & Woody, 1995; Shafran, Thordarson, & Rachman, 1996). Moral TAF refers to believing that thoughts are morally equivalent to actions; likelihood TAF refers to believing that thoughts can increase the probability of bad events actually occurring. Thus, TAF can be seen as two special cases of believing and interpreting negative intrusive thoughts as being overly important; one can believe thoughts are important because they are morally unacceptable, and one can believe thoughts are important because they increase the risk of real-life negative events. In our development of a measure of TAF (Shafran, Thordarson, & Rachman, 1996), we found that TAF-Likelihood (holding beliefs that thoughts about unacceptable or disturbing events increases the probability of those events occurring) was associated with obsessional compulsive symptoms. We suggested that this belief could be a precursor to a responsibility appraisal: if you believe your thought has increased the chances of a bad event happening, you are likely to feel an increased sense of responsibility for preventing the event (e.g., by performing compulsions).

In their work on cognitive therapy for OCD patients without overt compulsions, Freeston, Rhéaume, and Ladouceur (1996) found that a common feature of their patients was the importance they attached to the presence or content of their obsessions. They described three ways in which their patients appeared to be overestimating the importance of their obsessions. First, some patients tended to interpret the presence (and presumably persistence) of their intrusion as meaning it must be important, a form of ex-consequentia reasoning: If I think it all the time, it must be important. Second, some patients interpreted their obsession as meaning that it must reflect their true nature, or that their thoughts mean that they are a morally bad person; this could be considered a form of moral TAF. Third, some patients made interpretations consistent with likelihood TAF, namely, that thinking about a bad event makes the event more likely to happen.

In a recent paper, Rachman (1997) proposed that "obsessions are caused by catastrophic misinterpretations of the significance of one's thoughts, images, and impulses. The obsessions persist as long as these misinterpretations continue and diminish when the misinterpretations are weakened" (p. 793). Rachman considered that misinterpretations of the significance of thoughts fall into three main categories: "mad, bad and dangerous." Examples of attaching undue importance to the occurrence of intrusive thoughts include:

- This thought reflects my true evil nature.
- Having this thought means I'm a bad person.
- If I think this, I must really want it to happen.
- Thinking this can make the event more likely to happen.
- If others knew I thought this, they would think I was an evil person.
- Having this thought means I am likely to lose control over my mind or my behavior.

According to Rachman's cognitive theory of obsessions, people who make these interpretations are likely to become distressed by their intrusive thoughts and seek to neutralize them. On the other hand, people who interpret their negative intrusive thoughts as normal and meaningless should not be overly distressed by such thoughts. One of the goals of cognitive therapy for people with OCD is to change dysfunctional interpretations about intrusive thoughts, and replace them with more helpful, normalizing, benign interpretations. The theory suggests that successful treatment requires the modification of such interpretations as a necessary precursor for reduction in the persistence of obsessions.

Measurement of Importance of Thoughts

Beliefs in the over-importance of thoughts have been assessed in a variety of ways, including questionnaires and laboratory methods. These are described below.

Thought–Action Fusion Scale

Originally, TAF was measured as part of the development of a questionnaire on general responsibility (Rachman *et al.*, 1995). The four-item TAF subscale had included only one item addressing moral TAF ("For me, having a mean thought is as bad as doing something mean"). Two items had addressed likelihood TAF ("If I have a thought about something happening to an acquaintance, it may bring them bad luck"; "My mean thoughts wishing a person harm can increase the chance of something harmful happening to him/her"). The fourth item was a mixture of both types of TAF ("My mean thoughts can have the same consequences as my mean actions"). We found that the TAF subscale was internally consistent, and that TAF was strongly associated with measures of obsessional compulsive symptoms and beliefs related to OCD.

The encouraging results of that study led to the development of a full TAF questionnaire, separating out the different types of TAF, and TAF for different types of thoughts. A series of studies led to the development of a 19–item measure, the TAF Scale (Shafran *et al.*, 1996). Twelve of these items assessed the moral component of TAF (e.g., "Having a blasphemous thought is almost as sinful to me as a blasphemous action"). Four items assessed likelihood TAF for events happening to other people (e.g., "If I think of a relative/friend being in a car accident, this increases the risk that he/she will have a car accident"), and three assessed likelihood TAF for events happening to oneself (e.g., "If I think of myself being in a car accident, this increases the risk that I will have a car accident"). In the student sample, three factors emerged — TAF-Moral, TAF-Likelihood-Others, and TAF-Likelihood-Self. In the obsessional group, two clear factors emerged, TAF-Moral and TAF-Likelihood. There was a significant association between TAF-Likelihood-Others and subscales of the MOCI for the obsessional sample and for the student sample, but the associations between obsessional symptoms and TAF-Moral and TAF-Likelihood-Self were not significant for the obsessional sample. It may be that TAF for thoughts of events happening to other people is more "magical" and dysfunctional than TAF for events happening to oneself. To some degree, TAF-Likelihood-Self can be endorsed on the basis of self-fulfilling prophecies or believing that one's thoughts may influence one's own behavior in ways that lead to the undesired outcome. Other studies have also shown an association between TAF and state and trait guilt (Shafran, Watkins, & Charman, 1996).

The TAF scale has been investigated by other researchers, particularly by Rassin and colleagues in the Netherlands (Rassin, Diepstraten, Merckelbach, & Muris, in press; Rassin, Merckelbach, Muris, & Schmidt, in press). Rassin *et al.* provided further evidence of the reliability and validity of the scale and its factor structure. Their work indicates that TAF promotes obsessional thinking, that elevated scores on thought-action fusion are not specific to OCD, and that TAF scores decrease after successful behavioral treatment of the disorder. In a recent study, Zucker, Craske, Barrios and Holguin (2000) conducted a confirmatory factor analysis on the TAF scores of over 1000 students. The resultant three–factor solution accounted for 60.9 percent of the variance, and resulted in a replication of the three factors previously found by Shafran *et al.* (1996), i.e., TAF-Moral, TAF-Likelihood-Self and TAF-Likelihood-Other. Internal consistency of the three-factor model was excellent for this sample. No significant differences were found between the TAF scores on this sample and the original sample (Shafran *et al.*, 1996) on any of the subscales.

Different versions of the TAF Scale have been used by various researchers. For example, a positive form of TAF (which had been dropped during the development of the original scale) has been re-investigated by Amir and colleagues (Amir, Freshman, Ramsey, & Brigidi, 1999). A similar questionnaire has been developed to investigate the related concept of thought-shape fusion (e.g., "Just thinking about eating a chocolate bar can make me gain weight"), which has been shown to be associated with eating difficulties (Shafran, Teachman, Kerry, & Rachman, 1999).

Other Questionnaires

Other questionnaires with subscales addressing the interpretations of intrusive thoughts have also appeared. These included the Inventory of Beliefs Related to Obsessions (Freeston, Ladouceur, Gagnon, & Thibodeau, 1993) and a subscale of the Meta-Cognitions Questionnaire (Cartwright-Hatton & Wells, 1997) that measures negative beliefs about thoughts, including superstition, punishment and responsibility (e.g., "It is bad to think certain thoughts"). Yet other self-report measures are in the process of development (e.g., the Personal Significance Scale which uses a visual analogue scale to assess the personal significance of an idiosyncratic obsession; Rachman, 2000).

Obsessive Beliefs Questionnaire and Interpretations of Intrusions Inventory

Some of the measures described here (e.g., the Thought–Action Fusion Scale; Shafran, Thordarson, & Rachman, 1996) were used in the development of the Importance of Thoughts subscales of the Obsessive Beliefs Questionnaire (OBQ) and Interpretations of Intrusions Inventory (III) developed by the OCCWG (1997, 2001). The OBQ subscale contains 14 items assessing general beliefs about the importance of thoughts. Examples include "Having nasty thoughts means I am a terrible person", "The more I think of something horrible, the greater the risk it will come true", and "Having a bad thought means I am weird or abnormal." The III subscale contains ten items assessing immediate interpretations of participant-generated intrusive thoughts regarding excessive importance attached to these intrusions. The items include questions involving TAF, as well as interpretations of the mere presence of thoughts and the triad suggested by Rachman (1997) that the thoughts mean that the person is "mad, bad and dangerous." Examples include "Having this intrusive thought means I am a terrible person", "Because I have this thought, it must be important", and "This intrusive thought could be an omen."

After initial development, two waves of testing were conducted, the first (stage two,

OCCWG, 2001) with 101 OCD participants, 374 students and 76 community controls, and the second (stage three, OCCWG, in preparation) based on 257 participants with OCD, 104 with other anxiety disorders, 85 community controls and 285 students. Importance of Thoughts subscales from both the OBQ and III showed excellent internal consistency and generally good test–retest reliability in the 0.8 range for stage two findings but somewhat lower in stage three, especially the OBQ subscale for the OCD sample. Other psychometric findings are given below.

Laboratory Manipulations

Laboratory-based measures of importance of thoughts also have been used and have provided some predictive validity for the concept of TAF. A laboratory measure to operationalize TAF was developed by Rachman and colleagues (Rachman, Shafran, Mitchell, Trant, & Teachman, 1996) as part of a study of the effects of covert neutralization. In this study, 63 participants were asked to write a sentence that would be likely to elicit TAF. Participants were selected on the basis of having high scores on the TAF Scale. Measures of morality and the likelihood of harm (and other variables of interest such as anxiety, guilt, and responsibility) were taken before and after the experimental manipulation. Participants were asked to think of a close friend or relative and to write out the sentence "I hope [name of friend or relative] is in a car accident" on a piece of paper, inserting the name of the person in the blank.

There was a strong significant correlation between TAF scores on the pre-existing self-report measure for events related to other people, and estimates of the probability of the adverse event occurring within the next 24 h ($r = 0.61$), indicating the TAF Scale has predictive validity. Likelihood-Others TAF was also significantly correlated with anxiety, estimates of control, and feelings of responsibility if the threatened event had occurred. TAF was not significantly correlated with evoked guilt, moral wrongness or the urge to neutralize.

In another study, TAF was operationalized using a paradigm in which naïve participants were informed that an EEG recording device could detect their thoughts of the word "apple" and that having the thought "apple" would result in an electric shock for another person (Rassin, Merckelbach, Muris, & Spaan, 1999). Participants in the control condition were told that the equipment could detect their thoughts but they were not told that any specific thought would have negative consequences. The researchers found that participants in the experimental condition (those who were told that their thoughts had real-world negative consequences for other people) had more than three times as many intrusions, felt more than three times the discomfort, and engaged in neutralizing behavior in about half of the intrusions. The authors concluded, "in principle, TAF may contribute to the transformation of normal intrusions into obsessive intrusions" (p. 235).

Overlap Between Importance of Thoughts and Other Domains

Overlap with Control of Thoughts

Beliefs in and appraisals of the Importance of Thoughts may be conceptualized as precursor to beliefs/appraisals of the need to control thoughts and of responsibility, especially for repugnant obsessions. The Control of Thoughts domain (see Chapter three) refers to beliefs and interpretations of the necessity for controlling one's thoughts, and consequences of failure to control. It seems logical that people who interpret their negative intrusions as highly important (e.g., that the intrusive thoughts mean something terrible about themselves or about the future) may be driven to attempt to control their thoughts, both to reduce distress, and to remove or reduce threat associated with the thoughts. On the other hand, people who generally believe that their negative intrusive thoughts are unimportant "mental flotsam" presumably would lack motivation to control them. Two recent studies showed that beliefs about Importance of Thoughts and Control of Thoughts are highly correlated in varying populations such as OCD patients, students, and community controls (OCCWG, 2001, in preparation). Similar results were found for the III in these studies. Thus, Importance of Thoughts and Control of Thoughts appear to be closely related concepts.

Are interpretations and beliefs in the importance of thoughts more fundamental in the experience of obsessional compulsive problems than interpretations and beliefs in the control of thoughts? In a recent study, Rassin and colleagues (Rassin, Muris, Schmidt, & Merckelbach, 2000) used a structural equation modeling approach to address this question. In a sample of undergraduate students, they found that TAF (one type of belief in the importance of unwanted intrusive thoughts) appears to lead to attempts to suppress thoughts, and that both likelihood TAF and thought suppression contribute to obsessive compulsive symptoms. Their findings suggest that control of thoughts may be secondary to importance of thoughts.

Overlap with Responsibility

Similarly, at least for some negative intrusive thoughts, the constructs of responsibility and importance of thoughts are intimately related. If an intrusive thought is appraised as increasing the chances of a bad event happening, then an increased sense of responsibility may ensue. For example, if a person appraises an intrusive image of his or her relative having a car accident as increasing the chance of an accident occurring (due to TAF), then he or she is likely to perceive an exaggerated sense of responsibility. On the other hand, if an intrusive thought is appraised directly as indicating that one may be responsible for harm (without TAF), then it will be perceived as important. To take the example above, if the person interprets his or her intrusive image as indicating that he or she must warn the relative of the possibility of an impending car accident, then the thought will be viewed as an important one.

Correlations between the Importance of Thoughts and Responsibility subscales for both the OBQ and III from stages two and three indicate a close association (OCCWG, 2001; in preparation). As measured by the OBQ, beliefs about Importance of Thoughts and

Responsibility were strongly correlated in the combined sample of non-OCD anxiety disorder patients, community controls and students, as well as for OCD patients alone (OCCWG, 2001; in preparation). Again, it appears that Importance of Thoughts and Responsibility are closely connected concepts. However, as yet we have no evidence as to which type of interpretation may be more fundamental in the experience of obsessional compulsive problems. Furthermore, the relationship between importance and responsibility may be different for different types of intrusive thoughts. For example, thoughts about contamination or doubting may lead directly to interpretations of responsibility; repugnant obsessions (e.g., aggressive or sexual obsessions) may require an initial interpretation of importance of the intrusive thought itself.

Summary

In summary, beliefs and interpretations involving excessive importance placed on thoughts were highly correlated with beliefs and interpretations of responsibility and the need to control thoughts. It is possible that the intercorrelations are due to overlap among the concepts, that they are all measures of the same underlying construct (such as Salkovskis' broadly construed concept of responsibility). Factor analyses of the stage three data suggest that the items in the OBQ Importance of Thoughts and Control of Thoughts subscales may be interrelated due to an underlying construct, the significance of intrusions. On the III, it appeared that items related to harm tended to load together, irrespective of the original scale. These items included ideas that thoughts can cause harm (Importance of Thoughts), that one would be responsible for preventing harm arising from these thoughts (Responsibility), and that harm could happen if these thoughts are not controlled (Control of Thoughts). Alternatively, if importance of thoughts causes or leads to responsibility and control of thoughts beliefs and interpretations, the constructs would be likely to be highly interrelated, but it would still be important to have separable measures of the constructs for research into, for example, the origins of obsessions.

Relationship to OCD Symptoms

Importance of Thoughts and the Severity of OCD

If importance of thoughts is a core belief system underlying the development and maintenance of obsessions, particularly repugnant obsessions involving harm, aggression, sex, and blasphemy, OCD patients should score more highly on a measure of these beliefs than anxious controls or normal participants. Findings from the validation studies (OCCWG, 2001, in preparation) show that the Importance of Thoughts subscale of the OBQ significantly discriminated OCD patients from the comparison groups (anxious controls, community adults, and students). The Importance of Thoughts subscale of the III significantly discriminated OCD patients from community adults, anxious controls, and students in the stage two study (OCCWG, 2001), but not from anxious controls in the stage three study (OCCWG, in preparation). This suggests that interpreting one's intrusive thoughts as highly important may be OCD-relevant, but not necessarily specific to OCD (also see discussion below on relationship to other disorders).

Within the OCD sample, the Importance of Thoughts subscale was significantly associated with subscales of Thoughts of Harm and Impulses to Harm on the Padua Inventory-Revised which measures OCD symptom severity; however, they were not associated with Contamination/Washing, Checking, or Dressing/Grooming subscales. Thus, for patients with OCD, beliefs that thoughts are highly significant and important may be specifically associated with harming obsessions in particular, rather than OCD symptoms in general. However, the same pattern of results was not found in the student sample. For the students, the Importance of Thoughts subscale was highly correlated with Checking ($r = 0.57$) and Contamination/Washing ($r = 0.50$), and only moderately correlated with Thoughts of Harm ($r = 0.35$), suggesting that within normal samples, the importance placed on intrusive thoughts may not be specifically associated with repugnant obsessions.

OCCWG researchers also examined whether interpreting one's intrusive thoughts as highly important was associated with the frequency and distress of the intrusive thoughts that participants reported on the III (OCCWG, in preparation). The ratings of frequency and distress were moderately correlated with the Importance of Thoughts subscale of the III in both the OCD group and the anxious clinical control group. In the student sample, this subscale correlated highly with frequency and moderately with distress ratings. In the community adult sample, Importance of Thoughts was not significantly associated with frequency of intrusions, but was moderately correlated with distress ratings.

In summary, these research results suggest that holding beliefs that bad thoughts are highly important is a significant domain of beliefs for OCD patients. In people with OCD, believing that one's intrusive thoughts are highly important is associated with the experience of harming obsessions. In addition, interpreting particular intrusive thoughts as being highly important is related to the frequency and distress associated these thoughts.

It is tempting to see these results as supporting, at least in part, the hypothesis that beliefs and interpretations of the importance of thoughts contribute to the formation and maintenance of obsessions. However, it is possible that exaggerating the importance of thoughts is a *consequence* of obsessions, and not a cause of them. People who experience recurrent disturbing obsessions may engage in a form of ex-consequentia reasoning (Arntz, Rauner, & van den Hout, 1995), believing that they would not be having so many obsessions if they did not mean something very important (see Freeston, Rhéaume, & Ladouceur, 1996). Seen in this way, the sense of responsibility and guilt could "be regarded as a 'normal response' to their abnormal experience" (Jakes, 1996, p. 40). Further research is required to demonstrate that beliefs in the importance of thoughts are a vulnerability or maintenance factor in the experience of obsessions. Experimental manipulations of perceived responsibility go some way towards addressing this concern (see Chapter 4 in this volume).

Importance of Thoughts and Cognitive Therapy

Case reports have described various techniques to modify obsessions by reducing the degree to which patients view them as significant and important. For example, Salkovskis and

Westbrook (1989) describe the case of a man who had obscene sexual thoughts, which he neutralised by stating a set of phrases to himself. A habituation technique was used in which the patient listened to his thoughts on a loop tape without performing compulsions or otherwise responding to them. Implicit in this methodology is the message that the intrusive thoughts are not important and the patient does not *need* to respond to them in any way. The intervention was effective for this case and three others (Salkovskis & Westbrook, 1989).

Other methods have been developed explicitly to change the overestimation of the importance of thoughts (Freeston *et al.*, 1996) and have been evaluated in a controlled treatment trial for obsessions (Freeston *et al.*, 1997). The treatment protocol consists of a detailed cognitive account of the maintenance of obsessions, providing patients with a rationale for treatment; tape-loop exposure and response prevention; cognitive restructuring using standard techniques such as Socratic questioning and identification of negative automatic thoughts; behavioral experiments; and relapse prevention. In the trial published by Freeston *et al.* the sample comprised 15 patients in the treatment group and 14 patients in the control group. For the treatment group, the mean score on the Y-BOCS fell from 25.1 (SD=5.0) to 12.2 (SD=9.6). In the wait-list control group, the mean score on the Y-BOCS increased from 21.2 (SD=6.0) to 22.0 (SD=6.0). These scores represent a clinically significant change in the treatment group and gains were maintained at 6-month follow-up, suggesting that treatments aimed at reducing the importance attached to obsessions can be effective in reducing obsessive compulsive symptoms. Additional cognitive therapy interventions based on Rachman's cognitive theory of obsessions similarly aim to change the personal significance placed on obsessions, with the view that decreasing the importance of the obsession will lead to a decrease in neutralization, a reduction in the frequency and intensity of thought and, ultimately, the elimination of obsessions (Rachman, 2000).

In order to change overestimation of the importance of thoughts, it is necessary to activate the meaning placed on the thoughts by the patient. For example, obsessional patients usually have good insight that thinking about something bad happening to someone else cannot cause a negative event to happen to them; this is reflected in the relatively low endorsement of TAF statements in self-report questionnaires (Shafran *et al.*, 1996). These beliefs are most likely to be activated if patients are exposed to a feared stimulus and prevented from carrying out a response. If this is the case, then cognitive work challenging beliefs about the importance of thoughts should be done when the patient is carrying out exposure in vivo, as well as when he or she is sitting calmly, depending on the extent of the TAF and associated anxiety levels.

Relationship to Other Disorders

Based on Lazarus' cognitive appraisal theory (see Lazarus & Folkman, 1984), Beck (1976) developed a general cognitive theory of anxiety, suggesting that anxiety disorders involve the persistent misinterpretation of particular stimuli as threatening, and/or the underestimation of one's ability to cope effectively with the threat (see also Beck & Emery, 1985). According to the cognitive approaches to anxiety, normal fear and anxiety are caused by correctly appraising dangerous stimuli as threatening; pathological anxiety is caused by repeatedly misinterpreting benign stimuli as threatening. For some of the anxiety disorders, we may consider that part of the misappraisal of benign phenomena (such as intrusive thoughts) as threatening involves an exaggeration of the importance of the stimuli. In other words, we can think of Importance of Thoughts as a special case of misinterpreting normal, benign stimuli (namely, one's own thoughts) as being excessively important and significant, in a way that makes the thoughts themselves seem threatening. The concept of misinterpreting the Importance of Thoughts may play a role in other anxiety disorders for which recurrent, negative thoughts are a major feature. These include posttraumatic stress disorder (PTSD) and generalized anxiety disorder (GAD).

In their recent cognitive model of PTSD, Ehlers and Clark (2000) suggested that people with PTSD may make a number of misinterpretations that lead to a sense of current and persistent threat. One such misinterpretation is the appraisal of posttraumatic mental phenomena, such as intrusive recollections, as indicating a current threat to one's physical or mental well being. For example, a person who misinterprets the occurrence of intrusive memories as indicating "I'm going mad," is likely to experience anxiety (p. 322). Thus, according to the cognitive model, PTSD can be maintained by misinterpreting normal sequelae of trauma as being excessively important and significant.

Wells (1999) has recently proposed a cognitive model of GAD that focuses on the cognitive processes that may maintain abnormal worry. He distinguishes between two types of worry. Type 1 worry, or worry about external events, may lead to the activation of negative beliefs about worry. Once activated, these beliefs produce Type 2 worry, or "metaworry," which Wells described as "worry about one's own thinking" (p. 529). Examples of negative beliefs about worry include "Worrying could make me go crazy," "Worrying is harmful," "It's abnormal to worry," (p. 532). Such negative beliefs about worry could be seen as forms of overestimating the importance of thoughts, in this case, the importance and significance of worries.

A recent theory takes the view that auditory hallucinations in patients with a diagnosis of schizophrenia are maintained by the misinterpretation of normal, benign stimuli (Morrison, 1998). In a review of the existing literature, it is suggested that auditory hallucinations are normal phenomena and that it is the misinterpretation of such phenomena as significant that causes distress and disability. As with OCD and the other anxiety disorders, it is also proposed that these interpretations of auditory hallucinations are maintained by safety seeking behaviors (including hypervigilance) (Morrison, 1998).

Based on this analysis of current cognitive-behavior theories of PTSD, GAD, and auditory hallucinations in schizophrenia, we would expect to see elevated beliefs in the Importance of Thoughts in these patients, who, like OCD patients, are plagued by negative thoughts.

Summary

The Importance of Thoughts domain has been defined as comprising beliefs and interpretations in which negative intrusive thoughts are seen to have an exaggerated and negative importance (OCCWG, 1997). The thoughts are misinterpreted as overly important in any of three domains: (1) intrusive thoughts indicate something significant about oneself; (2) having negative intrusive thoughts increases the risk of bad things happening; and (3) negative intrusive thoughts must be important merely because they have occurred. We reviewed earlier writings that referred to similar concepts, and discussed the possible role of beliefs and interpretations involving the importance of thoughts in cognitive theories of OCD. The closely related concept of thought-action fusion (TAF) may be seen as a subset of the more general category of importance of thoughts. TAF refers to the idea that thoughts are morally equivalent to actions, or that thoughts themselves can cause negative events. Several researchers have developed laboratory manipulations of TAF, and the TAF Scale has been used in several studies. However, the Importance of Thoughts construct (and the OBQ and III scales) may turn out to be more useful and comprehensive.

We reviewed the relationships between Importance of Thoughts and the domains of Responsibility and Control of Thoughts. We suggested that, at least for repugnant obsessions, interpretations involving Importance of Thoughts may be a necessary precursor to Responsibility and Control appraisals; however, this hypothesis has yet to be examined empirically. The data analyses reviewed in this chapter suggest that Importance of Thoughts beliefs may be specifically related to obsessions about harm rather than obsessional compulsive symptoms in general. Finally, we suggested two anxiety disorders, in addition to OCD, in which beliefs in the Importance of Thoughts may be prominent: PTSD and GAD. We hope that the development of the concept of Importance of Thoughts in OCD and the Importance of Thoughts subscales of the OBQ and III will facilitate several useful lines of research, leading us ultimately to an improved understanding of cognition in OCD and other anxiety disorders.

References

Amir, N., Freshman, M., Ramsey, B., & Brigidi, B. (1999, November). Harm reduction and thought-action fusion in individuals with OCD symptoms. In T. Deckersbach & G. Steketee (Chairs), *Cognition and metacognition in subtypes of OCD*. Symposium conducted at the Annual Convention of the Association for Advancement of Behavior Therapy, Toronto.

Arntz, A., Rauner, M., & van den Hout, M. (1995). "If I feel anxious, there must be danger": Ex-consequentia reasoning in inferring danger in anxiety disorders. *Behaviour Research and Therapy*, *33*, 917–925.

Beck, A. T. (1976). *Cognitive therapy and the emotional disorders*. New York: International Universities Press.

Beck, A. T., & Emery, G. (1985). *Anxiety disorders and phobias: a cognitive perspective*. New York: Basic Books.

Bleuler, E. (1934). *Textbook of psychiatry* (A. A. Brill, Trans.). New York: Macmillan. (Original work published 1916).

Cartwright-Hatton, S., & Wells, A. (1997). Beliefs about worry and intrusions: The Meta-Cognitions Questionnaire and its correlates. *Journal of Anxiety Disorders*, *11*, 279–296.

Conolly, J. (1830). *An inquiry concerning the indications of insanity with suggestions for the better protection and care of the insane*. Reprinted in 1964 by Dawsons of Pall Mall, London.

Ehlers, A., & Clark, D. M. (2000). A cognitive model of posttraumatic stress disorder. *Behaviour Research and Therapy*, *38*, 319–345.

Freeston, M. H., Ladouceur, R., Gagnon, F., & Thibodeau, N. (1993). Beliefs about obsessional thoughts. *Journal of Psychopathology and Behavioral Assessment, 15*, 1–21.

Freeston, M. H., Ladouceur, R., Gagnon, F., Thibodeau, N., Rhéaume, J., Letarte, H., & Bujold, A. (1997). Cognitive–behavioral treatment of obsessive thoughts: a controlled study. *Journal of Consulting and Clinical Psychology, 65*, 405–413.

Freeston, M. H., Rhéaume, J., & Ladouceur, R. (1996). Correcting faulty appraisals of obsessive thoughts. *Behaviour Research and Therapy, 34*, 443–446.

Jakes, I. (1996). *Theoretical approaches to obsessive–compulsive disorder.* New York: Cambridge University Press.

Lazarus, R. S., & Folkman, S. (1984). *Stress, appraisal, and coping.* New York: Springer.

Maudsley, H. (1895). *The pathology of the mind* (Revised ed.). London: Macmillan.

Morrison, A. P. (1998). A cognitive analysis of the maintenance of auditory hallucinations: are voices to schizophrenia what bodily sensations are to panic? *Behavioural and Cognitive Psychotherapy, 26*, 289–302.

Obsessive Compulsive Cognitions Working Group (1997). Cognitive assessment of obsessive–compulsive disorder. *Behaviour Research and Therapy, 37*, 667–681.

Obsessive Compulsive Cognitions Working Group (2001). Development and initial validation of the Obsessive Beliefs Questionnaire (OBQ) and the Interpretation of Intrusions Inventory (III). *Behaviour Research and Therapy, 39*, 997–1006.

Obsessive Compulsive Cognitions Working Group (in preparation). *Psychometric validation of the Obsessive Beliefs Questionnaire and the Interpretation of Intrusions Inventory: findings from stage 3 data.* Unpublished manuscript.

Rachman, S. (1971). Obsessional ruminations. *Behaviour Research and Therapy, 9*, 229–235.

Rachman, S. (1976). The modification of obsessions: a new formulation. *Behaviour Research and Therapy, 14*, 437–443.

Rachman, S. (1993). Obsessions, responsibility and guilt. *Behaviour Research and Therapy, 31*, 149–154.

Rachman, S. (1997). A cognitive theory of obsessions. *Behaviour Research and Therapy, 35*, 793–802.

Rachman, S. (2000). *Cognitive–behavioural treatment of obsessions: therapist manual.* Unpublished manuscript.

Rachman, S., Shafran, R., Mitchell, D., Trant, J., & Teachman, B. (1996). How to remain neutral: an experimental analysis of neutralization. *Behaviour Research and Therapy, 34*, 889–898.

Rachman, S., Thordarson, D. S., Shafran, R., & Woody, S. R. (1995). Perceived responsibility: structure and significance. *Behaviour Research and Therapy, 33*, 779–784.

Rassin, E., Diepstraten, P., Merckelbach, H., & Muris, P. (2001). Thought–action fusion and thought suppression in obsessive–compulsive disorder. *Behaviour Research and Therapy, 39*, 757–764.

Rassin, E., Merckelbach, H., Muris, P., & Schmidt, H. (in press). The Thought–Action Fusion Scale: further evidence for its reliability and validity. *Behaviour Research and Therapy.*

Rassin, E., Merckelbach, H., Muris, P., & Spaan, V. (1999). Thought–action fusion as a causal factor in the development of intrusions. *Behaviour Research and Therapy, 37*, 231–237.

Rassin, E., Muris, P., Schmidt, H., & Merckelbach, H. (2000). Relationships between thought–action fusion, thought suppression and obsessive–compulsive symptoms: a structural equation modeling approach. *Behaviour Research and Therapy, 38*, 889–897.

Salkovskis, P. M. (1985). Obsessional–compulsive problems: a cognitive–behavioural analysis. *Behaviour Research and Therapy, 23*, 571–583.

Salkovskis, P. M. (1989). Cognitive–behavioural factors and the persistence of intrusive thoughts in obsessional problems. *Behaviour Research and Therapy, 27*, 677–682.

Salkovskis, P. M. (1996). Cognitive–behavioural approaches to the understanding of obsessional problems. In R. M. Rapee (ed.), *Current controversies in the anxiety disorders* (pp. 103–133). New York: Guilford.

Salkovskis, P. M. & Westbrook, D. (1989). Behaviour therapy and obsessional ruminations: can failure be turned into success? *Behaviour Research and Therapy, 27*, 149–160.

Shafran, R., Watkins, E., & Charman, T. (1996). Guilt in obsessive–compulsive disorder. *Journal of Anxiety Disorders, 10*, 509–516.

Shafran, R., Teachman, B. A., Kerry, S., & Rachman, S. (1999). A cognitive distortion associated with eating disorders: thought–shape fusion. *British Journal of Clinical Psychology, 38*, 167–179.

Shafran, R., Thordarson, D. S., & Rachman, S. (1996). Thought–action fusion in obsessive compulsive disorder. *Journal of Anxiety Disorders, 10*, 379–391.

Tallis, F. (1994). Obsessions, responsibility, and guilt: two case reports suggesting a common and specific aetiology. *Behaviour Research and Therapy, 32*, 143–145.

Wells, A. (1999). A cognitive model of generalized anxiety disorder. *Behavior Modification, 23*, 526–555.

Zucker, B. G., Craske, M. G., Barrios, V., & Holguin, M. (2000, November). Thought–action fusion: can it be corrected? In M. G. Craske & M. J. Dugas (Chairs), *The fusion of thoughts, actions, and perceptions in psychopathology*. Symposium conducted at the Annual Meeting of the Association for the Advancement of Behavior Therapy, New Orleans.

Chapter 3

The Need to Control Thoughts

Christine Purdon and David A. Clark

Introducti

d to influence their operation is an important
4). In fact our very survival and ability to
es that we willfully and consciously direct
uli and accurately appraise and ignore
vert attention away from unwanted or
t to human adaptation. Most individuals
ol in most circumstances, and yet, our
no means perfect. Indeed, perceived
n several psychological disorders,

ho reported a "breakdown" in his
and images. A devout evangelical
daughters, he reported that two
". This homosexual thought was
onfession. Before long he was
trusive thoughts and images
ense against his children, and
, and were accompanied by
strategies to purge his mind
reading, thought stopping, and self-
proved very successful, and the escalation of the
ing to him. He believed that the intrusions were an attack by
Satan, ti   emanated from an evil side of his personality, and that if he were close to
God he could get rid of the disturbing thoughts. His greatest fear was that if he continued
to allow the intrusions into his mind, he would eventually act upon them. This would cause
him to act out sexually thereby leading to a break-up in his marriage and family. For Bill
these tortuous unwanted intruders of the mind had caused havoc and mayhem in an
otherwise calm and productive life.

There is now considerable evidence that our ability to prevent unwanted thoughts from
entering the stream of consciousness or to remove such thoughts once we are aware of

their presence is far from perfect. In fact the intentional and effortful suppression of unwanted thoughts and images may have untoward and insidious effects on our mental functioning and emotional state. Wegner and colleagues (e.g., Wegner, 1994; Wegner, Schneider, Carter, & White, 1987) have shown that the deliberate suppression of even neutral target thoughts can lead to a resurgence of the unwanted thought once deliberate suppression is relinquished or when attentional resources are taxed. Rachman and others have found considerable evidence that even non-clinical individuals report frequent and disturbing unwanted intrusive thoughts, images and impulses that are similar in content to clinical obsessions and are difficult to control, have an internal origin, and interrupt ongoing activity (Clark & de Silva, 1985; Freeston, Ladouceur, Thibodeau, & Gagnon, 1991; Purdon & Clark, 1993, 1994; Rachman & de Silva, 1978; Salkovskis & Harrison, 1984).

If intentional control over unwanted thoughts is problematic even in the best of situations, there are a number of psychopathological conditions where a breakdown in mental control is a key complaint. In disorders such as generalized anxiety disorder, post-traumatic stress disorder, and even depression we find that patients often report frequent, unwanted distressing thoughts that they cannot be easily dismissed from conscious awareness. However the problem of mental control is nowhere more evident than in OCD. As in the case of Bill, many OCD sufferers seek treatment because of the torment of their obsessions and their apparent inability to do anything about them. Obsessions are thoughts that give rise to immediate active internal and behavioral resistance. Active resistance is a defining feature of obsessions in the Diagnostic and Statistical Manual of Mental Disorders (DSM-IV; American Psychiatric Association [APA], 1994), and is an important criterion for distinguishing obsessions from other kinds of persistent, negative, unwanted thoughts such as worry and depressive rumination (Rachman & Hodgson, 1980; Turner, Beidel, & Stanley, 1992; Wells & Morrison, 1994). Phenomenological reports of OCD emphasize that in most cases of OCD, the significant complaint is that the subjective level of control over obsessional thoughts is inadequate, as assessed by thought frequency, intensity and duration. That is, the usual powers of exclusion and removal are weakened. Successful treatment is characterized by restoration of an appropriate degree of self-regulation by making the need to control and exclude thoughts obsolete (Rachman & Hodgson, 1980).

Thought Control in OCD

Why do obsessional thoughts give rise to active resistance? Cognitive–behavioral models maintain that negative appraisal of the obsessional thought is the key factor in thought escalation and persistence. Salkovskis (1985, 1989, 1998), Salkovskis, Richards, and Forrester (1995), and Salkovskis *et al.* (in press) argue that thoughts give rise to active resistance when they activate overvalued beliefs that: (a) thoughts can cause harm; and (b) the individual is honor-bound to prevent harm, even if his/her responsibility for harm or to the potential victim of harm is remote, minute and uncertain. Thus, the individual must control thoughts that signify potential harm in order to avert harm and the aversive sense that otherwise one may become responsible for harm. Rachman (1997, 1998) and Rachman and Hodgson (1980) suggest that active resistance to thoughts arises from beliefs that having a thought about an action that is immoral is akin, morally, to actually conducting that action ('moral thought–action fusion'), and that having thoughts about an event increases the likelihood of that event happening ('likelihood thought–action fusion'). The individual attempts to control the thought because it offends her/his moral sensibilities both by its occurrence and because it may potentiate the occurrence of morally objectionable events. (See Chapter two for a more thorough discussion of thought–action fusion). Clark and Purdon (Clark, 1989; Clark & Purdon, 1993, 1995; Purdon & Clark, 1999) offer an elaboration and extension of these core ideas, and suggest that beliefs about thoughts and thought processes in general (i.e., 'meta-cognitive' beliefs) also lead to active resistance. For example, individuals who believe that mental control is an important part of self-control will have a high stake in being able to control thoughts. Individuals who believe that unwanted thoughts represent a lapse in mental control and who strive for perfect control will be invested in regaining mental control after such a thought occurs.

The Obsessive Compulsive Cognitions Workgroup (OCCWG, 1997) has identified six domains of appraisal that appear to be of relevance to obsessional problems. These include appraisals of responsibility, overimportance of thoughts, threat estimation, tolerance for uncertainty, perfectionism, and control of thoughts. The latter domain is the focus of this chapter, and is perhaps most relevant to the issue of active resistance. In general, beliefs about the need to control thoughts are said to increase the individual's stake in thought control. In his seminal paper, Salkovskis (1985) suggests that individuals vulnerable to obsessional problems tend to have overvalued beliefs about responsibility, which include beliefs that thoughts can and should be controlled. Clark and Purdon (Clark, 1989; Clark & Purdon, 1993, 1995; Purdon & Clark, 1999) proposed that all individuals have beliefs about their own thought processes. In individuals prone to obsessional problems, these beliefs about thoughts, or, 'meta-cognitive beliefs' are rigid, unrealistic and overvalued (e.g., "I must control every thought that enters my mind, especially negative ones"; "Losing control of thoughts is as bad as losing control over behavior"; "I would be a better person if I could control unwanted thoughts"; "Control over thoughts is an important part of self-control"). These beliefs result in heightened vigilance for the occurrence of unwanted, unbidden thoughts and immediate active resistance to them. Failures in thought control result in escalating attempts at regaining control and serve to strengthen other types of beliefs about the thought (e.g., that the thought is meaningful and has consequences for the real world) (Clark & Purdon, 1993, 1995; Purdon & Clark, 1999; Rachman, 1997, 1998; Salkovskis, 1985, 1989, 1998; Salkovskis *et al.*, 1995; Wells, 1997).

Empirical Research on the Role of Thought Control in OCD

Thought Control Strategies

There is significantly more research on the role of specific thought control strategies in the development and persistence of obsessional problems than there is on the role of appraisals about the need to control thoughts. However, thought control strategies may be understood as the behavioral manifestation of beliefs about need to control thoughts, and so is of relevance to the appraisal domain of thought control. Active resistance to obsessional thoughts often occurs in the form of compulsive acts that have some kind of neutralizing, restorative, or ameliorative function and thereby serve to reduce the anxiety associated with the obsession. Individuals with OCD are notorious for the extreme effort they exert to try to control thought occurrences before the compulsive act becomes necessary (Clark & Purdon, 1993; Rachman & Hodgson, 1980; Salkovskis, 1985, 1989). Such control efforts can take many forms. Wells and Davies (1994) identified five distinct thought control strategies in individuals with anxiety disorders characterized by persistent, unwanted, uncontrollable thoughts, including OCD, and developed a measure called the Thought Control Questionnaire (TCQ) to assess the frequency with which specific types of strategies are used. The strategies identified were: distraction (think pleasant thoughts, call positive images to mind), social control (reassurance, assess the normality of the thought), worry (focus on different negative thoughts, on other worries), punishment (slap or pinch self, get angry at self) and re-appraisal (try to reinterpret the thought, analyze the thought rationally). Wells argues that strategy selection will depend on situational factors and the appraisal evoked by the thought in the specific instance (Wells, 1997; Wells & Matthews, 1994). Amir, Cashman, and Foa (1997) used the TCQ to identify thought control strategies used by a large sample of individuals with OCD and found that worry, punishment, and re-appraisal were most typically used by this group compared to non-anxious controls. Furthermore, use of punishment and worry predicted OCD symptomatology.

In a similar vein, Freeston and Ladouceur (1997) interviewed 29 individuals diagnosed with OCD but without overt compulsions about their responses to obsessional thoughts. They identified seven types of strategies, which included physical action (i.e., distraction), self-reassurance (i.e., convince self that the thought is not important), thought replacement, talking to someone else (i.e., as a form of distraction), doing nothing, analyzing the thought (i.e., trying to understand the thought), and thought stopping. These strategies were not applied at random, but were selected according to various features of the situation under which the thought occurred, such as mood state and emotional intensity of the thought and the viability of a specific strategy given the situational circumstances. Finally, Ladouceur *et al.* (2000) compared thought control strategies in individuals with OCD, individuals with another anxiety disorder and non-clinical volunteers. They found that individuals with OCD were more likely to use overt and covert compulsions to control their thoughts than others, and that the strategies they used were more closely tied to thought content than the other groups.

Insidious Effects of Thought Control

Two-Factor Theory of Fear/Avoidance and the Role of Mood State.   Why are these control efforts so ineffectual? Cognitive–behavioral models of OCD posit a number of reasons. First, thought control efforts terminate exposure to the thought, thereby disallowing emotional habituation and ensuring that the thought will continue to be source of threat (Rachman & Hodgson, 1980). Second, when the thought is actively resisted, the individual is unable to learn new information about its actual harm potential. Thus, the thought persists as a source of threat and, like any threat stimulus, will be a focus of attention and lead to vigilant monitoring that ensures that all thought cues will be particularly salient (Salkovskis, 1998; Salkovskis *et al.*, 1995; Wells, 1997). Third, if the control effort is temporarily successful, it is likely to result in some reduction in anxiety, and is thus likely to be repeated (Rachman & Hodgson, 1980; Salkovskis, 1989, 1998; Salkovskis *et al.*, 1995). Fourth, failures in thought control, which are inevitable given the above factors, will result in a decline in mood state, which will in turn make control of negative thoughts evermore difficult, and the individual may begin to feel as if their catastrophic predictions about the consequences of failing to control thoughts (e.g., insanity, complete loss of mental control, exhaustion) are starting to come true (Purdon & Clark, 1999; Rachman, 1997, 1998; Rachman & Hodgson, 1980; Salkovskis, 1985, 1998; Wells, 1997).

Ironic Effects on Frequency.   It has also been suggested that deliberate, effortful attempts at thought control may result in a paradoxical increase in their frequency. Wegner *et al.* (1987) found that deliberate suppression of a neutral ('white bears') thought was associated with an ironic increase in its frequency once suppression efforts had ceased. Since this seminal finding, suppression has been implicated by cognitive–behavioral models of OCD as a factor in the actual escalation of thought frequency (Clark & Purdon, 1993, 1995; Rachman, 1997, 1998; Salkovskis, 1989, 1998; Salkovskis *et al.*, 1995; Wells, 1997). Empirical studies investigating the effects of suppression on the frequency of exclusively obsessional thoughts have yielded mixed findings. Salkovskis observed a paradoxical effect of suppression on the frequency of obsessional thoughts in non-clinical individuals (Salkovskis & Campbell, 1994; Trinder & Salkovskis, 1994), whereas Purdon did not (Purdon, in press; Purdon & Clark, 2001). In an investigation using a clinical sample of individuals with OCD, Janeck and Calamari (1999) did not find that suppression led to more frequent obsessions. It is important to note, however, that in all these studies, suppression efforts seldom achieved perfect results, so failures in control were common.

Effects on Appraisal and Mood.   Purdon (1999, in press) and Purdon and Clark (2001) have argued that the most insidious effects of suppression may be on thought appraisal and mood state rather than frequency, suggesting that failures in thought control may serve to confirm individuals' negative beliefs that the thought is truly meaningful. This leads to increasing concerns about the meaning of failures in thought control, enhanced concern that some of the negative predictions about failing to control thoughts are being realized, and a subsequent decline in mood state. Purdon (2001) also suggested that thought suppression studies might have more validity if the variables of interest were assessed under conditions of *natural* active resistance rather than under conditions of imposed suppression instructions. Participants in a 'do not suppress' or a 'monitor only' (i.e., no instructions about suppression) control condition typically do appear to engage in significant suppression efforts (Purdon, in press; Purdon & Clark, 2001). Furthermore, natural suppression effort may be an interesting variable to assess on its own as a marker of OCD severity.

Thought Content.   Finally, it may be the unique aspects of the content and experience of obsessions themselves that make them more difficult to control. Purdon and Clark (1999) propose that concern about the need to control an obsessional thought may arise from the experience of the thought as being ego-dystonic, or, as being inconsistent and at odds with valued aspects of the self, such as morality, personality and sense of self as a rational person. A thought that is experienced as ego-dystonic may suggest to the individual that he/she possesses undesirable, repugnant personality characteristics (e.g., "maybe I am a homicidal maniac at heart"; "maybe I am an irrational person"; "maybe I am a careless, irresponsible person"). Because the thought is the sole piece of evidence that the un-desirable personality exists, its absence would afford relief that the abhorred characteristic does not exist. The individual becomes hypervigilant for such thoughts and is highly motivated to control them. At the same time, the individual may begin scrutinizing his/her motives and behavior for information consistent with the idea that undesirable character-istics exist. Purdon (1999) argues that thoughts that are more ego-syntonic may give rise to less active resistance and that active resistance may be context specific. For example, worries may give rise to active resistance only after the individual becomes concerned about the physical and mental consequences of worrying (see Wells, 1997). Depressive rumination may give rise to active resistance only when the individual is motivated to manage mood symptoms, such as when attending a social function.

Empirical Research on Appraisals/Beliefs About Thought Control Pre-OCCWG

Researchers interested in cognitive features of OCD have independently developed measures of cognitive appraisal of obsessions. Many of these questionnaires include items that assess beliefs about thought control. Beliefs about the necessity of thought control are said to be important because, of course, they lead to active attempts at thought control that are, at best, ineffective, and at worst, counterproductive, as discussed above. Sookman and Pinard (1995) developed the Obsessive Compulsive Cognitive Schemata Scale, a 208-item measure designed to assess the various schemata thought to drive obsessional symptomatology, including the need for control in general. This latter schema contains items about the need to control thoughts (e.g., "I should be able to completely control all my thoughts and feelings"; "Any loss of control over my thoughts and feelings is frightening"). Tallis' (1995) Obsessional Beliefs Questionnaire also contains a few items about the necessity of thought control, as does the Obsessive Compulsive Cognitions List by Hoekstra (1995). However, these items form a relatively small component of their respective questionnaires.

Freeston, Ladouceur, Gagnon, and Thibodeau (1993) developed the Inventory of Beliefs Related to Obsessions (IBRO) to test cognitive models of obsessional problems. This measure draws primarily on the theoretical work of Rachman and Salkovskis, and included items specifically to assess control of thoughts and actions and the possible consequences of not controlling thoughts. Item selection for the final version of the questionnaire was based on identification of items that distinguished individuals who did nothing in response to an intrusive thought from those who engaged in neutralizing strategies. Factor analysis revealed three factors, the second of which assessed concern about thought control (e.g., "One should always feel guilty if thoughts are not controlled"; "Not being able to control thoughts will harm no one"; "Enduring unpleasant thoughts without doing anything can lead to their disappearance"), and was labeled "overestimation of threat". Psychometric information on the scales separately is not available, but overall scores were found to predict OC symptomatology.

Salkovskis *et al.* (2000) have also developed a measure of appraisal in OCD entitled The Responsibility Interpretations Questionnaire. This measure was designed to assess the frequency of and belief in specific interpretations of intrusive thoughts about possible harm, and derives from Salkovskis' theoretical perspective that overvalued beliefs about responsibility play a pivotal role in the persistence of OCD. Salkovskis' model proposes that the need to control obsessional thoughts arises from beliefs that thoughts lead to harm, and the individual is wholly responsible to prevent harm. Thus, appraisals involving thought control are viewed as being one of several manifestations of beliefs about responsibility. This scale contains numerous items relevant to thought control, such as "I must regain control of my thoughts" and "There's nothing wrong with letting my thoughts come and go naturally," and several items include ideas relevant to both responsibility and control appraisals (e.g., "If I don't resist these thoughts it means I am being irresponsible"). Salkovskis *et al.* (2000) found that this measure was a unique predictor of obsessional symptomatology in individuals with OCD, even when anxiety and depressive symptoms were controlled.

Clark and Purdon (1995) developed a measure of beliefs about thoughts called the Meta-Cognitive Beliefs Questionnaire (MCBQ). This measure was developed to test Clark and Purdon's (Clark, 1989; Clark & Purdon, 1993; Purdon & Clark, 1999) assertions that general beliefs about the need to control thoughts (that is, meta-cognitive beliefs about thoughts and thought processes) play a central role in the development and persistence of obsessional problems. The final version of this self-report inventory consists of 42 items that assess the personal meaning of obsessional thoughts across four dimensions. The first dimension is the importance of thought control, and reflects the belief that one can and should have perfect control over the kinds of thoughts they experience, that one is fully responsible for the content of all thoughts, and that unwanted thoughts represent lapses in control that must be addressed (e.g., "I can and should control my intrusive thoughts"; "I am morally responsible for even the unwanted, unacceptable intrusive thoughts that enter my mind"; "When an unwanted, unacceptable thought pops into my mind it is important that I do something in order to counter it"). The rest of the dimensions tapped by the MCBQ reflect other content domains of thought appraisal, such as responsibility and thought–action fusion. Clark and Purdon (1995) found that the Control scale was the only scale that predicted obsessional symptomatology in non-clinical individuals, and individuals with OCD had significantly higher scores on this scale than did the non-clinical sample.

Purdon (2001) suggested that the individual's in vivo interpretation of *failures* in thought control might also be a central factor in the escalation and persistence of obsessional thoughts. She developed a questionnaire entitled the "Concern over Failures in Thought Control Questionnaire" which assesses participants' in vivo appraisal of the meaning of thought *recurrences* while control efforts are in operation. This measure includes appraisals reflecting concerns about the need to control thoughts (e.g., "The more I had the thought, the more important it seemed that I try to control it"; "I had the thought more often than I expected"; "The more I had the thought the more strategies I used to control it"), as well as appraisals relevant to the domains of responsibility and thought-action fusion. She found that the perceived need to control thoughts was a significant unique predictor of immediate and subsequent suppression effort, even after controlling for other domains of general thought appraisal.

Comparisons Across Domains of Belief/Appraisal. Few studies have actually examined the relative importance of domains of belief/appraisal in OCD. There is good reason to believe that there may be overlap between the domains. For example, it could be argued that certain types of control beliefs are the product of beliefs about responsibility or thought-action fusion beliefs (e.g., beliefs that the thought must be controlled, that control is desirable). Emmelkamp and Aardema (1999) compiled a large item pool based on a number of questionnaires assessing appraisals and beliefs in OCD (including many of those described above). They administered this large series of items to a non-clinical community sample and conducted a factor analysis of this item pool. Fourteen separate domains were identified, including beliefs about control (a four-item factor). The 14 scales were then entered as predictors of various OCD symptom clusters (e.g., washing, checking) as assessed by the Padua Inventory in a stepwise regression analysis, controlling for depressed mood. Beliefs about control, in addition to concern over mistakes, magical thinking rigidity/morality and decision making, were not found to predict OCD symptoms over and above the other domains. However, the 'Control' scale consisted of only four items, which together do not reflect the range of themes of the Control dimension as discussed by Clark and Purdon (Clark & Purdon, 1993, 1995; Purdon & Clark, 1999). Furthermore, the stepwise approach to identifying unique predictors is problematic as enormous power is required to reliably establish unique predictors when predictors are correlated (Tabachnick & Fudell, 1996). Thus, this preliminary exploration of the respective roles of domains of belief in OCD may have limited implications.

Steketee, Frost, and Cohen (1998) took a similar approach to developing a measure of beliefs in OCD. They pooled items from a variety of measures of belief/appraisal and developed a final 90-item self-report measure assessing responsibility for harm, control of thoughts, threat estimation, tolerance for uncertainty, beliefs about discomfort/anxiety and beliefs about coping. This measure was administered to a large sample of individuals with OCD, anxious controls and non-clinical controls. Total scores on the measure were found to predict OCD symptomatology over and above mood state and general anxiety, suggesting that cognitive appraisal of obsessions indeed plays a significant role in obsessional problems. All scales except the Coping scale, and including the Control scale, were strongly correlated with each other, affirming that there is significant overlap between the domains of belief/appraisal in OCD. The OCD sample showed higher scores than the control groups on all six scales. The anxious controls did not score higher than the non-clinical controls on the Control, Responsibility, and Threat Estimation scales, suggesting that these domains of belief are unique to OCD as opposed to general beliefs characteristic of anxiety.

Beliefs About Thought Control: OCCWG Definition and Content

At the first meeting of the OCCWG in June of 1996 at Smith College, a subgroup of members[1] met to formally define the domain of beliefs about thought control and to specify the content of that domain. This goal was achieved by reviewing cognitive–behavioral models of OCD and examining the range of control-relevant beliefs included in measures of appraisal of obsessional thoughts, as well as those implicated in leading cognitive-behavioral models of OCD. The following definition of Beliefs about Control was thus developed:

> *"Overvaluation of the importance of exerting complete control over intrusive thoughts, images or impulses, and the belief that this is both possible and desirable."*

Four dimensions of belief encompassed by this definition were identified, including: (a) tracking of mental events and hypervigilance; (b) moral consequences of failing to control intrusive thoughts, control as a virtue; (c) psychological and behavioral consequences of failing to control intrusive thoughts (e.g., insanity, decreased ability to function); and (d) efficiency of thought control (e.g., efforts should result in immediate and prolonged control, one's ability to control thoughts should never wax and wane).

Empirical Research on the Control Scales of the OCCWG Measures

As discussed in two previous publications (OCCWG, 1997, 2001), the OCCWG was formed in 1995 in order to coordinate the development of instruments for measuring key cognitive features of OCD. The collaborative and coordinated efforts of 26 researchers from eight countries resulted in the development of a 129-item measure of obsessional beliefs called the Obsessional Beliefs Questionnaire (OBQ) and a 43-item measure of appraisals associated with specific unwanted intrusive thoughts called the Interpretations of Intrusions Inventory (III). The OBQ was designed to assess categories of beliefs considered critical in OCD such as inflated responsibility, overimportance of thoughts, need to control thoughts, overestimation of threat, intolerance of uncertainty and perfectionism (OCCWG, 2001). The III was designed to assess three types of appraisals or interpretations of specific unwanted intrusive thoughts, images or impulses; inflated responsibility, importance of thoughts and control of thoughts.

The OCCWG has now collected two large datasets on the OBQ and III. The first dataset, referred to as stage two, involved 101 patients with OCD, 374 undergraduate student controls and 76 English-speaking adult community controls, 12 non-OCD anxious patients, and 35 Greek-speaking controls (OCCWG, 2001). Data were collected across ten sites in four different countries. Item and factor analysis of the original OBQ and III resulted in a reduction of the item composition of the measures. Based on these results an intermediate 87-item OBQ and a 31-item III were utilized in the stage two and subsequent

---

[1]The working group on Beliefs About Control consisted of David A. Clark, Paul Emmelkamp, Mark Freeston, Cheryl Carmin, and Christine Purdon.

analyses conducted on these measures. The findings from the stage two data are reported in OCCWG (2001), the stage three data are in the process of analysis (OCCWG, in preparation). The OBQ-87 and III-31, along with measures of OCD, depressive and anxious symptoms and cognitions, were administered to a large number of individuals across 17 different sites from Australia, Canada, France, Greece, Italy, Netherlands, and the United States. The stage three data included more than 250 individuals with OCD, over 100 non-OCD anxious patients, 85 non-clinical adult community controls and more than 250 undergraduate students. Because the focus of this chapter is on the control of thoughts, we will deal exclusively with this subscale of the OBQ-87 and III-31.

The Control of Thoughts items for the OBQ-87 and the III-31 were based on the definition of thought control beliefs and appraisals developed by the OCCWG at the Smith Conference (see previous discussion). This resulted in a 14 item OBQ-87 Control of Thoughts subscale and a 11 item III-31 Control of Thoughts subscale. The OBQ items deal with various types of thought control beliefs such as perceived negative consequences of failing to control one's thoughts, the importance of exercising good mental control, positive attributions associated with good mental control, need to track one's thoughts, and beliefs that thought control is not only possible but highly desirable. The thought control items of the III-31 refer to one or two specific intrusive thoughts recorded on the form. The participant is asked to indicate the degree of importance of gaining control over specific intrusions, the negative impact of partial or failed control of the intrusion, and imperatives about the importance of controlling the specific intrusive thought recorded on the III-31. Results from the stage two data indicate that both the OBQ-87 and III-31 Control of Thoughts subscales had good internal consistency (α= 0.92 and 0.91, respectively, based on the OCD subsample) and 12 day test-retest coefficients of 0.85 and 0.83, respectively (OCCWG, 2001). Data from the stage three dataset revealed similar levels of internal consistency, but somewhat lower test-retest correlations among the OCD sample.

How specific to OCD are the thought control beliefs and appraisals measured by the OBQ-87 and III-31? Group comparisons of the stage two data revealed that OCD patients scored significantly higher than the non-OCD anxious, adult community controls and students on the OBQ-87 and III-31 Control of Thoughts subscales. Moreover, there were no significant differences between the remaining groups. This suggests that the thought control beliefs and appraisals of the OBQ-87 and III-31 are associated specifically with the presence of obsessional symptomatology and not just distress or anxiety more generally. The non-obsessional anxious patients did not score significantly higher than the non-clinical groups on these two subscales. Preliminary comparisons among the stage three groups indicated that the groups differed significantly on all six subscales of the OBQ with the OCD scoring highest, followed by the non-OCD anxiety group, the student sample and finally the adult community control group. Analyses of the three III-31 subscales revealed the same pattern of results except that the OC group and AC group did not differ significantly on the III-31 Control of Thoughts subscale. Evidence that OCD patients actually scored significantly higher on the OBQ Control of Thoughts subscale is a stringent test of specificity given the close association that OCD has with other anxiety states at both the symptom and disorder levels. As well, the findings, which are based on very large samples of OCD patients, indicate that maladaptive beliefs and appraisals about the importance of controlling unwanted thoughts are most evident in OCD, although it may also be manifest to a lesser degree in generally anxious non-obsessional patients. As expected non-clinical individuals showed the lowest rates of endorsement for these types of beliefs.

How distinct are the beliefs and appraisals concerning the control of unwanted thoughts from the other cognitive domains measured by the OBQ-87 and III-31? The intercorrelation matrix for the stage two data suggests a high degree of overlap between the OBQ-87 and III-31 subscales (OCCWG, 2001). Based on a sample of OCD and non-OCD subjects, the OBQ Control of Thoughts subscale had its highest correlation with Importance of Thoughts ($r = 0.80$) and its lowest correlation with Perfectionism ($r = 0.60$). All three III-31 subscales were highly intercorrelated (rs ranged 0.85–0.88). These findings were again replicated with the stage three data. Correlations based exclusively on the OCD subsample indicated that again OBQ-87 Control of Thoughts was most highly correlated with Importance of Thoughts and less strongly associated with Perfectionism. Intercorrelations among the III-31 subscales were also very high. These results indicate that despite conceptual distinctions between the various cognitive domains in OCD, the actual items written to assess these domains exhibit a high level of overlap. There are three possible reasons for this lack of differentiation. First, one would expect a high rate of concordance between the different cognitive domains because they all deal with some aspect of OCD. Thus, patients with this disorder should show elevated levels across the various cognitive domains. Second, it is possible that the cognitive domains are distinct but that the items intended to capture these domains have lower construct validity. The concepts represented by the items are fairly abstract and complex. It may be that respondents failed to fully understand many of the items and so responded at a more superficial level. And finally, it is possible that the fine discriminations in the cognitive domains of OCD offered by the OCCWG (1997) are not valid. Possibly the maladaptive beliefs and appraisals associated with OCD operate at a more generic level than researchers realized.

A final question that we can address with the OCCWG data is the specific relation between OCD symptoms and maladaptive beliefs and appraisals of thought control. The stage two data indicated that the OBQ-87 and III-31 Control of Thoughts subscales correlated moderately with self-report measures of obsessions, compulsions, anxious and depressive symptoms (OCCWG, 2001). After controlling for the high correlation between symptom measures, the OBQ-87 control subscale showed a low but significant correlation with anxiety, depression and obsessional symptoms, whereas there was very clear evidence that III-31 Control of Thoughts scale had higher partial correlations with the Padua Inventory Total Score than with the Beck Depression or Beck Anxiety Total Score.

Analysis of the stage three OCD subsample revealed a more discouraging pattern of results (OCCWG, in preparation). Zero-order correlations indicated that the OBQ-87 and III-31 Control of Thoughts subscales had minimal association with the YBOCS Obsessions and Compulsions subscales that declined to practically zero when anxious and depressive symptoms were partialled out of the correlations. The zero-order correlations with the Padua Inventory Total Score were modest for both OBQ-87 Control and III-31 Control subscales, and when anxiety and depression were controlled, the OBQ-87 and III-31 correlations declined substantially. Other research also suggests that the specific appraisals identified as important to OCD may play a role in the persistence of other anxiety disorders. Rassin, Diepstraten, Merckelbach, and Muris (2001) examined pre- and post-treatment thought–action fusion (TAF) beliefs and suppression effort in a sample of individuals with OCD and a clinical sample of individuals with other anxiety disorders. They found that TAF beliefs were endorsed equally by both groups pre- and post-treatment, but that TAF correlated with psychopathology in both groups.

At the same time, however, when we based our analyses of construct specificity on the non-OCD patient and normal controls a different picture emerged. Zero-order correlations of the OBQ-87 and III-31 Control of Thoughts subscales with YBOCS and Padua Inventory total scores were moderate to strong for both subscales. When self-reported worry was partialled from the correlations, the OBQ-87 and III-31 Control of Thoughts subscales remained modestly correlated with YBOCS Obsessions and Compulsion but fell more substantially with the Padua Inventory Total Score (OCCWG, in preparation).

These mixed findings on the construct specificity of maladaptive thought control beliefs and appraisals suggest that there might be different pathways depending on whether the primary diagnosis is OCD or some other disorder. For OCD patients, presence of general anxiety or depression might elevate a tendency to hold to maladaptive notions about thought control. Certainly there is evidence that the presence of dysphoria makes thought control much more difficult (e.g., Sutherland, Newman, & Rachman, 1982; Wenzlaff, Wegner, & Klein, 1991; Wenzlaff, Wegner, & Roper, 1988). Thus, measures of maladaptive thought control beliefs and appraisals may not be specific to OCD samples. For non-OCD patients and non-patients, the types of beliefs and appraisals about thought control contained in the OBQ-87 and III-31 may be much more sensitive to the presence of obsessionality. In these groups, measures of thought control beliefs and appraisals would appear much more specific to OC phenomena.

Summary and Conclusion

An apparent breakdown in the ability to control unwanted, disturbing intrusive thoughts, images or impulses is a cardinal feature of OCD. Patients with obsessional ruminations exhibit near Herculean determination to rein in their tormenting cognitions. And yet, the harder they try to control these thoughts, the more elusive the goal of complete eradication of the obsession.

In this chapter we have explored various facets of the problem of thought control in OCD. We offered a more precise definition of thought control based on the work of the OCCWG (1997) and we discussed the possibility that the nature and content of the thought may influence the level of control that one can attain. However, in this chapter we propose that the most important aspect of pathological thought control in OCD centers on the types of beliefs and appraisals patients hold to with regard to the control of their unwanted, distressing intrusive thoughts. The 'acid test' of this proposition will be in evidence of improved outcome when such domains of belief/appraisal are targeted directly in treatment and symptom reduction is found to have a strong relationship with decreases in the conviction of these beliefs/appraisal. In the meantime, it would be worthwhile to examine the relative contribution of domains of belief in OCD. It may also be the case that different domains of belief may have particular relevance within different sub-types of OCD (e.g., washers vs. checkers vs. ordering/arranging).

References

American Psychiatric Association. (1994). *Diagnostic and statistical manual of mental disorders* (4th ed.). Washington, DC: Author.

Amir, N., Cashman, L., & Foa, E. B. (1997). Strategies of thought control in obsessive–compulsive disorder. *Behaviour Research and Therapy, 35*, 775–777.

Clark, D. A. (1989). *A schema-control model of negative thoughts.* Paper presented at the World Congress of Cognitive Therapies, Oxford, England.

Clark, D. A., & de Silva, P. (1985). The nature of depressive and anxious thoughts: distinct or uniform phenomena? *Behaviour Research and Therapy, 23*, 279–282.

Clark, D. A., & Purdon, C. (1993). New perspectives for a cognitive theory of obsessions. *Australian Psychologist, 28*, 161–167.

Clark, D. A., & Purdon, C. (1995). Meta-cognitive beliefs in obsessive–compulsive disorder. In S. Rachman, G. Steketee, R. O. Frost, & P. Salkovskis (Chairs) *Towards a better understanding of obsessive–compulsive problems.* Symposium conducted at the First World Congress of Behavioural and Cognitive Therapies, Copenhagen, Denmark.

Emmelkamp, P. M. G., & Aardema, A. (1999). Metacognition, specific obsessive–compulsive beliefs and obsessive–compulsive behaviour. *Clinical Psychology and Psychotherapy, 6*, 139–145.

Freeston, M. H., & Ladouceur, R. (1997). What do patients do with their obsessive thoughts? *Behaviour Research and Therapy, 35*, 335–348.

Freeston, M. H., Ladouceur, R., Thibodeau, N., & Gagnon, F. (1991). Cognitive intrusions in a non-clinical population: I. Response style, subjective experience and appraisal. *Behaviour Research and Therapy, 29*, 585–597.

Freeston, M. H., Ladouceur, R., Gagnon, F., & Thibodeau, N. (1993). Beliefs about obsessional thoughts. *Journal of Psychopathology and Behavioral Assessment, 15*, 1–21.

Hoekstra, R.J. (1995). *Obsessive–Compulsive Cognitions List.* Unpulished scale, Research Office, Faculty of Medicine, Limburg University, Maastricht, The Netherlands.

Janeck, A. S., & Calamari, J. E. (1999). Thought suppression in obsessive–compulsive disorder. *Cognitive Therapy and Research, 23*, 497–509.

Ladouceur, R., Freeston, M. H., Rhéaume, J., Dugas, M. J., Gagnon, F., Thibodeau, N., & Fournier, S. (2000). Strategies used with intrusive thoughts: a comparison of OCD patients with anxious and community controls. *Journal of Abnormal Psychology, 109*, 179–187.

Obsessive Compulsive Cognitions Working Group. (1997). Cognitive assessment of obsessive–compulsive disorder. *Behaviour Research and Therapy, 35*, 667–681.

Obsessive Compulsive Cognitions Working Group. (2001). Development and initial validation of the Obsessive Beliefs Questionnaire and the Interpretations of Intrusions Inventory. *Behaviour Research and Therapy, 39*, 987–1006.

Obsessive Compulsive Cognitions Working Group. (in preparation). *Psychometric validation of the Obsessive Beliefs Questionnaire and the Interpretation of Intrusions Inventory: Findings from stage 3 data.* Unpublished manuscript.

Purdon, C. (1999). Thought suppression and psychopathology. *Behaviour Research and Therapy, 37*, 1029–1054.

Purdon, C. (2001). Appraisal of obsessional thought *recurrences*: impact on anxiety, active resistance and mood state. *Behaviour Therapy, 32*, 47–64.

Purdon, C., & Clark, D. A. (1993). Obsessional intrusive thoughts in nonclinical subjects. Part I. Content and relation with depressive, anxious and obsessional symptoms. *Behaviour Research and Therapy, 31,* 713–720.

Purdon, C., & Clark, D. A. (1994). Perceived control and appraisal of obsessional intrusive thoughts: a replication and extension. *Behavioural and Cognitive Psychotherapy, 22,* 269–286.

Purdon, C., & Clark, D. A. (1999). Metacognition and obsessions. *Clinical Psychology and Psychotherapy, 6,* 102–110.

Purdon, C., & Clark, D. A. (2001). Suppression of obsession-like thoughts in nonclinical individuals. Impact on thought frequency, appraisal and mood state. *Behaviour Research and Therapy, 39,* 1163–1181.

Rachman, S. J. (1997). A cognitive theory of obsessions. *Behaviour Research and Therapy, 35,* 793–802.

Rachman, S. J. (1998). A cognitive theory of obsessions: elaborations. *Behaviour Research and Therapy, 36,* 385–401.

Rachman, S. J., & Hodgson, R. J. (1980). *Obsessions and compulsions.* Englewood Cliffs, NJ: Prentice Hall.

Rachman, S., & de Silva, P. (1978). Abnormal and normal obsessions. *Behaviour Research and Therapy, 16,* 233–248.

Rassin, E., Diepstraten, P., Merckelbach, H., & Muris, P. (2001). Thought–action fusion and thought suppression in obsessive–compulsive disorder. *Behaviour Research and Therapy, 39,* 757–764.

Salkovskis, P. M. (1985). Obsessional–compulsive problems: a cognitive–behavioural analysis. *Behaviour Research and Therapy, 23,* 571–583.

Salkovskis, P. M. (1989). Cognitive–behavioural factors and the persistence of intrusive thoughts in obsessional problems. *Behaviour Research and Therapy, 27,* 677–682.

Salkovskis, P. M. (1998). Psychological approaches to the understanding of obsessional problems. In R. P. Swinson, M. M. Antony, S. Rachman, & M. A. Richter (eds), *Obsessive–compulsive disorder: theory, research and treatment* (pp. 33–50). New York: Guilford.

Salkovskis, P. M., & Campbell, P. (1994). Thought suppression induces intrusions in naturally occurring negative intrusive thoughts. *Behaviour Research and Therapy, 32,* 1–8.

Salkovskis, P. M., & Harrison, J. (1984). Abnormal and normal obsessions — a replication. *Behaviour Research and Therapy, 22,* 1–4.

Salkovskis, P. M., Richards, H. C., & Forrester, E. (1995). The relationship between obsessional problems and intrusive thoughts. *Behavioural and Cognitive Psychotherapy, 23,* 281–299.

Salkovskis, P. M., Wroe, A. L., Gledhill, A., Morrison, N., Forrester, E., Richards, C., Reynolds, M., & Thorpe, S. (2000). Responsibility attitudes and interpretations are characteristic of obsessive compulsive disorder. *Behaviour Research and Therapy, 38,* 347–372.

Sookman, D., & Pinard, G. (1995, July). *The Cognitive Schemata Scale: a multidimensional measure of cognitive schemas in obsessive compulsive disorder.* Paper presented at the World Congress of Behavioural and Cognitive Therapies, Copenhagen, Denmark.

Steketee, G., Frost, R. O., & Cohen, I. C. (1998). Beliefs in obsessive–compulsive disorder. *Journal of Anxiety Disorders, 12,* 525–537.

Sutherland, G., Newman, B., & Rachman, S. (1982). Experimental investigations of the relations between mood and intrusive unwanted cognitions. *British Journal of Medical Psychology, 55,* 127–138.

Tabacnick, B. G., & Fudell, L. S. (1996). *Using multivariate statistics* (3rd ed.). New York: Harper Collins.

Tallis, F. (1995). *Obsessional Beliefs Scale.* Unpublished scale, Charter Nightingale Hospital, London, UK.

Trinder, H., & Salkovskis, P. M. (1994). Personally relevant intrusions outside the laboratory: long-term suppression increases intrusion. *Behaviour Research and Therapy, 32*, 833–842.

Turner, S. M., Beidel, D. C., & Stanley, M. A. (1992). Are obsessional thoughts and worry different cognitive phenomena? *Clinical Psychology Review, 12*, 257–270.

Wegner, D. M. (1994). Ironic processes of mental control. *Psychological Review, 101*, 34–52.

Wegner, D. M., Schneider, D. J., Carter, S. R., & White, T. L. (1987). Paradoxical effects of thought suppression. *Journal of Personality and Social Psychology, 53*, 5–13.

Wells, A. (1997). *Cognitive therapy of anxiety disorders: a practice manual and conceptual guide.* Chichester: Wiley.

Wells, A., & Davies, M. (1994). The Thought Control Questionnaire: a measure of individual differences in the control of unwanted thoughts. *Behaviour Research and Therapy, 32*, 871–878.

Wells, A., & Matthews, G. (1994). *Attention and emotion: a clinical perspective.* Hove: Lawrence Erlbaum.

Wells, A., & Morrison, A. P. (1994). Qualitative dimensions of normal worry and normal obsessions: a comparative study. *Behaviour Research and Therapy, 32*, 867–870.

Wenzlaff, R. M., Wegner, D. M., & Klein, S. B. (1991). The role of thought suppression in the bonding of thought and mood. *Journal of Personality and Social Psychology, 60*, 500–508.

Wenzlaff, R. M., Wegner, D. M., & Roper, D. W. (1998). Depression and mental control: the resurgence of unwanted negative thoughts. *Journal of Personality and Social Psychology, 55*, 882–892.

Chapter 4

Responsibility

Paul M. Salkovskis and Elizabeth Forrester

Importance of Meaning and Specificity in Cognitive Theories of Anxiety Disorders

A defining feature of recent cognitive approaches to the understanding and treatment of anxiety disorders is the way in which some presentations (i.e., patients who are suffering from particular anxiety disorders) are differentiated by characteristic beliefs in the form of negative meanings triggered by anxiety-relevant stimuli. The focus of such appraisals determines the pattern of factors maintaining that disorder. More generalized "upstream" beliefs are involved in determining the way in which stimuli and situations are interpreted or appraised; the focus of some of these beliefs tends to be considerably less specific. Cognitive vulnerability to making appraisals ranges from the very general to the highly specific. The identification of beliefs and appraisals that are specific to a particular type of anxiety problem has the advantage of allowing the relatively straightforward identification of the way the person suffering from anxiety responds to their experience, particularly in terms of the focus of attention and behavioral reactions. Such responses are regarded as crucial, because they can, in vulnerable individuals (vulnerable by virtue of their general beliefs), augment both the appraisals and sometimes the extent and intensity of negatively appraised stimuli themselves. It is thus the understanding of the interrelationship of belief and appraisal factors and the person's responses to them that is the key to understanding the maintenance of the problem. Such an approach, concentrating on the *specific* beliefs and meanings that drive and/or motivate psychological factors involved in the maintenance of the disorder, has been central to the advances made in the treatment of anxiety disorders (Salkovskis, 1996a).

This type of cognitively-based analysis has allowed the identification of key treatment targets, and the development of very focused treatments that can greatly differ in the therapy procedures used to bring about change for different anxiety disorders. Although, by definition, the treatment targets vary systematically from problem to problem (and from person to person), they nevertheless tend to follow a general pattern. Cognitive–behavioral treatment for anxiety usually seeks to help the patient identify and change: (a) the main negative appraisals (interpretations) that occur in situations associated with their anxiety; (b) attention focused on the perceived source of such threat, and/or the possibility of reducing or preventing feared outcomes; (c) safety-seeking behaviors motivated by the perception of threat; (d) general beliefs (attitudes or assumptions) that give rise to misinterpretations of triggering stimuli; and (e) current circumstances or situations that confirm or strengthen negative interpretations and assumptions.

Cognitive analyses of anxiety therefore depend on a clear understanding of the way patients with a particular problem interpret key situations and stimuli. Early in the development of cognitive–behavioral approaches to emotional problems, Beck (1976) proposed that the experience of intense anxiety was associated with the perception that danger was relatively likely, would be particularly severe or serious, that the person would not be able cope and that external "rescue" factors were unlikely to be present. This can be expressed as a quasi-mathematical equation, viz.:

$$\text{Anxiety} = \frac{\text{perceived probability of danger X perceived cost/awfulness}}{\text{perceived ability to cope with danger} + \text{perceived rescue factors}}$$

Perceived probability *interacts* with the specific meaning, which the person assigns to the danger concerned. For example, the person may think it is very unlikely that intrusive images of violence mean that he/she will lose control and attack loved ones. However, if the person did so, that would be perceived as so extremely awful that it results in extremely intense anxiety. These two factors are thus regarded as multiplicative and synergistic. This conceptualization of cognitive factors in anxiety can account for the common obsessional phenomenon whereby the person believes that a particular negative outcome is extremely unlikely and/or unbelievable but nevertheless shows extreme fear of it. The person believes that, although unlikely, the threat is too awful to risk. The combination of risk and cost is further modulated by the extent to which the person feels they would be able to cope or not cope with the danger should it materialize and the extent to which factors extraneous to their own coping would be involved. Clinical and research evidence suggests that people who suffer from anxiety problems can show distortions involving each of these factors singly or in combination. Different combinations are likely across individuals and probably between disorders.

Beck (1976) also hypothesized that people are likely to interpret situations as more dangerous than they really are because of particular assumptions or beliefs they learned during an earlier period in their life. Such beliefs may have been useful during that earlier stage of life, but may become problematic when new situations arise that call for a different type of understanding. Many such assumptions are anxiety related, but not necessarily disorder specific. Examples of this kind of belief would be, "It is important to be perfectly calm at all times"; "If I don't control myself then I are in danger of losing control"; "I must not show my feelings"; "If I don't worry about things, then everything will go wrong for me." Other assumptions tend to be characteristic of specific disorders such as panic, social phobia, obsessive compulsive disorder (OCD), hypochondriasis and so forth. In some instances, such assumptions can be strong enough to mean that almost any situation will trigger an anxious response, resulting in a generalized tendency to experience anxiety in such situations (or even across a wide range of situations). In other instances, relatively intense life events or other "critical incidents" can result in the activation of assumptions resulting in an enduring tendency to react to particular situations with anxiety as indicating threat and/or danger.

Cognitive Aspects of Psychopathology of OCD: Specific Beliefs and Relevant Beliefs

A cognitive–behavioral analysis allows the classification of negative beliefs involved in obsessional problems into two broad groups: (a) beliefs specific to OCD; and (b) beliefs relevant to OCD. The first of these categories refers to those beliefs that occur more frequently in OCD patients than in other people suffering from anxiety disorders. This leads to the presumption that such beliefs are important in the *specific* psychopathology of OCD. Of course, such a presumption is not always justified, and can be misleading. The second category recognizes that there may be beliefs that feature in the psychopathology of anxiety and related psychological disturbances, but that are not unique to OCD, as they may occur in one or more of the other anxiety disorders, in depression and so on. Some such beliefs may not be specific to OCD, but may be important in the psychopathology of the problem. The fact that the same beliefs are relevant to other anxiety disorders simply indicates the unsurprising fact that different disorders have some mechanisms in common.

In research terms, disentangling these two categories presents a great deal of difficulty. The two most obvious approaches are either pragmatic (identify those beliefs that occur in OCD and do not occur, or occur at lower intensity, in other anxiety disorders) or theory driven. The first of these two is the least consistent with psychological approaches, as the underlying assumption is that some kind of nosology (most commonly a diagnostic system such as DSM) should be the driving principle in research. In contrast, the theory driven approach starts with a theoretical view of OCD not as a diagnosis, but as a way of operationally defining the more extreme manifestations of particular psychological processes. It is assumed that such processes can and do transcend diagnostic boundaries. Psychological theory (based both on an understanding of clinical phenomenology and research findings) helps the researcher and clinician to identify those beliefs likely to be specific to severe obsessional problems and those likely to be more general.

The boundary between these two ways of addressing the specific versus relevant issue is, in fact, less than precise, as a pragmatic approach has to start somewhere. When available theories are weak, it can be helpful to pool ideas gleaned from a range of theories in order to guide research strategies. Criterion group comparisons (based on diagnosis) allows theory to be developed iteratively. Our group has strongly favored the theory-driven approach because it has the further advantage of being able to progress to yet stronger tests of theory. Thus, having identified particular beliefs as likely to be specific to OCD, the next step is to design and conduct experimental studies focusing on the maintaining factors identified in studies of criterion groups and individual differences.

The advantage of a theory-driven approach is that it reduces the initial likelihood of identifying beliefs that are specific to OCD but are not involved in either producing or maintaining it. For example, it is possible that a belief such as "OCD is a brain disease" might be specific to people suffering from OCD, but not directly relevant to the maintenance of the problem. Thus, although the division into OCD-specific and OCD-relevant beliefs is helpful, it should not be assumed that, if a belief is specific to OCD it is necessarily relevant. To establish that a belief is relevant requires an integrated theoretical, psychometric and experimental research strategy; the experimental research can include treatment research, but only in a relatively limited way (see below). In terms of being both

OCD-specific and OCD-relevant, beliefs concerning responsibility are particularly well validated. In the remainder of this chapter, we will describe key aspects of the cognitive theory that sparked interest in the examination of beliefs related to OCD, discuss the present status of the concept of responsibility and consider the relationship between responsibility and other cognitive factors that have been related to OCD.

The Cognitive Approach to Understanding Obsessional Problems

People suffering from OCD characteristically experience thoughts, images and impulses that are intrusive, distressing, and personally unacceptable to them. The occurrence of such unacceptable intrusive thoughts about possible harm coming to oneself or others is not confined to people suffering from obsessional problems, but is a universal phenomenon (Rachman & de Silva, 1978; Salkovskis & Harrison, 1984). The last few years has seen the development of cognitive conceptualizations of OCD (Freeston, Rhéaume, & Ladouceur, 1996; Rachman, 1997, 1998; Salkovskis, 1985, 1989, 1999). These approaches are closely based on Beck's cognitive theorizing on anxiety as described above. Specifically, the cognitive theory of OCD emphasizes the importance of the way in which the occurrence and content of intrusive cognitions are interpreted. The meaning that patients attach to such intrusions both triggers adverse mood and motivates neutralizing behavior. Salkovskis (1985) suggested that the unique feature of obsessional problems lies not in the occurrence of ideas of danger or threat, although such threat perception is a necessary component of the cognitive theory of the way obsessional problems occur in the ways described above, but rather in the motivation of the compulsive component of the problem. It is certainly striking that the occurrence of some form of neutralizing appears to be always present in obsessional problems. The cognitive theory of obsessional problems accounts for neutralizing by specifying that the occurrence and/or content of intrusions (thoughts, images, impulses and/or doubts) are interpreted (appraised) as indicating that the person may be responsible for harm to themselves or others. The definition of responsibility has, at times, been a source of some confusion. Salkovskis, Rachman, Ladouceur, and Freeston, (1992), cited in Salkovskis, (1996b) produced a definition that was revised by a subgroup of the international working group as:

> *The belief that one has power which is pivotal to bring about or prevent subjectively crucial negative outcomes. These outcomes are perceived as essential to prevent. They may be actual, that is, having consequences in the real world, and/or at a moral level (Salkovskis, 1996b; p. 110–111).*

The cognitive–behavioral theory specifies that the origin of particular negative appraisals will usually lie in learned assumptions. Such assumptions often form as adaptive ways of coping with problematic aspects of early (earlier) experience, but have usually outlasted their initial usefulness, thereby being transformed from protective to vulnerability factors. Such assumptions may trigger an obsessional disorder, particularly when activated by critical incidents (origins). The cognitive theory of OCD specifies that assumptions may include not only tightly specified beliefs about harm and responsibility, but also about the nature and implications of intrusive thoughts themselves, as in the religious notion of sin by thought (e.g., "Thinking something wicked is as bad as doing it"). The occurrence of an intrusive thought or impulse concerning some extreme and unacceptable action would, for someone holding this belief, result in very negative appraisals and consequent efforts to undo such thoughts or prevent their recurrence. Other assumptions focus on the harm itself (e.g., "If one *can* have any influence over a harmful outcome, then one is responsible for it.") and on both the harm itself and the significance of intrusive thoughts about such harm (e.g., "If I don't act when I can foresee danger, then I am to blame for any consequences if it happens"). When someone who holds such general beliefs experiences intrusive cognitions concerning possible danger, the intrusions tend to be interpreted as indicating an imperative for preventative action.

Thus, this type of responsibility assumption makes it more likely that the person will react to intrusions with responsibility appraisals, which in turn increase the likelihood that the person will decide to seek to do things they believe will diminish their perceived risk of causing harm by their action or inaction. Threat and responsibility appraisals also trigger other reactions, such as selective attention, thought suppression and reassurance seeking that can play a further role in the maintenance of an obsessional beliefs and the re-occurrence of intrusions.

From Appraisals to Core Beliefs and Back Again: A Worthwhile Journey?

If the way in which intrusions are interpreted are indeed at the heart of the psychopathology of OCD, then it is crucial that the nature, scope and impact of the beliefs involved are clarified. In order to do this, we first need to consider which beliefs should form the focus of such consideration. From the broad theoretical perspective of cognitive–behavioral approaches, it is clear that these should involve both interpretations/appraisals (usually referred to clinically as negative automatic thoughts) and the assumptions that form the basis of such interpretations. What is much less clear is how important higher levels of meaning and meaning structures should be considered. Current writing in the field of cognitive approaches refers to core beliefs and schemas. Core beliefs are often regarded by clinicians writing in the field as being the closest cognitive correlate of schemas, probably because of their presumed depth. We remain somewhat skeptical of this view, preferring the view that higher-order belief factors conform to the structural complexity of the concept of schema rather than "boil down" to the relative unidimensionality of core beliefs. The attraction of core beliefs lies in the fact that the simple theoretical (nearly atheoretical) view they afford suggests that they should be measurable. On the other hand, the theoretical basis of the concept of schema means that, by definition, schematic structures have to be inferred and cannot be more directly measured. This is further complicated by the fact that there are several different theories concerning the nature of schemas. Most commonly, previous attempts at measurement have involved considering clusters of linked assumptions. Given these considerations, and the fact that our primary focus is on the maintenance and treatment of obsessional problems, we have chosen to confine the consideration of beliefs here to interpretations and assumptions, and their impact.

Responsibility Appraisals and the Maintenance of OCD

Neutralizing behavior is a result of the way in which vulnerable individuals misinterpret the occurrence and content of intrusions as indicating personal responsibility for some avoidable harm to themselves or others. Neutralizing includes both overt behaviors (such as washing and checking), (Rachman, 1976a, b; Salkovskis, 1985, 1989) or mental checking and restitution activity, (such as "putting right" by saying prayers, thinking good thoughts in response to bad thoughts, repeatedly running over details of events in memory) (Rachman, 1971; Salkovskis & Westbrook, 1989). Thus, the problem behaviors in obsessions include not only obvious compulsive activities such as repeated checking and washing and their mental equivalents, but also attempts at thought suppression which can have the effect of paradoxically increasing intrusions and preoccupation. These responsibility-motivated neutralizing efforts reduce discomfort in the short term but have the longer-term effect of increasing preoccupation and triggering further intrusions.

Intrusive cognitions acquire emotional significance as a result of the way in which they are interpreted. Intrusions are initially experienced as emotionally neutral, but can take on positive, negative or no emotional significance, depending on the person's prior experience (assumptions) and the context in which intrusions occur (Edwards & Dickerson, 1987; England & Dickerson, 1988). An intrinsic part of the appraisal of an intrusion concerns the need for further action. If the intrusion is interpreted as having no implications, further processing is unlikely. If the appraisal suggests a specific reaction (including attempts to suppress or avoid the thought), then further processing (particularly controlled processing) is extremely likely. Overt or covert behavioral reactions occurring as a response to intrusive cognitions result in such cognitions becoming salient and therefore acquiring priority of processing. Thus, when an intrusive cognition or its content have some direct implications for the reactions of the individual experiencing it, processing priority will increase and further appraisal and elaboration become more likely. Such a reaction is particularly likely if the person interprets the occurrence and/or content of the intrusion as making them responsible for preventing or undoing some kind of harm. Responsibility interpretations tend to lead the person to try too hard in several respects. Such efforts are particularly likely to focus on control of mental activity, including attempts to be sure of the accuracy of one's memory, to take account of all factors in one's decisions, to prevent the occurrence of unacceptable material, to ensure that an outcome has been achieved when the difference between achieving it and not achieving it is imperceptible (as in deciding that one's hands are sufficiently clean after washing to remove contamination).

Once neutralizing and related responses to intrusive thoughts are established, they are maintained by the association with the perception of reduced responsibility for harm and discomfort. However, responsibility beliefs are, at best, maintained by the occurrence of such safety-seeking behaviors (Salkovskis, 1991, 1996c), while the recurrence of the intrusive cognitions themselves becomes more likely. Thus, obsessional problems will occur in individuals who are distressed by the occurrence of intrusions, who believe the occurrence of such cognitions indicates personal responsibility for serious and distressing harm unless corrective action is taken, and who respond accordingly.

An obsessional pattern would be particularly likely in vulnerable individuals when intrusions are regarded as self-initiated (e.g., resulting in appraisals such as "these thoughts might mean I want to harm the children; I must guard against losing control"). In this respect, thought–action fusion (TAF; Rachman, 1993; Rachman, Thordarson, Shafran, & Woody, 1995) is a particularly powerful type of responsibility belief; ideas such as "thinking about causing harm is as bad as causing harm"; "only evil people think evil thoughts"; "thinking about harm can make harm happen" are particularly likely to trigger appraisals concerning responsibility for harm when intrusive thoughts occur.

In summary, responsibility beliefs have the effect of making the patient try too hard to exert control over both mental activity and potentially harmful events in the real world. They do so in variety of counter-productive and therefore anxiety-provoking ways. Efforts at overcontrol increase distress because: (a) direct and deliberate attention to mental activity can modify the contents of consciousness; (b) efforts to deliberately control a range of mental activities apparently and actually meet with failure and even opposite effects; (c) attempts to prevent harm and responsibility for harm increase the salience and accessibility of the patients' concerns about harm; and (d) neutralizing directed at preventing harm also prevents disconfirmation (i.e., prevents the patient from discovering that the things he or she is afraid of will not occur). This means that exaggerated beliefs about responsibility and harm do not decline.

Cognitive Factors Theoretically Linked to Responsibility

Concerns about Omission and Responsibility

Salkovskis (1985) suggested that some obsessional concerns might be related to beliefs concerning the consequences of omissions. Wroe and Salkovskis (2000) linked this aspect of the cognitive theory to social psychological research in decision making. Spranca, Minsk, and Barron (1991) have demonstrated what they refer to as "omission bias" in non-clinical subjects. They showed that normal subjects judge responsibility for negative consequences to be diminished when an omission is involved as opposed to when some specific action was involved in bringing about the negative consequence. This is true in normal subjects even when the element of intention (i.e. the extent to which the person wishes the "negative" outcome to occur) is controlled for. Thus, most people appear to regard themselves as more responsible for what they actively do than what they fail to do. Clinical experience and research suggests that obsessional patients are less likely to show omission bias.

Wroe and Salkovskis (2000) suggested that beliefs characteristic of OCD, such as "any influence over outcome = responsibility for outcome" could be expected to increase concern with omissions. Consideration of the phenomenology of obsessional problems suggests several other ways in which omissions may become relatively more important. An important factor in judgements concerning responsibility is the perception of agency, meaning that one has chosen to bring something about. Particular importance is usually given to *premeditation* in the sense of being able to foresee possible harmful outcomes. Thus,

> "responsible means 'to some extent culpable (either morally or in law according to the context) for* one's own *acts or omissions'. The ascription

of responsibility in this sense is based on what we believe to have been the person's mental state at or before the time of the act or omission. 'Premeditation' usually makes an objectionable act seem more culpable. If the actor foresaw a real possibility of his causing harm — *for example by his way of driving — his act or omission will be called 'reckless' and blamed accordingly." (emphasis added).*

and

"More often it is the actor's state of mind at the time of the act ... that determines the degree to which he is regarded as blameworthy. If the act seems to have been — quite accidental — if for instance he knocks over a child whom he did not see in — his path — he is not blamed, unless we think that he should have been aware of this as a real possibility." (**Oxford Companion to the Mind**, 1987).

One of the problems experienced by patients with obsessions is that it is often in the nature of the condition that they frequently foresee a wide range of possible negative outcomes (Wroe, Salkovskis, & Richards, 2000). That is, the intrusive thoughts often concern things that could go wrong unless dealt with (such as passing on contamination, hurting someone accidentally, leaving the door unlocked or the gas turned on). Sometimes it is not even permissible for the person to try not to foresee problems/disasters, because this would mean that he or she had deliberately chosen this course, again increasing responsibility. When aware of this, some patients regard it as a duty to try to foresee negative outcomes. However, if in any case a negative outcome is foreseen even an intrusive thought, responsibility is established, because to do nothing requires the person to decide not to act to prevent the harmful outcome. That is, deciding not to act despite being aware of possible disastrous consequences becomes an active decision, making the person a causal agent in relation to those disastrous consequences. Thus, the occurrence of intrusive/obsessional thoughts transforms a situation where harm can only occur by omission into a situation where the person has actively chosen to allow the harm to take place. This might mean that the apparent absence of omission bias in obsessive patients is mediated by the occurrence of obsessional thoughts.

Deciding not to do something results in a sense of agency; thus, a patient will not be concerned about sharp objects he or she has not seen, and will not be concerned if he or she did not consider the possibility of harm. However, if something is seen and it occurs to them that they could or should take preventative action, the situation changes because NOT acting becomes an active decision. In this way, the actual occurrence of intrusive thoughts of harm — and/or responsibility for it — come to play a key role in the perception of responsibility for their contents. Suppression, as described above, will further increase this effect by increasing the thoughts. Thus, having locked the door, the person tries not to think that it could be open, experiences the thought again, and is therefore constrained to act or risk being responsible through having chosen not to check. The motivation to suppress will increase, but it is very difficult to suppress a thought that is directly connected to an action just completed, so the action serves as a further cue for intrusion/suppression and so on.

Thought Occurrence and Perceived Responsibility

Wroe, Salkovskis, and Richards (2000) conducted an interview study to examine the hypothesis that the occurrence of an intrusion about possible harm in an otherwise responsibility-free situation has the effect of putting the person in the position of having to make a decision they would not otherwise face (whether or not to seek to prevent the harm suggested by the intrusion). In particular, Wroe *et al.* sought to address the question of whether there are generalized or specific differences between obsessional patients and non-clinical controls in terms of how frequently they are confronted with the decision to act to prevent harm by the occurrence of intrusions. Overall, obsessionals did not experience more frequent intrusions concerning harm than non-obsessionals. Harm intrusions specifically clustered on obsession-relevant situations for the obsessionals. Higher levels of harm intrusion were found in controls for obsession-irrelevant situations. This may indicate that, for non-obsessionals, the situations chosen are more likely to elicit harm intrusions, but that obsessional patients are not sensitive to these situations. Overall, the results of this study indicate that obsessionals are more likely to act following the occurrence of any intrusive thought concerning harm than are the non-obsessionals, and that obsession-relevant situations are more likely to elicit action in all individuals.

Although situations probed in the interview were designated obsession-relevant or irrelevant, the full range of apparently obsession-relevant situations seldom activates individual patients' concerns. A subsidiary analysis was therefore carried out focusing on the specific situations each individual reported to be most and least problematic. For 15 of the 34 obsessionals interviewed there was no intrusive thought concerning harm on which they never decided not to act (i.e., these participants always acted following an intrusive thought). This was significantly different from non-obsessionals. Ten out of the 19 obsessionals who did experience intrusions on which they did not act in such situations stated that the reasons for their decision not to act was that acting may itself cause further harm. For example, removing glass from a path to prevent someone cutting himself or herself may result in the participant becoming contaminated from touching the glass. So in these cases, the decision to not act actually involved preventing other potential harm, arising from an intrusion about the possibility of such harm.

Trying Too Hard: Links Between Responsibility, Elevated Evidence Requirements and Criteria for Stopping an Action

Many problematic areas for obsessional patients concern activities that, in others, require little conscious effort. For example, deciding when to stop washing, recalling what has been said during a conversation, deciding whether a door is locked or the gas has been turned off. When such things are the focus of their obsessional problems, patients suffering from OCD appear to be trying too hard in ways that actually interfere with the decision-making process itself. This problem may again be mediated by the occurrence of intrusions; to disregard intrusions concerning harm would be to actively disregard threat, as described above. Obsessionals tend to use two main solutions to the problem of how to decide when to stop or when they have done enough. These are: (a) repeat the action until it feels right; or (b) conducting the activity in such a way as to ensure some feeling or token of completeness.[1] The latter involves introducing some distinctive sequence to ensure that the neutralizing is recalled clearly enough "to be sure". Unfortunately, the frequency with which ordinary activities are carried out tends to result in difficulties remembering any particular instance. The greater the repetition the less distinctive any particular instance becomes. Patients adopt sequences to overcome this, but these become subject to the same doubts.

In the first instance, obsessionals use their affective state to confirm their decision to stop neutralizing activity. The basis for such judgements varies from person to person, but most commonly involves feeling comfortable to a particular level, having "the right attitude", or carrying out the neutralizing without experiencing the obsessional thought. In the first two of these instances, pre-existing mood disturbance (depression or anxiety) makes finishing particularly difficult, as the obsessional needs to a achieve the sense of rightness regardless of general mood. Trying not to have the obsessional thought while ritualizing is a particularly difficult version of thought suppression, in that there is almost invariably a link between the obsession and the neutralizing activity. If someone washes because they think they may be contaminated, terminating washing without thoughts of contamination presents special difficulties.

Work carried out by our group (particularly by Karina Wahl) has highlighted the impact of using internal and subjective criteria in the decision to stop an activity (i.e., to stop checking, washing and so on). Preliminary evidence suggests that obsessional patients make simple decisions (such as whether or not the light switch is off, or whether or not one's hands are clean) using the type of criteria that would be typical of non-obsessionals when they are making a particularly important decision. For example, when trying to decide whether or not to buy a new house, most of us would consider how big it is, its main features, the garden, the cost, its location relative to facilities we might need, the neighborhood and so on. Having considered all such factors available to us, it is still likely that we would finally interrogate our feelings. Did it feel right? If we bought it, would that be the correct decision? This final emotionally based criterion could potentially sway the decision. The stronger our "just right" feeling, the less we would subsequently doubt our decision. Interestingly, most people would also continue to gather information that may be relevant to buying the house until they achieved some emotional closure of this kind. Similarly, if they had to make the decision despite feeling that it might not be right, they are much more likely to be beset by doubts about the correctness of their decision. How can a set of phenomena that apply to "life and death" decisions be applied to the kind of

---

[1]There is an additional set of strategies available for use to ensure completeness. These involve introducing some distinctive sequence which ensures that the neutralizing is recalled clearly enough "to be sure". Unfortunately, the frequency with which ordinary activities are carried out tends to result in difficulties in remembering any particular instance. The greater the repetition the less distinctive any particular instance becomes. Patients adopt sequences to overcome this, but these become subject to the same doubts.

decisions OCD patients make, such as whether or not the gas is off, whether their hands are sufficiently free of contamination? The cognitive theory suggests that, for the obsessional patient, such decisions have taken on the proportions of life or death decisions (or at least having more serious implications than they actually have).

Thus, OCD patients misinterpret the gravity of certain decisions they have to make, often because they have experienced an intrusion concerning the possibility of negative consequences in a situation that would otherwise not have involved any decision. For the obsessional patient, stopping a compulsive behavior can become the type of important decision usually made on the basis of as wide a range of evidence as is available. Given that the evidence may be relatively complicated (and possibly even somewhat contradictory), they are more likely to use difficult to achieve internal states (being sure of something, feeling certain and so on) as the criteria for ceasing repetition (see also Salkovskis *et al.*, 1998; Salkovskis, Forrester, Richards, & Morrison, 1998). They therefore set elevated evidence requirements for their decision, most commonly for the decision that they have done enough to ensure that they are making the correct choice (to stop washing, that they do not need to check something).

The elevated evidence requirement means that the otherwise automatic decision would become a strategic one, and that multiple criteria have to be fulfilled in order to stop the compulsive activity. Initially, multiple external criteria (where these are available) would have to be fulfilled. Towards the end of the compulsion, if the person continues to be troubled by ideas of severely negative outcomes, additional internally referenced criteria become the criterion required for the decision. Note also that, when a decision is regarded as extremely important (such as a stop decision with high perceived negative consequences of being mistaken) and there are few or no external criteria available, then internal criteria and just right feelings may be the only way available to the person to make a strategic decision. There is one further instance in which internal criteria are likely to be deployed. Some decisions that enough has been done are made on the basis of one's memory of how much has in fact been done. If one: (a) makes efforts to try to recall what one has done (mental checking); and (b) either cannot clearly recall this, or is not confident in the memory, then repeating may again become important. In other words, the pattern in obsessionals could be a hierarchical one in which external criteria are important most of the time and internal criteria become more and more important when the compulsion progresses. For each of these criteria, it is assumed that they have to meet an increased threshold compared to thresholds involved in decision making for non-compulsive behavior.

The decision-making process involved in compulsive behavior is therefore not necessarily qualitatively different from that in non-compulsive behavior if the full range of decisions are considered. Under certain conditions every decision-making process can be based on elevated evidence requirements. An analysis derived from the cognitive theory suggests that these conditions may be characterized by the perception of harm threatening self or others and the belief that by acting in a certain way one can prevent or reduce this harm. OCD patients thus make use of strategic decision-making processes in order to stop a compulsion. These processes are assumed to require mental capacity and conscious awareness, and they can be voluntarily started and finished. By contrast, in order to initialize or terminate brief non-compulsive behavior, less mental effort is required, and it can occur without awareness, although subject to voluntary control.

Recent Research on Responsibility Beliefs

A considerable body of research has now been conducted on the measurement of excessive responsibility in obsessionality, although few of these studies have included samples of obsessional patients and fewer still have included anxious controls as a comparison group. A common problem in investigations of the link between beliefs and specific psychopathology is criterion contamination. That is, the measures of cognition used may include items that are actually ratings of the intensity of symptoms specific to the disorder under investigation. For example, an item phrased "I am greatly troubled by unwanted upsetting thoughts" is very likely to be selectively endorsed by obsessional patients because it embodies one of the most common symptoms experienced by obsessional patients.

Rachman *et al.* (1995) conducted two psychometric studies in non-clinical participants to develop a reliable self-report scale for measuring responsibility, and found four factors: responsibility for harm, responsibility in social contexts, a positive outlook toward responsibility, and thought–action fusion (TAF). Rhéaume, Ladouceur, Freeston, and Letarte (1994) developed a semi-idiographic questionnaire measuring responsibility and found satisfactory reliability and validity using non-clinical participants. Freeston, Ladouceur, Gagnon, and Thibodeau (1993) developed a questionnaire about beliefs concerning intrusive thoughts and responsibility; the control of such thoughts and their possible consequences; and appropriateness of guilt and neutralizing behavior as a response. A significant relationship between obsessive compulsive symptoms and beliefs about obsessions were found in 87 non-clinical participants and 14 patients. Bouvard, Harvard, Ladouceur, and Cottraux (1997) also found responsibility beliefs as measured by a French translation of the Responsibility Attitudes Scale (RAS) (Salkovskis, Wroe, *et al.* 2000) to be important in a comparison between obsessionals and non-obsessionals. These researchers also found that the consequences imagined by the two groups were similar, differing in terms of the evaluation of severity and probability of the consequences and the influence they can have on them.

In another study that included both OCD patients and anxious controls, Steketee, Frost, and Cohen (1998) used several belief measures, including one of those used here (the RAS) and Freeston *et al.*'s Inventory of Beliefs Related to Obsessions (IBRO). Findings are consistent with the hypothesis that obsessional problems are associated with beliefs including responsibility, control, threat estimation, tolerance of uncertainty, concern about anxiety and coping. However, there was very little evidence of specificity in the beliefs measured; for example, threat estimation was elevated in OCD but not in anxious controls, an extremely surprising result. However, the results of that study are difficult to interpret for a number of reasons. Items for all scales on the beliefs measure devised for this study were selected specifically because they correlated with the YBOCS, a specific measure of obsessional symptoms. There was considerable criterion contamination in many of the items used (Steketee, personal communication, 1/18/99). For example, at least ten of the threat estimation items (from a total of 16) referred to risk associated with obsessional symptoms, accounting for the specificity of this scale to OCD. We understand that there were similar problems in the other scales. There was also a problem in the way participants were diagnosed (self-report of having a particular diagnosis).

Salkovskis *et al.* (2000) recently reported studies that investigated responsibility assumptions and appraisals in OCD patients, patients suffering from other anxiety disorders and healthy controls. The measures of inflated responsibility were found to have good test–retest reliabilities and internal consistency. The results of these studies were consistent with the hypothesis that people suffering from obsessional problems are characterized by and experience an inflated sense of responsibility for possible harm, linked to the occurrence and/or content of intrusive cognitions. Obsessional patients were found to be more likely to endorse general responsibility beliefs and assumptions than were non-obsessionals and were also more likely to make responsibility-related appraisals of intrusive thoughts about possible harm. There was also evidence of an association between responsibility cognitions and the occurrence of compulsive behavior and neutralizing. The data suggest specificity of responsibility cognitions in OCD, as obsessional patients differed not only from the non-clinical group but also from the clinically anxious comparison group who had very similar levels of anxiety and depression.

There was evidence of a strong association between the measures of responsibility and of obsessionality. Multiple regression analyses indicated that both types of responsibility measures made unique and substantial contributions to the prediction of scores on measures of obsessional symptoms. Further analyses indicated that the responsibility measures were less strongly associated with measures of symptoms of depression and anxiety. As depression and anxiety symptoms are themselves associated with obsessional symptoms, this result suggests that the responsibility measures used may be tapping something other than general dysfunction and dysphoria. Consistent with this view, responsibility measures did not make a unique contribution to the prediction of depression symptoms, and made only a very minor contribution to clinical anxiety symptoms.

In that study, the SCID-defined clinical groups had demonstrably comparable and high levels of anxiety and depression, and all were current patients. The inclusion of such anxious controls in the analyses tests the possibility that any difference between obsessionals and non-obsessionals is a general effect of anxiety, depression or clinical patient status. The differences found between OCD patients and both non-clinical controls and anxious patients suggest specificity to OCD.

The finding that responsibility assumptions and appraisals are significantly elevated in obsessionals compared to controls is consistent with the cognitive–behavioral theory. However, the presence of such an association could also be interpreted as indicating that such beliefs might arise as a consequence of having OCD. Evidence consistent with a causal role for responsibility beliefs comes from experimental studies on the impact of responsibility manipulations. Ladouceur *et al.* (1995) asked non-clinical participants to complete a manual classification task and manipulated responsibility by giving participants different reasons for the study. The high-responsibility group was informed that the research group was "specialized in the perception of colors and had recently been mandated by a pharmaceutical company for a project concerning the explorations for medication for a virus that was presently very widespread in a South-East Asian country." The low-responsibility group was told that the researchers were "only interested in the perception of colors and that this was only a practice before the real experiment began." Differences were found between the groups in perceived severity of the outcome. Lopatka and Rachman (1995) tested 30 obsessive compulsive checkers and ten obsessive compulsive cleaners and demonstrated that a decrease in perceived responsibility was followed by decreased discomfort and by a decline in the urge to carry out compulsive checking. Shafran (1997) found that these effects were not confined to checkers, but occurred in obsessional patients with a range of symptoms.

Belief Domains and OCD: Apparent Theoretical Convergence

The OCCWG (1997) has focused on a number of belief domains including: (a) inflated responsibility; (b) overimportance of thoughts; (c) beliefs about the importance of controlling one's thoughts; (d) overestimation of threat; (e) intolerance of uncertainty; and (f) perfectionism. Although discussion has resulted in some polarization so that these domains have been treated as distinct, this distinctness is largely illusory, as a careful consideration of the constructs reveals. The belief assessment effort has largely arisen from the desire to refine, extend and ultimately apply cognitive approaches to OCD. The belief domain that forms the focus of this chapter, responsibility, was given a central place in cognitive theories because, when this type of appraisal occurs, it is particularly likely to motivate neutralizing behavior. Other belief domains in fact overlap considerably with responsibility. In most instances, the perceived responsibility for harm linked to the occurrence or content of intrusive thoughts, images, impulses and doubts represent a subset of beliefs characterized by the domain in question. Taking the main constructs that form the focus of the 1997 OCCWG paper, the relationships are mostly clear. Cognitive theories that focus on misinterpretations clearly identify the overimportance of thoughts. This construct has been identified as beliefs in which the mere presence of a thought gives it status, and has the implication of responsibility for one's thoughts and for their consequences (OCCWG, 1997). This concept encompasses thought-action fusion (see Chapter two in this volume), including variants on "if I think something this means I want to do it/have done it/am the kind of person who will do it". Not entirely unrelated are beliefs about the importance of controlling one's thoughts. Note that such beliefs concern something one has to do (control one's thoughts). Theorizing in this area tends to focus on metacognitive beliefs, that is, the beliefs concerning the meaning of thoughts and the way in which they are interpreted. This view is *de facto* indistinguishable from cognitive theories of obsessions, encompassing as it does "excessive monitoring for the presence of mental intrusions; belief that intrusions portend some catastrophe; belief that one is responsible for this harm because of the thoughts; belief that one must control the thoughts to avoid harm and reduce distress" (OCCWG, 1997, p. 672).

As described above, cognitive theories of anxiety (including, but not confined to, obsessional problems) have at their core the tendency towards overestimation of threat. As already discussed, the perception of threat involves a number of dimensions beyond just the notion that danger is particularly likely. For example, Salkovskis (1996b) argues that the cost and awfulness of a perceived threat has a synergistic relationship with perceived probability. This framework suggests that the overestimation of threat is a necessary condition for the experience of obsessional problems, but is not sufficient. Salkovskis (1985) pointed out that the negative interpretation of intrusions could and would result in mood disturbance (both anxiety and depression), and that when they were taken as indicating likely harm or danger, anxiety would be the consequence. However, the perception of responsibility was necessary for harm to generate obsessional phenomena. By the same token, perceived responsibility for harmless or beneficial consequences is not relevant to obsessional problems.

Intolerance of uncertainty has been linked to decision-making problems, particularly excessive caution. This phenomenon is characterized by greater doubt about the correctness of decisions (see section above on elevated evidence requirements). The motivation to "do no harm" by gaining certainty represents another facet of personal responsibility appraisals. Again, it is clear that this concept goes beyond the realms of responsibility, but we would argue that it is seldom relevant to obsessional problems when it does so, merging imperceptibly into generalized anxiety disorder. Similar notions apply to perfectionism where concern over mistakes made by the person himself or herself is likely to be highly correlated with an inflated sense of responsibility. Perfectionism is the net sum of the notion of "trying too hard" described above.

Thus, an inflated sense of responsibility, the overimportance of thoughts and beliefs about the importance of controlling one's thoughts are so closely linked as to tap a single construct linked to the idea of causing harm through things that one does, things that one does not do or by things that one thinks or does not think. All three are relevant to obsessional symptoms because they are likely to lead to the appraisal of intrusions in ways that motivate preventative or restitutive reactions. Intolerance of uncertainty and, in particular, overestimation of threat, are more likely to be general vulnerability factors likely to contribute to the misinterpretation and negative appraisal of intrusions in important but less specific ways (Beck, Emery, & Greenberg, 1985). These beliefs are likely to occur in a range of psychological problems other than OCD; however, theoretically, they are likely to be OCD relevant. Perfectionism is usually defined in terms suggesting more enduring personality-type characteristics that might be expected to interact with the appraisal of intrusions, particularly when such intrusions concern the completion (or non-completion) of particular actions.

References

Beck, A. T. (1976). *Cognitive therapy and the emotional disorders.* New York: International Universities Press.

Beck, A. T., Emery, G., & Greenberg, R. L. (1985). *Anxiety disorders and phobias.* New York: Basic Books.

Bouvard, M., Harvard, A., Ladouceur, R., & Cottraux, J. (1997). Le trouble obsessionel-compulsif et al responsabilité excessive. *Revue Francophone de Clinique Comportementale et Cognitive, 2,* 9–16.

Edwards, S., & Dickerson, M. (1987). Intrusive unwanted thoughts: A two stage model of control. *British Journal of Medical Psychology, 60,* 317–328.

England, S. L., & Dickerson, M. (1988). Intrusive thoughts: Unpleasantness not the major cause of uncontrollability. *Behaviour Research and Therapy, 26,* 279–282.

Freeston, M. H., Ladouceur, R., Gagnon, F., & Thibodeau, N. (1993). Beliefs about obsessional thoughts. *Journal of Psychopathology and Behavioral Assessment, 15,* 1–21.

Freeston, M. H., Rhéaume, J., & Ladouceur, R. (1996). Correcting faulty appraisals of obsessional thoughts. *Behaviour Research and Therapy, 34,* 433–446.

Ladouceur, R., Rhéaume, J., Freeston, M. H., Aublet, F., Jean, K., Lachance, S., Langlois, F., & de Pokomandy-Morin, K. (1995). Experimental manipulations of responsibility: An analogue test for models of obsessive–compulsive disorder. *Behaviour Research and Therapy, 33,* 937–946.

Lopatka, C., & Rachman, S. J. (1995) Perceived responsibility and compulsive checking: An experimental analysis. *Behaviour Research and Therapy, 33,* 673–684.

Obsessive Compulsive Cognitions Working Group [OCCWG]. (1997). Cognitive assessment of obsessive–compulsive disorder. *Behaviour Research and Therapy, 35,* 667–681.

Rachman, S. J. (1971). Obsessional ruminations. *Behaviour Research and Therapy, 9,* 229–235.

Rachman, S. J. (1976a). The modification of obsessions: A new formulation. *Behaviour Research and Therapy, 14,* 437–443.

Rachman, S. J. (1976b). Obsessive–compulsive checking. *Behaviour Research and Therapy, 14,* 269–277.

Rachman, S. J. (1993). Obsessions, responsibility, and guilt. *Behaviour Research and Therapy, 31,* 149–154.

Rachman, S. J. (1997). A cognitive theory of obsessions. *Behaviour Research and Therapy, 35,* 793–802.

Rachman, S. J. (1998). A cognitive theory of obsessions: Elaborations. *Behaviour Research and Therapy, 36,* 385–401.

Rachman, S. J., & de Silva, P. (1978). Abnormal and normal obsessions. *Behaviour Research and Therapy, 16,* 233–238.

Rachman, S. J., Thordarson, D. S., Shafran, R., & Woody, S. (1995). Perceived responsibility: Structure and significance. *Behaviour Research and Therapy, 33,* 779–784.

Rhéaume, J., Ladouceur, R., Freeston, M. H., & Letarte, H. (1994). Inflated responsibility in obsessive–compulsive disorder: Psychometric studies of a semi-idiographic measure. *Journal of Psychopathology and Behavioral Assessment, 16,* 265–276.

Salkovskis, P. M. (1985). Obsessional–compulsive problems: A cognitive–behavioural analysis. *Behaviour Research and Therapy, 23,* 571–583.

Salkovskis, P. M. (1989). Cognitive–behavioural factors and the persistence of intrusive thoughts in obsessional problems. *Behaviour Research and Therapy, 27,* 677–682.

Salkovskis, P. M. (1991). The importance of behavior in the maintenance of anxiety and panic: A cognitive account. *Behavioural Psychotherapy, 19,* 6–19.

Salkovskis, P. M. (1996a). The cognitive approach to anxiety: Threat beliefs, safety seeking behaviour, and the special case of health anxiety and obsessions. In P. M. Salkovskis (ed.), *Frontiers of cognitive therapy* (pp. 48–75). New York: Guilford.

Salkovskis, P. M. (1996b). Cognitive–behavioral approaches to the understanding of obsessional problems. In R. Rapee (ed.), *Current controversies in the anxiety disorders* (pp. 103–133). New York: Guilford.

Salkovskis, P. M. (1996c). Resolving the cognition–behaviour debate. In P. M. Salkovskis (ed.), *Trends in cognitive–behaviour therapy.* Chichester: Wiley.

Salkovskis, P. M. (1998). Psychological approaches to the understanding of obsessional problems. In R. P. Swinson, M. M. Antony, S. J. Rachman, & M. A. Richter (eds), *Obsessive–compulsive disorder: Theory, research and treatment* (pp. 33–50). New York: Guilford.

Salkovskis, P. M. (1999). Understanding and treating obsessive–compulsive disorder. *Behaviour Research and Therapy, 37,* S29–S52.

Salkovskis, P. M., & Harrison, J. (1984). Abnormal and normal obsessions: A replication. *Behaviour Research and Therapy, 22,* 549–552.

Salkovskis, P. M., & Westbrook, D. (1998). Behaviour therapy and obsessional ruminations: Can failure be turned into success? *Behaviour Research and Therapy, 27,* 149–160.

Salkovskis, P. M., Forrester, E., Richards, H. C., & Morrison, N. (1998). The devil is in the detail:

Conceptualizing and treating obsessional problems. In N. Tarrier (ed.), *Cognitive therapy with complex cases* (pp 46–80). Chichester: Wiley.

Salkovskis, P. M., Rachman, S. J., Ladouceur, R., & Freeston, M. (1996). Defining responsibility in obsessional problems. *Proceedings of the the Toronto cafeteria.*

Salkovskis, P. M., Wroe, A. L., Gledhill, A., Morrison, N., Forrester, E., Richards, C., Reynolds, M., & Thorpe, S. (2000). Responsibility attitudes and interpretations are characteristic of obsessive compulsive disorder. *Behaviour Research and Therapy, 38*, 347–372.

Shafran, R. (1997). The manipulation of responsibility in obsessive–compulsive disorder. *British Journal of Clinical Psychology, 36*, 397–407.

Spranca, M., Minsk, E., & Baron, J. (1991). Omission and commission in judgment and choice. *Journal of Experimental Social Psychology, 27*, 76–105.

Steketee, G., Frost, R. O., & Cohen, I. (1998). Beliefs in obsessive–compulsive disorder. *Journal of Anxiety Disorders, 12*, 525–537.

Wroe, A. L., & Salkovskis, P. M. (2000). Causing harm and allowing harm: A study of beliefs in obsessional problems. *Behaviour Research and Therapy, 38*, 1141–1162.

Wroe, A. L., Salkovskis, P. M., & Richards, H. C. (2000). "Now I know it could happen, I have to prevent it": A clinical study of the specificity of intrusive thoughts and the decision to prevent harm. *Behavioural and Cognitive Psychotherapy, 28*, 63–70.

Chapter 5

Overestimation of Threat and Intolerance of Uncertainty in Obsessive Compulsive Disorder

Debbie Sookman and Gilbert Pinard

Introduction

This chapter will review the literature on dysfunctional beliefs and information processing biases related to overestimation of threat and intolerance of uncertainty in obsessive compulsive disorder (OCD). These domains of cognition have been identified by expert consensus to be among those relevant to OCD (Obsessive Compulsive Cognitions Working Group [OCCWG], 1997). Overestimation of threat has been defined as "exaggeration of the probability or severity of harm" (OCCWG, 1997, p. 678). Intolerance of uncertainty refers to "beliefs about the necessity of being certain, about the capacity to cope with unpredictable change, and about adequate functioning in situations which are inherently ambiguous." (OCCWG, 1997, p. 678). There is evidence these domains are highly interrelated. Intolerance of uncertainty may be one factor that influences estimation of threat in OCD (OCCWG, 2001; Sookman, Pinard, & Beauchemin, 1994; Steketee, Frost, & Cohen, 1998).

Cognitive processes and content related to threat or danger have been hypothesized to be a central characteristic of anxiety disorders (Beck & Clark, 1997; Beck, Emery, & Greenberg, 1985; McNally, 1994). These encompass selective attention, memory, appraisal, and beliefs related to specific internal and external events. Internal events or stimuli that may be perceived as dangerous include sensations, thoughts, images, impulses, and feelings. Rachman (1980) suggested several stimulus factors that contribute to difficulties in emotional processing, including sudden, intense, or uncontrollable stimulation, unpredictable stimuli, and signals of danger. Beck et al. (1985) proposed that anxiety develops when the number or cost of perceived threats is greater than perceived ability to cope with them.

Explanatory cognitive models of anxiety disorders, including OCD, share several common features which involve overestimation of threat (see Clark, 1997; OCCWG, 1997; Steketee, Frost, Rhéaume, & Wilhelm, 1998): (a) Individuals become anxious in response to specific stimuli which are appraised or processed as more dangerous to the self or significant others than they really are; (b) maladaptive cognitive and behavioral strategies are utilized to reduce anxiety or to prevent feared events from occurring; (c) these

Cognitive Approaches to Obsessions and Compulsions – Theory, Assessment, and Treatment
Copyright © 2002 by Elsevier Science Ltd.
All rights of reproduction in any form reserved.
ISBN: 0-08-043410-X

maladaptive strategies perpetuate/worsen anxiety because they prevent disconfirmation of unrealistic appraisals; and (d) symptoms of anxiety may be perceived as dangerous, escalating attempts at anxiety reduction or avoidance. These aspects are to some extent diagnosis specific, as will be elaborated below. Although the focus of this chapter is on OCD, some findings pertinent to threat estimation and intolerance of uncertainty in other anxiety disorders will be briefly reviewed.

Theoretical Background and Conceptualization of Overestimation of Threat

Catastrophic Interpretations of Intrusive Thoughts

One central aspect of overestimation of threat postulated in OCD is faulty appraisals or interpretations of intrusive thoughts. Intrusive cognitions, whose content is often indistinguishable from that of obsessions, are normal phenomena (e.g., Salkovskis & Harrison, 1984). Salkovskis (1985, 1989) and Salkovskis and Kirk, (1999) hypothesized that it is faulty appraisals of intrusions (e.g., "Having this unwanted thought means I will act on it"), and not occurrence of intrusions, which differentiate OCD from other populations. Unrealistic appraisals are commonly associated with feelings of anxiety, guilt, or dysphoric mood. Dysfunctional responses include hypervigilance, reassurance seeking, avoidance of external precipitants, and attempts at thought suppression and neutralization, that is, attempts to undo the harmful effects of obsessions or to reduce discomfort (e.g., Freeston, Rhéaume, & Ladouceur, 1996; Rachman, 1997, 1998). Attempts to suppress or neutralize spontaneously occurring intrusions increase their occurrence (Salkovskis & Campbell, 1994; Trinder & Salkovskis, 1994). Freeston *et al.* (1996) and others have discussed the role of dysphoric mood in activating intrusive thoughts, dysfunctional appraisals, and neutralization.

In his cognitive theory of obsessions, Rachman (1997, 1998) underlines the importance of threat appraisals on the development and persistence of symptoms. Catastrophic appraisals increase the range and perceived seriousness of threatening stimuli, so that previously neutral stimuli become significant: "If a person catastrophically misinterprets his unwanted intrusive thoughts about harming other people as signifying that he is potentially dangerous, then a range of formerly neutral stimuli are turned into potential threats (e.g. sharp objects are transformed into potential weapons)" (Rachman, 1998, p. 384). As a result, intrusions are provoked by an increased number of feared external stimuli. Faulty information processing, such as "ex-consequentia reasoning" or assuming from feelings of anxiety that danger is present, contribute to sense of danger (e.g., "I feel scared so I must be in danger") (Arntz, Rauner, & van den Hout, 1995). Avoidance or neutralization prevent disconfirmation of threat-related perceptions. Rachman emphasizes the importance of inner as well as external threat cues, including the person's view of self as dangerous. The idiosyncratic meaning given to specific thoughts is influenced by more general beliefs and cognitive biases about the self and world (e.g., Beck *et al.*, 1985; Rachman, 1998).

Dysfunctional Beliefs About Threat

Overestimation of threat has been hypothesized to include beliefs about the likelihood or probability of aversive events, and their severity and consequences (OCCWG, 1997; Steketee, Frost & Cohen, 1998). Examples are "I believe that the world is a dangerous place"; "Bad things are more likely to happen to me than to other people"; or "When anything goes wrong in my life, it is likely to have terrible effects" (Obsessive Beliefs Questionnaire, OCCWG, 2001). Beliefs about coping and emotional discomfort have also been linked to overestimation of threat (e.g., Beck *et al.*, 1985; Steketee, Frost, & Cohen, 1998). Sookman *et al.* (1994) proposed that vulnerability schemas influence processing and perception of danger in OCD (see section on level of cognition below). Although not the focus of this chapter, it has been suggested that physiological susceptibilities may lead to "false-alarm" reactions (Barlow, 1991) and shape the development of unrealistic thoughts (Warren & Zgourides, 1991). This section will summarize the theoretical background related to overestimation of threat beliefs in OCD.

In an early model, Carr (1971, 1974) emphasized the importance in OCD of unrealistic threat appraisals, with rituals seen as attempts to reduce perceived danger. Based on this work and that of Lazarus (1966), McFall and Wollersheim (1979) elaborated on the importance of perceived coping skills in the face of threat. According to these authors, underestimation of capacity to cope leads to anxiety, uncertainty and fear of loss of control accompanied by repetitive thinking and rituals to cope with discomfort. Guidano and Liotti (1983) suggested that several irrational beliefs described by Ellis are relevant to OCD, including excessive need for competence, certainty, need to avoid criticism, and concerns about potential danger.

Kozak, Foa, and McCarthy (1987) postulated that OCD patients tend to perceive situations as dangerous until proven safe, creating a bias toward fear of harm. Exposure to feared situations in which no harm occurs does not result in an assumption of general safety, so rituals do not provide sustained reassurance and are repeated. In discussing the meaning of possessions to hoarders, Frost and Hartl (1996) hypothesized that these may also represent safety and comfort in an environment perceived as threatening. In contrast, non-clinical individuals may be more likely to assume safety unless there is realistic evidence of danger. Other authors have proposed that people with OCD symptoms tend to overestimate the likelihood and severity of aversive events, exaggerate the risk of negative consequences of a variety of actions (i.e., presume worse outcomes), and be overly cautious (e.g., Foa & Kozak, 1986; Freeston *et al.*, 1996; Rasmussen & Eisen, 1989; Salkovskis, 1985; Steketee & Frost, 1994; van Oppen & Arntz, 1994). Butler and Mathews (1983) suggested that available heuristics for specific events, such as recency, frequency of occurrence, ease of recall, and salience, may influence estimates of the probability these events will occur. For example, frequent thoughts about harm, combined with catastrophic appraisals (salience), may contribute to overestimation of the probability that harm will actually occur.

Beliefs about threat overlap conceptually and statistically with other cognitive domains: intolerance of uncertainty, perfectionism and particularly doubts about actions (Frost, Marten, Lahart, & Rosenblate, 1990), importance and control of thoughts, and beliefs and information processing distortions related to thought–action fusion (Rachman, 1993).

Studies of information processing reveal attentional and memory biases related to threat (see sections on measurement and laboratory studies below).

Intolerance of Uncertainty

In describing "la folie du doute", clinicians have highlighted uncertainty and doubt in OCD since the 1800s (e.g., Janet, 1908; cited in Ey, Bernard, & Brisset, 1963). Intolerance of uncertainty and difficulty making decisions are commonly observed features of this disorder (Beech & Liddell, 1974; Carr, 1974; Guidano & Liotti, 1983; Kozak, *et al.*, 1987; Rasmussen & Eisen, 1989). Several conceptualizations have linked intolerance of uncertainty with symptoms, and with beliefs about threat estimation, perfectionism, and need for control. It has been suggested that OCD patients have an excessive need for certainty in order to control and predict events (Makhlouf-Norris & Norris, 1972). Beech and Liddell (1974) proposed that need for certainty about when to end an activity, as well as anxiety reduction, are factors that maintain ritualistic behavior. Reed (1985) considered doubt about one's experience and actions to be a hallmark of OCD that leads to uncertainty about capacity to cope with or avert danger. Patients may feel uncertain about their capacity to reduce risk when there are no perfect solutions (Guidano & Liotti, 1983). Sookman and Pinard (1995) hypothesized a close association between beliefs about one's personal susceptibility to danger and unpredictability, newness, and change. Langlois, Freeston, and Ladouceur (2000) suggested that uncertainty or doubt about the meaning of intrusions as potentially dangerous leads to anxiety.

Level and Specificity of Dysfunctional Beliefs: From Appraisals to Core Beliefs

Different levels of cognitive content have been postulated (for a review of level of cognition in OCD, see OCCWG, 1997), including domains of appraisals of intrusive thoughts or images. An appraisal is the interpretation given to a specific event, and the content may be highly syndrome specific. For example, overestimation of the potential importance and danger of an aggressive thought is particularly characteristic of OCD (e.g., "Thinking this thought could make it happen"). Assumptions or beliefs are more general than appraisals of particular events and are held across contexts. Specific assumptions are hypothesized to be highly characteristic of OCD, and perhaps also of people at risk of developing the disorder. General assumptions are considered related to, but not exclusive to OCD, and may be found in other clinical disorders such as anxiety or mood disorders (Beck *et al.*, 1985; Beck, Rush, Shaw, & Emery, 1979). Beliefs pertaining to threat and uncertainty may fall into both categories. For example, a belief such as "If I do not take extra precautions, I am more likely than others to have or cause a serious disaster" may be more characteristic of OCD than a general belief such as "Small problems always seem to turn into big one's in my life."

In their integrative conceptual and treatment model of OCD, Sookman and Pinard focused on multidimensional core beliefs and schemas. Core beliefs refer to an individual's basic beliefs about self and world. These authors (Sookman & Pinard, 1995, 1997, 1999;

Sookman, Pinard, & Beauchemin, 1990, 1994; Sookman, Pinard, & Beck, 2001) proposed that dysfunctional vulnerability schemas are characteristic of OCD, and that these are a central underlying mechanism of excessive threat appraisals to a variety of internal and external stimuli. Vulnerability schemas are comprised of core beliefs about danger, with emotional, interpersonal, and behavioral aspects emanating in part from significant developmental and attachment experiences. They selectively influence attention, memory, and appraisal of specific stimuli perceived/processed as threatening. This conceptualization built on the previous work of several authors, especially Beck and colleagues (e.g., Beck *et al.*, 1985), as well as Carr, and McFall and Wollersheim.

Sookman and Pinard (1995) proposed four classes of dysfunctional beliefs (assumptions or core beliefs) to comprise vulnerability schemas in OCD: Perceived vulnerability; view of/response to unpredictability, newness and change; view of strong affect; and need for control. Perceived vulnerability was defined as "an excessive sense of personal susceptibility to danger from internal (e.g., thoughts, feelings) as well as from external (illness, accidents, interpersonal) sources." We hypothesized that OCD patients experience as particularly threatening situations involving unpredictability, newness, or change that require flexible coping and adaptation. Beliefs about a variety of strong feelings (e.g., anger, sadness) and one's capacity to tolerate and cope with these were considered integral to the notion of perceived vulnerability from inner sources. Excessive need for control of inner and external events was considered a dysfunctional response to perceived vulnerability.

Measurement of Overestimation of Threat and Intolerance of Uncertainty

Four self-report psychometric measures will be reviewed, including the Obsessive Beliefs Questionnaire (OBQ; OCCWG, 1997, 2001), Obsessive Compulsive Beliefs Questionnaire (OCBQ, Steketee, Frost, & Cohen, 1998), the Vulnerability Schemata Scale (VSS; Sookman & Pinard, 1995; Sookman *et al.*, 2001), and the Inventory of Beliefs Related to Obsessions (IBRO; Freeston, Ladouceur, Gagnon, & Thibodeau, 1993). Although predominantly a measure of responsibility, this last scale also includes beliefs about threat and uncertainty. Other more general measures not reviewed here include the Tridimensional Personality Questionnaire (Cloninger, Przybeck, & Svrakic, 1991) which assesses novelty seeking, harm avoidance, and reward dependence. A study with this scale showed that only harm avoidance distinguished OCD patients from non-clinical participants (Richter, Summerfeldt, Russell, & Swinson, 1996). In addition, the Intolerance of Uncertainty Questionnaire was developed to assess beliefs about uncertainty in generalized anxiety disorder (Freeston, Rhéaume, Letarte, Dugas, & Ladouceur, 1994).

Obsessive Beliefs Questionnaire

Because the development and psychometric properties of the OBQ (OCCWG, 1997, 2001) are described in Chapter seven, only selected findings about Threat Estimation and Tolerance for Uncertainty subscales are summarized here. Items were selected or modified from existing cognitive instruments, or were generated by OCCWG members (OCCWG, 1997). The first set of data (identified as stage two) was based on following samples: 101 OCD participants, 76 community controls, 374 student controls, 12 participants with other anxiety disorders, and 35 Greek-speaking community controls. Data from these subjects were used to reduce the OBQ Threat Estimation and Tolerance for Uncertainty subscales to 14 and 13 items respectively.

Overall, the initial data supported the internal consistency, stability, and discriminant validity for both subscales. For the OCD group, Threat Estimation and Tolerance for Uncertainty subscales showed excellent internal consistency; Cronbach alphas were 0.91 and 0.88 respectively. Test–retest reliability coefficients for 22 OCD subjects were 0.89 and 0.90, indicating excellent stability over time. Comparisons among the groups indicated that OCD patients had significantly higher scores than all other groups on both subscales. Students scored higher than community controls on Threat Estimation. Correlational analyses indicated that the Threat and Uncertainty subscales correlated moderately to highly with OCD symptoms on the Padua Inventory (PI) and on the self-report Yale–Brown Obsessive Compulsive Scale (YBOCS) (range 0.38–0.74). When partial correlations controlling for the Beck Anxiety Inventory and Beck Depression Inventory were calculated, the Threat and Uncertainty subscales remained significantly correlated with OCD symptoms. The strongest partial correlation of Threat was with the thoughts of harming self/others and the checking subscales of the PI. For Uncertainty, the strongest relationship occurred with PI checking. With respect to the relationship among belief domains, Threat Estimation correlated highly with Tolerance for Uncertainty ($r = 0.81$) and also with Perfectionism ($r = 0.79$); correlations for other cognitive domains ranged from 0.63 to 0.73. These high correlations indicate considerable overlap among the constructs, which are examined further in stage three data analyses (OCCWG, in preparation).

Stage three findings for these domains generally confirmed the above results with some exceptions for generally larger samples (257 OCD participants, 104 anxious controls, 85 community controls, and 285 students). Internal consistency remained very high and test–retest was good for the student sample, but poor for the OCD one. Group comparisons indicated that OCD participants scored higher on Threat Estimation and Tolerance for Uncertainty than all other groups except anxious controls. Again, the two scales were highly correlated (0.8 range) for both the OCD sample and the combined comparison groups. Correlations with the Padua Inventory and YBOCS were moderately high for both OCD and comparison samples (0.4–0.6 range), but these correlations were generally not stronger than those for other forms of psychopathology (anxiety, depression, worry). Findings suggest that these two domains are not exclusive to OCD, but also pertain to other emotional disorders.

Obsessive Compulsive Beliefs Questionnaire

The OCBQ (Steketee, Frost, & Cohen, 1998) is a 90-item scale which assesses six cognitive domains, including Threat Estimation (18 items) and Tolerance for Uncertainty (15 items). Items were modified from existing cognitive instruments or were generated by the first two authors. The sample consisted of 62 patients with OCD, 45 patients with other anxiety disorders (AD, 13 panic disorder, 11 agoraphobia, 11 generalized anxiety disorder, seven social phobia, seven agoraphobia), and 34 non-clinical participants.

Internal consistency of the two subscales was very good at 0.88 for Threat Estimation and 0.87 for Tolerance for Uncertainty. Convergent validity included a comparison with the IBRO (Freeston *et al.*, 1993), and these scales were found to be highly related; $rs = 0.69$ and 0.70 respectively. OCD patients scored significantly higher than AD subjects and non-clinical controls on both subscales, and AD subjects scored higher than non-clinical controls on Tolerance for Uncertainty. The authors interpreted these findings as indicating that this domain, although endorsed strongly by OCD patients, may also be relevant to other anxiety disorders. Correlational analyses indicated that Threat Estimation and Tolerance for Uncertainty respectively were significantly related to measures of depression (0.42 and 0.47), anxiety sensitivity (0.48 and 0.53) and especially worry (0.56 and 0.58). They were only somewhat more strongly related to OCD symptoms (0.56–0.68). The correlation among the two domains was very high at 0.82. An important finding of this study was that only beliefs about uncertainty predicted scores for OCD symptoms beyond mood and worry, suggesting that threat estimation may not be specific to OCD.

Vulnerability Schemata Scale

The Vulnerability Schemata Scale (VSS; Sookman & Pinard, 1995) is an 81-item scale designed to measure dysfunctional vulnerability beliefs in OCD. The following four cognitive domains are assessed: Perceived Vulnerability (24 items); View of/Response to Unpredictability, Newness, and Change (16 items); View of/Response to Strong Affect (21 items); and Need for Control (20 items). The items comprising these domains were retained on a theoretical basis from a larger pool of multiple dysfunctional beliefs in OCD generated by the first two authors (Sookman, Pinard, & Beauchemin, 1994). Two classes of beliefs were included: Beliefs at the assumption or core level hypothesized to be specific to OCD and beliefs hypothesized to be related, but not exclusive to, this disorder.

The Perceived Vulnerability domain includes beliefs about: (a) general overestimation of the probability of danger; (b) personalized overestimation of the occurrence of danger; (c) exaggeration of the seriousness of danger to the self or significant others; (d) danger to self-percept; and (e) belief that one's coping skills are deficient. The Unpredictability, Newness, and Change domain was defined as comprising beliefs about: (a) situations which are unforeseen, unexpected, or unfamiliar; (b) potential change or novelty; (c) uncertainty; and (d) experiences to which it is difficult to assign a single meaning (ambiguity).

VSS internal consistency and test–retest reliability calculated for a heterogeneous sample were excellent: Cronbach alpha for the total scale was 0.97, and for the domains this ranged from 0.91 to 0.94; the test–retest reliability coefficient for the total scale (mean interval 14 days) was 0.95. In a recently reported study with 111 subjects (Sookman *et al.*, 2001), OCD patients ($n = 32$) more strongly endorsed these beliefs compared with patients with other anxiety disorders (50 percent agoraphobia and/or panic disorder; social phobia, and generalized anxiety disorder), mood disorders, and normal controls. When the effect of anxiety and depression was controlled, group differences were maintained, except for the difference between the OCD and anxious clinical groups on the View of Affect domain. Consistent with the authors' conceptualization, beliefs about perceived vulnerability and unpredictability were highly related ($r = 0.78$).

Sensitivity to change of the VSS following Integrative CBT that targeted dysfunctional vulnerability beliefs was reported with a series of 22 patients (Sookman & Pinard, 1999, 2000). Most were treatment resistant; mean duration of previous unsuccessful CBT was over two years. In the first study, six out of seven patients who showed clinically significant improvement in OCD symptoms (mean YBOCS reduction from 21.7 to 4.7) were also reliably changed on Perceived Vulnerability after an average of ten months of weekly outpatient treatment. Cognitive and symptomatic improvement was maintained up to a two-year follow-up. In the second study, ten responders (OCD symptoms improved more than 33 percent) reported significant change on the VSS following an average of six months of CBT. Five non-responders were unchanged on the VSS at reassessment.

Selected items from the VSS domains Perceived Vulnerability and View of/Response to Unpredictability, Newness, and Change were included in the Threat Estimation and Tolerance for Uncertainty subscales respectively, of the Obsessive Beliefs Questionnaire (OCCWG, 1997, 2001).

Inventory of Beliefs Related to Obsessions

The 20-item IBRO (Freeston, Ladouceur, Gagnon, & Thibodeau, 1993) measures harm avoidance and uncertainty but focuses mostly on responsibility. Findings from a series of six experiments with non-clinical and clinical samples indicated its reliability and validity. Three factors were identified: (a) Responsibility, guilt, blame, punishment and loss; (b) Overestimation of Threat; and (c) Intolerance of Uncertainty. The IBRO showed good reliability (Cronbach alpha = 0.82; test–retest after 4 weeks, $r = 0.70$), and distinguished OCD patients ($n = 14$) from students. Significant correlations were found between beliefs about obsessions and symptomatology. Regression analyses showed that the IBRO Total score remained a significant predictor of OCD symptoms even when the effect of negative mood was controlled.

Idiographic and Other Self-Report Measures

Dysfunctional beliefs can also be assessed using idiographic, self-report, and experimental methodology, which can valuably supplement psychometric scales. For example, Rhéaume, Ladouceur, Freeston, and Letarte (1994) developed a semi-idiographic assessment tool to assess beliefs using personal narratives and self-scenarios. Although predominantly a measure of responsibility, it included items related to estimation of threat by asking subjects to describe a personal situation in which they assessed probability of occurrence and seriousness of danger. Record keeping by patients of specific, idiosyncratic dysfunctional beliefs can be used to assess different aspects of these beliefs (e.g., intellectual versus emotional believability) which may show a differential response to treatment (Freeston, Todorov, Fournier, & Gareau, 2000; Sookman & Pinard, 2000).

Relationship to Other Cognitive Domains

Beliefs About Coping

As stated above, beliefs about coping ability have also been related to overestimation of threat. Guidano and Liotti (1983) and Carr (1971, 1974) suggested that OCD patients devalue or underestimate their ability to deal adequately with threatening situations and view rituals and avoidance as their only available coping strategy. McFall and Wollersheim (1979) described the obsessional's need for perfect coping. Steketee, Frost, and Cohen (1998) found that OCD patients endorsed more negative beliefs about coping than non-patients, but not than other anxious patients. In a study by Woods, Frost, and Steketee (2000, see below), regression results indicated that the only predictor of patients' OCD symptoms was coping ability. Actual or perceived inadequate coping may augment fears of being overwhelmed (harmed) emotionally or physically, and thus constitute a general component of threat estimation. There is some evidence that perceived vulnerability to danger is greater in situations where occurrence of danger and capacity to cope are unpredictable (Sookman *et al.*, 2001). General beliefs about coping are likely relevant to, but not specific to, OCD.

Anxiety Sensitivity

The extensively studied construct of Anxiety Sensitivity (AS) refers to fears of anxiety symptoms based on beliefs that these symptoms have harmful consequences. This construct is measured by The Anxiety Sensitivity Index (ASI; Peterson & Reiss, 1992; Reiss, Peterson, Gursky, & McNally, 1986), a 16-item measure of the extent to which a person experiences anxiety-related sensations as fearful or catastrophic (Peterson & Reiss, 1992). Emphasis is on fear of physical sensations (e.g., feeling shaky or faint, experiencing a rapid heartbeat, being nauseated or short of breath), although a few items assess fear of loss of mental control or interpersonal evaluation. Reiss (1991) and Reiss and Havercamp (1996) proposed that AS is comprised of several fundamental fears, including illness, injury, death, and fear of negative evaluation. While trait anxiety denotes a general tendency to respond fearfully to stressors, AS refers to a specific tendency to respond fearfully to one's own anxiety-related sensations (Lilienfeld, Turner, & Jacob, 1996; McNally, 1989). Related to AS is the extent to which fearful individuals overpredict the amount of anxiety they will experience when facing a feared situation (e.g., Taylor & Rachman, 1994). This construct has been studied largely with clinical populations other than OCD (see Taylor 1999, for review).

Beliefs about anxiety have been hypothesized to play a role in the development and maintenance of OCD symptoms for some patients (Freeston *et al.*, 1996). When asked to predict their anxiety level during exposure, OCD patients may also anticipate higher levels than they actually experience. Some patients report they perceive anxiety as threatening or intolerable, with feared consequences such as losing control, doing something abhorrent, or going crazy. Overestimation of threat from anxiety itself can lead to neutralization and avoidance of precipitants, and impede adaptive coping (Foa & Kozak, 1986; Freeston *et al.*, 1996; Salkovskis, 1985). Arntz, Hilderbrand, and van den Hout (1994) found that strength of fear reported prior to an exposure task was related to anxiety predictions, as well as dysfunctional beliefs (danger expectations), in a mixed group of anxiety disorder patients (*n* = 37) including those with OCD (*n* = 8). Reduction of fear following exposure was influenced by the experience of anxiety, change in the believability of dysfunctional beliefs, and by a more general emotional evaluation (degree to which the exercise was an "unpleasant experience").

Beliefs About Strong Emotions

A few authors have proposed that anxiety disorder patients, including those with OCD, view strong emotion in general as threatening. This could include a lower threshold for emotional pain, and less ability to cope with (tolerate, regulate, problem solve) emotions, compared with non-clinical individuals. Taylor and Rachman (1992) reported that students' fear of anxiety and fear of sadness, as assessed on a modified version of The Fear Survey Schedule-III, loaded on separate factors and promoted avoidance of specific stimuli (i.e., anxiety or sadness related). There is some evidence that beliefs about a variety of strong affects are relevant to, but not specific to, OCD (Sookman *et al.*, 2001). Attempts at overcontrol of emotion may be more characteristic of OCD, whereas different strategies are more typical of other groups (e.g., escape in phobias).

Williams, Chambless, and Ahrens (1997) and Berg, Shapiro, Chambless, and Ahrens (1998) suggested that anxiety disorder patients have greater fear of emotion than those without anxiety disorders because of concerns about losing control over emotions or because of behavioral reactions, even to strong positive emotions. To test this hypothesis, Williams *et al.* (1997) developed the Affective Control Scale (ACS), a self-report measure of fear of loss of control during the experience of anxiety, positive emotion, depressed mood, and anger. The authors found that students with higher ACS scores became more anxious and fearful after induction of panic-like bodily sensations than low-scoring students. Fear of emotion predicted fear of bodily sensations even when anxiety items were excluded from the ACS (Williams *et al.*, 1997). The capacity of patients to cope with strong emotions would seem important to address in treatment for OCD.

Laboratory Studies

Several researchers (e.g., Macleod, 1999) have described the limitations of studying internal processes solely with self-report measures, which rely on introspective methodology. Experimental paradigms from the field of cognitive psychology have been used to elucidate information processing difficulties or biases in areas such as decision making, attention, and memory. These paradigms permit examination of implicit or automatic (not in conscious awareness) as well as explicit (accessible to awareness) processes in psychopathology. For example, evidence of hypervigilance for (or avoidance of) threat could be reflected in selective attention (or inattention) to threat cues compared with neutral cues, and by differences in response to the same stimulus by patients compared with non-clinical individuals. Specificity of response could be examined during exposure to threat stimuli hypothesized to be disorder specific versus nonspecific. Detection, encoding (learning), and retrieval (accessing the stored representation from memory) phases of information processing may be affected. Relatively few studies have been carried out with OCD patients. Because this literature is the focus of Chapter nine, only a sampling of these studies are summarized here. For theoretical background relevant to information processing in anxiety, see Rachman (1998), Beck's (1996) description of primary modes postulated to underlie basic processing related to survival, and Ledoux's (1996) neurophysiological model of the danger detecting system of the brain.

Attention

In modified Stroop (1935) experiments subjects are shown words on a screen or cards that convey threat (e.g. bacteria) or that are neutral (table, desk), written in different colors. The task is to name the color while ignoring the word meaning. If an attentional bias exists for threat related information, patients should take longer to color-name threat as compared with neutral words (i.e., processing is slowed by interference of attention to threat stimuli). In the Dot Probe task, attentional bias for threat related information is inferred if subjects localize a probe on a computer screen faster when it is situated close to where threat words have been flashed. This is taken to indicate that they have paid greater attention to this area of the screen because of the presence of the threat word. In dichotic listening paradigms, different prose passages are presented to each ear. Subjects are asked to repeat one passage, to ignore the other, or to detect presentations of neutral or fear-related words that occur in either passage.

Several studies have reported that OCD patients, in particular those with contamination fears, demonstrate attentional biases to specific threat stimuli. Foa and McNally (1986) reported attentional biases to threat relevant material using a dichotic listening paradigm with 11 OCD patients, seven of whom had contamination fears. The finding that these biases were not evident after successful behavior therapy suggests they resulted from fear of, rather than familiarity with, the stimuli. In a later study using modified Stroop paradigm, OCD subjects with washing rituals were compared to those without washing rituals, and to non-clinical participants (Foa, Ilai, McCarthy, Shoyer, & Murdock, 1993). OCD subjects showed longer latencies for contamination words than non-clinical individuals, and washers had longer response latencies for contamination compared with neutral words. Only the non-washer group showed significantly more interference to general threat words compared with the non-clinical group.

Lavy, van Oppen, and van de Hout (1994) examined the question of whether attentional biases operate only for threat stimuli related to patients' specific concerns, or whether these occur for emotional cues in general. In a modified Stroop task, the emotional words presented were positive ("happy"), negative ("hate") and neutral ("square"). The study also examined relatedness of threat stimuli to specific OCD sub-groups of checkers ("precise, wrong") and washers ("filthy, neat"). OCD subjects showed evidence of selective attention to threat words specifically associated with their fears, but not to positive OCD words. There was also a trend for OCD subjects to be slower in processing the disorder-unrelated emotional stimuli.

Tata, Leibowitz, Prunty, Cameron, and Pickering (1996) compared 13 OCD patients with contamination fears to 18 non-clinical controls with high or low trait anxiety on a dot probe task that presented neutral words and words related to contamination or social anxiety. Although both OCD and high trait anxiety subjects showed increased vigilance for threat words, OCD patients selectively focused on contamination content whereas the high anxious subjects preferentially focused on the social anxiety content.

In contrast, McNally and colleagues reported several studies with inconsistent results. In one, ten OCD patients with contamination fears did not show significant interference for relevant threat words (e.g., feces, germs) on a Stroop task (McNally, Kaspi, Reimann, & Zeitlin, 1990). McNally, Reimann, Luro, Lukach, and Kim (1992) found that OCD patients (subgroup unspecified) showed interference to words thought to be characteristic of panic disorder (e.g., breathless or choking). However, in a subsequent study no interference was found for somatic or for general threat words, and OCD patients showed significantly greater interference for positive compared with panic-threat words (McNally *et al.*, 1994). As pointed out by the OCCWG (1997), considerable heterogeneity of obsessive fears could influence studies of attentional biases to specific threats in OCD. Patients with somatic concerns might be expected to selectively attend to health related cues, whereas this would not be expected with patients whose contamination fears do not involve fear of becoming ill. Attentional biases associated with the content or emotional valence of verbal information may be more characteristic of patients with contamination fears than of other subgroups such as checkers (Summerfeldt & Endler, 1998).

Memory

It is a common clinical observation that OCD patients have an unusually detailed memory for threat cues (e.g., "I can never seem to find my keys but I can sure tell you where the germs are in my home", Radomsky & Rachman, 1999, p. 614). Examination of memory in OCD has yielded mixed results. Some studies suggest difficulty with encoding and retrieval of non-verbal memory (see Savage, 1998, for a review of the neuropsychological literature), while others have not found this to be the case (e.g., Constans, Foa, Franklin, & Mathews, 1995; Radomsky & Rachman, 1999).

In some studies, checkers (subclinical OCD or non-OCD psychiatric patients) displayed worse recall of their own actions, or of words from a study list, compared with non-checkers (Sheffler-Rubenstein, Peynircioglu, Chambless, & Pigott, 1993; Sher, Frost, Kushner, Crews, & Alexander, 1989; Sher, Frost, & Otto, 1983). In contrast, Maki, O'Neill, and O'Neill (1994) found no differences in recall (directed forgetting) of performance in college students with high versus low OCD symptom scores. In two studies with clinical samples, OCD patients did not differ from controls in their ability to recall words presented through visual or auditory channels (Brown, Kosslyn, Breiter, Baer, &

Jenike, 1994), and memory of checkers did not differ from non-checkers and normals on a recognition task (MacDonald, Anthony, MacLeod, & Richter, 1997). McNally and Kohlbeck (1993) found that OCD patients doubted their memory (for real versus imagined performance of a task) more than controls, even though the memory accuracy of the groups did not differ. These results suggest that uncertainty rather than actual memory deficit may be related to checking.

There is some evidence for enhanced recall of threatening situations in OCD. In a study of recall for real versus imagined actions categorized as neutral versus distressing, OCD patients showed no overall memory impairment but had better recall of anxiety provoking situations than controls (Constans *et al.*, 1995). In this study as well, patients reported more dissatisfaction with their recall compared with normals. Wilhelm, McNally, Baer, and Floring (1996) found that OCD patients had more difficulty forgetting negative material compared with positive and neutral material, whereas this was not the case for normal controls. Radomsky and Rachman (1999) examined memory for contaminated objects in OCD patients ($n = 10$) with contamination fears, compared with a group of anxious controls ($n = 10$) or students ($n = 20$). One of the strengths of this elegant study was the use of clinically salient stimuli. Recall of the OCD group was better for contaminated objects than for clean ones, and neither control group showed this bias. Neuropsychological test scores indicated these results were not due to group differences in general memory ability. There was evidence of an implicit memory bias: Patients recalled a greater number of contaminated objects even though they were unable to remember which objects were "contaminated" versus "clean".

Summary

The laboratory studies reviewed provide some evidence of an attentional bias for processing of OCD threat-relevant stimuli, particularly in patients with contamination fears. There are mixed results with respect to memory. A few studies with non-clinical checkers suggested an action-memory deficit, but this was not replicated with patients. There is evidence of enhanced memory for threat cues in OCD, and support for the hypothesis that patients experience uncertainty about the accuracy of their memory despite unimpaired performance. A methodological limitation of many studies of attentional and memory biases in anxiety is use of words as threat cues. Words may not have sufficient emotional salience to activate explicit (elaborative) memory (Williams, Watts, MacLeod, & Mathews, 1997). Further research with specific, clinically relevant, and emotionally salient stimuli (e.g., contamination objects for washers, stoves or switches for checkers) are needed to elucidate the role of uncertainty beliefs versus actual memory ability in OCD (Radomsky & Rachman, 1999). Bouvard and Cottraux (1997) reported that while checkers showed visual processing deficits on neuropsychological testing, washers did not show any deficit, underlining the need to study the differential response of OCD subgroups.

Relationship to OCD Symptoms

Overestimation of Threat

Several studies, some with clinical samples, have demonstrated the relationship of overestimation of threat to OCD symptoms (for other reviews see OCCWG, 1997; Steketee, Frost, Rhéaume, & Wilhelm, 1998). The self-report variables in the studies reviewed here were: (a) willingness to take risks; (b) threat perceptions or beliefs; and (c) the relation of risk taking, or threat perceptions/beliefs, to OCD symptoms.

In an early study by Steiner (1972), obsessive patients gave more cautious responses than other groups on a self-report questionnaire about risk taking in various real-life situations. Steketee and Frost (1994) developed a 32-item scale, the Everyday Risk Inventory, to assess avoidance of potentially harmful ordinary activities (e.g., leaving a car unlocked briefly or driving in poor weather). Non-clinical individuals with obsessive symptoms, as well as patients diagnosed with OCD, reported they would avoid taking daily risks more than normal controls. This was the case even when items that could overlap with OCD fears were removed from the analyses (e.g., drinking from a cup used by a friend).

Frost and Sher (1989) demonstrated a link between perception of personally relevant threat and checking behavior. Students who scored high on the checking subscale of the MOCI, or who reported high levels of daily checking behavior, checked more in a personally relevant and potentially threatening situation (a graded exam) compared with students who scored low on these measures. The authors suggested indecisiveness/ uncertainty about the quality of their performance may also have been salient in the checking group; however, the design did not allow examination of this hypothesis. Freeston, Ladouceur, Thibodeau, and Gagnon (1992) reported that overestimation of threat was a feature of volunteer subjects with OCD symptoms. Measures of perceived danger also correlated with OCD severity for non-clinical subjects in a later study (Rhéaume, Ladouceur, & Freeston, 1996, cited in Steketee, Frost, Rhéaume, & Wilhelm, 1998).

A study by Woods, Frost, and Steketee (1998) indicated that students' beliefs about threat on a preliminary version of the OBQ, and about every-day risk taking, were significantly correlated with OCD symptoms but not, as suggested by Carr (1971, 1974), with estimates of the probability of future negative events. Subjects rated the probability of specific negative events that they worried might happen in the future on the Future Events Questionnaire constructed by the authors. While probability estimates were not related to general beliefs about threat, Woods *et al.* reported that a manipulation of availability heuristics did effect probability ratings. High OCD participants who wrote reasons their feared negative events would occur rated these as more likely to actually happen compared with subjects who wrote reasons their events would not occur. Findings by Riskind, Abreu, Strauss, and Holt (1997) suggest that probability ratings may be greater for threatening events that are specific to participants' concerns. Undergraduate students scoring high in contamination fear rated the probability of contamination in specific situations as significantly higher than students who scored low on this fear. Consistent with this possibility, an earlier study by Simos, Vaiopoulos, Giouzepas, and Parasehos (1995) found that estimations of the likelihood of general classes of dangerous events (e.g., traffic accidents, earthquakes) did not correlate with scores on the revised Maudsley Obsessional Compulsive Inventory.

In a recent study, Woods, Frost, and Steketee (2001) examined the relationship between estimates of subjective probability and severity of idiographic future negative events, anticipated coping ability, and OCD symptoms in a sample of 18 OCD patients and 73 students. Previous research by this group had also suggested that individuals may overestimate the probability only of personally salient negative events (Woods, Frost, Rubeck, & Steketee, 1997). As predicted by cognitive models, as OCD symptoms increased, severity estimation increased and ratings of coping ability decreased for both patients and students. However, estimates of the probability of negative events were related to OCD symptoms for students, but for OCD patients. Results were consistent with Salkovskis' (1996) hypothesis that anxiety relates to the product of probability and severity, divided by coping ability. The authors proposed that OCD patients may have underreported (or already modified) their probability estimates, but not severity or coping ability, or that expected severity of feared consequences may overwhelm probability estimates. It is also possible that patients may overestimate the probability of obsession-related events, but not other negative events. In this study data on participant's obsessions were not collected.

Intolerance of Uncertainty

As noted by Steketee, Frost, and Cohen (1998), there is little empirical research on beliefs about uncertainty in OCD. Most research to date has focused on symptoms, rather than on beliefs. For example, compared with other psychiatric patients or normal controls, individuals with OCD symptoms are slower to categorize objects, request more repetition of information, have more difficulty making decisions, and show more doubt about their decisions (Frost, Lahart, Dugas, & Sher, 1988; Frost & Shows, 1993; Milner, Beech, & Walker, 1971; Persons & Foa, 1984; Volans, 1976). Frost and Steketee (1997) found that doubt about one's actions was the only dimension of perfectionism that distinguished OCD from panic disorder patients. The role of beliefs about uncertainty versus reluctance to take perceived risks in explaining symptoms in OCD requires further study (Steketee, Frost, Rhéaume, & Wilhelm, 1998).

Summary

Individuals with OCD symptoms overestimate the severity of negative events, and show less willingness to take risks than normals. The relation between symptoms and probability estimates has not yet been demonstrated. Symptoms may be associated with overestimation of probability of personal (and idiosyncratic) harm, rather than with general classes of negative events. Estimates of probability are likely to vary with subgroup and the content of the feared threat (e.g., checkers overestimate the likelihood of being responsible for harm). Several authors (e.g., Frost *et al.*, 1988; Rachman, 1998; Rachman & Hodgson, 1980) have suggested different processes for checking compared to washing behaviors, noting for example, that slowness, indecisiveness, and concerns about memory are more characteristic of checkers than cleaners. While the relation between uncertainty beliefs and symptoms has been demonstrated in psychometric studies, experimental studies are needed to further examine their contribution.

Overestimation of Threat and Intolerance of Uncertainty in Other Disorders

Overestimation of Threat

Dysfunctional beliefs and information processing biases related to threat are prevalent across diagnostic groups. Anxiety disorder patients overestimate the threat of specific negative events: an aggressive thought in OCD; a physical sensation in panic disorder or hypochondriasis; or perceived interpersonal rejection or failure in social phobia (e.g., Butler & Mathews, 1983, 1987; Foa, Franklin, Perry, & Herbert, 1996; Lucock & Salkvoskis, 1988; McNally & Foa, 1987). Laboratory studies have demonstrated that information processing is influenced by the emotional significance of the threat to the individual, the degree of subjects' anxiety, and whether subjects are anxious or depressed (see Clark & Fairburn, 1997; Mogg & Bradley, 1999 for reviews). For example, panic disorder patients show an attentional bias for physical stimuli matching their fears, but not for socially threatening stimuli (Mathews, 1997). Panic patients have shown enhanced recall for threat related words, while speech phobic patients have shown impairment of recall (Cloitre & Liebowitz, 1991; McNally, Foa, & Donnell, 1989). These findings seem to reflect different responses to perceived threat: In this case, hypervigilance (panic) versus avoidance (speech). Similar findings have been reported for a group of students facing the same situation (an exam), but differing in level of trait anxiety. High trait anxious students showed selective attention to threatening words, whereas low anxious students not only did not show this effect but seemed at times to avoid attending (Mogg, Bradley, & Hallowell, 1994). Anxiety seems to be associated predominantly with a selective attention bias; and depression with a negative recall bias, especially for self-referential material (Mogg & Bradley, 1999). It is a normal phenomenon that stimuli having emotional significance elicit attention. Words chosen to reflect the emotional concerns of normals result in more interference compared with matched control words in Stroop color-naming tasks (e.g., Riemann & McNally, 1995). There is evidence that interference due to threat cues in patients diminishes following therapy (Mathews, Mogg, Kentish, & Eysenck, 1995; Mattia, Heimberg, & Hope, 1993). However, as stated above, reliance on words as stimuli is an important methodological limitation of many studies.

The cognitive models of other anxiety disorders recognize the role of past experiences on current information processing, appraisals, and beliefs. For example, susceptibility to panic disorder has been theoretically linked to specific learning experiences such as observing parents appearing overwhelmed by anxiety or illness (Ehlers, 1993). The cognitive model of social phobia postulates that, on the basis of early experience, social phobics develop dysfunctional assumptions about themselves and interpersonal situations that effect current appraisals (Clark & Wells, 1995). Thus, as in OCD, anticipatory anxiety and dysfunctional beliefs include expectations about the future colored by perceptions of past experiences. Several self-report scales have been developed to assess dysfunctional beliefs characteristic of other anxiety disorders (e.g., Agoraphobic Cognitions Questionnaire by Chambless, Caputo, Bright, & Gallagher, 1984; Panic Belief Questionnaire by Greenberg, 1988; Panic Appraisal Inventory by Telch, Brouillard, Telch, Agras, & Taylor,1989).

In this section, the role of overestimation of threat will be briefly summarized for Panic Disorder, Generalized Anxiety Disorder (GAD), and Social Phobia in order to illustrate some commonalities and differences (for a review of this literature, see Clark, 1997). Overestimation of threat to trauma-related stimuli is also a central feature of Post Traumatic Stress Disorder. A review of the extensive literature from experimental and laboratory studies carried out with disorders other than OCD is beyond the scope of this chapter.

Panic Disorder. Just as intrusions are normal phenomena, up to a quarter of the normal population have experienced at least one panic attack (Clark, 1997). However, only three to five percent of the general population develop panic disorder (Wittchen & Essau, 1991). The available evidence suggests that recurrent panic attacks occur in individuals who catastrophically appraise bodily sensations that accompany anxiety, such as palpitations, breathlessness, or dizziness. These symptoms are misinterpreted as indicative of imminent physical or mental disaster, such as loss of consciousness or heart attack (Clark, 1988). This overestimation of threat leads to a further increase in anxiety and physical symptoms, which may escalate to the point of panic (Clark, 1988). External stimuli that provoke anxiety (e.g., crowds) are also perceived as dangerous.

Two additional processes are hypothesized to contribute to symptom maintenance: Hypervigilance and safety behaviors (Clark, 1999; Salkovskis, 1991). A hypervigilant individual typically scans his/her body for signs of sensations perceived as threatening, which become the center of attention. This internal focus, or narrowing of attention, augments perception of these sensations. Safety behaviors are carried out to avert/ protect against the feared danger. For example, physical exercise may be avoided to prevent a heart attack. Safety behaviors maintain anxiety by preventing disconfirmation of the original overestimation of threat. For example, non-occurrence of a heart attack is appraised as due to the safety behavior rather than to the overestimation of threat.

Social Phobia. A central feature of social phobia is overestimation of the threat of negative interpersonal evaluation, such as ridicule, loss of respect, or rejection (see Clark, 1997; Clark & Wells, 1995). Social interactions are perceived as more negative than they really are. For example, during a conversation, if the other person excuses himself to go to the washroom, the social phobic may think: "He doesn't like me." Perception of threat is associated with feelings of anxiety and other physiological responses such as blushing or difficulty concentrating. Appraisal of symptoms as threatening increases both symptoms and sense of danger. For example, patients may appraise (and assume others appraise) blushing or shaking as meaning they have appeared anxious, foolish, or out of control. Attention becomes centered on self- observation and thinking about what others think. Dysfunctional safety behaviors, such as censoring during conversations or avoiding eye contact, are attempts to reduce social threat and prevent feared outcomes from occurring.

Hypervigilance for negative evaluation, faulty processing of positive evaluation, predominance of internal focus, mental reviewing of social failures, and safety behaviors all contribute to perpetuation of faulty threat appraisals.

Generalized Anxiety Disorder.   Worrying is a component of most emotional disorders, viewed in part as a coping strategy for threat and as preparation for potential negative events. While worry is the predominant symptom in GAD, the content of worry in GAD and normal populations may to some extent be similar (for a review of a cognitive model of this disorder, see Wells & Butler, 1999). There is some evidence that GAD patients worry more about illness and injury compared with normals (Craske, Rapee, Jackel, & Barlow, 1989) and worry more about remote future events compared with other anxiety disorder patients (Dugas *et al.*, 1998). The content of these ruminations is likely more variable than automatic thoughts found in other anxiety disorders, perhaps reflecting differences in information processing. Patients with GAD also negatively appraise their own thoughts; that is, they overestimate the threat of worry itself (Wells, 1995). Similarities between OCD and GAD include repetitive intrusions perceived as threatening and difficult to dismiss, dysfunctional meta-cognition (thinking about thinking), and perceived loss of mental control (Langlois *et al.*, 2000; Wells & Matthews, 1994).

GAD individuals also avoid specific external threats (e.g., media, hospitals) and emotional arousal in an attempt to avoid provoking worry. Borkovec and colleagues (e.g., Borkovec & Inz, 1990; Borkovec, Shadick, & Hopkins, 1991) suggested that worry may constitute avoidance of cognition such as images which are perceived as threatening because they are strongly associated with emotion. Langlois *et al.* (2000) found that worry is more often experienced in verbal form, whereas obsessions are more often experienced as images. However, as these authors suggest, there may be a relationship between content and form of intrusions: It may be easier to create mental images of aggressive themes (OCD) than of everyday or remote future problems (GAD). Again, hypervigilance for cues which provoke symptoms, avoidance and other safety behaviors, narrowing of attention on the content of worry, worry about being out of control of worry, and attempts at thought control all contribute to perpetuation of anxiety and prevent disconfirmation of dysfunctional beliefs (Barlow, 1988; Borkovec *et al.*, 1991; Craske *et al.*, 1989; Rapee, 1991; Wells, 1994).

Intolerance of Uncertainty

Intolerance of uncertainty is a feature of disorders other than OCD, especially GAD (Dugas, Gagnon, Ladouceur, & Freeston, 1998). It may also be found in Axis II diagnoses such as obsessive compulsive personality disorder and dependent personality disorder (Steketee, Frost & Cohen, 1998). Several studies indicate that intolerance of uncertainty is a central characteristic of individuals who worry, in both clinical (GAD) and non-clinical populations, even when the effect of anxiety and depression is controlled (e.g., Dugas, Freeston, & Ladouceur, 1997; Freeston *et al.*, 1994). Ladouceur *et al.* (1995) reported that GAD patients showed greater intolerance of uncertainty than a mixed group of patients suffering from other anxiety disorders including OCD, panic disorder with or without agoraphobia, and social phobia. Some evidence indicates that worriers take longer to categorize ambiguous stimuli than non-worriers, and tend to interpret ambiguous material as threatening (Butler, 1993; Metzger, Miller, Cohen, Sofka, & Borkovec, 1990; Tallis, Eysenck, & Mathews, 1991).

Using an elegant experimental task, Ladouceur, Talbot, and Dugas (1997) found that normal subjects scoring high on intolerance of uncertainty required more information before responding to a moderately ambiguous task, but not to an unambiguous task (regardless of level of difficulty). The authors suggested that intolerance of uncertainty may be associated with a lower threshold for perception of ambiguity. Interestingly, intolerance of uncertainty was not related to performance on a highly ambiguous task, suggesting that high levels of ambiguity may lead to uncertainty for most people. The authors cite Krohne's (1993) model of anxiety, which proposed that intolerance of uncertainty is associated with a lower perceptual threshold and stronger emotional reaction to ambiguity, and importantly, with anticipation of threatening future consequences of uncertainty.

Several studies have shown that worry is strongly related to intolerance of uncertainty, poor problem-solving confidence, and perceived control (i.e., poor "problem orientation"), but not to problem-solving ability (Blais, Freeston, Dugas, & Ladouceur, 1994; Dugas, Letarte, Rhéaume, Freeston, & Ladouceur, 1995). Dugas *et al.* (1997) suggested that GAD patients may selectively attend to ambiguous or uncertain aspects of a problem situation and perceive threat at minimal levels of uncertainty.

Overall Summary and Conclusions

The literature reviewed indicates that overestimation of threat is a central characteristic of OCD that should be included in a comprehensive cognitive model of the disorder. While highly characteristic of OCD, overestimating threat is a predominant feature of all anxiety disorders. The stage two studies carried out by the OCCWG (2001), and earlier studies, found that OCD patients endorsed selected beliefs in this domain more strongly than other anxiety disorders and normal subjects. These beliefs were significantly related to OCD symptoms even when the effect of anxiety and depression was controlled. Growing empirical evidence indicates that intolerance of uncertainty is also relevant to OCD. The pattern of results found for threat and uncertainty was similar, and these domains are highly interrelated.

The results from the OCCWG stage three study based on larger samples (OCCWG, in preparation) further substantiate the importance of threat estimation and tolerance of uncertainty in this disorder. Patients with OCD were again found to endorse these dysfunctional beliefs, as assessed on the OBQ, significantly more strongly compared to two groups of normal controls. Further, factor analyses supported the centrality of overestimation of threat in OCD-related beliefs. As in previous studies, these domains were highly related. However, in contrast to stage two findings and other studies reviewed in this chapter, at stage three no significant difference was found between OCD and other anxiety disorder groups in endorsement of these beliefs. These subscales correlated almost as highly with measures of general distress as with OCD symptoms. The stage three results suggest that although the dysfunctional beliefs examined are relevant to OCD, they are shared by other anxiety disorders as well.

The possibility that differences among studies could be related in part to methodological factors should also be considered. For example, heterogeneity and degree of co-morbidity in the psychiatric groups examined, and type of anxiety disorders included in comparative groups, could effect degree of overlap of symptoms and related beliefs. Of the other anxiety disorder participants at stage three testing, 25 percent were diagnosed with post traumatic stress disorder (PTSD) and 17 percent with generalized anxiety disorder. These diagnoses may be more similar to OCD in terms of content of threat and uncertainty beliefs respectively, compared to patients with panic disorder/agoraphobia, social phobia, or hypochondriasis. Previous studies that found a significant difference between OCD and other anxiety disorder groups did not include PTSD patients (Steketee *et al.*, 1998) and excluded comorbid Axis I participants (Sookman *et al.*, 2001). The question of which threat and uncertainty beliefs may be specific to OCD, and which are relevant but not specific to this disorder, might be best examined with homogeneous samples. Also, the relation between these beliefs and symptoms may vary with OCD subgroup (e.g., washers, checkers, hoarders).

The relative contribution and role of the cognitive domains identified as relevant to OCD requires further study. Consistent with clinical observation, the available evidence indicates that dysfunctional beliefs about threat and uncertainty are moderately to highly related to beliefs about importance of thoughts, control of thoughts, responsibility, and perfectionism, that also discriminate OCD from other groups (OCCWG, 2001). Overestimation of threat from inner phenomena such as thoughts is associated with exaggeration of their importance and attempts at overcontrol. Individuals who are intolerant of uncertainty may have a lower threshold for perceiving a variety of ambiguous situations as threatening. Difficulty with unpredictability, newness, and change could increase the range of situations in which "degree of danger" is overestimated and "capacity to cope" is underestimated. Freeston, Leger, Rhéaume, and Ladouceur (1996, cited in Steketee, Frost, Rhéaume, & Wilhelm, 1998) have suggested that overestimating threat may be a necessary precursor to overestimating responsibility. An important question that awaits further research is to what extent overestimation of threat is such a central aspect of OCD that it is a necessary condition to the development and maintenance of symptoms.

References

Arntz, A., Hildebrand, M., & van den Hout, M. A. (1994). Overprediction of anxiety, and disconfirmatory processes, in anxiety disorders. *Behaviour Research and Therapy, 32,* 709–722.

Arntz, A., Rauner, M., & van den Hout, M. A. (1995). "If I feel anxious, there must be a danger": Ex-consequentia reasoning in inferring danger in anxiety disorders. *Behaviour Research and Therapy, 33,* 917–925.

Barlow, D. H. (1988). *Anxiety and its disorders: The nature and treatment of anxiety and panic.* New York: Guilford.

Barlow, D. H. (1991). Disorders of emotion. *Psychological Inquiry, 2,* 58–71.

Beck, A. T. (1996). Beyond belief: A theory of modes, personality, and psychopathology. In P. M. Salkovskis (ed.), *Frontiers of cognitive therapy* (pp. 1–25). New York: Guilford.

Beck, A. T., & Clark, D. A. (1997). An information processing model of anxiety: Automatic and strategic processes. *Behaviour Research and Therapy, 35,* 49–58.

Beck, A. T., Emery, G., & Greenberg, R. L. (1985). *Anxiety disorders and phobias: A cognitive perspective*. New York: Basic Books.

Beck, A. T., Rush, A. J., Shaw, B. R., & Emery, G. (1979). *Cognitive Therapy of Depression*. New York: Guilford.

Beech, H. R., & Liddell, A. (1974). Decision-making, mood states and ritualistic behavior among obsessional patients. In H. R. Beech (ed.), *Obsessional States* (pp. 143–160). London: Methuen.

Berg, C. Z., Shapiro, N., Chambless, D. L., & Ahrens, A. H. (1998). Are emotions frightening? II: An analogue study of fear of emotion, interpersonal conflict, and panic. *Behaviour Research and Therapy, 36*, 3–15.

Blais, F., Freeston, M. H., Dugas, M. J., & Ladouceur, R. (1994, November). *Problem orientation and problem-solving skills in clinical and nonclinical worriers*. Paper presented at the annual meeting of the Association for Advancement of Behavior Therapy, San Diego, CA.

Borkovec, T. D., & Inz, J. (1990). The nature of worry in generalized anxiety disorder: A predominance of thought activity. *Behaviour Research and Therapy, 28*, 153–158.

Borkovec, T. D., Shadick, R. N., & Hopkins, M. (1991). The nature of normal and pathological worry. In R. M. Rapee & D. H. Barlow (eds), *Chronic anxiety: Generalized anxiety disorder and mixed anxiety–depression* (pp. 29–51). New York: Guilford.

Bouvard, M., & Cottraux, J. (1997). Étude comparative chez le sujet normal et le sujet obsessif-compulsif des pensées intrusives et de la mémoire. [A comparative study of intrusive thoughts and memory in normal subjects and obsessive-compulsive patients]. *L'Encéphale, 23*, 175–179.

Brown, H. D., Kosslyn, S. M., Breiter, H. C., Baer, L., & Jenike, M. A. (1994). Can patients with obsessive–compulsive disorder discriminate between percepts and mental images? A signal detection analysis. *Journal of Abnormal Psychology, 103*, 445–454.

Butler, G. (1993). Predicting outcome after treatment for GAD. *Behaviour Research and Therapy, 31*, 211–213.

Butler, G., & Mathews, A. (1983). Cognitive processes in anxiety. *Advances in Behaviour Research and Therapy, 5*, 51–62.

Butler, G., & Mathews, A. (1987). Anticipatory anxiety and risk perception. *Cognitive Therapy and Research, 11*, 551–565.

Carr, A. T. (1971). Compulsive neurosis: Two psychological studies. *Bulletin of the British Psychological Society, 24*, 256–257.

Carr, A. T. (1974). Compulsive neurosis: A review of the literature. *Psychological Bulletin, 81*, 311–318.

Chambless, D. L., Caputo, G. C., Bright, P., & Gallagher, R. (1984). Assessment of fear of fear in agoraphobics: The Body Sensations Questionnaire and the Agoraphobic Cognitions Questionnaire. *Journal of Consulting and Clinical Psychology, 52*, 1090–1097.

Clark, D. M. (1988). A cognitive model of panic attacks. In S. Rachman & J. Maser (eds), *Panic: Psychological Perspectives* (pp. 71–89). Hillsdale, NJ: Erlbaum.

Clark, D. M. (1997). Panic disorder and social phobia. In D. M. Clark & C. G. Fairburn (eds), *Science and practice of cognitive behaviour therapy* (pp. 121–153). New York: Oxford University Press.

Clark, D. M. (1999). Anxiety disorders: Why they persist and how to treat them. *Behaviour Research and Therapy, 37*, 5–27.

Clark, D. M., & Fairburn, C. G. (eds). (1997). *Science and practice of cognitive behaviour therapy*. Oxford: Oxford University Press.

Clark, D. M., & Wells, A. (1995). A cognitive model of social phobia. In R. Heimberg, M. Liebowitz, D. A. Hope, & F. R. Schneier (eds), *Social Phobia: Diagnosis, Assessment and Treatment* (pp. 69–93). New York: Guilford.

Cloitre, M., & Liebowitz, M. R. (1991). Memory bias in panic disorder: An investigation of the cognitive avoidance hypothesis. *Cognitive Therapy and Research, 15*, 371–386.

Cloninger, C. R., Przybeck, T. R., & Svrakic, D. M. (1991). The Tridimensional Personality Questionnaire: U. S. normative data. *Psychological Reports, 69*, 1047–1057.

Constans, J. I., Foa, E. B., Franklin, M. E., & Mathews, A. (1995). Memory for actual and imagined events in OC checkers. *Behaviour Research and Therapy, 33*, 665–671.

Craske, M. G., Rapee, R. M., Jackel, L., & Barlow, D. H. (1989). Qualitative dimensions of DSM-III-R generalized anxiety disorder subjects and nonanxious controls. *Behaviour Research and Therapy, 27*, 397–402.

Dugas, M. J., Freeston, M. H., & Ladouceur, R. (1997). Intolerance of uncertainty and problem orientation in worry. *Cognitive Therapy and Research, 21*, 593–606.

Dugas, M. J., Freeston, M. H., Ladouceur, R., Rhéaume, J., Provencher, M., & Boisvert, J.-M. (1998). Worry themes in primary GAD, secondary GAD and other anxiety disorders. *Journal of Anxiety Disorders, 12*, 253–261.

Dugas, M. J., Gagnon, F., Ladouceur, R., & Freeston, M. H. (1998). Generalized anxiety disorder: a preliminary test of a conceptual model. *Behavior Research and Therapy, 36*, 215–226.

Dugas, M. J., Letarte, H., Rhéaume, J., Freeston, M. H., & Ladouceur, R. (1995). Worry and problem solving: Evidence of a specific relationship. *Cognitive Therapy and Research, 19*, 109–120.

Ehlers, A. (1993). Interoception and panic disorder. *Advances in Behaviour Research and Therapy, 15*, 3–21.

Ey, H., Bernard, P., & Brisset, C. (1963). *Manuel de Psychiatrie.* (2nd ed.). Paris: Libraires de l'académie de médecine.

Foa, E. B., & Kozak, M. J. (1986). Emotional processing of fear: Exposure to corrective information. *Psychological Bulletin, 99*, 20–35.

Foa, E. B., & McNally, R. J. (1986). Sensitivity to feared stimuli in obsessive-compulsives: A dichotic listening analysis. *Cognitive Therapy and Research, 10*, 477–486.

Foa, E. B., Franklin, M. E., Perry, K. J., & Herbert, J. D. (1996). Cognitive biases in generalized social phobia. *Journal of Abnormal Psychology, 105*, 433–439.

Foa, E. B., Ilai, D., McCarthy, P. R., Shoyer, B., & Murdock, T. (1993). Information processing in obsessive compulsive disorder. *Cognitive Therapy and Research, 17*, 173–189.

Freeston, M. H., Ladouceur, R., Gagnon, F., & Thibodeau, N. (1993). Beliefs about obsessional thoughts. *Journal of Psychopathology and Behavioral Assessment, 15*, 1–21.

Freeston, M. H., Ladouceur, R., Thibodeau, N., & Gagnon, F. (1992). Cognitive intrusions in a non-clinical population. II. Associations with depressive, anxious and compulsive symptoms. *Behaviour Research and Therapy, 30*, 263–271.

Freeston, M. H., Rhéaume, J., & Ladouceur, R. (1996). Correcting faulty appraisals of obsessional thoughts. *Behaviour Research and Therapy, 34*, 433–446.

Freeston, M. H., Rhéaume, J., Letarte, H., Dugas, M. J., & Ladouceur, R. (1994). Why do people worry? *Personality and Individual Differences, 17*, 791–802.

Freeston, M. H., Todorov, C., Fournier, S., & Gareau, D. (2000, March). *Changing assumptions and interpretations during the treatment of obsessive thoughts.* Paper presented at the annual meeting of the Anxiety Disorders Association of America, Washington, DC.

Frost, R. O., & Hartl, T. L. (1996). A cognitive–behavioural model of compulsive hoarding. *Behaviour Research and Therapy, 34*, 341–350.

Frost, R. O., & Sher, K. J. (1989). Checking behavior in a threatening situation. *Behaviour Research and Therapy, 27*, 385–389.

Frost, R. O., & Shows, D. L. (1993). The nature and measurement of compulsive indecisiveness. *Behaviour Research and Therapy, 31*, 683–692.

Frost, R. O., & Steketee, G. (1997). Perfectionism in obsessive-compulsive disorder patients. *Behaviour Research and Therapy, 35*, 291–296.

Frost, R. O., Lahart, C. M., Dugas, K. M., & Sher, K. J. (1988). Information processing among non-clinical compulsives. *Behaviour Research and Therapy, 26*, 275–277.

Frost, R. O., Marten, P., Lahart, C. M., & Rosenblate, R. (1990). The dimensions of perfectionism. *Cognitive Therapy and Research, 14*, 449–468.

Greenberg, R. L. (1988). Panic disorder and agoraphobia. In J. M. G. Williams & A. T. Beck (eds), *Cognitive therapy in clinical practice: An illustrative casebook* (pp. 25–49). London: Routledge.

Guidano, V. F., & Liotti, G. (1983). Obsessive–compulsive patterns. In V. F. Guidano (ed.), *Cognitive processes and emotional disorders* (pp. 243–275). New York: Guilford.

Krohne, H. W. (1993). Vigilance and cognitive avoidance as concepts in coping research. In H. W. Krohne (ed.), *Attention and avoidance strategies in coping with aversiveness*. Seattle, MA: Hogrefe & Huber.

Kozak, M. J., Foa, E. B., & McCarthy, P. (1987). Assessment of obsessive–compulsive disorder. In C. Last & M. Hersen (eds), *Handbook of anxiety disorders*. New York: Pergamon Press.

Ladouceur, R., Freeston, M. H., Dugas, M. J., Rhéaume, J., Gagnon, F., Thibodeau, N., Boisvert, J.-M., Provencher, M., & Blais, F. (1995, November). *Specific association between Generalized Anxiety Disorder and intolerance of uncertainty among anxiety disorder patients*. Poster session presented at the annual meeting of the Association for Advancement of Behavior Therapy, Washington, DC.

Ladouceur, R., Talbot, F., & Dugas, M. J. (1997). Behavioral expressions of intolerance of uncertainty in worry. *Behavior Modification, 21*, 355–371.

Langlois, F., Freeston, M. H., & Ladouceur, R. (2000). Differences and similarities between obsessive intrusive thoughts and worry in a non-clinical population: study 2. *Behaviour Research and Therapy, 38*, 175–189.

Lavy, E., van Oppen, P., & van den Hout, M. (1994). Selective processing of emotional information in obsessive–compulsive disorder. *Behaviour Research & Therapy, 32*, 243–246.

Lazarus, R. (1966). *Psychological stress and the coping process*. New York: McGraw Hill.

Ledoux, J. E. (1996). *The emotional brain: The mysterious underpinnings of emotional life*. New York: Simon & Schuster.

Lilienfeld, S. O., Turner, S. M., & Jacob, R. G. (1996). Further comments on the nature and measurement of anxiety sensitivity: A reply to Taylor. *Journal of Anxiety Disorders, 10*, 411–424.

Lucock, M., & Salkovskis, P. M. (1988). Cognitive factors in social anxiety and its treatment. *Behaviour Research and Therapy, 26*, 297–302.

MacDonald, P., Anthony, M. M., MacLeod, C., & Richter, M. A. (1997). Memory and confidence in memory judgments among individuals with obsessive compulsive disorder and non-clinical controls. *Behaviour Research and Therapy, 35*, 497–505.

MacLeod, C. (1999). Anxiety and anxiety disorders. In T. Dalgleish & M. Power (eds), *Handbook of cognition and emotion* (pp. 447–477). Chichester, England: Wiley.

Makhlouf-Norris, F., & Norris, H. (1972). The obsessive–compulsive syndrome as a neurotic device for the reduction of self-uncertainty. *British Journal of Psychiatry, 121*, 277–288.

Maki, W. S., O'Neill, H. K., & O'Neill, G. W. (1994). Do nonclinical checkers exhibit deficits in cognitive control? Tests of an inhibitory control hypothesis. *Behaviour Research and Therapy, 29*, 147–160.

Mathews, A. (1999). Information-processing biases in emotional disorders. In D. M. Clark & C. G. Fairburn (eds), *Science and practice of cognitive behaviour therapy* (pp. 47–66). New York: Oxford University Press.

Mathews, A., Mogg, K., Kentish, J., & Eysenck, M. (1995). Effect of psychological treatment on cognitive bias in generalized anxiety disorder. *Behaviour Research and Therapy, 33*, 293–303.

Mattia, J. I., Heimberg, R. G., & Hope, D. A. (1993). The revised Stroop color-naming task in social phobics. *Behaviour Research and Therapy, 31*, 305–313.

McFall, M. E., & Wollersheim, J. P. (1979). Obsessive–compulsive neurosis: A cognitive–behavioral formulation and approach to treatment. *Cognitive Therapy and Research, 3*, 333–348.

McNally, R. J. (1989). Is anxiety sensitivity distinguishable from trait anxiety? A reply to Lilienfeld, Jacob, and Turner (1989). *Journal of Abnormal Psychology, 98*, 193–194.

McNally, R. J. (1994). *Panic disorder: A critical analysis.* New York: Guilford.

McNally, R. J., & Foa, E. B. (1987). Cognition and agoraphobia: Bias in the interpretation of threat. *Cognitive Therapy and Research, 11*, 567–581.

McNally, R. J., & Kohlbeck, P. A. (1993). Reality monitoring in obsessive-compulsive disorder. *Behaviour Research and Therapy, 31*, 249–253.

McNally, R. J., Amir, N., Louro, C. E., Lukach, B. M., Riemann, B. C., & Calamari, J. E. (1994). Cognitive processing of idiographic emotional information in panic disorder. *Behaviour Research and Therapy, 32*, 119–122.

McNally, R. J., Foa, E. B., & Donnell, C. D. (1989). Memory bias for anxiety information in patients with panic disorder. *Cognition and Emotion, 3*, 27–44.

McNally, R. J., Kaspi, S. P., Riemann, B. C., & Zeitlin, S. B. (1990). Selective processing of threat cues in panic disorder. *Behaviour Research and Therapy, 28*, 407–412.

McNally, R. J., Riemann, B. C., Luro, C. E., Lukach, B. M., & Kim, E. (1992). Cognitive processing of emotional information in panic disorder. *Behaviour Research and Therapy, 30*, 143–149.

Metzger, R. L., Miller, M. L., Cohen, M., Sofka, M., & Borkovec, T. D. (1990). Worry changes decision making: The effect of negative thoughts on cognitive processing. *Journal of Clinical Psychology, 46*, 78–88.

Milner, A., Beech, R., & Walker, V. (1971). Decision processes and obsessional behavior. *British Journal of Social Clinical Psychology, 10*, 88–89.

Mogg, K., & Bradley, B. P. (1999). Selective attention and anxiety: A cognitive–motivational perspective. In T. Dalgleish & M. Power (eds), *Handbook of cognition and emotion* (pp. 145–170). Chichester, England: Wiley.

Mogg, K., Bradley, B. P., & Hallowell, N, (1994). Attentional bias to threat: Roles of trait anxiety, stressful events, and awareness. *Quarterly Journal of Experimental Psychology, 47A*, 841–864.

Obsessive Compulsive Cognitions Working Group (1997). Cognitive assessment of obsessive-compulsive disorder. *Behaviour Research and Therapy, 35*, 667–681.

Obsessive Compulsive Cognitions Working Group (2001). Development and initial validation of the Obsessive Beliefs Questionnaire and the Interpretation of Intrusions Inventory. *Behaviour Research and Therapy, 39*, 987–1006.

van Oppen, P., & Arntz, A. (1994). Cognitive therapy for obsessive-compulsive disorder. *Behaviour Research and Therapy, 32*, 79–87.

Persons, J. B., & Foa, E. B. (1984). Processing of fearful and neutral information by obsessive-compulsives, *Behaviour Research and Therapy, 22*, 259–265.

Peterson, R. A., & Reiss, S. (1992). *Anxiety Sensitivity Index Manual* (2nd ed.). Worthington Hills, OH: International Diagnosis Services.

Rachman, S. (1980). Emotional processing. *Behaviour Research and Therapy, 18*, 51–60.

Rachman, S. (1993). Obsessions, responsibility, and guilt. *Behaviour Research and Therapy, 31*, 149–154.

Rachman, S. (1997). A cognitive theory of obsessions. *Behaviour Research and Therapy, 35*, 793–802.

Rachman, S. (1998). A cognitive theory of obsessions: Elaborations. *Behaviour Research and Therapy, 36*, 385–401.

Rachman, S., & Hodgson, R. J. (1980). *Obsessions and compulsions.* Englewood Cliffs, NJ: Prentice Hall.

Radomsky, A. S., & Rachman, S. (1999). Memory bias in obsessive–compulsive disorder (OCD). *Behaviour Research and Therapy, 37,* 605–618.

Rasmussen, S. A., & Eisen, J. L. (1989). Clinical features and phenomenology of obsessive compulsive disorder. *Psychiatric Annals, 19,* 67–73.

Rapee, R. M. (1991). Generalized anxiety disorder: A review of clinical features and theoretical concepts. *Clinical Psychology Review, 11,* 419–440.

Reed, G. F. (1985). *Obsessional experience and compulsive behavior: A cognitive-structural approach.* Orlando, FL: Academic Press.

Reiss, S. (1991). Expectancy model of fear, anxiety, and panic. *Clinical Psychology Review, 11,* 141–153.

Reiss, S., & Havercamp, S. H. (1996). The sensitivity theory of motivation: Implications for psychopathology. *Behaviour Research and Therapy, 34,* 621–632.

Reiss, S., Peterson, R. A., Gursky, D. M., & McNally, R. J. (1986). Anxiety sensitivity, anxiety frequency and the prediction of fearfulness. *Behaviour Research and Therapy, 24,* 1–8.

Rhéaume, J., Ladouceur, R., Freeston, M. H., & Letarte, H. (1994). Inflated responsibility in obsessive–compulsive disorder: Psychometric studies of a semiideographic measure. *Journal of Psychopathology and Behavioral Assessment, 16,* 265–276.

Richter, M. A., Summerfeldt, L. J., Russell, T. J., & Swinson, R. P. (1996). The Tridimensional Personality Questionnaire in obsessive–compulsive disorder. *Psychiatry Research, 65,* 185–188.

Riemann, B. C., & McNally, R. J. (1995). Cognitive processing of personally relevant information. *Cognition and Emotion, 9,* 325–340.

Riskind, J., Abreu, K., Strauss, M., & Holt, R. (1997). Looming vulnerability to spreading contamination in subclinical OCD. *Behaviour Research and Therapy, 35,* 405–414.

Salkovskis, P. M. (1985). Obsessional-compulsive problems: A cognitive–behavioural analysis. *Behaviour Research and Therapy, 23,* 571–583.

Salkovskis, P. M. (1989). Cognitive–behavioral factors and the persistence of intrusive thoughts in obsessional problems. *Behaviour Research and Therapy, 27,* 677–682.

Salkovskis, P. M. (1991). The importance of behaviour in the maintenance of anxiety and panic: A cognitive account. *Behavioural Psychotherapy, 19,* 6–19.

Salkovskis, P. M. (1996). *Frontiers of cognitive therapy.* New York: Guilford.

Salkovskis, P. M., & Campbell, P. (1994). Thought suppression induces intrusion in naturally occurring negative intrusive thoughts. *Behaviour Research and Therapy, 32,* 1–8.

Salkovskis, P. M., & Harrison, J. (1984). Abnormal and normal obsessions: A replication. *Behavior Research and Therapy, 22,* 549–552.

Salkovskis, P. M., & Kirk, J. (1999). Obsessive–compulsive disorder. In D. M. Clark & C. G. Fairburn (eds), *Science and practice of cognitive behaviour therapy* (pp. 179–208). New York: Oxford University Press.

Savage, C. R. (1998). Neuropsychology of obsessive–compulsive disorder: research findings and treatment implications. In M. A. Jenike, L. Baer, & W. E. Minichiello (eds), *Obsessive–compulsive disorders: Practical management* (pp. 254–275). St. Louis, MO: Mosby.

Sheffler-Rubenstein, C. S., Peynircioglu, Z. F., Chambless, D. L., & Pigott, T. A. (1993). Memory in sub-clinical checkers. *Behaviour Research and Therapy, 31,* 759–765.

Sher, K. J., Frost, R. O., Kushner, M., Crews, T., & Alexander, J. (1989). Memory deficits in compulsive checkers: Replication and extension in a clinical sample. *Behaviour Research and Therapy, 27,* 65–69.

Sher, K. J., Frost, R. O., & Otto, R. (1983). Cognitive deficits in compulsive checkers: An exploratory study. *Behaviour Research and Therapy, 4,* 357–364.

Simos, G., Vaiopoulos, C., Giouzepas, I., & Parasehos, A. (1995, July). *Worry and obsessionality: Do they predict non significant personal concerns?* Paper presented at the World Congress of Behavioural and Cognitive Therapies, Copenhagen, Denmark.

Sookman, D., & Pinard, G. (1995, July). *The Cognitive Schemata Scale: Reliability and validity.* Paper presented at the World Congress of Behavioural and Cognitive Therapies, Copenhagen, Denmark.

Sookman, D., & Pinard, G. (1997, September). *Vulnerability and response to unpredictability, newness, and change in obsessive compulsive disorder: Measurement and implications for treatment.* Paper presented at the Congress of European Association for Behavioral and Cognitive Therapies, Venice, Italy.

Sookman, D., & Pinard, G. (1999). Integrative cognitive therapy for obsessive compulsive disorder: A focus on multiple schemas. *Cognitive and Behavioral Practice, 6,* 351–361.

Sookman, D., & Pinard, G. (2000, March). *Assessing change in core beliefs in the treatment of resistant obsessive compulsive disorder.* Paper presented at the annual meeting of the Anxiety Disorders Association of America, Washington, DC.

Sookman, D., Pinard, G., & Beauchemin, N. (1990, September). *Multidimensional conceptualization and treatment of obsessions.* Presented at the European Congress on Behavioral Therapy, Paris, France.

Sookman, D., Pinard, G., & Beauchemin, N. (1994). Multidimensional schematic restructuring treatment for obsessions. Theory and practice. *Journal of Cognitive Psychotherapy, 8,* 175–194.

Sookman, D., Pinard, G., & Beck, A. T. (2001). Vulnerability schemas in obsessive compulsive disorder. *Journal of Cognitive Psychotherapy, 15(2),* 109–130.

Steiner, J. (1972). A questionnaire study of risk-taking in psychiatric patients. *British Journal of Medical Psychology, 45,* 365–374.

Steketee, G., & Frost R. O. (1994). Measurement of risk-taking in obsessive–compulsive disorder. *Behavioural and Cognitive Psychotherapy, 22,* 269–298.

Steketee, G., Frost, R. O., & Cohen, I. (1998). Beliefs in obsessive–compulsive disorder. *Journal of Anxiety Disorders, 12,* 525–537.

Steketee, G., Frost, R. O., Rhéaume, J., & Wilhelm, S. (1998). Cognitive theory and treatment of obsessive–compulsive disorder. In M. A. Jenike, L. Baer, & W. E. Minichiello (eds), *Obsessive–compulsive disorders: Practical management* (pp.369–399). St. Louis, MO: Mosby.

Stroop, J. R. (1935). Studies of interference in serial verbal reactions. *Journal of Experimental Psychology, 18,* 643–661.

Summerfeldt, L. J., & Endler, N. S. (1998). Examining the evidence for anxiety-related cognitive biases in obsessive–compulsive disorder. *Journal of Anxiety Disorders, 12,* 579–598.

Tallis, F., Eysenck, M. W., & Mathews, A. (1991). Elevated evidence requirements and worry. *Personality and Individual Differences, 12,* 21–27.

Tata, P. R., Leibowitz, J. A., Prunty, M. J., Cameron, M., & Pickering, A. D. (1996). Attentional bias in obsessional compulsive disorder. *Behaviour Research and Therapy, 34,* 53–60.

Taylor, S. (1999). *Anxiety sensitivity. Theory, research, and treatment of the fear of anxiety.* London: Erlbaum.

Taylor, S., & Rachman, S. J. (1992). Fear and avoidance of aversive affective states: Dimensions and causal relations. *Journal of anxiety disorders, 6,* 15–25.

Taylor, S., & Rachman, S. (1994). Stimulus estimation and the overprediction of fear. *British Journal of Clinical Psychology, 33,* 173–181.

Telch, M. J., Brouillard, M., Telch, C. F., Agras, W. S., & Taylor, C. B. (1989). Role of cognitive appraisal in panic related avoidance. *Behaviour Research and Therapy, 27,* 373–383.

Trinder, H., & Salkovskis, P. M. (1994). Personally relevant intrusions outside the laboratory: long term suppression increases intrusion. *Behaviour Research and Therapy, 32,* 833–842.

Volans, P. J. (1976). Styles of decision making and probability appraisal in selected obsessional and phobic patients. *British Journal of Social Clinical Psychology, 15*, 305–317.

Warren, R., & Zgourides, G. D. (1991). *Anxiety disorders: A rational–emotive perspective.* New York: Pergamon Press.

Wells, A. (1994). Attention and control of worry. In G. C. L. Davey & F. Tallis (eds), *Worrying: Perspectives on theory, assessment and treatment* (pp. 91–114). Chichester, England: Wiley.

Wells, A. (1995). Meta-cognition and worry: A cognitive model of generalized anxiety disorder. *Behavioural and Cognitive Psychotherapy, 23*, 301–320.

Wells, A., & Butler, G. (1999). Generalized anxiety disorder. In D. M. Clark & C. G. Fairburn (eds), *Science and practice of cognitive behaviour therapy* (pp. 155–178). New York: Oxford University Press.

Wells, A., & Matthews, G. (1994). *Attention and emotion: A clinical perspective.* Hove, England: Erlbaum.

Wilhelm, S., McNally, R. J., Baer, L., & Florin, I. (1996). Directed forgetting in obsessive–compulsive disorder. *Behaviour Research and Therapy, 34*, 633–641.

Williams, K. E., Chambless, D. L., & Ahrens, A. (1997). Are emotions frightening? An extension of the fear of fear construct. *Behaviour Research and Therapy, 35*, 239–248.

Williams, J. M. G., Watts, F. N., MacLeod, C., & Mathews, A. (1997). *Cognitive psychology and emotional disorders* (2nd ed.). Chichester, England: Wiley.

Wittchen, H. A., & Essau, C. A. (1991). The epidemiology of panic attacks, panic disorder and agoraphobia. In J. R. Walker, G. R. Norton, & C. A. Ross. *Panic Disorder and Agoraphobia* (pp. 103–149). Pacific Grove, CA: Brooks/Cole.

Woods, C. M., Frost, R. O., Rubeck, J., & Steketee, G. (1997, November). *The faulty appraisal of event specific and general threat in obsessive compulsive disorder (OCD).* Paper presented at the annual meeting of the Association for Advancement of Behavior Therapy, Miami, FL.

Woods, C. M., Frost, R. O., & Steketee, G. (1998, November). *Cognitive phenomena underlying threat over-estimation in obsessive–compulsive disorder.* Paper presented at the annual meeting of the Association for Advancement of Behavior Therapy, Washington, DC.

Woods, C. M., Frost, R. O., & Steketee, G. (2000). Subjective severity, probability, and coping ability estimations of future negative events. Submitted for publication.

Chapter 6

Perfectionism in Obsessive Compulsive Disorder

Randy O. Frost, Caterina Novara and Josée Rhéaume

Introduction

Theorists have linked perfectionism with obsessive compulsive disorder (OCD) for nearly a century. The association has been suggested by authors from diverse theoretical perspectives including psychoanalytic and cognitive behavioral models of human behavior. Only in the last 10 years, however, have refinements in the conceptualization and measurement of perfectionism allowed for empirical testing of this association. In this chapter we review the theoretical perspectives on this relationship, recent developments in the conceptualization and measurement of perfectionism, and the existing research on the association of perfectionism and OCD. In addition, we review the limited research on the relationship between perfectionism and other OCD beliefs.

Theoretical Background

In the early 1900s, Janet (1903; as cited in Pitman, 1987) suggested that a form of perfectionism initiates the development of OCD. He proposed that early precursors of OCD involved a sense of never having performed actions in exactly the right way. This sense of imperfection subsequently leads to a need for perfection in perceptions and behavior to overcome feelings of uncertainty. Over time, these early stages give way to full-blown obsessions and compulsions. Other early theorists also emphasized perfectionism as central to the development of OCD. Jones (1918) suggested that OCD was a "pathological intolerant insistence on the absolute necessity of doing things in exactly the 'right' way." (p. 417). Similarly, Straus (1948) suggested that obsessionals avoid uncertainty by striving to make their behavior perfect. Recent analytic theorists have emphasized the importance of perfectionism as a means of attaining control over their environment by people with OCD (Mallinger, 1984; Mallinger & DeWyze, 1992; Salzman, 1979). By being perfect or having perfect control over one's behavior, the obsessional eliminates the risk of harm. Events that cannot be perfectly controlled lead to anxiety and superstitious behavior.

Cognitive theorists have also emphasized the importance of perfectionism in

Cognitive Approaches to Obsessions and Compulsions – Theory, Assessment, and Treatment
Copyright © 2002 by Elsevier Science Ltd.
ISBN: 0-08-043410-X

understanding OCD. Guidano and Liotti (1983) proposed that OCD results from a combination of perfectionism, a need for certainty, and a belief in the existence of perfect solutions. McFall and Wallersheim (1979) hypothesized several assumptions or beliefs that lead to the appraisal of threat and are at the core of OCD. These include the belief that "one should be perfectly competent, adequate, and achieving in all possible respects" (p. 335), and that "making mistakes or failing to live up to one's perfectionistic ideals should result in punishment or condemnation" (p. 335). They argue that people with OCD believe they must be perfect to feel good about themselves and to avoid criticism, similar to Mallinger (1984), Mallinger and DeWyze (1992), and Salzman (1979), and that people with OCD assume that mistakes and failure are catastrophic. More recently, Freeston and colleagues have included perfectionism as one of five faulty beliefs characterizing OCD (Freeston & Ladouceur, 1997; Freeston, Rhéaume, & Ladouceur, 1996). Following from this work, the Obsessive Compulsive Cognitions Working Group (OCCWG) included perfectionism as one of the six major domains of obsessional beliefs (OCCWG, 1997).

Despite the differing origins of theorizing about the role of perfectionism in OCD, a predominant theme is that perfectionism represents an attempt to avoid something unpleasant (i.e., criticism, disaster, uncertainty, lack of control). Some theorists suggest that perfectionism develops in an attempt to avoid uncertainty or in an attempt to establish control, while others suggest that perfectionism produces uncertainty and the desire for control over ones' environment. In either case, the major feature is the avoidance of mistakes (negative perfectionism), rather than the achievement of goals.

Conceptualizations of Perfectionism

While the term perfectionism and related ideas have been mentioned frequently with respect to OCD, little work has been devoted to the construct of perfectionism until recently. In 1984, Pacht argued that perfectionism was a widespread and debilitating problem. Other theorists emphasized the importance of perfectionism in general psychopathology as well (Burns, 1980; Hollender, 1965). In one of the first attempts to describe the phenomena, Hamachek (1978) drew a distinction between "normal" and "neurotic" perfectionism. Normal perfectionism involves the setting of high standards, accompanied by a flexible self-evaluation that is sensitive to constraints on one's performance. Neurotic perfectionism also involves the setting of high standards, but these are accompanied by a rigid self-evaluation that allows little latitude for mistakes. Until recently, these conceptualizations suffered from a lack of any adequate definition or measures of perfectionism. Early in the 1990s, however, two elaborate multidimensional models of perfectionism were generated (Frost, Marten, Lahart, & Rosenblate, 1990; Hewitt & Flett, 1991). The Hewitt and Flett model used the locus or target of excessively high expectations to define three primary dimensions: self-oriented, socially prescribed, and other-oriented perfectionism. Self-oriented perfectionism involves the tendency to set excessively high standards and to worry about failure to meet those standards. Socially prescribed perfectionism reflects excessive concern with the expectations of other people. The third dimension, other-oriented perfectionism, involves the setting of excessively high standards for other people. The model of Frost *et al.* (1990) model distinguished the setting of high personal standards from maladaptive evaluation of performance. This model comprises six dimensions distinguished by aspects of the nature of perfectionistic thoughts and evaluations. The dimensions include personal standards, concern over mistakes, doubts about actions, parental expectations, parental criticism, and organization. Personal standards reflects the extent to which people set excessively high standards for themselves. Concern over mistakes involves the interpretation of mistakes as an indication of failure. Doubts about actions reflects the level of confidence people have about their ability to complete tasks. The concern over mistakes and doubts about actions dimensions were drawn heavily from the work of Hamachek (1978) who emphasized the experience of dissatisfaction with performance and from the work of Reed (1985), tying feelings of uncertainty regarding task completion to obsessional experiences. Parental expectations and parental criticism comprise the perception that parents set excessive high standards and are or were overly critical. Finally, organization reflects the tendency to place importance on order and organization.

Other investigators studying the factor structure of the Frost Multidimensional Perfectionism Scale (MPS) have suggested three (Purdon, Antony, & Swinson, 1999) or four (Stöber, 1998) factors in lieu of the six dimensions originally described. The factors in the Purdon *et al.* (1999) three-factor structure included fear of mistakes (concern over mistakes and doubts about actions), goal/achievement orientation (personal standards, organization), and perceived parental pressures (parental expectations and parental criticism). Stöber's (1998) four-factor model was similar in that concern over mistakes and doubts about actions formed one factor, parental expectations and criticisms formed a second factor, but personal standards and organization each formed separate factors.

Attempts to further examine the interrelationships among these dimensions have led to further clarification of the construct of perfectionism. Frost, Heimberg, Holt, Mattia, and Neubauer (1993) conducted a factor analysis of all nine subscales from the Hewitt and Flett (1991) and Frost *et al.* (1990) perfectionism measures and found two clear factors: positive achievement striving and maladaptive evaluation concern. The positive achievement striving dimensions included personal standards, organization, and self-oriented perfectionism, while the maladaptive evaluation concern factor consisted of concern over mistakes, doubts about actions, parental expectations, parental criticism, and socially prescribed perfectionism.

Slade and Owens (1998) have gone further to suggest a new model of perfectionism based on the distinction between these two factors which they refer to as positive and negative perfectionism (Terry-Short, Owens, Slade, & Dewey, 1995). Their model draws this distinction based on the function of the perfectionistic behavior. Specifically, positive perfectionism involves cognitions and behaviors designed to achieve goals to obtain positive reinforcement, while negative perfectionism involves cognitions and behaviors designed to achieve goals to avoid or escape failure (i.e., negative consequences). Positive perfectionism corresponds to the dimensions of personal standards and organization from the Frost *et al.* MPS and self-oriented perfectionism from the Hewitt and Flett MPS. Negative perfectionism includes dimensions of concern over mistakes, doubts about actions, parental expectations, parental criticism, and socially prescribed perfectionism. A growing literature generally supports this dual process model in that positive perfectionism dimensions have been found to correlate with success orientation (see Slade & Owens, 1998), while negative perfectionism is more closely associated with psychopathology (Frost *et al.*, 1993). The dimensions comprising negative perfectionism are those of most interest with respect to OCD.

Measurement of Perfectionism

Subscales in Measures of Dysfunctional Thinking

A variety of measures have been used to operationally define perfectionism in recent years. The earliest of these included perfectionism as one among a broad array of theoretical concepts. Over time, measures of perfectionism became more specific and more multi-dimensional. Perfectionism was first operationalized as a subscale in several measures of general beliefs related to psychopathology. In the Irrational Beliefs Test (Jones, 1968), the perfectionism subscale was heavily weighted on personal standard setting, while in the Eating Disorder Inventory (Garner, Olmsted, & Polivy *et al.*, 1983), and the Dysfunctional Attitude Scale (DAS; Weissman & Beck, 1978), the perfectionism subscales emphasized parental expectations, as well as personal standard setting. All of these instruments have been reported to possess adequate reliability and validity for assessing general dysfunctional cognitive patterns, but the perfectionism subscales were not clearly defined.

Independent Measures of Perfectionism

Burns (1980) modified a portion of the DAS to create the first independent measure of perfectionism. The Burns' Perfectionism Scale was heavily weighted toward personal standards setting and concerns over mistakes. It required subjects to rate ten statements on a five-point scale. Pyschometric properties were mixed. Hewitt and Dyck (1986) obtained a test–retest coefficient of 0.63 for college students over a two-months period. Additionally, Hewitt, Mittelstaedt, and Wollert (1989) found a standardized item-alpha coefficients of 0.70 and significant correlations of 0.70 and 0.65 with the convergent measures of the Attitudes Towards Self (High Standards) Scale and the Irrational Beliefs Test (High Self-Expectations), respectively. The Burns scale was unidimensional and mixed positive and negative perfectionism items.

By far the most widely used measures of perfectionism have been based on the multidimensional conceptualizations of perfectionism. Two different scales, with the same name, were created to measure the multidimensional aspects of perfectionism. Hewitt and Flett's (1991) Multidimensional Perfectionism Scale consists of 45 items subdivided into three subscales: Self-Oriented Perfectionism, Socially Prescribed Perfectionism and Other Oriented Perfectionism. Each subscale is scored by summing its 15 items. Coefficient alphas were 0.86 for Self-Oriented Perfectionism, 0.82 for Other-Oriented Perfectionism, and 0.87 for Socially-Prescribed Perfectionism. The MPS subscales showed acceptable test–retest reliability over a three-month interval with coefficients of 0.88 for Self-Oriented Perfectionism, 0.85 for Other-Oriented Perfectionism and 0.75 for Socially Prescribed Perfectionism.

The Frost *et al.* measure includes six subscales measured by 35 items of the

Multidimensional Perfectionism Scale. The coefficients of internal consistency for these subscales range between 0.77 and 0.93. The reliability of the total perfectionism scale is 0.90. The six scales are correlated with one another and have good concurrent validity.

More recently several additional measures of perfectionism have been developed. Rhéaume, Freeston, and Ladouceur (1995) developed the Perfectionism Questionnaire (PQ) based on the distinction between functional and dysfunctional perfectionism. The PQ contains 64 items divided into three subscales: perfectionistic tendencies, domains affected by perfectionism and negative consequences of perfectionism. The coefficients of internal consistency range between 0.82 and 0.96, and the scale has good convergent validity. Terry-Short *et al.* (1995) developed a 40-item measure of perfectionism called the Positive and Negative Perfectionism Scale (PANPS), which was designed to measure these two aspects of perfectionism. The PANPS is a revision of the authors' attempts to measure perfectionism in eating disorder populations (Mitzman, Slade, & Dewey, 1994; Waller, Wood, Miller, & Slade, 1992). This measure has shown promise in samples of eating disorder patients, but no information is yet available on its relationship to OCD symptoms.

Measures of Perfectionistic Cognitions

The measures reviewed thus far have focused on perfectionism as a global trait and not on ongoing cognitive activity reflecting perfectionistic thought. Flett, Hewitt, Blankstein, and Gray (1998) developed the Perfectionistic Cognitions Inventory as a measure of the frequency of perfectionistic rumination. Respondents are asked to indicate the frequency of occurrence of each of 25 perfectionistic thoughts during the past week. The scale has good internal and test–retest reliability, and mounting evidence for its validity has been reported (Ferrari, 1995; Flett *et al.*, 1998).

Finally, in 1997 the OCCWG published the first description of an attempt to develop a measure of perfectionism relevant to OCD via expert consensus (OCCWG, 1997). In this context, "perfectionism was defined as the tendency to believe there is a perfect solution to every problem, that doing something perfectly (i.e. mistake free) is not only possible, but also necessary, and that even minor mistakes will have serious consequences." (OCCWG, 1997, p. 678). This definition emphasized the role of a belief in perfect solutions and excessive concern over mistakes. Doubts about actions, a central component in the maladaptive evaluative concern dimension of perfectionism, was de-emphasized since it was believed to be more closely related to a different OCD belief (tolerance for uncertainty). Doubting the quality of one's actions is likely to be a strong characteristic of people with concerns about being certain. Subsequent study revealed that the 16-item perfectionism subscale of the OBQ-87 has adequate reliability across a number of different samples (OCCWG, 2001).

The many and varied measures of perfectionism hamper our ability to draw conclusions about the relationship between perfectionism and OCD. Nevertheless, a number of studies have indicated significant overlap among the measures, especially those reflecting maladaptive evaluative concern, negative perfectionism or dysfunctional perfectionism.

Research on Perfectionism and Obsessive Compulsive Phenomena

Until recently, most of the literature examining the link between perfectionism and OCD consisted of clinical observations. In these studies, perfectionism was only loosely defined if at all. Nonetheless, these reports demonstrate a consistent pattern of evidence. A number of individual case reports and case series have indicated that OCD patients see imperfections everywhere and attempt to cope by engaging in compulsive behavior (Adams, 1973; Anonymous & Tiller, 1989; Rasmussen & Tsuang, 1986).

Perfectionism in OCD Families

Other clinical studies have reported elevated levels of perfectionism in the families of OCD patients. Allsopp and Verduyn (1990) reported that perfectionism and precision were the most frequently noted characteristics of the parents of 44 adolescent OCD patients. Lo (1967) also noted a higher frequency of perfectionism among parents of OCD patients compared to parents of schizophrenics. Hoover and Insel (1984) concluded that perfectionism characterized a large number of the family members of OCD patients in their study. Others have made similar observations (Clark & Bolton, 1985; Rasmussen & Eisen, 1989).

Lo (1967) theorized that perfectionism in parents leads to perfectionism in offspring and subsequently OCD symptoms. He suggests that the child feels pressure to meet the perfectionistic demands of the parents. Seeking security and acceptance from the parents, the child will strive to meet these demands. In time the child internalizes these standards and becomes perfectionistic. The perfectionistic demands intensify and when they can no longer be met, the child becomes anxious. Compulsive behavior develops in an attempt to control the mistakes and criticism perceived when the perfectionistic demands are not met. Such theorizing is similar to Janet's early speculation regarding OCD, but evidence regarding this model has been inconsistent. While parents (fathers) of subclinical compulsives have been reported to be more perfectionistic (Frost, Steketee, Cohn, & Greiss, 1994), and perfectionism in parents (especially mothers) is correlated with perfectionism in daughters (Frost, Lahart, & Rosenblate, 1991), Frost and Steketee (1997) failed to find higher levels of parental criticism or parental expectations among OCD patients compared to controls or panic disorder patients.

Perfectionism and OCD in Nonclinical Samples

A number of empirical studies have demonstrated a link between perfectionism and OCD symptoms/traits among nonclinical samples. Frost *et al.* (1990) found Concern Over Mistakes and Doubts about Actions to be positively correlated with the Maudsley Obsessive Compulsive Inventory and a measure of everyday checking behavior. Likewise, Rhéaume, Freeston, Dugas, Letarte, and Ladouceur (1995) found Concern Over Mistakes and Doubts About Actions to be positively correlated with the Padua Inventory among college students. Frost *et al.* (1994) found subclinical compulsives to score higher on Concern Over Mistakes,

Doubts About Actions and Personal Standards than controls in both student and community samples. Ferrari (1995) found significant positive correlations between the Perfectionistic Cognitions Inventory and the Lynfield Obsessive Compulsive Questionnaire as well as the Compulsive Activity Checklist among college students.

Rhéaume *et al.* (2000) examined a large number of students using the PQ and selected functional and dysfunctional perfectionists for a laboratory study. Functional perfectionists were those who "reported perfectionistic tendencies but few negative consequences" (p. 121), while dysfunctional perfectionists were those who "reported strong perfectionistic tendencies and a high level of negative consequences associated with these tendencies" (p. 121), similar to the distinction drawn earlier between positive achievement striving (positive perfectionism) and maladaptive evaluative concern (negative perfectionism). Dysfunctional perfectionists scored higher on the Padua Inventory and took more time to complete a precision task than functional perfectionists. However, contrary to expectations, functional perfectionists needed more certainty before making a decision than dysfunctional perfectionists in a probabalistic inference task.

Kawamura, Hunt, Frost, and DiBartolo (2001) administered the Frost Multidimensional Perfectionism Scale and measures of social anxiety, worry, OCD, trait anxiety, posttraumatic stress disorder, anxiety sensitivity, and depression in an attempt to determine which features of anxiety were related to maladaptive and adaptive perfectionism, independent of depression. A factor analysis of the anxiety measures resulted in three anxiety disorder factors: OCD, social/trait anxiety/worry, and PTSD. All three factors were significantly and positively correlated with maladaptive evaluative concern. However, only the social/trait anxiety/worry factor was related to maladaptive perfectionism independent of depression. This study raises important questions about the role of mood in mediating the relationship between perfectionism and OCD.

In a similar attempt, Wade, Kyrios, and Jackson (1998) tested a vulnerability model of obsessive compulsive symptoms among a nonclinical sample. Perfectionism, as well as guilt and trait anxiety, was hypothesized to be a vulnerability factor related to obsessive compulsive symptoms and mediated by negative mood. Structural equation modeling revealed that perfectionism (as measured by a composite of self-oriented and other-oriented perfectionism from the Hewitt & Flett measure) predicted checking and cleaning symptoms, but not obsessional activity, independent of negative mood. The socially prescribed dimension contributed to a neurotic factor whose relationship to compulsive behavior and obsessional activity was mediated by negative mood.

Perfectionism and Specific Obsessive Compulsive Symptoms

In addition to these studies, a number of reports link perfectionism with specific obsessive compulsive symptoms (i.e. washing, checking, hoarding, and "not-just-right" experiences). Gershuny and Sher (1995) found higher perfectionism (Frost MPS) scores among a group of subclinical compulsive checkers compared to noncheckers, and hypothesized that perfectionism leads some people to try to exert control over events through checking rituals (similar to early theorizing about control). Likewise, Ferrari (1995) found significant positive correlations between the Perfectionistic Cognitions Inventory and compulsive checking from the Compulsive Activity Checklist, but not with compulsive washing. Tallis (1996), however, has suggested that there may be a specific form of washing compulsion that is closely tied to perfectionism. Specifically, Tallis reported that some patients use washing rituals not to remove contamination, but to achieve a perfect state of cleanliness.

Jones and Menzies (1997) examined the role of various cognitive mediators in response to a contamination behavioral avoidance test (BAT) among OCD washers. They found no association between a global measure of perfectionism (total score from the Frost MPS) and four measures of OCD severity in response to the BAT. Unfortunately, they did not report correlations with the maladaptive dimensions (especially concern over mistakes and doubts about actions). Combining maladaptive and adaptive dimensions of perfectionism may have obscured potential relationships.

Frost and Gross (1993) found predicted dimensions of perfectionism (concern over mistakes, doubts about actions, and socially prescribed perfectionism) to be correlated with hoarding symptoms among college students. In a community sample, concern over mistakes, doubts about actions, and parental criticism from the Frost MPS and socially prescribed perfectionism and other-oriented perfectionism from the Hewitt and Flett MPS were correlated with hoarding symptoms. Further, compared to a nonclinicial community control, people reporting a problem with hoarding behavior scored higher on five perfectionism dimensions from the Frost MPS (concern over mistakes, doubts about actions, personal standards, parental expectations, and parental criticism) and two dimensions from the Hewitt and Flett MPS (self-oriented and socially prescribed perfectionism).

Concern over mistakes and doubts about actions have also been associated with compulsive indecisiveness (Frost & Shows, 1993; Gayton, Clavin, Clavin, & Broida, 1994), although Ferrari (1995) failed to find a significant correlation between decisional procrastination (i.e., indecisiveness) and perfectionistic cognitions among college students. Finally, Coles, Rhéaume, Frost, and Heimberg (2000) found positive correlations between various dimensions of perfectionism and "not-just-right" experiences among college students. They suggest that "not-just-right" experiences (NJREs) are a form of "sensory" perfectionism that may be associated with certain kinds of OCD symptoms like symmetry and exactness. Coles *et al.* (2000) report that NJREs were highly correlated with OCD symptoms and only moderately or slightly correlated with other anxiety disorder symptoms.

Perfectionism and OCD in Clinical Samples

A small but growing number of studies have shown associations between perfectionism and OCD in clinical populations. Among 123 psychiatric outpatients, Norman, Davies, Nicholson, Cortese, and Malla (1998) found the maladaptive evaluative concern composite measure from the Frost MPS to be significantly and positively correlated with the Maudsley Obsessive Compulsive Inventory and the Padua Inventory, whereas the positive achievement striving composite revealed few significant correlations. Most of the correlations with the maladaptive evaluative concern were substantial in magnitude (up to 0.61). Interestingly, the correlations with cleaning/washing and slowness subscales tended to be smaller than those with checking, rumination, doubting, impulses and precision.

Ferrari (1995) reported a significant relationship between the Perfectionistic Cognitions Inventory (PCI) and the obsessions and compulsions subscales of the Lynfield Obsessive/ Compulsive Questionnaire, as well as a significant correlation between the PCI and indecisiveness. It was not clear, however, whether the subjects in this study had OCD or obsessive compulsive personality disorder.

Frost and Steketee (1997) compared 34 patients diagnosed with OCD, 14 diagnosed with panic disorder with agoraphobia, and 35 community controls on the Frost *et al.* (1990) MPS. Both OCD and panic disorder patients scored higher on concern over mistakes and doubts about actions than community controls. However, panic patients did not differ from the OCD patients on concern over mistakes. However, OCD patients had higher doubts about actions scores than panic disorder patients.

Antony, Purdon, Huta, and Swinson (1998) examined perfectionism as measured by the Frost MPS and the Hewitt and Flett MPS across four groups of anxiety disorder patients (OCD, panic, social phobia, specific phobia) and a nonclinical control. While OCD patients had higher scores on Concern Over Mistakes and Doubts About Actions than the nonclinical controls, comparison of the OCD group with the other patient groups revealed only more doubts about actions than the panic and specific phobia patients, and less concern over mistakes than social phobia patients. On the Hewitt and Flett MPS, the OCD patients scored higher than the nonclinical controls on socially prescribed perfectionism, but there were no differences among the patient groups on any of the other dimensions.

Mavissakalian, Hamann, Haider, and de Groot (1993) reported that OCD patients scored significantly higher than panic disorder and generalized anxiety disorder patients on the perfectionism items from the Personality Disorders Questionnaire.

As part of the development and validation of the Obsessive Beliefs Questionnaire, the OCCWG recruited volunteers at ten sites to complete the OBQ, measures of anxiety, depression and obsessive compulsive symptoms (OCCWG, 2001). Five groups of subjects were tested: 101 patients with a diagnosis of OCD, 374 English speaking college student controls, 76 English speaking community (non-clinical) controls, 12 anxious controls, and 35 Greek speaking community (non-clinical) controls. Data from these subjects were used to reduce the OBQ Perfectionism subscale to 16 items. The internal and test–retest reliabilities were good across all samples (alphas = 0.87 to 0.93; test–retest = 0.85). Comparisons among the groups indicated that OCD patients had significantly higher perfectionism scores than student, community and Greek nonclinical control groups, but did not differ significantly from the anxious controls, though the differences in means were in the predicted direction. Correlational analyses indicated that perfectionism correlated moderately to strongly with Beck Anxiety Inventory, Beck Depression Inventory, and Padua Inventory subscales ($r = 0.39$–0.63). Among a subset of subjects who completed the YBOCS ($n = 63$), perfectionism was significantly and positively correlated with YBOCS scores ($r = 0.32$ to 0.40). When partial correlations controlling for BAI and BDI were conducted, perfectionism remained significantly correlated with all PI subscales, though the magnitudes declined substantially. The smallest partial correlation with perfectionism occurred for the contamination subscale of the PI ($r = 0.19$). The strongest partial correlation was with the mental control subscale ($r = 0.42$). Partial correlations with the BAI and BDI controlling for Padua Inventory scores dropped substantially (prs = 0.06 and 0.20 respectively). Similar findings were apparent in a recent validation study of the OBQ (OCCWG, in preparation). Internal reliabilities of the Perfectionism subscale were high, though the test–retest reliabilities were somewhat lower than in the earlier study (OCCWG, 2001). Both OCD and anxiety disorder control groups had higher Perfectionism scores than community and student controls. Perfectionism was correlated with measures of anxiety, depression, and worry at levels that approached, and sometimes exceeded, those with OCD symptom measures.

Despite general support for the association of perfectionism and OCD, there is no convincing evidence that any identified dimension of perfectionism is more closely tied to OCD than to other disorders. Doubts about Actions has shown the strongest and most consistent association with OCD symptoms, but it may overlap with other domains identified by the OCCWG. Sensory perfectionism (or NJREs) may turn out to be more specifically associated with OCD, that is, it may constitute a sort of OCD perfectionism. In particular, ordering and arranging compulsions as well as symmetry obsessions, can be conceptualized as forms of sensory perfectionism in which the belief is that one's experience is not quite right and must be somehow "perfected." However, almost nothing has been written about this construct and more research is needed to draw firm conclusions.

Perfectionism and OCPD

Perfectionism is one of eight characteristics comprising the obsessive compulsive personality disorder (OCPD) diagnosis in DSM-IV (American Psychiatric Association [APA], 1994). Early theorists assumed that OCPD was a precursor to OCD, but recent empirical research has failed to support such an association (see Baer & Jenike, 1998 for a review). Empirical work linking recent measures of perfectionism to OCPD has been limited. While perfectionism correlates with certain OCPD characteristics like hoarding (Frost & Gross, 1993), contemporary measures of perfectionism do not appear to be any more closely related to OCPD than to other personality disorders in the anxious/avoidant cluster (Hewitt, Flett, & Turnbull, 1992). Furthermore, socially prescribed perfectionism appears to be most closely related to traits of paranoid and schizotypal personality disorder than to OCPD (Hewitt *et al.*, 1992).

Overlap With Other Domains

Perfectionism is one of six belief domains identified by expert consensus as relevant to OCD (OCCWG, 1997). The other belief domains (tolerance for uncertainty, importance of thoughts, responsibility, control over thoughts, and probability overestimation) are reviewed elsewhere in this volume. While each domain was conceptualized as distinct, there is significant overlap among them. For instance, doubts about actions have been conceptualized as a component of perfectionism (Frost *et al.*, 1990) and is closely related to the domain of tolerance for uncertainty. Several studies have examined the overlap of perfectionism with these other domains. Rhéaume *et al.* (1995) administered the Frost MPS (Frost *et al.*, 1990), the Responsibility Scale (RS; Salkovskis, 1992), the Responsibility Questionnaire (RQ; Rhéaume, Ladouceur, Freeston, & Letarte, 1995) and the Padua Inventory (PI; Sanavio

1988) to a student population. Concern over mistakes, doubts about actions and personal standards were significantly correlated with both responsibility measures, while parental expectations and parental criticism were significantly correlated only with Salkovskis' RS. The magnitude of the correlations of concern over mistakes and doubts about actions with Salkovskis' RS (r's = 0.53 and 0.50, respectively) suggest considerable overlap. Hierarchical regression indicated that responsibility accounted for more of the variance in PI scores and was a better predictor of OC symptoms than perfectionism. However, perfectionism still accounted for significant variance in PI scores after the contribution of responsibility was removed. Similarly, Rhéaume *et al.* (2000) found that dysfunctional perfectionists scored higher on Salkovskis' RS than functional perfectionists.

In an attempt to better understand the links between perfectionism and responsibility, Bouchard, Rhéaume, and Ladouceur (1999) selected nonclinical subjects either high in perfectionism (above the 90th percentile on the PQ) or low in perfectionism (below the 40th percentile). Subjects were further divided into high and low responsibility conditions based on an experimental manipulation. In the high responsibility condition the subjects were told that they were part of a pharmaceutical company project. The aim of the project was to develop a system of colors that would make the distribution of the medications in a very poor region safer. The subjects were also told that they had great responsibility because each result could influence the color of the medication. In the low responsibility condition the subjects were told that they were in a practice trial and that each result had no importance. Aspects of performance measured included hesitations, checking, modifications, number of errors and time taken to complete the task. Subjective variables were doubts, preoccupations, need to check, desire additional time, and anxiety. Results did not show any intergroup effect both in behavioral and subjective dependent variables: high perfectionistic subjects did not differ from low perfectionistic subjects. However, after completing the task high perfectionistic subjects reported more influence and responsibility for negative consequences than low perfectionistic subjects. This result suggests that perfectionism may predispose individuals to feel responsible and that, according to the authors, perfectionism in OCD could be conceptualized as a factor that leads to the perception of responsibility.

Finally, based on a large number of subjects, findings from the recent OCCWG study validating the OBQ-87 (OCCWG, 2001) revealed strong correlations between perfectionism and each of the other five belief domains. Magnitudes of these correlations ranged from 0.59 (Importance of Thoughts) to 0.79 (Tolerance for Uncertainty). The high correlation with Tolerance for Uncertainty is understandable in that perfectionism has been conceptualized as containing doubts about the quality of one's actions (Frost *et al.*, 1990). Correlations among the subscales of the subsequent investigation (OCCWG, in preparation) again revealed substantial overlap with the tolerance for uncertainty domain.

Summary

Despite differences in the measurement of perfectionism, it is clear from the research to date that perfectionism is related to obsessive compulsive symptoms and obsessive compulsive disorder. However, as suggested previously (OCCWG, 1997), high levels of perfectionism may not be unique to obsessive–compulsive disorder. The literature suggests high levels of negative perfectionism in most of the anxiety disorders, depression (Blatt, 1995), eating disorders (Bastiani, Rao, Weltzin, & Kaye, 1995), as well as other forms of psychopathology (Pacht, 1984). Its contribution to understanding OCD may be as a general vulnerability factor (Wade *et al.*, 1998) rather than a cognitive orientation that is specific to OCD, though to date there is little data on this possibility. Further, the contribution of perfectionism to OCD symptoms may operate through its influence on mood (Kawamura *et al.*, 2001; Wade *et al.*, 1998) and on responsibility (Bouchard *et al.*, 1999). Further research on the role of perfectionism in OCD and other forms of psychopathology will help to elucidate these issues.

Thus far, the usefulness of research linking perfectionism and OCD has been limited. As of yet, no studies have examined how differing levels of perfectionism (or its dimensions) influence treatment, nor whether addressing perfectionism directly in therapy would be beneficial. Such evidence has been collected with respect to other disorders such as eating disorders (Bastaini *et al.*, 1995) and depression (Blatt, 1995) and suggests that specifically addressing perfectionistic thinking may be an important component of treatment. It would not be surprising to find that higher levels of perfectionism may interfere with OCD patients' ability to endure exposure and carefully examine evidence regarding their beliefs about intrusive thoughts. Treatments specifically designed to modify perfectionistic thinking may be a useful adjunct to OCD treatment (Freeston *et al.*, 1996).

References

Adams, P. (1973). *Obsessive children.* New York: Brunner/Mazel.

Allsop, M., & Verduyn, C. (1990). Adolescents with obsessive–compulsive disorder: A case note review of consecutive patients referred to a provincial regional adolescent unit. *Journal of Adolescence, 13*, 157–169.

American Psychiatric Association. (1994). *Diagnostic and statistical manual of mental disorders* (4th ed.). Washington, DC: Author.

Anonymous & Tiller, J. (1989). Obsessive compulsive disorder: A sufferer's viewpoint. *Australia and New Zealand Journal of Psychiatry, 23*, 279–281.

Antony, M. M., Purdon, C. L., Huta, V., & Swinson, R. P. (1998). Dimensions of perfectionism across the anxiety disorders. *Behaviour Research and Therapy, 36*, 1143–1154.

Baer, L., & Jenike, M. A. (1998). Personality disorders in obsessive–compulsive disorder. In M. A. Jenike, L. Baer, & W. E. Minichiello. *Obsessive–compulsive disorders: Practical management.* St. Louis: Mosby.

Bastaini, A. M., Rao, R., Weltzin, T., & Kaye, W. H. (1995). Perfectionism in anorexia nervosa. *International Journal of Eating Disorders, 17*, 147–152.

Blatt, S. J. (1995). The destructiveness of perfectionism: Implications for the treatment of depression. *American Psychologist, 50*, 1003–1020.

Bouchard, C., Rhéaume, J., & Ladouceur, R. (1999). Responsibility and perfectionism in OCD: An experimental study. *Behaviour Research and Therapy, 37*, 239–248

Burns, D. (1980). The perfectionist's script for self-defeat. *Psychology Today*, 34–52.

Clark, D. A., & Bolton, D. (1985). Obsessive–compulsive adolescents and their parents: A psychometric study. *Journal of Child Psychology and Psychiatry, 26*, 267–276.

Coles, M. E., Rhéaume, J., Frost, R. O., & Heimberg, R. G. (2000, November). Paper presented at the annual meeting of the Association for the Advancement of Behavior Therapy, New Orleans.

Ferrari, J. R. (1995). Perfectionistic cognitions with nonclinical and clinical samples. *Journal of Social Behavior and Personality, 10,* 143–156.

Flett, G., Hewitt, P., Blankstein, K. R., & Gray, L. (1998). Psychological distress and frequency of perfectionistic thinking. *Journal of Personality and Social Psychology, 75,* 1363–1381.

Freeston, M. H., & Ladouceur, R. (1997). *The cognitive behavioral treatment of obsessions: A treatment manual.* Quebec, Canada: University of Laval.

Freeston, M. H., Rhéaume, J., & Ladouceur, R. (1996). Correcting faulty appraisals of obsessional thoughts. *Behaviour Research and Therapy, 34,* 433–446.

Frost, R. O., & Gross, R. (1993). The hoarding of possessions. *Behaviour Research and Therapy, 31,* 367–381.

Frost, R. O., Heimberg, R., Holt, C., Mattia, J., & Neubauer, A. (1993). A comparison of two measures of perfectionism. *Personality and Individual Differences, 14,* 119–126.

Frost, R. O., Lahart, C. M., & Rosenblate, R. (1991). The development of perfectionism: A study of daughters and their parents. *Cognitive Therapy and Research, 15,* 469–489.

Frost, R., Marten, P., Lahart, C., & Rosenblate, R. (1990). The dimensions of perfectionism. *Cognitive Therapy and Research, 14,* 449–468

Frost, R., & Shows, D. (1993). The nature and measurement of compulsive indecisiveness. *Behaviour Research and Therapy, 35,* 291–296.

Frost, R. O., & Steketee, G. (1997). Perfectionism in obsessive–compulsive disorder patients. *Behaviour Research and Therapy, 35,* 291–296.

Frost, R. O., Steketee, G., Cohn, L., & Greiss, K. (1994). Personality traits in subclinical and non-obsessive–compulsive volunteers and their parents. *Behaviour Research and Therapy, 32,* 47–56.

Garner, D. M., Olmstead, M. P., & Polivy, J. (1983). Development and validation of a multidimensional eating disorder inventory for anorexia nervosa and bulimia. *International Journal of Eating Disorder, 2,* 15–34.

Gayton, W. F., Clavin, R. H., Clavin, S. L., & Broida, J. (1994). Further validation of the indecisiveness scale. *Psychological Reports, 75,* 1631–1634.

Gershuny. B., & Sher, K. (1995). Compulsive checking and anxiety in a nonclinical sample: differences in cognition, behavior, personality, and affect. *Journal of Psychopathology and Behavioral Assessment, 17,* 19–38.

Guidano, V., & Liotti, G. (1983). *Cognitive processes and emotional disorders.* New York: Guilford.

Hamacheck, D. E. (1978). Psychodynamics of normal and neurotic perfectionism. *Psychology, 15,* 27–33.

Hewitt, P. L., & Dyck, D. G. (1986). Perfectionism, stress, and vulnerability to depression. *Cognitive Therapy and Research, 10,* 137–142.

Hewitt, P. L., & Flett, G. L. (1991). Perfectionism in the self and social contexts: Conceptualization, assessment, and association with psychopathology. *Journal of Personality and Social Psychology, 60,* 456–470.

Hewitt, P. L., Flett, G. L., & Turnbull, W. (1992). Perfectionism and multiphasic personality inventory (MMPI) indices of personality disorder. *Journal of Psychopathology and Behavioral Assessment, 14,* 323–335.

Hewitt, P. L., Mittelstaedt, W., & Wollert, R. (1989). Validation of a measure of perfectionism. *Journal of Personality Assessment, 53,* 133–144.

Hollender, M. H. (1965). Perfectionism. *Comprehensive Psychiatry, 6,* 94–103.

Hoover, C. F., & Insel, T. R. (1984). Families of origin in obsessive–compulsive disorder. *The Journal of Nervous and Mental Disease. 172,* 207–215.

Jones, E. (1918). The anal-erotic character traits. In *Papers on psycho-analysis*. London: Baillere, Tindall and Cox.

Jones, M. K., & Menzies, R. G. (1997). The cognitive mediation of obsessive–compulsive handwashing. *Behaviour Research and Therapy, 35*, 843–850.

Jones, R. G. (1968). *A factored measure of Ellis's irrational beliefs systems with personality and maladjustment correlated*. Wichita, KS: Test Systems.

Kawamura, K. Y., Hunt, S., Frost, R. O., & DiBartolo, P. (2001). Perfectionism, anxiety, and depression: Are the relationships independent? *Cognitive Therapy and Research, 25*, 291–301.

Lo, W. H. (1967). A follow-up study of obsessional neurotics in Hong Kong Chinese. *British Journal of Psychiatry, 113*, 823–832.

Mallinger, A. E. (1984). The obsessive's myth of control. *Journal of the American Academy of Psychoanalysis, 12*, 147–165.

Mallinger, A. E., & DeWyze, J. (1992). *Too perfect: When being in control gets out of control*. New York: Clarkson Potter Pub.

Mavissakalian, M. R., Hamann, M. S., Haidar, S. A., & de Groot, C. M. (1993). DSM-III personality disorders in generalized anxiety, panic/agoraphobia, and obsessive–compulsive disorders. *Comprehensive Psychiatry, 34*, 243–248.

McFall, M., & Wallersheim, J. (1979). Obsessive compulsive neurosis: A cognitive-behavior formulation and approach to treatment. *Cognitive Therapy and Research, 3*, 333–348.

Mitzman, S. F., Slade, P., & Dewey, M. E. (1994). Preliminary development of a questionnaire designed to measure neurotic perfectionism in the eating disorders. *Journal of Clinical Psychology, 50*, 516–529.

Norman, R. M. G., Davies, F., Nicholson, L. C., & Malla, A. K. (1998). The relationship of perfectionism with symptoms in a psychiatric outpatient population. *Journal of Social and Clinical Psychology, 17*, 50–68.

Obsessive Compulsive Cognitions Working Group. (1997). Cognitive assessment of obsessive–compulsive disorder. *Behaviour Research and Therapy, 35*, 667–681.

Obsessive Compulsive Cognitions Working Group. (2001). Development and initial validation of the Obsessive Beliefs Questionnaire (OBQ) and the Interpretation of Intrusions Inventory (III). *Behaviour Research and Therapy, 39*, 987–1006.

Obsessive Compulsive Cognitions Working Group. (in preparation). *Psychometric validation of the Obsessive Beliefs Questionnaire and the Interpretation of Intrusions Inventory: Findings from stage three data*. Unpublished manuscript.

Pacht, A. (1984). Refelections on perfection. *American Psychologist, 39*, 386–390.

Pitman, R. (1987). Pierre Janet on obsessive–compulsive disorder (1903): Review and commentary. *Archives of General Psychiatry, 143*, 317–322.

Purdon, C. L., Antony, M. M., & Swinson, R. P. (1999). Psychometric properties of the Frost Multidimensional Perfectionism Scale in a clinical anxiety disorders sample. *Journal of Clinical Psychology, 55*, 1271–1286.

Rasmussen, S., & Eisen, J. L. (1989). Clinical features and phenomenology of obsessive compulsive disorder. *Psychiatric Annals, 19*, 67–73.

Rasmussen, S., & Tsung, M. (1986). Clinical characteristics and family history in DSM-III obsessive–compulsive disorder. *American Journal of Psychiatry, 143*, 317–322.

Reed, G. F. (1985). *Obsessional experience and compulsive behavior: A cognitive-structural approach*. New York: Academic Press.

Rhéaume, J., Freeston, M. H., Dugas, M. J., Letarte, H., & Ladouceur, R. (1995). Perfectionism, responsibility and obsessive–compulsive symptoms. *Behaviour Research and Therapy, 33*, 785–794

Rhéaume, J., Freeston, M. H., & Ladouceur, R. (1995, June). *Functional and dysfunctional perfectionism: construct validity and a new instrument.* Paper presented at the World Congress of Behavioural and Cognitive Therapy, Copenhagen, Denmark.

Rhéaume, J., Freeston, M. H., Ladouceur, R., Bouchard, C., Gallant, L., Talbot, F., & Vallières, A. (2000). Functional and dysfunctional perfectionists: Are they different on compulsive-like behaviors? *Behaviour Research and Therapy, 38,* 119–128.

Rhéaume, J., Ladouceur, R., Freeston, M. H., & Letarte, H. (1995). Inflated responsibility in obsessive–compulsive disorder. Validation of an operational definition. *Behaviour Research and Therapy, 33,* 159–169.

Salkovskis, P. M. (1992). *Cognitive models and therapy of obsessive compulsive disorder.* Communication presented at Word Congress of Cognitive Therapy, Toronto, Ontario, Canada

Salzman, L. (1979). Psychotherapy of the obsessional. *American Journal of Psychotherapy, 33,* 32–40.

Sanavio, E. (1988). Obsessions and compulsions: The Padua Inventory. *Behaviour Research and Therapy, 26,* 169–177

Slade, P. D., & Owens, R. G. (1998). A dual process model of perfectionism based on reinforcement theory. *Behavior Modification, 22,* 372–390.

Stöber, J. (1998). The Frost Multidimensional Perfectionism Scale revisited: More perfect with four (instead of six) dimensions. *Personality and Individual Differences, 24,* 481–491.

Straus, E. W. (1948). On obsession: A clinical and methodological study. *Nervous and Mental Disease Monograph, 73,* 1948.

Tallis, F. (1996). Compulsive washing in the absence of phobic and illness anxiety. *Behaviour Research and Therapy, 34,* 361–362.

Terry-Short, L. A., Owens, G. R., Slade, P. D., & Dewey, M. E. (1995). Positive and negative perfectionism. *Personality and Individual Differences, 18,* 663–668.

Wade, D., Kyrios, M., & Jackson, H. (1998). A model of obsessive–compulsive phenomena in a nonclinical sample. *Australian Journal of Psychology, 50,* 11–17.

Waller, G., Wood, A., Miller, J., & Slade, P. (1992). The development of neurotic perfectionism: A risk factor for unhealthy eating attitudes. *British Review of Bulimia and Anorexia Nervosa, 6,* 57–62.

Weissman, A. N., & Beck, A. T. (1978). *Development and validation of the Dysfunctional Attitude Scale.* Paper presented at the annual meeting of the Association for the Advancement of Behavior Therapy, Chicago.

Commentary on Cognitive Domains Section

David A. Clark

If Austin Powers, the fictitious British spy agent of recent movie fame who returned to life after being frozen in the 1960s, were to read the recent developments in cognitive theory and treatment of *obsessive compulsive disorder* (OCD), he might exclaim "Yeah, baby, you've come a long ways". Certainly there has been a renewed fervour in theory and research on OCD after a relatively dormant period during the 1980s and early 1990s. The late 1960s and 1970s saw unprecedented developments in behavioral research and treatment of OCD. This highly productive and innovative period ended with the publication of Rachman and Hodgson's (1980) seminal book *Obsessions and Compulsions*. But then little further work was conducted on OCD until Salkovskis (1985) published his paper on a cognitive–behavioral theory and treatment for OCD which advocated a synthesis of Aaron T. Beck's cognitive therapy of depression with the behavioral treatment of exposure and response prevention (ERP). Salkovskis' paper stimulated renewed interest in OCD among behavioral researchers by providing a fresh perspective on previously overlooked cognitive mechanisms that may underlie this disorder.

The present volume, and in particular the chapters that comprise this section, provide an excellent overview of current progress on the key developments in cognitive theory of OCD. After reading these chapters, it is apparent that much progress has been made in understanding the cognitive basis of OCD. Researchers, especially those that comprise the Obsessive Compulsive Cognitions Working Group (OCCWG), have ferreted out key cognitive constructs of the disorder and have sharpened our understanding of these concepts. In many respects the collaborative work of the OCCWG has taken the cognitive perspective on OCD to a new level and future possibilities. The contributors in this section each take a specific aspect of the cognitive formulation of OCD and present a critical, empirically based analysis of the role the domains may play in the pathogenesis of obsessions. Many interesting possibilities for future research and the development of a better understanding of OCD are presented along with a historical overview of the antecedents of these constructs. As well, the contributors provide a glimpse into the empirical work of the OCCWG referencing to findings from two large data sets. Together, the chapters in this section of the book present a comprehensive and detailed review of the key components of cognitive theory of OCD.

Although one can be encouraged by the progress made on the cognitive basis of OCD, it is also clear from these chapters that many gaps remain in our knowledge. Cognitive research on obsessions and compulsions has produced a number of inconsistencies and confusing findings. Rather than critique each chapter in turn, I organize this brief commentary around three themes. First, I draw out some of the key findings that cut across the various chapters. Then I highlight some of the critical issues that are apparent in the cognitive research. And finally, I conclude with a statement on the future of cognitive theory and research in OCD.

Findings on Cognition in OCD

It is clear from these chapters that we have learned much about the cognitive structures, processes and products of OCD. The research reviewed in this section has brought with it greater elaboration and clarification of the nature and function of cognition in OCD. In fact a number of conclusions listed below can be reached about the cognitive basis of OCD.

1. We now have a much better understanding of the key cognitive constructs of OCD. Each chapter began with a specific definition of a particular cognitive domain that then guided measurement and experimentation on that construct. Responsibility is defined in terms of belief in one's influence to cause harm. Importance is characterized by beliefs that intrusive thoughts indicate personal significance, that these thoughts have significance by their mere occurrence in the stream of consciousness, and that they increase the risk of bad things happening. Control is defined as the overvaluation of the importance of attaining complete control over intrusions and the belief that this is possible and desirable. Overestimation of threat is considered the exaggeration of the probability and severity of harm or danger. Intolerance of uncertainty refers to the necessity of being certain, the capacity to cope with unpredictable change and the importance of adequate functioning in ambiguous situations. Finally, perfectionism, at least in OCD, is defined as belief that there is a perfect solution to every problem, that it is necessary to do things without making mistakes, and that even minor mistakes will have serious consequences. These definitions provide greater precision to cognitive constructs that were ill defined and quite tangential in past OCD writings.

2. New self-report measures and experimental manipulations have been developed that appear to have considerable construct validity. This indicates that the cognitive domains of OCD can be empirically investigated in a reliable and systematic fashion. The greatest advances have been made in measurement and experimentation of inflated responsibility, thought–action fusion (i.e., importance of thoughts), threat estimation, and possibly perfectionism. The authors of these chapters present excellent examples of fairly sophisticated and innovative experimental procedures for manipulating these constructs.

3. Recently McNally (2001) identified two tracks in cognitive–clinical research, one that focuses on problematic beliefs and appraisals and the other that deals with information-processing abnormalities. Both research traditions are evident in OCD, although the chapters in this section deal mainly with the beliefs and appraisal side of the cognitive perspective (see also Chapter nine in this volume). However the research to date suggests that dysfunctional beliefs and appraisals may play a greater role in the etiology and persistence of obsessions and compulsions than specific information-processing biases or deficits. For example, in their chapter Sookman and Pinard (2002) review

information processing studies on attentional and memory biases in OCD. A series of recent studies indicates that individuals with OCD do not have actual memory deficits, but instead appraise their memory performance differently in terms of lower confidence and certainty ratings. In fact, Radomsky and Rachman (1999) have shown that for symptom-related information, individuals with OCD may show enhanced recall. Clearly, then, thoughts, beliefs and appraisals or interpretations, the core foci of cognitive therapy, are critically important in OCD.

4. The cognitive research reviewed in these chapters highlights an obvious but often overlooked fact; the dysfunctional beliefs and appraisals involved in the pathogenesis of obsessions are complex, involving a number of different yet overlapping cognitive constructs or domains. Simply defining the cognitive basis of OCD in terms of single constructs will obfuscate the true complex, interactive and multidimensional nature of cognition in OCD. However, many cognitive–clinical studies in OCD still focus on single cognitive domains (e.g., responsibility, perfectionism, thought–action fusion) in isolation from other constructs, thereby offering a distorted and one-sided view on the cognitive basis of OCD. Researchers need to investigate multiple cognitive domains in order to capture the richness of the cognitive nature of this disorder.

5. Dysfunctional beliefs and appraisals are very closely tied to the obsessional content and current concerns of patients. Sookman and Pinard (2002) conclude that OCD patients overestimate the probability of harm only in relation to their particular symptom concerns (i.e., contamination for washers, mistakes for checkers, etc.) rather than for all negative events. More global measures of responsibility have produced inconclusive results whereas responsibility measures that target the specific OC-related concerns of patients have shown greater specificity to OCD. Thordarson and Shafran (2002) note that one aspect of thought–action fusion (TAF), that one's thoughts might increase the likelihood of bad things happening to others, may be more related to OCD than more general TAF because it is closer to the magical thinking one often sees in OCD. Purdon and Clark (2002) argue that the thought content of an unwanted intrusion (that is, its ego-dystonic nature) may make it more difficult to exert mental control. Frost, Novara, and Rhéaume (2002) provide some evidence that concern over mistakes and doubt about actions may be more specific to OCD than global perfectionism measures because they are closer to the actual symptomatology of OCD. These results indicate that researchers must use cognitive measures that are relevant to the disorder-specific concerns of OCD patients.

6. There is an emerging research basis to conclude that beliefs and appraisals of importance of thoughts, mental control, responsibility, perfectionism, threat estimation, and intolerance of uncertainty are highly relevant concepts for understanding OCD. Each of the contributors to this section have shown that these cognitive domains are linked to OCD symptoms and that OCD patients endorse more of this dysfunctional thinking style than non-clinical controls. However, it is also clear that these constructs are not OCD specific (see discussion below). In fact all of the contributors noted that these cognitive domains are evident in other disorders such as GAD, PTSD and the like. Nevertheless, non-specific constructs can still play a critical role in the etiology and persistence of a disorder, an observation made by Garber and Hollon (1991) in reference to the causal status of cognitive variables in depression.

7. Finally, threat or danger is clearly a core feature of OCD. It is difficult, if not impossible, to define or measure other cognitive domains in isolation from threat. It is the centrality of threat or danger that makes OCD an anxiety disorder. Again, Sookman and Pinard (2002) make a convincing argument for the central role of overestimation of threat in OCD.

Critical Issues

On mere appearance Austin Powers, and anyone else who has been out-of-touch for 30 years, might easily be fooled into thinking that a paradigmatic shift has occurred in our approach to OCD. While fresh insights have been offered, the advances in the cognitive perspective on OCD may not be nearly as deep as may seem from first impression. As most of the contributors to this section point out, perfectionism, overestimation of threat, intolerance of uncertainty, responsibility and control of thoughts have long been postulated as important constructs in OCD. Moreover, many fundamental issues remain unresolved, thereby precluding any firm conclusion on whether cognitive factors play a critical role in the treatment of OCD. The following are some key questions that remain for further research.

1. To date cognitive researchers have been unable to identify distinct dimensions of maladaptive thinking in OCD. All the contributors have reviewed a number of studies, including the two data sets collected by the OCCWG, that show a high degree of association and overlap across the six cognitive domains. There are a number of reasons for this high level of association. First, certain features of one domain may be also relevant for another domain. Frost *et al.* (2002), for example, point out that doubt over one's actions was assigned to intolerance of uncertainty even though this feature has been traditionally associated with perfectionism. Thus, it is not surprising that the Perfectionism and Intolerance of Uncertainty subscales of the Obsessive Beliefs Questionnaire (OBQ) correlated 0.79. Second, more specific elements of a construct may show a distinct relationship with OCD symptoms whereas the more general concept may lack specificity. As noted previously, it is quite possible that this criticism is particularly relevant for global indices of perfectionism. Third, it is possible that some constructs are precursors to other domains, which would inflate the correlation between the two constructs. Thordarson and Shafran (2002) have argued that importance of thoughts may be a precursor to mental control and responsibility beliefs. A certain level of personal significance must first be attributed to the intrusive thought before beliefs in responsibility and control will be activated. Finally, it could be that certain cognitive domains are more relevant for one subtype of OCD than for another subtype. Thordarson and Shafran (2002) suggest that importance of thoughts beliefs may be more relevant for obsessions dealing with harm and aggression. At the very least, the high overlap among the cognitive domains reviewed in this section will present difficult challenges to researchers interested in the investigation of multiple cognitive constructs.

2. At this point, the nature of the relationship between various levels of cognitive conceptualization remains unclear. Sookman and Pinard (2002) present the classic cognitive formulation where general vulnerability schemas lead to specific assumptions

that then result in context-specific appraisals. However the relationship between beliefs and appraisals is not well-understood, particularly in light of the overlap between the OBQ that was designed to measure beliefs, and the Interpretations of Intrusions Inventory that was constructed to measure appraisals.

3. The search for OCD-specific cognitive constructs has so far eluded researchers. None of the six cognitive domains reviewed in these chapters can claim to be specific to OCD, although Salkovskis and Forrester (2002) argue the case for responsibility. All can be found in various forms in other anxiety disorders like GAD or PTSD. Some of the reasons cited under my first point are applicable to this lack of disorder specificity. It may be that cognitive specificity will be found but finer-grained measures are needed that are linked to the idiosyncratic, threat-related concerns of patients.

4. Another issue raised by many of the contributors concerns subtyping in OCD. A number of the cognitive domains may be more applicable to certain types of obsessions or compulsions than others. For example, Thordarson and Shafran (2002) suggest that a tendency to interpret intrusive thoughts as highly important may be particularly evident with harming or repugnant obsessions. Sookman and Pinard (2002) raise the possibility that uncertainty beliefs may be more germane for checkers than washers. Questions have been raised about whether inflated responsibility is more salient in checking as opposed to cleaning compulsions (Rachman & Shafran, 1998). This suggests that research on the cognitive basis of OCD may have to concentrate on different subtypes of the disorder rather than lumping together everyone with a primary Axis I diagnosis of OCD.

5. Most research on the cognitive domains of OCD has relied on retrospective self-report measures and correlational research designs. While informative, these studies cannot ferret out the cause and effect relations between cognition and symptoms. Instead laboratory-based and naturalistic experimental studies are needed that can manipulate key elements of a cognitive domain and then measure this effect on a dependent variable such as manifest symptoms, mood state, or the like. The chapters in this section review some very promising experimental approaches to mental control (i.e., thought suppression), responsibility, thought–action fusion, and threat estimation.

6. Finally, research on the cognitive domains is too new to determine whether changes in dysfunctional beliefs and appraisals play a significant role in the treatment of OCD. Some of the initial cognitive behavioral treatment studies suggest that the combination of cognitive restructuring and ERP is not more effective than ERP alone (Kozak, 1999). However it may be that targeting OCD-relevant cognitive domains during treatment will improve maintenance of treatment gains or it may be more critical for some OCD subtypes, like obsessional ruminators, than for other subtypes like those with cleaning compulsions. Now that specific self-report measures are available for most of the cognitive domains, this type of treatment process and outcome research is possible.

Conclusion

In many respects the groundwork has been set for a very fruitful investigation of the cognitive basis of OCD over the next few years. Certainly progress has been made, and our understanding of the richness and complexity of the maladaptive thinking style in OCD has been advanced. However, in some ways the initial findings from the OCCWG have been disappointing. There is considerable overlap across cognitive constructs originally thought to be distinct cognitive characteristics of OCD. Our conceptualization of the six cognitive domains was more precise than previous attempts, and yet our measures may not be sufficiently fine-grained to detect critical differences. Because of the heterogeneity of OCD symptom expression, research strategy may need to focus on more homogeneous obsessional subtypes. Valid psychiatric comparison groups will be difficult to obtain because of high comorbidity in OCD and many of these cognitive constructs have relevance for other forms of negative thought such as worry, depressive rumination and trauma-related unwanted intrusions.

Despite these challenges, research into the cognitive basis of OCD is a promising endeavor. In future, researchers would be wise to adopt more experimental, laboratory-based approaches where various aspects of OCD-related cognition can be manipulated within an ecologically valid context. Self-report measures of OCD cognitive domains are now available to make these research designs feasible. Ultimately we may be in a position to begin to understand the interplay among various facets of maladaptive thinking in OCD, and how this relates to the persistence of the disorder. This should provide a solid theoretical and empirical basis to offer new cognitive innovations in the treatment of obsessions in particular. Within a few years, we may be more inclined to embrace Austin Powers' enthusiasm about cognitive behavioral research in OCD.

References

Frost, R. O., Novara, C., & Rhéaume, J. (2002). Perfectionism in obsessive–compulsive disorder. In R. O. Frost & G. Steketee (eds), *Cognitive approaches to obsessions and compulsions: Theory, assessment and treatment.* (pp. 91–105). Oxford: Elsevier.

Garber, J., & Hollon, S. D. (1991). What can specificity designs say about causality in psychopathology research? *Psychological Bulletin, 110,* 129–136.

Kozak, M. J. (1999). Evaluating treatment efficacy for obsessive–compulsive disorder: Caveat practitioner. *Cognitive and Behavioral Practice, 6,* 422–426.

McNally, R. J. (2001). On the scientific status of cognitive appraisal models of anxiety disorders. *Behaviour Research and Therapy, 39,* 513–521.

Purdon, C., & Clark, D. A. (2002). The need to control thoughts. In R. O. Frost & G. Steketee (eds), *Cognitive approaches to obsessions and compulsions: Theory, assessment and treatment.* (pp. 29–43). Oxford: Elsevier.

Rachman, S. J., & Hodgson, R. J. (1980). *Obsessions and compulsions.* Englewood Cliffs, NJ: Prentice-Hall.

Rachman, S. J., & Shafran, R. (1998). Cognitive and behavioral features of obsessive–compulsive disorder. In R. P. Swinson, M. M. Antony, S. Rachman, & M. A. Richter (eds), *Obsessive–compulsive disorder: Theory, research and treatment* (pp. 51–78). New York: Guilford.

Radomsky, A. S., & Rachman, S. (1999). Memory bias in obsessive–compulsive disorder (OCD). *Behaviour Research and Therapy, 37,* 605–618.

Salkovskis, P. M. (1985). Obsessional–compulsive problems: A cognitive–behavioural analysis. *Behaviour Research and Therapy, 23,* 571–583.

Salkovskis, P. M., & Forrester, E. (2002). Responsibility. In R. O. Frost & G. Steketee (eds),

Cognitive approaches to obsessions and compulsions: Theory, assessment and treatment. (pp. 45–61). Oxford: Elsevier.

Sookman, D., & Pinard, G. (2002). Overestimation of threat and intolerance of uncertainty in obsessive–compulsive disorder. In R. O. Frost & G. Steketee (eds), *Cognitive approaches to obsessions and compulsions: Theory, assessment and treatment.* (pp. 63–89). Oxford: Elsevier.

Thordarson, D. S., & Shafran, R. (2002). Importance of thoughts. In R.O. Frost & G. Steketee (eds), *Cognitive approaches to obsessions and compulsions: Theory, assessment and treatment.* (pp. 15–28). Oxford: Elsevier.

Section B

Measurement of Cognition in Obsessive Compulsive Disorder

Chapter 7

Development and Validation of Instruments for Measuring Intrusions and Beliefs in Obsessive Compulsive Disorder

Steven Taylor, Michael Kyrios, Dana S. Thordarson, Gail Steketee and Randy O. Frost

Introduction

Recently, theoreticians interested in etiology, assessment, and treatment of obsessive compulsive disorder (OCD) have focused their attention on cognitive factors that may be central to this disorder. These factors include both cognitive processing (attention, memory, and information processing) and cognitive appraisals or interpretations of internal and external events. The latter aspect of cognition is the focus of the present chapter, specifically appraisals or beliefs associated with negative emotions like anxiety, embarrassment, and guilt for individuals with OCD. Theoretical models (especially those of Salkovskis, 1985, 1989; Rachman, 1997) detailing cognitive appraisals in OCD are described in Chapters 1–6 of this volume. As these chapters indicate, various cognitive models identified several cognitive domains considered especially relevant to OCD.

Interestingly, descriptions of standard behavioral treatments for OCD that included exposure to feared obsessive situations and response prevention of associated rituals (ERP) have also contained some discussion of cognitive factors. At least partly addressed in relation to ERP treatments are such cognitive features as overestimates of threat (exaggerated beliefs about danger) and faulty epistemological reasoning (e.g., belief that situations are dangerous until proven safe) (e.g., Foa & Kozak, 1985). In addition, the problem of overvalued ideation or absence of insight into the irrational nature of obsessive fears has also been discussed (see Kozak & Foa, 1994 and Chapter 10 in this volume). Newer cognitive models of OCD have led to specific treatment strategies that target faulty thinking (e.g., Freeston *et al.*, 1997; van Oppen & Arntz, 1994) and to the development of measures assessing appraisals and beliefs associated with obsessive intrusions. These assessment methods are discussed below, along with a description of the process and procedures employed by an international working group of OCD researchers to develop two new measures of cognition, the Obsessional Beliefs Questionnaire (OBQ) and the Interpretation of Intrusions Inventory (III).

Instruments Assessing Cognition in OCD

Measures of Cognition Used in Cognitive Therapy Studies of OCD

The first studies to examine the effects of cognitive treatments for OCD used Rational Emotive Therapy (RET) to alter irrational beliefs about obsessions. Emmelkamp and colleagues conducted two studies in the Netherlands comparing Rational Emotive Therapy (RET) to conventional Exposure and Response Prevention (ERP) treatment (Emmelkamp & Beens, 1991; Emmelkamp, Visser, & Hoekstra, 1988). To assess cognitive change these studies both employed a Dutch version of the Irrational Beliefs Test (IBT), originally developed by Jones (1968) to assess 10 types of irrational beliefs associated with Ellis' RET. Although evidence for reliability and validity of this measure is generally good, Robb and Warren (1990) reported that this scale, like a number of other general measures of irrational beliefs, included a large percentage of items that describe general symptoms of emotional or behavioral maladjustment rather than beliefs. Further, the IBT does not assess a number of beliefs and attitudes considered representative of or specific to OCD. Interestingly, in the earlier study, irrational beliefs changed marginally with treatment and did not differ between RET and ERP. In the later Emmelkamp and Beens study, irrational beliefs changed more with cognitive plus exposure therapy than with exposure alone. In both studies, the amount of change evident on this general cognitive measure was small.

Another test of cognitive therapy from the Netherlands by van Oppen, de Haan, van Balkom, Spinhoven, Hoogduin, and van Dyck (1995) employed Beck's model for cognitive therapy and assessed change in beliefs with the Irrational Beliefs Inventory (Koopmans, Sanderman, Timmerman, & Emmelkamp, 1994). This 50-item questionnaire based on the IBT and on the Rational Behavior Inventory (Shorkey & Whitman, 1977) is another general measure of beliefs and attitudes, not specifically linked to cognitive theories about OCD. In this study, cognitive therapy led to significant improvement in irrational beliefs, whereas exposure treatment did not, but once again, the average reduction in scores for cognitive therapy was small.

More recent studies of cognitive therapy have employed measures of beliefs that were more closely tied to models of cognition in OCD. McLean *et al.* (2001) used three measures of OCD beliefs to assess cognitive change following group treatment of either Cognitive-Behavior Therapy (CBT) or ERP compared to waitlist control. These measures were the Responsibility Attitude Scale devised by Salkovskis *et al.* (2000), the Intrusive Beliefs Related to Obsessions developed by Freeston, Ladouceur, Gagnon, and Thibodeau (1993), and the Thought–Action Fusion scale by Shafran, Thordarson, and Rachman (1996). They are described in the next section of this chapter. Findings indicated that only on the responsibility measure was significant change detected in active treatments compared with control treatment, and that cognitive treatment did produce more change in beliefs than exposure therapy. Cottraux *et al.* (2000) also compared cognitive therapy and exposure treatments, assessing cognitive change using the Intrusive Thoughts and Interpretations Questionnaire (Yao, Cottraux, & Martin, 1999). This measure indicated significant and substantial change in frequency and interpretation of thoughts, but no differences were detected between treatment conditions; that is, cognitive therapy did not produce more cognitive change than exposure at posttest or at one-year follow-up.

Some case studies have also assessed the cognitive outcomes of cognitive therapy for OCD. Ladouceur, Leger, Rhéaume, and Dube (1996) used a Responsibility Questionnaire developed by Rhéaume and colleagues (described below) to assess cognitive change. All four of their OCD clients showed a clinically significant decrease on this measure of responsibility after treatment that targeted inflated responsibility and awareness and correction of negative automatic thoughts. Sookman, Pinard, and Beauchemin (1994) reported on three cases successfully treated with cognitive therapy who were assessed using an idiographic belief rating for dysfunctional schemas related to obsessions. Other examples of the use of idiographic ratings of the strength of target beliefs to assess cognitive change can be found in the case study literature (e.g., Salkovskis & Warwick, 1985).

As we have noted, however, most early studies assessed changes in cognitive appraisals or beliefs using standardized questionnaires that were not designed for OCD beliefs. Thus, along with extensive cognitive theory development and testing of cognitive therapies for OCD came a pressing need for adequate instruments to assess the types and severity of cognitive aspects of OCD. Not surprisingly, as evident from recent studies of cognitive therapy described above, several researchers began to develop mainly self-report measures intended to capture key elements of interpretations and beliefs thought to be linked to OCD symptoms. These measures are briefly described below.

Measures Assessing General Beliefs in OCD

Several self-report instruments were developed in different centers during approximately the same time period in the 1990s to assess general beliefs and specific domains of beliefs considered pertinent to the development and maintenance of OCD symptoms. Many of these are multidimensional, attempting to measure several different domains of beliefs linked to OCD symptoms. Instruments we are aware of are described briefly below.

Freeston and colleagues developed a brief 20-item scale, the Inventory of Beliefs Related to Obsessions (Freeston *et al.* 1993) to identify problematic thoughts and beliefs. This scale generates a total OC belief score and subscales for inflated responsibility, overestimation of threat, and intolerance of uncertainty. Tests of its psychometric properties indicated satisfactory reliability and evidence of criterion, convergent, discriminant, and factorial validity (see also Steketee, Frost, & Cohen, 1998). However, the IBRO was not more strongly related to OCD symptoms than to other forms of psychopathology (Steketee *et al.*, 1998).

Clark and Purdon (1995) developed a 67-item Metacognitive Beliefs Questionnaire to assess multiple domains of OCD cognition: positive beliefs about worry; uncontrollability and danger; confidence in memory and attention; superstition, punishment and responsibility; and cognitive self-consciousness. A series of psychometric studies demonstrated adequate to good internal consistency and test–retest reliability and concurrent and discriminant validity. Attempting to capture very similar domains, Cartwright-Hatton and Wells (1997) reported on the Meta-Cognitions Questionnaire to measure beliefs about worry and intrusive thoughts. Designed mainly to assess worry in generalized anxiety disorder, this instrument also has relevance for OCD. Of five dimensions identified in factor analyses, four pertain to beliefs (positive beliefs about worry, negative beliefs about controllability of thoughts and danger, cognitive confidence, and negative beliefs about thoughts in general) and one to metacognitive processes (cognitive self-consciousness or monitoring of thinking). This measure showed good psychometric properties on several tests of reliability and validity and predicted other measures of proneness to obsessive symptoms.

Steketee *et al.* (1998) developed a 90-item Obsessive Compulsive Beliefs Questionnaire to assess responsibility for harm, control of thoughts, threat estimation, tolerance for uncertainty, and beliefs about anxiety and coping. Initial findings comparing OCD, anxiety disordered and non-psychiatric control subjects suggested that all of these subscales discriminated among groups and that all except anxiety and coping beliefs correlated highly with measures of OCD symptoms and with other measures of OCD beliefs. However, inclusion of OCD symptoms in some items and the overlap among belief domains presented problems.

Sookman and Pinard's (1995) 208-item Obsessive Compulsive Cognitive Schemata Scale assesses OCD core beliefs or schemas about the self and the world. Subscales cover 12 domains, including vulnerability, responsibility, magical thinking, doubt/indecision, response to ambiguity, need for control, response to affect, perfectionism, perseveration, overinclusion, generalization, and self-perceptions. This instrument demonstrated good internal consistency, test–retest reliability and convergent validity and discriminated OCD patients from psychiatric and non-psychiatric controls. Like other measures of beliefs in OCD, some items appear to assess OCD symptoms (especially contamination) and high correlations among some of the subscales indicated that hypothesized dimensions overlapped substantially, especially responsibility, generalization and magical thinking. Further, the length of this measure may render it unfeasible in some assessment contexts.

Hoekstra (1995) developed a 60-item Obsessive Compulsive Cognitions List that assessed several dimensions of OCD beliefs, including perfectionism, threat estimation, thought–action fusion, importance of thoughts, doubt, and responsibility. Psychometric properties were not reported, but some items from this scale appear problematic in that they assess OCD symptoms as well as beliefs. Tallis (1995) began the development of a 29-item Obsessional Beliefs scale containing items pertinent to beliefs about uncertainty, tolerance for discomfort, risk, thought–action fusion and superstitious beliefs, control over thoughts and actions, perfectionistic standards, and memory.

Other scales were developed after the Obsessive Compulsive Cognitions Working Group (OCCWG) began its work. Hedlund and Oppelt (1998) reported on a 58-item OCD Meta-Inventory to assess intermediate level beliefs in OCD that included subscales similar to other measures: thought–action fusion, inflated responsibility, risk aversion, guilt and shame, perfectionism, obsessive doubt, acceptance of thoughts and feelings, control, moralism, and fear avoidance. Preliminary testing indicated OCD subjects scored higher than healthy controls on all scales but moralism, but scored higher than depressed patients only on control and perfectionism. Finally, Yao *et al.* (1999) developed a French language instrument, the Intrusive Thoughts and Interpretations Questionnaire, to assess the frequency of four types of intrusive thoughts and the degree of irrational interpretation of these thoughts on three dimensions: inferiority, responsibility, and guilt. Some evidence for known-groups and convergent validity of this measure has been published, along with findings suggesting that some cognitive domains are more closely linked to certain types of intrusive thoughts than others (e.g., responsibility and aggressive thoughts, inferiority, and perfectionism).

Measures Assessing Specific Belief Domains for OCD

In addition to the above-described questionnaires that assess multiple domains of beliefs thought related to OCD, several instruments have been developed to measure single domains. These include measures of responsibility, thought–action fusion, interpretations or appraisals of intrusive thoughts, tolerance for anxiety and insight into the irrationality of obsessive fears and compulsive behaviors.

Three instruments have been developed to assess irrational beliefs about responsibility associated with OCD. Salkovskis *et al.*'s (2000) Responsibility Appraisal Scale (identified as the R-Scale in some studies) has been tested in several studies. This 26-item questionnaire focuses on general beliefs about responsibility for causing or failing to prevent harm. It showed good evidence of stability, internal consistency, and criterion related validity, and correlated more highly with measures of OCD symptoms than other forms of psychopathology (Salkovskis *et al.*, 2000; Steketee *et al.*, 1998). It also showed strong correlations with other measures of OCD beliefs, including the OCBQ subscales of responsibility, control, threat estimation, and uncertainty and the Inventory of Beliefs Related to Obsessions described above (Steketee *et al.*, 1998).

Kyrios and Bahr's (1995) 60-item Responsibility Questionnaire assessed inflated responsibility. In testing with university students, four factors emerged: safety of others, blame for faults and negative outcomes, compensation for negative outcomes, and control over thoughts and actions. Internal consistency and convergent validity with measures of OCD symptoms were generally good. Finally, Rhéaume and colleagues assessed responsibility by asking participants to answer several questions about their degree of personal influence over and responsibility for expected negative outcomes for a series of OCD-relevant situations (Rhéaume, Ladouceur, Freeston, & Letarte, 1994). This instrument demonstrated good reliability and validity. It is clear from the proliferation of measures of this construct and its regular inclusion in general measures of OCD beliefs that responsibility is considered by many to be a critical construct for OCD.

A method to assess thought-action fusion, closely related to constructs of over-importance of thoughts, responsibility for harm and overestimation of threat from thoughts, was developed by Shafran, Thordarson, and Rachman (1996). This 20-item questionnaire assessed beliefs that thinking unacceptable thoughts is morally equivalent to doing the action (Moral Thought-Action Fusion) and that thinking about negative outcomes makes them more likely to happen (Likelihood Thought-Action Fusion). It proved internally consistent and discriminated between OCD subjects and controls.

Several investigators have sought to measure the degree to which individuals with OCD misinterpret the meaning and importance of intrusive thoughts. Salkovskis and colleagues (2000) developed the 22-item Responsibility Interpretations Questionnaire to assess the frequency and strength of interpretations of recently occurring intrusive thoughts, images, or impulses about responsibility (including thought-action fusion, importance and control of thoughts). Like its companion measure, the Responsibility Appraisal Scale, this instrument performed well in studies of reliability and validity, with the exception of positively worded (low responsibility) items which had low reliability. The Responsibility Interpretations Questionnaire has served as a template for the development of the Interpretation of Intrusions Inventory described later in this chapter.

The Cognitive Intrusions Questionnaire (Freeston, Ladouceur, Thibodeau, & Gagnon, 1991) was partly derived from two earlier instruments about distressing and intrusive thoughts. This measure first determines whether intrusive thoughts, images, or impulses have occurred recently and rates these on emotional, behavioral, and cognitive dimensions. The latter include belief strength, self-disapproval, responsibility, and insight. Reports on non-clinical samples indicated some association of these variables with efforts to escape or avoid intrusive thoughts. Thus, although not originally intended as a primary measure of cognitive domains for OCD, this questionnaire contains several relevant items. Clark and Purdon (1995) also sought to determine the frequency with which 52 different intrusive thoughts, images, and/or urges occurred using their Obsessional Intrusions Inventory. Similar to Freeston and colleagues' measure, Part II of the inventory inquires about emotional distress, strength of belief, difficulty eliminating the intrusion, and responsibility for the thought. Both questionnaires also assess in a very similar fashion what the individual does in response to intrusions.

To date, at least three instruments have been developed to assess the degree of insight that individuals with OCD have about the irrationality of their obsessive fears. These include Kozak's unpublished five-item Fixity of Beliefs Questionnaire, Neziroglu, McKay, Yaryura-Tobias, Stevens, and Todaro's (1999) Overvalued Idea Scale rated for each of three main OCD-related beliefs, and Eisen, Philips, Baer, Beer, Atala, and Rasmussen's (1998) more detailed Brown Assessment of Beliefs Scale. All are interviewer-rated instruments since the concept of insight is considered difficult for clients to assess independently because the patient may lack the necessary objectivity to complete the ratings. The Brown Assessment of Beliefs Scale provides detailed instructions to raters for identifying the relevant beliefs and for rating conviction, perception of others' views, explanation for discrepancies from others' beliefs, fixity of ideas, efforts to disprove ideas, and insight. Additional items help distinguish obsessions associated with schizophrenia from typical obsessions. Chapter 11 contains a description of these instruments and related concepts about insight.

Tolerance for anxiety associated with obsessions has been assessed by selected items from an early instrument called the Exposure Thought Inventory (Steketee & Foa, 1985) designed for use in conjunction with behavioral treatment sessions. Twenty-two items inquired about beliefs about the effects of anxiety experienced during exposure, and 22 items refer to thoughts about specific feared consequences or catastrophes during exposure. Unfortunately, this instrument was not subjected to psychometric testing. Apart from the subscale included in Steketee *et al.*'s Obsessive Compulsive Beliefs Questionnaire, other scales have not assessed feared consequences associated with obsessive anxiety.

Measures of Cognitive Constructs Pertinent to OCD

Perfectionism, guilt, and superstitious beliefs are considered closely associated with OCD but by no means specific to this disorder. Here we mention a few self-report measures developed to assess these dimensions. Two instruments have been widely used to measure perfectionism in a variety of disorders. Frost and colleagues' 35-item Multidimensional Perfectionism Scale is particularly pertinent for OCD because its subscales cover concern over mistakes, personal standards, doubts about actions, order and organization, and parental expectations and criticism (Frost, Marten, Lahart, & Rosenblate, 1990). Hewitt and Flett's (1991) Multidimensional Perfectionism Scale measures self-oriented, socially prescribed, and other-oriented perfectionism. Both of these instruments have demonstrated good reliability and validity. Finally, Rhéaume, Freeston, Dugas, Letarte, and Ladouceur (1995) developed a multidimensional Perfectionism Questionnaire, also pertinent for OCD, which includes sections on perfectionistic attitudes and standards, general ratings of perfectionistic tendencies in various life domains (work, sports, etc.), negative consequences of perfectionistic actions, and concern about mistakes, standards, criticism, risk taking, and control. These measures of perfectionism have generally been found to be related to OCD and OCD symptoms (see Chapter six).

Guilt is the emotion most closely related to beliefs about responsibility and may be especially relevant for OCD. Existing instruments that assess guilt include Kugler and Jones' (1992) 45-item Guilt Inventory and Klass' (1987) Situational Guilt Scale in which 22 items identify guilt anticipated in a range of commonly occurring situations. These instruments contain some questions that assess beliefs, but generally refer mainly to emotional experiences and actions. Although superstitious beliefs are not necessarily characteristic of individuals with OCD, they may be relevant for some individuals. Frost *et al.* (1993) developed a 22-item Lucky Beliefs Questionnaire that assesses the strength of typical superstitious beliefs in the U.S. (e.g., beliefs about black cats, ladders, the number 13) was found to be related to OCD symptoms.

The Need for a Comprehensive Measure of Beliefs in OCD

In earlier sections, we have documented the development of an array of instruments to assess beliefs in OCD, designed and partially tested by individual investigators working independently. More than 15 such measures have been developed, representing diverse aspects of OCD and creating a confusing picture of the role of cognitive phenomena in this disorder. Several problems are evident in these measures. Many overlap considerably, making it difficult to choose among them. None has received comprehensive psychometric evaluation on large samples that included individuals diagnosed with OCD, as well as clinical and healthy control groups. Further, at the time of their development, researchers had not reached a consensus regarding the types of cognitive content considered most important for evaluating cognitions in OCD. Continuing development of many measures in separate sites would inevitably bring confusion to the field and make it very difficult for researchers to select appropriate measures and eventually to compare findings about intrusive thoughts and beliefs across studies. Thus, coordinated research on assessment, including standardization of definitions for domains of study, could save considerable time and expense in advancing the study of cognition in OCD. Collaborative research efforts would facilitate more rapid identification of possible etiologic mechanisms, development of novel interventions, and consistent evaluation of the effects of cognitive, behavioral, and pharmacological therapies. Such collaborative research across multiple settings is relatively rare in psychopathology and psychotherapy research, but in several cases has considerably advanced the field, witness U.S. government-sponsored multi-site research on epidemiology and comorbidity in psychiatric disorders and on cognitive treatments for depression.

The international Obsessive Compulsive Cognitions Working Group (OCCWG) was born of a small group of researchers who met following a symposium on OCD-related beliefs at the World Congress of Behavioural and Cognitive Therapies in Denmark in 1995. Following a discussion of problems in the current status of cognitive assessment of OCD, this group agreed to engage in a coordinated effort to develop and evaluate assessment strategies, including both self-report and laboratory methods, and to involve other researchers in studying beliefs in OCD in this effort. As an initial step, the organizers scheduled a first large meeting in Northampton, MA, with 26 OCCWG participants from eight countries. For this meeting, participants collected existing self-report instruments pertinent to cognition in OCD and identified and provided definitions for multiple domains of OCD-related beliefs. These instruments (described above) were judged to assess 19 different domains of beliefs (see Table 7.1) considered important in the development and maintenance of OCD. The group then reduced these domains to a manageable subset for purposes of assessment. The scales from which these domains were obtained are listed in Table 7.2.

Working subgroups then generated potential items to assess selected domains and modeled the formats for proposed measures on Brown, Craske, and Rassovsky's (1995) Anxiety Attitude and Belief Scale, the Dysfunctional Attitude Scale by Weissman (1980) and on Salkovskis' Responsibility Appraisal Questionnaire. The group planned procedures for developing a first instrument and testing it for psychometric adequacy. Extensive communication among members who organized themselves into working teams and subsequent meetings of the full OCCWG group have resulted in two waves of psychometric testing of two self-report instruments. These measures are the Obsessive Beliefs Questionnaire (OBQ) intended to assess beliefs associated with OCD and the Interpretation of Intrusions (III) questionnaire designed to capture appraisals that immediately follow intrusive experiences. The advantages of such collective efforts in measurement development have been abundantly clear in the Working Group's capacity to utilize expert consensus for instrument development and to access large samples in a very short period of time for instrument testing.

Methodological Development of OCCWG Instruments

Level of Measurement

In preparing to develop measures of OCD beliefs, the OCCWG reviewed the levels at which these measurements might be made (OCCWG, 1997). This review relied heavily on

Table 7.1. Belief Domains Associated with OCD.

OC Belief Domain	Description
Overestimation of severity or probability of danger	Overestimation of the probability or severity of threat or harm.
Inflated responsibility	The belief that one has power, which is pivotal to bring about or prevent subjectively crucial negative outcomes. They may be actual, that is, having consequences in the real world, and/or at the moral level.
Omissions/commission	Belief that not preventing something harmful from happening is as bad as actually doing something harmful.
Thought–action fusion	Belief that: (a) thinking about something increases its likelihood of occurrence, or (b) thoughts are (almost) morally equivalent to actions.
Superstitions/magical thinking	Beliefs that defy normal laws of cause and effect.
Overimportance given to thoughts	Beliefs that "I think about it because it's important" and "The thought is important because I think about it."
Consequences of having thoughts — Emotional cost	Belief that one will become very anxious as a consequence of having unwanted thoughts, and that this will impair one's functioning.
Control over thoughts	Importance of control over one's thoughts.
Perfectionism	Belief that a perfect state exists that one should try to attain.
High personal standards for one's performance	Beliefs that one needs to perform according to some very high standard.
Concern over mistakes	Belief that making mistakes is very bad.
Rigidity: follow rules strictly	Belief that it is important to follow rules in a strict manner. Includes scrupulousness, and excessive concerns with one way of doing things.
Control over life circumstances	Belief that one must exercise complete control over one's life circumstances.
Intolerance of anxiety and discomfort	Belief that feeling anxiety or discomfort is bad and may have harmful consequences.
Intolerance for uncertainty, newness, and change	Belief that uncertainty, newness, and change are intolerable because they are potentially dangerous.
Decision-making, doubting	Belief that it is possible to find perfect choices or solutions.
Beliefs about coping	Beliefs about one's ability to cope with anxiety or discomfort.
Lack of confidence in memory and other senses.	Beliefs about the reliability of one's memory and other senses.
Overgeneralization	Beliefs reflecting an excessive tendency to derive a general conception or principle from insufficient particulars; e.g. "If I do something dangerous once, then that means I can't trust my judgement."

Table 7.2: Measures relevant to the assessment of OCD-related beliefs.

Author(s)	Instrument	Subscales
Brown et al. (1995)	Attitude and Belief Scale	
Clark and Purdon (1995a)	Meta-cognitive Beliefs Questionnaire	1. Importance of thought control 2. Fusion of thought and action (consequences) 3. Shame and embarrassment about intrusive thoughts 4. Positive attributes of unwanted intrusive thoughts
Freeston et al. (1995)	Typical Interpretation of Thoughts	
Freeston et al. (1993)	Irrational Beliefs Regarding Obsessions	1. Responsibility, guilt, blame, punishment and loss 2. Overestimation of threat 3. Intolerance of uncertainty
Frost et al. (1990)	Multidimensional Perfectionism Scale	1. Concern over mistakes 2. Personal standards 3. Parental expectations 4. Parental criticism 5. Doubting of actions 6. Order and organization
Frost et al. (1993)	Lucky Beliefs Questionnaire	
Hoekstra (1995)	obsessive compulsive Cognitions List	
Kozak (1996)	Fixity of Beliefs Scale	
Kugler and Jones (1992)	Guilt Inventory	1. Trait guilt 2. State guilt 3. Moral standards
Kyrios and Bhar (1995)	Responsibility Questionnaire	
Shafran et al. (1996)	Thought–Action Fusion Scale	1. Moral thought–action fusion 2. Likelihood thought–action fusion

Table 7.2: (Continued)

Author(s)	Instrument	Subscales
Rhéaume *et al.* (1995)	Responsibility Questionnaire	
Salkovskis (1992)	Responsibility Scale (Versions I & II)	
Sookman and Pinard (1995)	Obsessive Compulsive Disorder Cognitive Schemata Scale	1. Vulnerability 2. Responsibility 3. Confusion of thought and action/magical thinking 4. Pathological doubting/indecision 5. View of/response to ambiguity, newness, and change 6. Need for control 7. View of/response to strong affect 8. Perfectionism 9. Perseveration 10. Overinclusion/underinclusion 11. Generalization 12. Self-percept
Steketee *et al.* (1996)	Obsessive Compulsive Beliefs Questionnaire	1. Responsibility for harm 2. Controllability of thoughts and actions 3. Estimation of risk 4. Tolerance for uncertainty
Tallis (1995b)	Obsessional Beliefs	

a framework for classifying cognitive contents relevant to OCD developed by Freeston, Rhéaume, and Ladouceur (1996) and based on the theoretical work of Salkovskis (1985, 1989) and Rachman (1997). Three levels of cognitive content were hypothesized. The first consists of cognitive intrusions defined as unwanted thoughts, images, and impulses that intrude on consciousness. These intrusions are experienced by nearly everyone (Rachman, 1997), but people with OCD experience them as more intense, frequent, and distressing. When experienced this way, intrusive thoughts are commonly referred to as obsessions.

The second level of cognitive content, appraisals (akin to automatic thoughts in Beck's model), concerns the process by which intrusions are evaluated, that is, the meaning given to intrusive thoughts. The process of appraisal is instrumental in converting an intrusive thought into an obsession (Rachman, 1997). Intrusions are hypothesized to become obsessions when people with OCD appraise them as threatening and attempt to remove or suppress them, or to prevent or undo negative consequences they believe might result. Appraisals may be expectations or interpretations which frequently fall into several dimensions (OCCWG, 1997). These dimensions include appraisals of the importance of the intrusion. In this type of appraisal, the person assumes that the mere occurrence of the thought gives it importance (e.g., "Having this thought means that it is true."). A second dimension of appraisal is judgment about personal responsibility for an imagined event. For instance, having the thought "If I don't check the stove again, the house might burn down" leads the person with OCD to believe that if this event happened, it would be his/her fault.

The third dimension of appraisal of an intrusive thought concerns the necessity of stopping the thought from occurring. Controlling the intrusive thought is an attempt to avoid the discomfort produced by appraisals of importance and responsibility. These appraisals are strong enough to override logical reality-based judgments of the association between an action and consequence. Therefore, individuals with OCD know their actions have no influence over the outcome (e.g., rechecking), but nonetheless feel compelled to perform them. One way to measure such appraisals is by inventories of thoughts that occur in response to intrusions, probability judgments of the occurrence of the feared consequences, and ratings of perceived responsibility for negative consequences.

The third level of cognitive content related to OCD concerns more enduring assumptions or beliefs that are global rather than specific to a particular event. Typically, these beliefs are defined as dysfunctional attitudes or irrational beliefs. Such beliefs have been implicated as potential causal and maintaining features of a number of anxiety and depressive disorders (Beck & Emery, 1985). Whereas some general dysfunctional beliefs may characterize many disorders, including OCD, others may be specifically related to OCD. These more specific beliefs may be instrumental in how intrusive thoughts are interpreted and subsequently in the development of OCD.

Measuring each level of cognitive content may reveal important information about the nature of OCD. However, a number of challenges exist to developing a measurement scheme. The first concerns what measurement strategy to employ. The OCCWG identified three potential strategies: self-report, idiographic measurement, and laboratory tasks. After discussing each of these types of measurement, the group decided to begin by developing self-report instruments to assess appraisals and specific beliefs related to OCD and later to work on other methods. A second challenge is whether distinctions among levels of cognitive content can be made. The outcome of this challenge awaits empirical testing once suitable measures are generated. A third challenge concerns the extent to which measures at each level can discriminate people with OCD (or OCD symptoms) from other populations. Symptom measures (i.e., measures of intrusions) already have a high degree of discriminability as they make up the diagnostic criteria for OCD. In addition, some evidence exists for the discriminability of appraisal measures and measures of specific beliefs (Freeston *et al.*, 1993; Sookman & Pinard, 1995; Sookman, Pinard, & Englesmann, 1997).

Development and psychometric evaluation of the cognitive measures have gone through three stages. Stage one (OCCWG, 1997) involved consensus meetings on the types of beliefs and appraisals to assess, and the development of the first versions of the scales. Stage two (OCCWG, 2001) consisted of further revision of the scales and preliminary evaluation of their reliability and validity. Stage three (OCCWG, in preparation) involved a replication and extension the stage three findings regarding reliability and validity of the final version of the scales.

Development of a Measure of Beliefs in OCD: Stage One

The first task in creating a self-report measure of the content of OCD cognitions was the determination of relevant domains. A review of the literature identified 16 different measures of cognitive domains relevant to OCD that tapped 19 separate types of beliefs (OCCWG, 1997). Most of these measures were described earlier in this chapter. These 19 domains were ranked independently by members of the group (all experts in assessing and treating OCD) based on their relevance to OCD. One ranking was made for the extent to which the domain was specific to OCD in contrast to other disorders, and may constitute a vulnerability factor for the development of OCD. The second ranking was of the etiological significance of the domain, independent of its association with other disorders. As can be seen in Table 7.1, several domains were combined to form six major domains and a few were classified as minor because they were judged to be related to anxiety disorders generally but not uniquely to OCD (OCCWG, 1997).

The major domains identified by this procedure were inflated responsibility, over-importance of thoughts, excessive concern about controlling one's thoughts, overestimation of threat, intolerance of uncertainty, and perfectionism. Working subgroups for each domain provided formal definitions and presented these to the full group for consensus; the following definitions were developed. Inflated responsibility refers to the belief that one has pivotal power to cause or prevent outcomes that are believed to be catastrophic. Overimportance of thoughts refers to the belief that the mere presence of a thought gives it importance. The control domain involves the belief that one must have complete control over intrusive thoughts. Exaggeration of the probability and cost of harmful events is reflected in the overestimation of threat domain. The sixth domain, perfectionism, involves beliefs about the existence of a perfect solution and the consequences of even minor mistakes.

The subgroups then identified at least 15 items to represent the domain (OCCWG, 1997). Items from existing relevant measures (over 500 items) were used as a potential item pool, as well as new items generated by subgroup members. Each item had to meet the following criteria: (1) representation of the domain in question; (2) not considered a symptom of OCD; (3) not an emotional reaction; and (4) not phrased as a double negative. Approximately 25 percent of the items selected for the initial item pool were worded positively and reverse scored. Item format followed that of existing scales such as Brown, *et al.*'s (1995) Anxiety Attitude and Belief Scale and Weissman's (1980) Dysfunctional Attitude Scale using a seven-point rating scale. All items were worded in the present tense with a preference for items using "I" or "me" in order to insure relevance for the person completing the questionnaire. Wording such as "I feel" or "I worry that . . ." were avoided to avoid confusing beliefs with emotions. Simple language was used with only one idea per item so that the full seven-point range of responses would be used. The anchors were "disagree very much" and "agree very much." All Working Group members reviewed the resulting item pool and submitted modifications to the co-chairs who developed revisions. Working Group members again reviewed and revised the final set of items. The resulting 129-item OBQ was subjected to empirical testing described further below and in OCCWG (2001).

Development of a Measure of Appraisal of Intrusions: Stage One

The Interpretation of Intrusions Inventory (III) was designed to measure appraisals of intrusive thoughts using a format similar to earlier scales (e.g., Salkovskis *et al.*, 2000). Respondents were asked to recall intrusions occurring during the previous two weeks and to respond to the items in the scale while thinking of those intrusions. Working Group members concluded that appraisals occurred in three of the six domains described above: responsibility, importance of thoughts, and control of thoughts. The other three domains (overestimation of threat, tolerance for uncertainty, and perfectionism) were thought to represent beliefs relevant across contexts but not typically used to evaluate a particular intrusive thought, image or impulse. Items from the OBQ were altered to fit the format for measuring appraisals and new ones were generated to complete the 43 items in the first version of this scale.

Some beliefs related to OCD are likely to be held across a wide variety of situations and mood states. However, people with anxiety disorders have been hypothesized to display different danger-related beliefs during threatening situations (Beck & Emery, 1985). For the OBQ, the group agreed to retain items without priming instructions and to await further research on the effects of priming these beliefs. However, since the purpose of the III was to measure appraisals of recent intrusions, priming was considered necessary (see also Salkovskis *et al.*, 2000). The instructions for the III therefore provided a brief description of intrusive experiences and several examples of what was meant by intrusions and what was not meant (i.e., worries). These instructions were designed to allow the use of this instrument with non-clinical populations. The priming instructions provided examples of intrusive thoughts and asked respondents to record two of their own recent intrusions on blank lines and to keep these in mind when responding to items. Response categories ranged from zero ("I did not believe this idea at all") to 100 ("I was completely convinced this idea was true"). The instrument was kept relatively brief to facilitate recall of the two personal intrusions while answering items. In order to assess the importance of the mental intrusions, three questions about the experience of these thoughts were asked. These questions concerned the recency ("When did you last experience an intrusion of this kind?"), frequency ("In the last six months, how frequently did you experience an intrusion of this kind?"), and distress ("On average, how much distress do you usually experience when you have an intrusion of this kind?").

Scale Reduction: Stage Two

The newly created OBQ (127 items) and III (43 items) were given to 101 people with OCD, 374 student controls, and 76 English-speaking non-clinical controls to provide initial validation and to reduce the number of items on each measure (OCCWG, 2001). Additional instruments administered included the Yale–Brown Obsessive Compulsive Scale (Goodman *et al.*, 1989), the Padua Inventory (Sanavio, 1988), the Beck Anxiety Inventory (Beck, Epstein, Brown, & Steer, 1988) and the Beck Depression Inventory (Beck & Emory, 1985). Three stages of scale construction followed: (1) separate factor analysis of each subscale; (2) examination of internal consistency with resulting item reduction; and (3) examination of deleted items. Factor analyses of subscales revealed a pattern in which positively worded items loaded on a separate factor for each subscale. Thus, these items did not elicit responses like those for the negatively worded ones they were intended to represent, and they were therefore removed from the scales. Corrected item–total correlations and item intercorrelations resulted in further reduction of the scales to 87 items for the OBQ and 31 for the III. Finally, examination of all deleted items was undertaken to insure that no important information was lost. The reverse-scored and other eliminated items did not consistently discriminate among OCD and control groups, suggesting that little useful information had been lost in removing these items. The resulting scales (87-item OBQ and 31-item III) were then used to compare different subject samples to provide initial evidence regarding the reliability and validity of the revised OBQ and III. Results suggest the scales perform reasonably well on tests of internal consistency, criterion-related (known groups) validity, convergent validity, and discriminant validity (OCCWG, 2001).

Stage Three Findings Regarding the OBQ and III

The purpose of stage three was to replicate and extend the stage two findings. Detailed description of the data collection, analysis, and results are presented in a manuscript currently in preparation by the OCCWG. Below we present a summary of the results from stage three data collected from fresh samples of clinical and nonclinical participants. These participants completed the English-language version of the OBQ and III administered in Australia, Canada, and the United States. Findings are presented below on the test–retest reliability, internal consistency, criterion-related (known groups) validity, and convergent and discriminant validity of the scales.

Method

Participants

Four groups of participants completed the English-language scales: patients with DSM-IV obsessive–compulsive disorder as their most severe problem (OC, n=248), anxious controls (AC, n=105), community controls (CC, n=87), and student controls (SC, n=291). ACs consisted of patients without OCD who met criteria for a DSM-IV anxiety disorder other than specific phobia. CCs resided in the United States or Canada and included acquaintances or family members of OCCWG members, teachers, and community service organization members. SCs were university or college students.

Measures

In addition to completing the OBQ and III, participants at most sites completed the following scales: Padua Inventory — Washington State University revision (Burns, Keortge, Formea, & Sternberger, 1996); Beck Anxiety Inventory (Beck & Steer, 1993a); Beck Depression Inventory (Beck & Steer, 1993b); Penn State Worry Questionnaire (Meyer, Miller, Metzger, & Borkovec, 1990); and State-Trait Anxiety Inventory, trait anxiety scale (Spielberger, 1983).

Results

Internal Consistency

The OBQ and III scales had good internal consistency in all four samples (OC, AC, CC, and SC). The values of Cronbach alpha for the subscales ranged from 0.79 to 0.93.

Test–retest Reliability

Test–retest reliability correlations were computed for each scale in the OC and SC samples. In the OC sample, the test–retest correlations were moderate-to-large for most OBQ subscales (range 0.39 to 0.70) and large for III subscales (range 0.69 to 0.77). In the SC sample, correlations were large for both the OBQ subscales (0.67 to 0.82) and III subscales (0.64 to 0.68). This suggests that the OBQ and III subscales have adequate test–retest reliability as measures of enduring cognitive dispositions.

Criterion-related (Known Groups) Validity

To test criterion-related validity, the mean scores on the OBQ and III scales were compared among the four groups. On each scale, OCs scored significantly higher than CCs and SCs based on Student–Newman–Keuls post hoc comparisons. OCs also consistently scored higher than ACs, although the comparisons only reached statistical significance for the OBQ control of thoughts, importance of thoughts, and responsibility scales, and the III measures of control of thoughts and responsibility. In addition, on the III, OCs scored higher than ACs, CCs, and SCs on the single-item measures of recent, frequency and distress associated with the intrusive thoughts listed. The OBQ and III scales appear to have adequate criterion-related validity.

Convergent and Discriminant Validity

Analyses of the correlates of the OBQ and III were conducted separately within the OC and SC groups only. The OBQ and III scales tended to be highly correlated with one another. In addition, the mean *r* between corresponding OBQ and III subscales (e.g., OBQ Responsibility and III Responsibility) was 0.64 for the OCs and 0.55 for the SCs, supporting the convergent validity of the OBQ and III. For non-corresponding subscales (e.g., OBQ Responsibility and III Control of Thoughts), the mean *r* was 0.44 for the OCs and 0.49 for the SCs. Thus, the correlations between corresponding scales were only slightly higher than the correlations between non-corresponding scales, providing only modest support for the discriminant validity of the OBQ and III.

The OBQ and III scales were also correlated with the scales from the Revised Padua Inventory and measures of anxiety, worry, and depression. Each OBQ and III scale was significantly correlated with at least one of the Padua scales. However, for both the OCs and SCs, the correlations with the Revised Padua Inventory total score tended to be no bigger than the mean correlation with the measures of anxiety, worry, and depression. In other words, the OBQ and III are as strongly correlated with anxiety, worry, and depression, as they are with obsessions and compulsions. These findings raise concerns about the discriminant validity of the OBQ and III.

Discussion

The results of stage three analyses are broadly consistent with those of stage two; the OBQ and III generally performed well on indices of internal consistency, criterion-related validity, and convergent validity. Stage three findings suggest that the scales have moderate-to-high test–retest correlations. However, unlike the earlier findings the results of more recent analyses on a larger sample raise concerns about the discriminant validity of the OBQ and III scales.

The comparisons among groups support the criterion-related validity of the OBQ and III. In both sets of analyses, the OBQ and III scales discriminated OCs from normal controls (CCs and SCs), supporting the conclusion that the scales measure OC relevant beliefs and appraisals. As might be expected, some of the scales (in particular OBQ intolerance for uncertainty, overestimation of threat, and perfectionism) did not discriminate OCs from ACs. This suggests that rather than measuring OC-specific beliefs (i.e., beliefs specifically important in the genesis and maintenance of OCD rather than other anxiety disorders), these subscales of the OBQ measure beliefs common to anxiety disorders in general. Intrusive thoughts do occur in anxiety disorders other than OCD (e.g., catastrophic thoughts during panic attacks, worries in GAD, intrusive memories in post-traumatic stress disorder; see Ehlers & Clark, 2000; Taylor, 2000). Appraising such thoughts as highly important and significant, as well as holding general beliefs involving the overestimation of threat and perfectionism, could well play a role in non-OCD anxiety disorders. See Chapters five and six in this volume for more extensive reviews of this issue.

Readers who are interested in more detailed description of the results presented here, as well as additional information on the factor structure and other analyses, are referred to an article, currently in preparation by the OCCWG (in preparation).

Summary and Comment

The OBQ and III were developed by a large group of researchers and experts in the field and appear to show initial evidence of good psychometric properties. The collaborative endeavor undertaken by the OCCWG is unusual in several ways, and appears to offer considerable advantages for instrument development and assessment. Certainly, several such collaborations among researchers have been reported previously. Examples include U.S. government sponsored epidemiology and treatment studies, as well as projects such as the Harvard/Brown Anxiety Research Project funded by pharmaceutical companies and the U.S. government. Somewhat unique to the OCCWG is its international character, with researchers from nine countries participating at present. This international character will permit cross-cultural investigations to determine needed modifications in the instructions and/or items of instruments to suit other cultures. These studies are currently in progress (see Chapter 20 in this volume).

Because the group contained most of the leading theorists and researchers on cognition in OCD (e.g., D. A. Clark, Emmelkamp, Freeston, Rachman, Salkovskis), the instruments that resulted were largely theory driven and therefore fairly inclusive of hypothesized domains of beliefs and interpretations in OCD. Putting many theorists and clinical researchers of OCD in the same room permitted extensive dialogue regarding what aspects of cognition to study and how to study them. Obtaining consensus among these experts on definitions, item wording, and wording of instructions, especially for the priming of the III, required constant e-mail communication of co-chairs with members. It nonetheless proved a very workable strategy that resulted in two new instruments with exceptional face validity across experts.

The next challenge of testing the measures for psychometric properties also benefited from the size and range of skill among group members. After the entire group developed a basic plan for data collection, analyses and publication of results, within months subsets of members had collected data, developed a central database, identified specific steps for cleaning and processing data, and determined what analytical strategies would be employed and by whom. This process led to a remarkably rapid collection of a large pool of diagnosed subjects and non-clinical controls who completed a basic instrument package for initial analysis. Thus, the collaborative plan among multiple sites resulted in more rapid data collection and larger sample than would have been possible for individual or even small groups of investigators. In three stages of psychometric work on these instruments to date, it is clear that large groups of researchers can work collaboratively to advance assessment in newly developing fields. While it may not be feasible in some cases, collaborative instrument development and testing appears to have distinct advantages over individual investigations.

Author note: Preparation of this chapter was supported in part by grants to the first author from the British Columbia Health Research Foundation and from the Obsessive Compulsive Foundation.

References

Beck, A. T., & Emery, G. (1985). *Anxiety disorders and phobias: A cognitive perspective.* New York: Guilford.

Beck, A. T., Epstein, N., Brown, G., & Steer, R. A. (1988). An inventory for measuring clinical anxiety: Psychometric properties. *Journal of Consulting and Clinical Psychology, 56,* 893–897.

Beck, A. T., & Steer, R. A. (1993a). *Manual for the Beck Anxiety Inventory.* San Antonio, TX: Psychological Corporation.

Beck, A. T., & Steer, R. A. (1993b). *Manual for the Beck Depression Inventory.* San Antonio, TX: Psychological Corporation.

Brown, G. P., Craske, M. G., & Rassovsky, Y. (1995, July). *A new scale for measuring cognitive vulnerability to anxiety disorders: The Anxiety Attitude and Belief Scale.* Paper presented at the World Congress of Behavioural and Cognitive Therapies, Copenhagen, Denmark.

Burns, G. L., Keortge, S. G., Formea, G. M., & Sternberger, L. G. (1996). Revision of the Padua Inventory for obsessive compulsive disorder symptoms: Distinctions between worry, obsessions, and compulsions. *Behaviour Research and Therapy, 34,* 163–173.

Cartwright-Hatton, S., & Wells, A. (1997). Beliefs about worry and intrusions: The Meta-Cognitions Questionnaire and its correlates. *Journal of Anxiety Disorders, 11,* 279–96.

Clark, D. A., & Purdon, C. (1995, July). *Meta-cognitive beliefs in obsessive–compulsive disorders.* Paper presented at the World Congress of Behavioural and Cognitive Therapies, Copenhagen, Denmark.

Cottraux, J., Yao, S. N., Mollard, E., Bouvard, M., Note, I., Dartigues, J. F., Sauteraud, A., Lafont, S., Dubroca, B., & Bourgeois, M. (2000, March). *A multi-center controlled trial of cognitive therapy versus intensive behavior therapy.* Paper presented at the annual meeting of the Anxiety Disorders Association of America, Washington, D.C.

Ehlers, A., & Clark, D. M. (2000). A cognitive model of posttraumatic stress disorder. *Behaviour Research and Therapy, 38,* 319–345.

Eisen, J. L., Phillips, K. A., Baer, L., Beer, D. A., Atala, K. D., & Rasmussen, S. A. (1998). The Brown Assessment of Beliefs Scale: Reliability and validity. *American Journal of Psychiatry, 155,* 102–108.

Emmelkamp, P. M. G., & Beens, I. (1991). Cognitive therapy with OCD. A comparative evaluation. *Behaviour Research and Therapy, 29,* 293–300.

Emmelkamp, P. M. G., Visser, S., & Hoekstra, R. J. (1988). Cognitive therapy vs. exposure in vivo in the treatment of obsessive–compulsives. *Cognitive Therapy and Research, 12,* 103–114.

Foa, E. G., & Kozak, M. J. (1985). Treatment of anxiety disorders: Implications for psychopathology. In H.A. Tuma and J. D. Maser (eds), *Anxiety and the anxiety disorders.* Hillsdale, NJ: Lawrence Erlbaum Associates.

Foa, E. G., & Kozak, M. J. (1986). Emotional processing of fear: Exposure to corrective information. *Psychological Bulletin, 99*, 20–35.

Freeston, M. H., Rhéaume, J., & Ladouceur, R. (1996). Correcting faulty appraisals of obsessive thoughts. *Behaviour Research and Therapy, 34*, 443–446.

Freeston, M. H., Ladouceur, R, Gagnon, F., & Thibodeau, N. (1993). Beliefs about obsessional thoughts. *Journal of Psychopathology and Behavioral Assessment, 15*, 1–21.

Freeston, M. H., Ladouceur, R., Thibodeau, N., & Gagnon, F. (1991). Cognitive intrusions in a non-clinical population: I. Response style, subjective experience, and appraisal. *Behaviour Research and Therapy, 29*, 585–597.

Frost, R. O., Krause, M. S., McMahon, M. J., Peppe, J., Evans, M., McPhee, A. E., & Holden, M. (1993). Compulsivity and superstitiousness. *Behaviour Research and Therapy, 31*, 423–425.

Frost, R. O., Marten, P., Lahart, C., & Rosenblate, R. (1990). The dimensions of perfectionism. *Cognitive Therapy and Research, 14*, 449–468.

Goodman, W. K., Price, L. H., Rasmussen, S. A., Mazure, C., Fleischmann, R. C., Hill, C. L., Heninger, G. R., & Charney, D. S. (1989). The Yale–Brown Obsessive–Compulsive Scale: I. Development, use, and reliability. *Archives of General Psychiatry, 46*, 1006–1011.

Hedlund, S., & Oppelt, B. (1998, November). *Intermediate-level beliefs in OCD: A new instrument to evaluate cognitive specificity — "OCD Meta-Inventory".* Paper presented at the annual meeting of the Association for Advancement of Behavior Therapy, Washington, DC.

Hewitt, P. L., & Flett, G. L. (1991). Perfectionism in the self and social contexts: Conceptualization, assessment, and association with psychopathology. *Journal of Personality and Social Psychology, 60*, 456–470.

Hoekstra, R. J. (1995). *Obsessive–Compulsive Cognitions List.* Unpublished scale, Research Office, Faculty of Medicine, Limburg University, Maastricht, The Netherlands.

Jones, R. (1968). *A factored measure of Ellis' irrational belief system with personality and maladjustment correlates.* Unpublished doctoral dissertation, Texas Technical College, Lubbock, TX.

Klass, E. (1987). Situational approach to assessment of gulit: development and validation of a self-report measure. *Journal of Psychopathology and Behavioral Assessment, 9*, 35–48.

Koopmans, P. C., Sanderman, R., Timmerman, I., & Emmelkamp, P. M. G. (1994). The Irrational Beliefs Inventory: Development and psychometric evaluation. *European Journal of Psychological Assessment, 10*, 15–27.

Kozak, M., & Foa, E. (1994). Obsessions, overvalued ideas, and delusions in obsessive–compulsive disorder. *Behaviour Research and Therapy, 32*, 343–353.

Kugler, K., & Jones, W. H. (1992). On conceptualizing and assessing guilt. *Journal of Personality and Social Psychology, 62*, 318–327.

Kyrios, M., & Bahr, S. S. (1995, July). *A measure of inflated responsibility: its development and relationship to obsessive–compulsive phenomena.* Paper presented at the World Congress of Behavioural and Cognitive Therapies, Copenhagen, Denmark.

Ladouceur, R., Leger, E., Rhéaume, J., & Dube, D. (1996). Correction of inflated responsibility in the treatment of obsessive–compulsive disorder. *Behaviour Research and Therapy, 34*, 767–774.

McLean, P. D., Whittal, M. L., Thordarson, D. S., Taylor, S., Söchting, I., Koch, W. J., Paterson, R., & Anderson, K. W. (2001). Cognitive versus behavior therapy in group treatment of obsessive compulsive disorder. *Journal of Consulting and Clinical Psychology, 69*, 205–214.

Meyer, T. J., Miller, R. L., Metzger, R. L., & Borkovec, T. D. (1990). Development and validation of the Penn State Worry Questionnaire. *Behaviour Research and Therapy, 28*, 487–495.

Neziroglu, F., McKay, D., Yaryura-Tobias, J. A., Stevens, K. P., & Todaro, J. (1999). The overvalued ideas scale: development, reliability and validity in obsessive–compulsive disorder. *Behaviour Research and Therapy, 37,* 881–902.

Obsessive Compulsive Cognitions Working Group. (1997). Cognitive assessment of obsessive–compulsive disorder. *Behaviour Research and Therapy, 35,* 667–681.

Obsessive Compulsive Cognitions Working Group (2001). Development and initial validation of the Obsessive Beliefs Questionnaire and the Interpretation of Intrusions Inventory. *Behaviour Research and Therapy, 39,* 987–1006.

Obsessive Compulsive Cognitions Working Group (in preparation). *The Obsessive Beliefs Questionnaire and the Interpretation of Intrusions Inventory: Findings of stage 3.* Unpublished manuscript.

Rachman (1997). A cognitive theory of obsessions. *Behaviour Research and Therapy, 35,* 793–802.

Rhéaume, J., Freeston, M. H., Dugas, M. J., Letarte, H., & Ladouceur, R. (1995). Perfectionism, responsibility and obsessive–compulsive symptoms. *Behaviour Research and Therapy, 33,* 785–794.

Rhéaume, J., Ladouceur, R., Freeston, M. H., & Letarte, H. (1994). Inflated responsibility in obsessive–compulsive disorder: psychometric studies of a semi-idiographic measure. *Journal of Psychopathology and Behavioral Assessment, 16,* 265–276.

Robb, H. B., & Warren, R. (1990). Irrational belief tests: New insights, new directions. *Journal of Cognitive Psychotherapy, 4,* 303–311.

Salkovskis, P. M. (1985). Obsessional-compulsive problems: A cognitive-behavioural analysis. *Behaviour Research and Therapy, 23,* 571–583.

Salkovskis, P. M. (1989). Cognitive-behavioural factors and the persistence of intrusive thoughts in obsessional problems. *Behaviour Research and Therapy, 27,* 677–682.

Salkovskis, P. M., & Warwick, H. (1985). Cognitive therapy of obsessive–compulsive disorder: Treating treatment failures. *Behavioural Psychotherapy, 13,* 243–255.

Salkovskis, P. M., Wroe, A. L., Gledhil, A., Morrison, N., Forrester, E., Richards, C., Reynolds, M., & Thorpe, S. (2000). Responsibility attitudes and interpretations are characteristic of obsessive compulsive disorder. *Behaviour Research and Therapy, 38,* 347–372.

Sanavio, E. (1988). Obsessions and compulsions: The Padua Inventory. *Behaviour Research and Therapy, 26,* 169–177.

Shafran, R., Thordarson, D. S., & Rachman, S. (1996). Thought–action fusion in obsessive compulsive disorder. *Journal of Anxiety Disorders, 10,* 379–391.

Shorkey, C. T., & Whiteman, V. L. (1977). Development of the Rational Behavior Inventory: Initial validity and reliability. *Educational and Psychological Measurement, 37,* 527–534.

Sookman, D., & Pinard, G. (1995, July). *The Cognitive Schemata Scale: A multidimensional measure of cognitive schemas in obsessive compulsive disorder.* Paper presented at the World Congress of Behavioural and Cognitive Therapies, Copenhagen, Denmark.

Sookman, D. Pinard, G., & Beauchemin, N. (1994). Multidimensional schematic restructuring treatment for obsessions: Theory and practice. *Journal of Cognitive Psychotherapy, 8,* 175–194.

Sookman, D., Pinard, G., & Engelsmann, F. (1995, unpublished). The Obsessive Compulsive Disorder Cognitive Schemata Scale: Reliability and validity.

Spielberger, C. D. (1983). *Manual for the State-Trait Anxiety Inventory (Form Y).* Palo Alto, CA: Consulting Psychologists Press.

Steketee, G., & Foa, E. B. (1985). Obsessive compulsive disorder. In D. H. Barlow (ed.), *Clinical handbook of psychological disorders.* New York: Guilford.

Steketee, G., Frost, R. O., & Cohen, I. (1998). Beliefs in obsessive–compulsive disorder. *Journal of Anxiety Disorders, 12,* 525–537.

Tallis, F. (1995). *Obsessional Beliefs Scale.* Unpublished scale, Charter Nightingale Hospital, London, UK.

Taylor, S. (2000). *Understanding and treating panic disorder: Cognitive-behavioural approaches.* New York: Wiley.

Van Oppen, P., & Arntz, A. (1994). Cognitive therapy for obsessive compulsive disorder. *Behaviour Research and Therapy, 32,* 79–87.

van Oppen, P., de Haan, E., van Balkom, A. J. L. M., Spinhoven, P., Hoogduin, K., & van Dyck, R. (1995). Cognitive therapy and exposure in vivo in the treatment of obsessive–compulsive disorder. *Behaviour Research and Therapy, 33,* 379–390.

Weissman, A. N. (1980). *Assessing depressogenic attitudes: A validation study.* Paper presented at the annual meeting of the Eastern Psychological Association, Hartford, CT.

Yao, S.-N., Cottraux, J., & Martin, R. (1999). Une étude contrôlee sur les Interprétations Irrationnelles des Pensées Intrusives dan le trouble obsessionel compulsif. *L'Encéphale, 25,* 461–469.

Chapter 8

Experimental Methods for Studying Cognition

John H. Riskind, Nathan L. Williams and Michael Kyrios

Introduction

Obsessive compulsive disorder (OCD) is associated with some of the worst impairments observed among the anxiety disorders and is rated as the tenth leading cause of disability by the World Health Organization (WHO, 1996). Recent research advances have increased our understanding of the cognitive phenomenology of OCD, as well as its information-processing correlates, and approaches to assessment and treatment. While much research has used correlational data based on questionnaire responses, issues relating to the nature and direction of causal relations between cognition and OCD symptoms or phenomena (e.g., checking, neutralization, hoarding) may be better dealt with through the use of experimental manipulations (Garber & Hollon, 1991). Experimental methods for studying cognition can also provide a wealth of information that could improve our ability to design useful clinical interventions and to assess treatment outcomes.

In this chapter we present a review of experimental methods for studying cognition in OCD. The first section of the chapter provides a conceptual foundation and addresses experimental methods used to study the six domains of cognition that have been identified by the Obsessive Compulsive Cognitions Working Group (OCCWG, 1997). These domains include responsibility, over importance of thoughts, control of thoughts, overestimation of threat, tolerance for uncertainty, and perfectionism. The second section describes experimental methods for studying related domains of cognition and dysfunctional personality processes that may influence or overlap with the six central OCD domains. These related domains are categorized into cognitive–behavioral variables (e.g., looming vulnerability) and affective variables (e.g., guilt). The third section reviews experimental methods that may be used in clinical interventions and in the assessment of treatment outcomes and thus has a more applied focus. The fourth section briefly reviews neuropsychological assessment of OCD as it pertains to the domains of cognition. In the final section, we present recommendations for future research on OCD. While the present review is by no means comprehensive, we aim to highlight the most commonly employed and/or promising methodologies for studying cognition in OCD. We hope that readers will find this chapter useful in conceptualizing future research, synthesizing past research methodologies, and refining measurement techniques and operationalizations of OCD-relevant concepts.

Cognitive Approaches to Obsessions and Compulsions – Theory, Assessment, and Treatment
Copyright © 2002 by Elsevier Science Ltd.
All rights of reproduction in any form reserved.
ISBN: 0-08-043410-X

Methods Used in Studying Domains of Beliefs Related to OCD

Responsibility

Conceptual considerations and general assessment. Distorted appraisals of responsibility have received attention in OCD research and cognitive theories for over 15 years and are reviewed in detail in Chapter four of this volume. Briefly, Salkovskis (1985, 1989) proposed that individuals who experience an exaggerated sense of personal responsibility to prevent intrusive thoughts, or the outcomes such thoughts imply, feel an increased urgency that impels them to neutralize and/or suppress thoughts, which can paradoxically increase their occurrence. The definition of inflated responsibility, as it relates to OCD, has undergone a number of refinements since Salkovskis' pivotal 1985 paper (e.g., Salkovskis *et al.*, 1996).

Inflated responsibility has been examined using a variety of methods, including self-report questionnaires, experimental methods aimed at increasing or decreasing subjects' sense of personal responsibility, and clinical treatment studies that target responsibility. Evidence to support the connection between distorted appraisals of responsibility and OCD is provided by clinical findings (e.g., Lopatka, 1994; Salkovskis, 1985; Tallis, 1994; van Oppen & Arntz, 1994), correlational studies (e.g., Freeston, Ladouceur, Thibodeau, & Gagnon, 1992; Rhéaume, Freeston, Dugas, Letarte, & Ladouceur, 1995; Rhéaume, Ladouceur, Freeston, & Letarte, 1995; Salkovskis, 1989; Salkovskis, Shafran, Rachman, & Freeston, 1999) and experimental manipulation studies (e.g., Ladouceur *et al.*, 1995; Lopatka & Rachman, 1995; Shafran, 1997).

While the majority of studies provide support for the expected associations between distorted appraisals of responsibility and OCD symptoms (e.g., Salkovskis *et al.*, 2000), other studies have found only minimal (e.g., Steketee, Frost, & Cohen, 1998) or non-significant relationships (e.g., Frost, Steketee, Cohen, & Griess, 1994). These discrepant findings indicate the need for a more tightly defined operational definition of responsibility. Recently, Salkovskis and colleagues have proposed such a definition in terms of exaggerated "beliefs that one has power which is pivotal to bring about or prevent subjectively crucial negative outcomes" that are "perceived as essential to prevent" (Salkovskis *et al.*, 1996).

There is also evidence that distorted appraisals of OCD-related responsibility may represent a multidimensional construct, and that it may hold greater significance for obsessional symptoms associated with compulsive checking in OCD (Rachman, 1998) than for those associated with compulsive washing or fears of contamination (Riskind & Williams, 2000). Thus, while correlational studies generally support the expected associations between responsibility and OCD, they also highlight the importance of establishing an accepted operationalization of responsibility and examining its generality across obsessive and compulsive domains.

Experimental investigations. Experimental investigations of inflated responsibility have addressed whether direct manipulations of beliefs about responsibility lead to corresponding changes in OCD symptomatology or task performance. Responsibility appraisals have been manipulated in a variety of ways. For example, a typical manipulation involves directly varying the degree of personal responsibility taken by the subject or experimenter during a personally threatening task. A typical indirect manipulation of personal responsibility involves varying the absence or presence of the experimenter during a personally threatening task. A third approach has involved directly varying instructions during a cognitive task (e.g. memory and classification task) to assess changes in performance. The two former methodologies have been conducted using predominantly clinical samples with positive results, while the latter methodology has been applied to both clinical and non-clinical cohorts with mixed results.

Lopatka and Rachman (1995) assessed the influence of directly varying levels of perceived responsibility on compulsive checking and cleaning behavior. All subjects participated in a control condition in which cleaning or checking urges were provoked. The experimental manipulation involved increasing or decreasing subjects' perceived responsibility for an anticipated negative event. For example, in the high responsibility condition subjects were told: "You are responsible for anything that happens or anything that is not perfect as a result of not checking." Conversely, participants in the low responsibility condition were told that the experimenter would take complete responsibility if anything undesirable happened. Following the experimental manipulation, subjects took part in an individually tailored behavioral approach test that involved exposing the individual to an object/situation where s/he usually cleans or checks (e.g. "We would like you to lock the door and then walk away from it without checking it at all."). Consistent with expectations, results suggested that subjects with OCD experienced a steep decline in compulsive checking urges when they transferred their sense of responsibility for the anticipated consequences of their actions to the experimenter (i.e., the low responsibility condition). Likewise, increased responsibility was followed by increased urges to check, but this effect was not as large perhaps due to the result of a ceiling effect for responsibility. Similar results were reported by Shafran (1997) who manipulated responsibility indirectly by varying the absence or presence of the experimenter during a behavioral task.

In a study that manipulated responsibility by varying instructions during a cognitive task, the Laval group found that increased responsibility was associated with more checking and slower completion times on a classification task in a nonclinical sample (Ladouceur *et al.*, 1995). The induction of responsibility consisted of informing participants that their responses on a color classification task (for various pills) had potentially serious consequences, as it could directly influence the manufacture of an anti-viral medication for distribution in a poor Southeast Asian country. As expected, participants in the high responsibility condition exhibited increased hesitation and checking behavior during the task, as well as increased preoccupation with avoiding errors and greater anxiety. A second experiment, however, only partially replicated these findings using a different sound recognition task; investigators found similar results for increases in anxiety in the high responsibility condition, but no effects for the experimental manipulation of responsibility on checking behavior.

Using a variation of the Laval group's manipulation, Kyrios and Bhar (1997) examined the effects of responsibility on a memory classification task. This study highlights an important complication in the experimental manipulation of responsibility appraisals. Contrary to expectations, and despite confirming an increased sense of personal responsibility and anxiety following the manipulation, participants in the high responsibility condition exhibited improved performance on a number of computer-based measures. These included decreased frequency and time spent checking, decreases in total time taken to complete the task, increased number of correct versus incorrect responses, and decreased number of unsure responses. Moreover, this improvement in performance after the high responsibility induction was found both in an OCD clinical sample and a non-clinical sample. These paradoxical findings suggest that responsibility manipulations may not invariably provoke behavior intended to prevent mistakes behavior, but rather, under certain circumstances, may help individuals to become more task focused. Further-more, laboratory manipulations of responsibility may be limited in their ecological validity, in that participants may not have related their responsibility to the task at hand in the same way as they might in a real life situation. Thus, some laboratory manipulation studies may instate a reasonable sense of responsibility, rather than the overvalued responsibility emphasized by theoretical discourse on OCD (e.g., Salkovskis *et al.*, 2000).

A further difficulty associated with experimental manipulations of responsibility is that some studies may not isolate responsibility beliefs, or relevant aspects of responsibility beliefs, with unalloyed purity. For example, it is often difficult to ascertain both which aspect of responsibility has been manipulated in experimental studies and which con-comitant domains of cognition have been affected by manipulations of responsibility. Given the multidimensional nature of responsibility in obsessional problems (e.g., Kyrios & Bhar, 1995; Rachman, Shafran, Mitchell, Trant, & Teachman, 1996; Shafran, Thordarson, & Rachman, 1995; Salkovskis *et al.*, 2000), researchers would be wise to provide evidence of subjects' experience during experimental manipulations, perhaps through the use of ratings of beliefs and appraisals during and after experimental procedures.

Treatment outcome studies that intervene specifically with one OCD-related belief (such as responsibility) may also be useful in exploring the relationship between specific beliefs and OCD symptoms. For instance, Ladouceur, Leger, Rhéaume, and Dube (1996) used cognitive therapy to correct responsibility beliefs in OCD patients with checking rituals without any exposure or response prevention. As expected, cognitively treated patients who experienced decreases in perceived responsibility showed corresponding reductions in checking rituals.

Summary. In general, there is compelling evidence to support an association between distorted appraisals of personal responsibility and OCD, particularly its association with obsessional phenomena and compulsive checking symptoms. Experimental manipulations of responsibility have provided support for the cognitive model advanced by Salkovskis (1985, 1989) and Rachman (1997, 1998), although these studies have demonstrated occasional, but revealing, difficulties. A more explicit and tightly defined operational definition of responsibility in OCD may facilitate more consistent findings.

Overall, five considerations appear warranted for future research: (a) the development of standardized responsibility manipulation methods that lead to more consistent results; (b) improved understanding of factors that influence success or failure of such manipula-tions; (c) assessments of which aspects of responsibility and concomitant domains of cognition have been affected by responsibility manipulations; (d) greater examination of the generalizability of responsibility-related findings to a range of OCD symptom types (e.g., obsessional fears of contamination and compulsive cleaning behaviors); and (e) longitudinal studies to address the vulnerability that distorted appraisals of responsibility may confer in real life situations.

Beliefs About the Nature and Control of Intrusions and Associated Cognitive Responses

Conceptual considerations and general assessment. A further spectrum of cognitive factors relating to obsessional problems includes: (a) the importance assigned to particular intrusions (i.e., thoughts, urges and images); (b) beliefs about the intrusions themselves (e.g., "sexual or violent thoughts are unacceptable and dangerous"; "having an unacceptable thought is morally equivalent to acting out the content of the thought"); (c) the conviction that particular intrusions must be controlled and kept out of conscious awareness; (d) strategies, often cognitive in nature, that are used to control unwanted intrusions (e.g., thought suppression) or mitigate the threat associated with them (e.g., mental checking, praying); and (e) perceptions about failure to control such intrusions (e.g., self-appraisals of oneself as a failure because of an inability to suppress unwanted thoughts). Such beliefs about intrusions and associated cognitive responses have most often been examined via questionnaire-based research methods focusing on intrusive thoughts in non-clinical cohorts. While some researchers are beginning to use idiographic or semi-idiographic measures of appraisals about a wider range of specific intrusions with clinical subjects, experimental methods with non-clinical cohorts have been used mostly in the study of responses to intrusions rather than beliefs per se.

Cognitive models of OCD emphasize distinct aspects of this spectrum of beliefs that are considered critical both to the experience of distress and to the motivation to engage in behaviors such as neutralizing, thought suppression, reassurance seeking, and avoidance as a response to the experience of unwanted intrusions (Salkovskis *et al.*, 1999; Rachman, 1997). Individuals who suffer from recurrent obsessions commonly attach exaggerated significance to intrusive thoughts and regard them as horrific, repugnant, threatening, and/ or dangerous (e.g., Freeston, Ladouceur, Gagnon, & Thibodeau, 1993). Rachman (1997) noted that such individuals commonly describe their intrusive thoughts as immoral, sinful, disgusting, dangerous, threatening, alarming, insane, bewildering and criminal. A related factor, thought–action fusion (TAF; Shafran *et al.*, 1995; Rachman *et al.*, 1996) is a cognitive bias towards the conviction that having abhorrent intrusive thoughts is the moral equivalent to endorsing the thoughts or carrying them out. TAF also involves a bias to believe that having such thoughts increases the probability that the implied repugnant actions or outcomes will reach fruition. A body of evidence is emerging to support the association between TAF and OCD (e.g., Freeston, Rhéaume, & Ladouceur, 1996). More recently, Clark, Purdon, and Byers (2000) reported that TAF was a significant unique predictor of the perceived controllability of university students' most upsetting sexual and non-sexual intrusive thoughts.

Purdon and Clark (1994a, b) have suggested that higher-order meta-cognitive beliefs about the importance and subjective meaning of obsessional thoughts are major predictors of both the development and persistence of obsessional thinking. For example, Purdon and Clark (1994b) provided evidence that the belief that one could act on a noxious thought or obsession and the perceived uncontrollability of the noxious thought were the two most important predictors of the frequency and/or persistence of distressing intrusions in a non-clinical sample. Moreover, intrusive thoughts that were rated difficult to control were associated with an increased belief that one could act on the intrusion, avoidance of situations that may trigger the intrusion, higher thought frequency, and reduced success with one's most typical thought control strategy. Further, using their Revised Obsessive Intrusions Inventory (ROII; Clark & Purdon, 1993; Purdon & Clark, 1994a), they found that individuals interpret intrusive thoughts as revealing important but usually hidden elements in their character.

Clark and Purdon have suggested that a more fine grained analysis of meta-cognitive beliefs about thought controllability (e.g., "I should be able to control my thoughts") and the associated urge to control thoughts is necessary to advance our understanding of thought controllability as an appraisal dimension (e.g., Clark & Purdon, 1995; Purdon, 1998; Purdon & Clark, 1994a). A similar point is supported by Wells and colleagues' findings that meta-beliefs about the efficacy of one's thought control strategies, the threat that different types of cognitions may represent, and the advantages of worry may all contribute to decreased controllability and increased frequency of worrisome thoughts (e.g., Wells & Davies, 1994; Wells & Papageoriou, 1997). Results from a recent study indicate that positive beliefs about worry predicted checking compulsions, whereas negative beliefs (e.g., "My worrying thoughts are uncontrollable") independently predicted washing compulsions (Wells & Papageoriou, 1997). These results suggest that more fine-grained measures of meta-cognitive beliefs may have utility in understanding the relevant cognitive appraisal dimensions in OCD.

Given that OCD is associated with a tendency to appraise intrusions as requiring control and preventative or compensatory action, it is not surprising that various researchers have examined the thought control strategies used in response to the experience of unwanted thoughts. However, there is little information about the relationships between specific thought control strategies and beliefs about thoughts. Although it is likely that various OCD-related belief systems may be responsible for attempts at thought control, little research has investigated specific associations. The lack of experimental research in this area is particularly evident. Nonetheless, questionnaire-based research has found that OCD patients seem to use more thought suppression, punishment, worry, reappraisal and social control strategies, while distraction strategies have been reported in non-clinical subjects (Amir, Cashman, & Foa, 1998). In a comparison of control strategies for upsetting thoughts, Clark *et al.* (2000) indicated that cognitive and behavioral distraction, cognitive restructuring, reassurance seeking from self and others, and thought stopping were used significantly more often in response to subjects' most upsetting sexual versus non-sexual intrusions. Interestingly, women were found to report engaging more often in thought control efforts to suppress their unwanted intrusions, contradicting earlier findings (Freeston, Ladouceur, Thibodeau, & Gagnon, 1991). Nonetheless, assessment of the frequency of intrusive thoughts has relied on self-report irrespective of whether the research is experimental or questionnaire-based. There is a need for researchers to seek out new technologies to assess cognitive activity with regard to the experience of intrusive thoughts.

Experimental investigations. In a rare experimental study, Salkovskis, Westbrook, Davis, Jeavons, and Gledhill (1997) compared the short- and long-term effects of neutralizing and distraction of personally relevant distressing thoughts in non-clinical subjects. They found that in the short-term neutralizing led to decreased distress, but in the longer-term high distress was maintained. Conversely, distraction from the distressing thought led to long-term decreases in distress, but relatively stable short-term distress ratings. However, to date, no published study has examined directly the underlying appraisal substrates of such effects during this type of experimental manipulation.

Experimental studies of thought suppression provide additional support for the role of control strategies (e.g., see Purdon, 1999 for a review; Wegner, Schneider, Carter, & White, 1987). Thought suppression is one of the most common control strategies employed to exclude unwanted thoughts (Amir *et al.*, 1998). Wegner (1994) suggests that the process of thought suppression itself is sufficient to maintain obsessions. There is growing theoretical unanimity that avoiding a stressful thought can lead to subsequent intrusions of the thought (Horowitz, 1975; Wegner *et al.*, 1987). Wegner and colleagues have termed this phenomenon the "rebound effect" and have successfully demonstrated its occurrence in nonclinical cohorts (e.g., Wegner *et al.*, 1987).

The rebound effect is one of two phenomena that have been linked to thought suppression. The "enhancement effect" refers to the paradoxical effect that thought suppression instructions have on increasing rather than decreasing target thought product. However, these phenomena have not been reliably replicated in research to date. Thus, Muris, Merckelbach, van den Hout, and de Jong (1992) reported initial enhancement, but not rebound, with neutral but not with emotional material. Clark, Ball, and Pape (1991) and Clark, Winton, and Thynn (1993) did not observe enhancement, but were successful in demonstrating a rebound effect. The variability in results could be a reflection of the great variability in the thought suppression paradigms utilized, in terms of stimuli (e.g. neutral, negative), measures (e.g., bell rings, verbalization) and design (suppression and expression only).

Recently, Salkovskis and Campbell (1994) argued that examining individuals' responses while they try to suppress personally relevant intrusive thoughts is more appropriate to the study of obsessionality than examining responses to suppression of experimenter-provided thoughts. In their study, Salkovskis and Campbell (1994) observed an enhancement effect when they asked subjects to suppress personally relevant, naturally occurring negative thoughts over time. Another study also observed an enhancement effect after four days outside the laboratory (Trinder & Salkovskis, 1994), demonstrating that such an effect is not confined to the laboratory setting. On the other hand, Janeck and Calamari (2000) failed to find either rebound or enhancement effects in their study of thought suppression of a personally relevant, naturally occurring intrusive thought over time. Several other studies investigating this paradigm also failed to observe true rebound/ enhancement (Ruthledge, 1996; Smari, Sigurjonsdottir, & Sacmundsdottir, 1994), although differences in success at suppression have generally been shown to relate to obsessionality. Despite a plethora of studies examining the effects of thought suppression, there is relatively little experimental research investigating the relationship of OCD-related beliefs about thoughts and thought suppression outcomes.

Summary. In sum, proponents of cognitive models of OCD have proposed that negative appraisals of intrusions cause significant distress/discomfort and are followed by subsequent control efforts (e.g., neutralization, thought suppression). Paradoxically, these may increase the frequency of the thoughts and maintain this maladaptive cycle. While many studies provide compelling evidence for an association between the perceived controllability of thoughts and variables related to intrusive thought frequency and obsessional symptoms, the generalizability or specificity of results is limited by the fact that few studies have examined clinical samples. Moreover, given the relationship between ineffective thought control strategies and other forms of psychopathology (e.g., depression), further studies are needed to examine the specific causal mechanisms by which suppression strategies confer specific vulnerability to OCD.

Experimental studies are also necessary to provide additional criterion-related validity for existing measures of thought control beliefs and strategies. Procedures implemented by Wegner (1989, 1994) and adapted by Salkovskis and colleagues (Reynolds & Salkovskis, 1991; Salkovskis & Campbell, 1994; Salkovskis *et al.*, 1997; Trinder & Salkovskis, 1994) provide useful methodological guidelines for evaluating the consequences of thought control strategies. However, experimental manipulation of beliefs, as distinct from control strategies, has proved difficult to achieve. Finally, experimental analyses that directly examine manipulations of the importance that people ascribe to intrusions are necessary. Useful methodologies for future studies may be drawn from the social-cognitive literature addressing the extent to which attitudes predict behaviors (e.g., Bonninger, Krosnick & Berent, 1995; Krosnick, 1988).

Overestimation of Threat

Conceptual considerations and general assessment. Another cognitive appraisal variable that has been implicated in the pathogenesis and maintenance of OCD is the extent to which individuals overestimate the amount and severity of threat in the environment and threat associated with noxious thoughts or obsessions (e.g., Beck, 1976; Beck & Emery, 1985; Rachman, 1998; Salkovskis, 1989, 1998). As with other domains of OCD-related beliefs, more fine-grained analyses of the concept of threat may be required. For example, some models focus on the role of overestimates of the probability and consequences of noxious outcomes (e.g., Beck & Emery, 1985; Salkovskis, 1996), whereas other models emphasize overestimates of the dynamic intensification of "looming danger" as the quintessential cognitive element of the phenomenology of threat (e.g., Riskind, 1997; Riskind & Williams, in press).

Cognitions about danger and potential catastrophic outcomes have been identified in many individuals with OCD (e.g., Emmelkamp, 1987: Foa, 1979; Frost *et al.*, 1994; Jones & Menzies, 1998a; Yaryura-Tobias & Neziroglu, 1983). Individuals with OCD or obsessive compulsive symptoms have been shown to overestimate the probability and consequences of threatening events (e.g., Yaryura-Tobias & Neziroglu, 1983), as well as the rate at which perceived risk is rapidly rising or "looming" (Riskind & Williams, 2000). For example, obsessional fears may be triggered by exaggerated beliefs about the speed with which contaminants can spread, or rate at which abhorrent outcomes are approaching.

Evaluations of individuals' perceptions of threat associated with noxious thoughts can be indirectly inferred via items that assess unpleasantness, unacceptability, disapproval, perceived harm or responsibility, and affective variables such as guilt, anxiety, and depression (e.g., Purdon & Clark, 1994a).

Many of the same instruments, methodologies, and studies that have been discussed in the preceding sections provide evidence for a significant association between the overestimation of threat and obsessional thinking or OCD. For example, Freeston and colleagues provide evidence for an association between disapproval ratings and more obsessional, anxious, and depressive symptoms in non-clinical cohorts (Freeston *et al.*, 1991). Likewise, the studies by Rachman and colleagues and Salkovskis and colleagues support associations between responsibility and OCD and/or obsessional thinking. The experimental analyses of responsibility may be further interpreted to suggest that higher levels of perceived threat are associated with increased discomfort, increased urges to engage in compulsive behavior, and increased probability and likelihood ratings of noxious thoughts reaching fruition (e.g., Lopatka & Rachman, 1995). However, two general limitations of this research include an over-reliance on indirect measures of threat estimation(s) and a focus on non-clinical cohorts.

Experimental investigations. While the majority of studies have inferred threat estimation indirectly or via verbal analogue or self-report ratings, several studies have examined the independent influence of threat estimation in OCD. For example, Jones and Menzies (1997) examined the roles of danger expectancies and other cognitive variables (i.e., responsibility, perfectionism, anticipated anxiety, and self-efficacy) in a sample of diagnosed OCD washers. In this study, they provide evidence that danger expectancies were the most likely mediator of compulsive behavior in OCD washers. In a second study, Jones and Menzies (1998a) examined the effects of experimental manipulations of perceived danger in a behavioral avoidance task (BAT) on OCD washers' levels of anxiety, avoidance, and compulsive behavior. The manipulation involved varying the instructions that participants were given prior to the BAT. Consistent with predictions, they found that individuals in the high danger condition report higher mean ratings of anxiety, avoidance, and the urge to engage in compulsive washing than did those in the low danger condition. Finally, Jones and Menzies (1998b) provide evidence in a treatment outcome study of danger ideation reduction therapy (DIRT) for compulsive washers that decreases danger-related expectancies related to contamination resulted in decreased obsessive compulsive symptomatology, anxiety, and depression compared to a control condition.

Several other experimental methodologies are relevant to an examination of threat-related cognitions and expectancies in obsessional thinking and OCD. While these studies do not directly address the overestimation of threat in OCD, they suggest useful methodologies for further consideration. For example, Taylor and Rachman (1994) have addressed the issue of over-prediction of fear in a series of experimental analyses that employed methodologies drawn from cognitive–experimental psychology. These investigators had spider-phobics participate in a fear-relevant priming task in which they were asked to provide a detailed written account of a fearful experience with a spider. Next, participants took part in a predict-report task in which they were told that the task required approaching a container that had a 50 percent chance of containing a spider, removing the cover and touching the inside base. Participants were asked to provide verbal analogue ratings of fear after hearing the instructions and while approaching the container. As predicted, spider-phobics reported significantly greater fear predictions and higher levels of fear as they approached the container. Other relevant experimental tasks include primed lexical decision tasks (e.g., Bradley, Mogg, & Williams, 1994), modifications of the Stroop Task (e.g., Foa, Ilai, McCarthy, Shoyer, & Murdock, 1993), and other implicit and explicit memory tasks for fear-relevant processing (e.g., Radomsky & Rachman, 1999; Riskind, Williams, Gessner, Chrosniak, & Cortina, 2000). However, inconsistencies from the results of such studies may indicate the limitations of some of these tasks for use in OCD research (e.g., Kyrios & Iob, 1998).

Summary. Considerable research evidence supports between the over-estimations of threat and obsessional thinking and OCD. The most pressing limitations of most studies on this relationship is that they indirectly infer individual's estimations of threat from other variables, are correlational in nature and do not address causality or directionality of the relationship, and are conducted on non-clinical populations. The findings of Jones and Menzies, using both experimental and correlational methodologies are promising in that they more directly assess the role of threat estimations in OCD. More fine-grained analyses of the relationship between threat estimations and other OCD-relevant domains of cognition (e.g., responsibility, importance and controllability of thoughts, etc.) seem essential to advancing our understanding of this construct. Information-processing tasks drawn from the cognitive–experimental literature may provide one method by which such fine-grained analyses might be achieved.

Tolerance for Uncertainty

Conceptual considerations and general assessment. According to cognitive models, beliefs that reflect an intolerance of uncertainty are associated with OCD and obsessional thinking. The importance of this domain is indicated by clinical evidence and research that highlights the phenomena of uncertainty and doubting (e.g., Antony, Purdon, Huta, & Swinson, 1998; Frost & Steketee, 1997; Summerfeldt, Huta, & Swinson, 1998). For example, using Cloninger's (1987) Tridimensional Personality Questionnaire, Richter, Summerfeldt, Joffe, and Swinson (1996) reported that individuals with OCD had a strong fear of uncertainty. Another study by Steketee, Frost, and Cohen (1998) found that OCD patients had higher scores on a self-report measure of beliefs associated with intolerance of uncertainty than other anxiety disorder patients or normal controls. Moreover, the beliefs about uncertainty measures afforded significant explanatory power beyond the effects of mood state and worry, and predicted severity of OCD symptoms beyond other beliefs that were measured.

A potentially important conceptual limitation of the existing research is that uncertainty may be a multidimensional construct. For instance, in constructing a general model of anxiety, Krohne (1989, 1993) distinguished between intolerance of uncertainty and intolerance of emotional arousal. While it is suggested that hypervigilance is triggered by uncertain or ambiguous situations, cognitive avoidance reactions are thought to result from an intolerance of emotional arousal. Previous work in the broader literature has indicated additional important distinctions between different types of uncertainty, including outcome uncertainty, temporal uncertainty, and outcome variability. For example, outcome uncertainty refers to ambiguity about whether a given outcome will occur (e.g., a clinical doctoral student might ask "Will I match for a clinical internship?"), while temporal uncertainty refers to ambiguity about when a given event will occur (e.g., "When will I hear about my internship placement?"). Finally, outcome variability refers to the degree of ambiguity in the possible range of outcomes that could occur (e.g., "I could receive my top choice of placements, I could receive my last choice of placements, or I could receive no placement at all."). While these distinct forms of uncertainty need not be equally relevant to OCD, finer-grained analysis of each component and investigation of their relevance to cognitive theories of OCD is warranted.

Experimental investigations. The expected link between an exaggerated need for certainty and OCD has been supported by several experimental studies (e.g., Steketee *et al.*, 1998; Rode, Cosmides, Hell, & Tooby, 1999). For example, over the past several decades, several studies have shown that individuals with OCD need more information before making decisions than do other people (Steketee *et al.*, 1998; Richter *et al.*, 1996). In early experiments on the uncertainty phenomenon, Milner, Beech, and Walker (1971) showed that individuals with OCD had equivalent performance to controls on a signal detection task, but required more information before making decisions (i.e., they needed significantly more repetitions of stimuli). This theme of an exaggerated need for information is also reflected in studies using a variety of other experimental methodologies, including lexical decision tasks (Frost, Lahart, Dugas, & Sher, 1988; Persons & Foa, 1984), and reasoning tasks (O'Connor & Robillard, 1995). For example, Kyrios and Bhar (1997) interpreted the unexpected result that clinical and non-clinical subjects in a low responsibility condition performed more poorly than those in a high responsibility condition in a memory classification task as indicative of the higher sense of uncertainty engendered by the low responsibility condition. In addition, intolerance for at least some types of uncertainty appear to have behavioral consequences for OCD individuals. For example Rode *et al.* (1999) found that individuals with OCD are more likely to avoid situations with high outcome variability, regardless of whether probabilities of the individual outcomes are explicitly stated or made otherwise available.

Direct manipulations of intolerance of uncertainty have not been conducted with a focus on OCD or with OCD clinical cohorts. A recent direct manipulation by Ladouceur, Gosselin and Dugas (2000) examined the effects of manipulating tolerance of uncertainty on worries. A gambling task was used to increase or decrease intolerance of uncertainty in student cohorts by varying the instructions given. Results were interpreted as indicating that increased intolerance was associated with higher levels of worry. However, the instructions could also be seen to be manipulating other OCD-related beliefs such as personal responsibility. In the absence of ratings of increases or decreases in a range of beliefs, such results remain inconclusive.

Summary. Echoing research suggesting the need to refine the broad construct of responsibility as it applies to OCD, research suggests a similar need for more fine-grained structural analyses of the construct of intolerance for uncertainty as it pertains to OCD. It is premature to assume that all aspects of uncertainty are equally relevant to OCD symptoms. Future experimental studies could examine these issues, as well as the possibility that there are multiple causal and/or developmental pathways to intolerance of uncertainty (cf., Salkovskis *et al.*, 1999). Current evidence indicates that outcome variability may be an important form of uncertainty that is feared and avoided by individuals with OCD. The degree to which this is related to high threat estimation, inflated personal responsibility and other important OCD-related beliefs such as perfectionism remains to be established.

Perfectionism

Conceptual considerations and general assessment. Perfectionism has been characterized as an overly self-critical tendency to judge the self against excessively high standards (e.g., Frost, Marten, Lahart, & Rosenblate, 1990). While sometimes considered an adaptive personality trait, perfectionism is usually regarded as a vulnerability factor for later pathology (e.g., Blatt, 1995). Early theories conceptualized perfectionism as a unidimensional personality style (e.g., Burns, 1980; Pacht, 1984), yet recent research has advanced our understanding of the multidimensional nature of this construct (e.g., Hewitt & Flett, 1991; Frost *et al.*, 1990). The validity of such multidimensional approaches has been supported by correlational studies using self-report assessments (Frost *et al.*, 1990). A further finding is that some dimensions of perfectionism are clearly related to OCD symptomatology (e.g., concerns and doubts about making mistakes), whereas others are not (e.g., other-oriented perfectionism).

Frost *et al.* (1990) found that concerns about mistakes and doubts about past actions, along with excessively high personal standards, distinguished between sub-clinical obsessive compulsive and non-compulsive subjects. This trend was also observed by Antony *et al.* (1998) both in a clinical sample, in that only the doubting dimension of perfectionism differentiated between the OCD group and a panic disorder (PD) comparison group, and in a clinical study of perfectionism across anxiety disorders. Likewise, Frost and Steketee (1997) found similar evidence for the importance of the doubting dimension in a study that compared perfectionism levels of individuals with diagnosed OCD, PD, and non-patient controls. Rasmussen and Eisen (1992) have described this component of perfectionism as the incompleteness phenomenon (which appears to be closely linked to intolerance of uncertainty) and have proposed that it is a core feature of OCD.

Studies assessing the relationship between OCD symptomatology and "other-oriented" components of perfectionism (i.e., the perception of other's high expectations and the associated risk of criticism) have yielded considerably more mixed results. Although some studies indicate a unique relationship between this other-oriented form of perfectionism and OC phenomena (Bhar & Kyrios, 1999; Chang & Rand, 1999), other studies do not (Frost *et al.*, 1990; Rhéaume *et al.*, 1995; Antony *et al.*, 1998). Moreover, other-oriented perfectionism and depressive symptoms appear to be closely related (e.g., Bhar & Kyrios, 1999; Enns, 1999). Thus, while other-oriented perfectionism may play a role in OCD, the relationship may be somewhat more complex than previously considered (Wade, Kyrios, & Jackson, 1998).

Experimental analysis. Several studies have used experimental methodologies to examine the relationship between perfectionism and OCD. One series of studies examined information-processing styles of obsessionals that may implicate perfectionistic tendencies. In an early experimental study, Reed (1969) asked subjects with diagnosed OCD and matched controls to sort blocks into classes according to shared features while attempting to create the smallest number of groups. As expected, subjects with OCD allocated fewer blocks to each class and required more "overly precise" classes to do so, prompting Reed (1969, 1991) to posit that existence of an underinclusive cognitive style in OCD. Pearsons and Foa (1984) obtained further support for this underinclusive style in a study in which OCD subjects and controls participated in a semantic card-sorting task. As predicted, OCD subjects required more time to complete the task and used a significantly greater number of piles to group semantically similar cards. Frost *et al.* (1988) partially replicated these results in a non-clinical sample, in that participants in the OC group required more time, but not more piles to complete a similar card-sorting task. Additionally, Goodwin and Sher (1992) found similar evidence in a study of cognitive "set-shifting" in non-clinical compulsive checkers using the Wisconsin Card Sorting Test. While such difficulties may be associated with perfectionism and related beliefs (e.g., poor confidence in task performance, intolerance of uncertainty), other factors may also play a role in poor performance (e.g., organizational and neuropsychological deficits). Hence, the results from such studies may be more closely related to the emerging neuropsychological literature discussed later in this chapter.

In a more targeted experimental analysis, Frost and Marten (1990) compared female perfectionists and non-perfectionists on a low or high threat evaluated-writing task. As expected, the two groups differed on cognitive, behavioral and affective responses to the task, although there was no significant effect for the threat value of the task. Perfectionists assigned greater importance to their performance from the outset, reported higher levels of negative affect, and reported that they should have performed better following the tasks. Perfectionism was also associated with poorer writing performance, although affect was not. In a further development of this methodology, Frost *et al.* (1995) compared the reactions of subjects high and low in perfectionistic concern over mistakes on tasks associated with either a high or low probability of mistakes. Subjects high in perfectionistic concern over mistakes reacted with more negative mood, a lowered sense of confidence in their performance, an inflated sense that they should have performed better, a reticence to share the results of their performance with others, and a perception that others would see them as less intelligent. These effects were almost exclusively seen in the high-mistake-prone and not the low-mistake-prone task.

In an experiment more closely associated with OCD, Bouchard, Rhéaume, and Ladouceur (1999) examined the effect of perfectionism and exaggerated beliefs about responsibility on checking behaviors during a classification task. Participants who were either moderately perfectionistic or highly perfectionistic were given a manipulation of responsibility and then participated in a classification task. As expected, more checking behaviors occurred in the highly perfectionistic group. Moreover, the highly perfectionistic group, when induced to experience greater personal responsibility, reported that they had more influence over and responsibility for negative consequences than less perfectionistic subjects during the classification task. These results provide evidence for a significant association, not just between perfectionism and checking behavior, but also between perfectionism and exaggerated responsibility.

Summary. Both correlational studies and experimental analyses support a relationship between perfectionism and OCD or related problems. These findings suggest that concerns over mistakes and doubts about actions may be the most strongly related dimensions of perfectionism in OCD, and provide more mixed evidence for the role of more other-oriented perfectionistic concerns. Future studies are needed to address the specific relationships between dimensions of perfectionism and OCD, with an emphasis on both causal directionality and potential mediators of this relationship. There is a need to examine, not only the role of depression and/or negative mood (e.g., Bhar & Kyrios, 1999) and negative life events (e.g., Chang & Rand, 1999) as potential mediators of this relationship, but also the interaction between perfectionism and other domains of OCD-related cognition (c.f., Bouchard *et al.*, 1999). It is also likely that research will need to assess the value of differentiating perfectionism dimensions such as doubting from beliefs about tolerance for uncertainty.

Experimental Methods in Studies of Related Domains

This section describes experimental methods in studies of related domains with an emphasis on their methodology. These related domains are divided into cognitive and affective variables.

Cognitive–Behavioral Variables

Cognitive variables that are not specific to OCD can play important roles in many cases of obsessional problems. Salkovskis *et al.* (1999) noted that "in some cases, there are general and enduring belief factors which may have made the patient prone to developing OCD, and which do not fully change in the course of treatment, and that it can be helpful to identify and deal with these" (p. 1069). It is likely that such cognitive factors could include anxiety sensitivity (e.g., Reiss, Peerson, Gursky, & McNally, 1986), beliefs about the importance of social approval (Bhar & Kyrios, 1999), self-identity and self-esteem (Bhar & Kyrios, 2000; Ehntholt, Salkovskis, & Rimes, 1999; Guidano & Liotti, 1983), and the looming maladaptive style (Riskind & Williams, in press, 2000; Riskind *et al.*, 2000).

Anxiety sensitivity refers to intolerance of anxiety and anxiety sensations and fearful appraisals of anxiety reactions (e.g., Reiss *et al.*, 1986). While it has mainly been identified as important to panic disorder (e.g., Schmidt, Lerew, & Tralowski, 1995; Schmidt & Woolaway-Bickel, in press), obsessional patients are frequently observed to experience anxiety sensitivity. It seems likely that anxiety sensitivity may influence the distress that unwanted intrusions create in such patients, particularly in terms of a psychophysiological vulnerability. Likewise, beliefs related to social approval (Bhar & Kyrios, 1999) and those that link self-worth to relationships with other people (Ehntholt *et al.*, 1999) seem to play a role in OCD. It seems likely that such beliefs could intensify the fear of intrusive thoughts about committing harm because they inflate the negative significance that individuals attach to the reactions of others. Furthermore, self-perceptions related to an ambivalent sense of identity and self-esteem have been linked to obsessive–compulsive symptoms both theoretically (Guidano & Liotti, 1983) and, more recently, through the use of self-report measures in non-clinical and clinical cohorts (Bhar & Kyrios, 2000).

The looming vulnerability model of anxiety assumes that the quintessential phenomenological theme in the threat-related ideation is the mental representation of rapidly intensifying danger (Riskind, 1997). For example, anxiety is likely to result from perceptions (or misperceptions) that a repugnant source of contamination is rapidly spreading or approaching, or that the risk of losing control of harmful interpersonal impulses is rapidly rising. From their learning histories (e.g., childhood experiences, insecure attachment relationships) certain individuals are assumed to develop an enduring maladaptive cognitive style to mentally represent and appraise self-environment relationships as rapidly rising in risk or danger. This looming maladaptive style (LMS) is postulated to be a distal, superordinate cognitive vulnerability factor that interacts with and affects the disorder-specific cognitive mechanisms that are central to each anxiety disorder (e.g., overestimating responsibility and negative significance in OCD). Research has provided evidence that the LMS is likely to impair mental control and the individual's capacity to suppress intrusive thoughts, is strongly associated with obsessional symptoms, and can lead to cognitively vulnerable individuals to feel heightened responsibility and imperative need for action for dealing with potential threats. Moreover, the LMS is likely to generate a schematic processing bias for threat-related information on both implicit and explicit memory tasks, even in individuals who are not currently anxious (Riskind & Williams, in press).

Finally, several variables related to general behavioral self-regulation also have potential implications for experimental studies of domains of cognition in OCD. For example, Frost, Meagher, and Riskind (2001) recently developed a ten-item questionnaire called the Impulsive Experiences Scale on which respondents rate the intensity of their urges to behave in inappropriate and harmful ways (e.g., to shout something inappropriate while surrounded by other people, to jump off of a high place, to steal or take something, and to strike or slap someone). The potential value of this scale is indicated by a recent study that revealed strong associations between the scale and OCD symptoms on the Yale–Brown Obsessive–Compulsive Scale.

Another set of variables that may have implications for domains of cognition in OCD are problem-solving orientation and problem-solving skills (e.g., Ladouceur, Blais, Freeston, & Dugas, 1998). The potential deficits in problem solving are implied by the wide agreement that intolerance for uncertainty, doubt, and indecisiveness are important domains of OCD cognition. Moreover, it may be useful to consider such deficits when designing clinical interventions for OCD-related cognitions.

Affective Variables

A set of related affective (cognitive–affective) variables can also be examined in research on domains of cognition in OCD. Shafran, Watkins, and Charman (1996) have shown that the experience of guilt is associated with OCD symptoms, as expected given the relation between guilt and responsibility. Moreover, research indicates that general states of neuroticism, trait anxiety, and depression are related to obsessions and other OCD symptoms (Summerfeldt *et al.*, 1998; Wade *et al.*, 1998). The unique contributions that the various domains of OCD cognition make to OCD symptoms need to be evaluated when these general states are *controlled*, and vice versa. Although experimental manipulations of affective variables have seldom been undertaken in OCD research, it may be useful to examine their implications for both symptomatology and domains of OCD cognition. Future studies could employ mood induction paradigms (e.g., Riskind, 1989), comparisons of cohorts under high and low levels of "cognitive load" (e.g., Wegner, 1994), or even comparisons of the same cohort under high- or low-stress conditions. Such methodologies may help to clarify the relative contributions of affective and cognitive factors to OCD symptomatology.

Summary

Measures of a variety of variables related to the domains of cognition are likely to be useful in future experimental research because these variables could contribute to a vulnerability to developing OCD, and not fully remit in the course of standard treatment. Moreover, in some cases such variables may overlap with domains of OCD cognition and potentially confound the effects of these domains. In other cases, the overlap might be inherent to the meaning of the domains of cognitions, rather than spurious, and add to our understanding of these domains. For example, there is a possibility that certain variables represent overarching meta-belief systems or distal and superordinate vulnerability factors that interact with the OCCWG belief domains in the development and maintenance of OCD.

Experimental Methods for Clinical Intervention or Treatment Outcome

Many of the experimental methods used in studies of OCD-related domains of cognition may be useful when designing clinical interventions. In general terms, many of these methods can be productively adapted to use as behavioral experiments in cognitive therapy to facilitate OCD patients' evaluations of their belief systems. Moreover, these methods may provide conceptual frameworks that might be useful for evaluating treatment efficacy and outcome research. Examples include thought suppression methods, experimental manipulations of responsibility, and/or manipulations of danger-related ideation.

One extension of experimental methods to clinical application involves demonstrating the mechanism(s) and/or effects of instructed thought suppression on subsequent intrusive thoughts. Borrowing from experimental methods for instructed suppression (e.g., Purdon, 1999; Purdon & Clark, 1994b; Salkovskis & Campbell, 1994; Wegner, 1994), the therapist can instruct patients to imagine a purple elephant and then instruct them to "not think about it" for a brief time interval. During this interval the patient is asked to indicate or record the number of intrusive thoughts that s/he experiences. Using this procedure, the therapist can demonstrate that intrusive thoughts can be readily elicited in ordinary individuals when they attach prohibitions to having such thoughts. Likewise, variants of the therapist's instructions can be employed to demonstrate the effects of specific beliefs on intrusive thinking. For example, the therapist could test the hypothesis that the inability to suppress thoughts is exacerbated when one believes that it must reveal underlying weakness in one's character or that most people are able to accomplish this task with ease. So variations on this task could be used to demonstrate the power of beliefs about the negative significance and/or over-importance of thoughts on obsessional thinking.

Therapists can also productively adapt responsibility inductions from experimental studies to use in behavioral experiments that test the impact of beliefs about inflated responsibility. For example, the behavioral experiments can examine the extent to which responsibility beliefs increase patients' urges to neutralize and engage in compulsive rituals, as well as exacerbate their distress. The therapist can use Shafran's (1997) indirect ploy of varying the presence/absence of the therapist during a behavioral task. Similarly, the therapist could set up a behavioral experiment using Lopatka and Rachman's (1995) more direct manipulation of responsibility. For example, the therapist can induce high responsibility by stating: "I want you to know that you will have to take complete responsibility if anything bad happens or anything is not perfect." Likewise, the therapist could induce low responsibility by stating: "I want you to know that I will take complete responsibility if anything bad happens or anything is not perfect. You are not responsible." Such behavioral experiments could test the hypothesis that OCD patients with inflated responsibility can increase their urges to neutralize, experience distress, and overestimate threat. Conversely, they could test the "therapeutic hypothesis" that a reduction in personal responsibility is likely to be accompanied by a decline in the belief that misfortunes will occur (see Lopatka & Rachman, 1995).

Analogous behavioral experiments can be used to test the validity of other links in the cognitive conceptualization of the problems of OCD patients. For example, the therapist can adapt the procedure of Salkovskis *et al.* (1997) who had non-clinical subjects listen to repeated recordings of one of their own intrusive thoughts, and then asked them to either neutralize the thought or distract themselves. Neutralizing thoughts led to significantly greater subsequent discomfort, as well as stronger urges to neutralize. Therapists can similarly gather evidence about whether neutralization of unwanted thoughts strengthens a patient's subsequent discomfort and urges to neutralize. The therapist can likewise adapt the procedure of Rachman *et al.* (1996) who asked patients to write sentences that would evoke anxiety (e.g., "my father will fall down the stairs and break his neck"), and examine the implications of such statements for symptomatology. During such tasks, the therapist could assess verbal reports of anxiety and other variables such as guilt, responsibility, and likelihood of harm, as well as negative automatic thoughts. Such behavioral experiments could help the OCD patient test the costs and benefits of engaging in neutralization, thought suppression, or compulsive rituals.

Experimental manipulations of mental representations of danger can also be adapted for clinical use. For example, a recent study (Riskind, Wheeler, & Picerno, 1997) used an experimental imagery-modification procedure to reduce fear of contamination in subclinical obsessionals. They found evidence with both self-report measures and a BAT that "freezing" contaminants in their place to reduce perceptions that they can spread rapidly was effective in reducing fears and overestimation of threat in a subclinical sample.

For other examples of "looming management" in the treatment of anxiety disorders see Riskind and Williams, 1999b). Further research can examine whether analogous experimental interventions can reduce the overestimation of threat and resultant fear in clinical patients with OCD.

The various experimental methods used in studies of the domains of belief in OCD can also be employed as measures of *treatment outcome*. For example, the presence or absence of the therapist would be expected to have less effect after a trial of successful cognitive–behavioral therapy. Likewise, cognitively treated patients would be expected to show reduced responsiveness when listening to recorded presentations of their intrusive thoughts or when writing sentences about events that would elicit anxiety. Furthermore, other experimental methods (e.g., classification tasks) could be used as adjunctive outcome measures or as probes of change in possible mediating processes (e.g., underinclusive cognitive style).

Neuropsychological and Related Methods

OCD subjects have been found to exhibit specific deficits (poorer spatial memory and spatial working memory, and slowed motor responses) not found in panic disorder, major depression and normal controls (Purcell, Maruff, Kyrios, & Pantelis, 1998). Equivocal results have emerged from studies investigating changes in neuropsychological performance associated with psychological treatment (see Chapter nine in this volume). A recent pilot study by Kyrios, Wainwright, Purcell, Pantelis, and Maruff, (1999) provided evidence that improvements on neuropsychological tasks were associated with cognitive–behavior therapy, although Bolton, Raven, Madronal-Luque, and Marks (2000) reported no such changes following behaviour therapy.

The origins of the neuropsychological deficits associated with OCD have been elusive. While such deficits are interpreted by some researchers as indicative of frontal–striatal dysfunction (Savage *et al.*, 2000), others have not been as ready to accept such assertions (Tallis, Pratt, & Jamani, 1999). Cognitive–behavioral models may also be useful in explaining such deficits. Recent studies from the cognitive–behavioral perspective have indicated a range of strategic cognitive factors, including metacognition, which influence performance on neuropsychological tasks. For instance, Richards (1997) concluded that memory problems in OCD mainly ensue from counterproductive unrealistic perfectionistic demands on memory that interfere with confidence in memory capacity (see also Deckersbach, Otto, Savage, Baer, & Jenike, 2000; MacDonald, Antony, MacLeod, & Richter, 1997). Frost and Steketee (1997) have also supported the etiological importance of perfectionism in OCD, although it's relationship to information processing and memory difficulties has only been investigated with hoarders (Steketee, Frost, & Kyrios, 2001). OCD-related deficits in memory confidence rather than memory abilities per se have been supported by a number of experimental investigations (e.g., MacDonald *et al.*, 1997). However, although OCD subjects with and without memory impairments have been found to doubt the accuracy of their memories, little is known about the interaction between memory and meta-memory and their relation to OCD symptoms. Furthermore, it is not known whether OCD severity and symptom type influences the relationship between memory accuracy and meta-cognition. For example, are checking symptoms, as distinct from washing or obsessional presentations, associated with different memory appraisals or a different pattern of relationships between neuropsychological deficits, metacognition and symptom severity? Moreover, the question of whether neuropsychological performance improves in OCD patients with the adoption of more adaptive meta-cognitive and related strategic processing styles has yet to be investigated.

Should it be established more convincingly that neuropsychological performance improves with treatment, it is possible that such improvements are closely related to the consistently reported adaptive changes in cognitive style associated with successful cognitive therapy outcomes. For instance, cognitive styles associated with OCD (e.g., perfectionistic tendencies, poor confidence in memory, apprehension due to self-doubts, inflated responsibility, thought–action fusion, etc.) may compromise cognitive strategies and motor response times on non-verbal memory tasks. There is an intriguing possibility that neuropsychological deficits are by-products of an OCD-related cognitive style, and that such deficits may be ameliorated with the improved thinking styles associated with treatment. Indeed, adaptive changes in cognitive style may influence the relationship between improved neuropsychological performance and symptom amelioration. Should this prove true, it may account for the improved neuropsychological performance reported by Kyrios *et al.* (1999) following cognitive–behavioral therapy.

Recommendations for Future Research

This chapter has provided an overview of some of the major experimental methods used in research on the domains of cognition in OCD. This chapter has also examined research in several related domains that may be potentially relevant to a fuller understanding the domains of cognition in OCD. Overall, significant methodological advances and resourcefulness have been evidenced in research addressing the relationship between the domains of cognition and OCD. Certainly these advances have contributed, at least in part, to the growing effectiveness and popularity of both cognitive theories and cognitive–behavioral treatment of OCD.

At the same time, there appear to be several general limitations of past research that could be addressed in future studies. First, past research on the domains of cognition in OCD has primarily examined non-clinical or subclinical cohorts, and the generalizability of past research to clinical populations and OCD subtypes may be somewhat limited. Second, because most past research has been correlational, relatively little is known about the causal influence of the domains of cognition on OCD. For example, are these belief domains causal psychological antecedents or psychogenic vulnerabilities to OCD, or are they the result OC symptomatology? Third, few studies have isolated belief domains, either experimentally or in correlational analysis, in assessing their pattern of associations with OCD, and relatively little is known about the validity and incremental value of differentiating between responsibility, the over-importance of thoughts, the controllability of thoughts, the over-estimation of threat, intolerance of uncertainty, and perfectionism. Finally, there is a paucity of information about the cognitive, behavioral, and affective consequences of these belief domains.

Based on these limitations and on the advances evidenced by some recent studies, we suggest that future research on the identified domains of cognition will be likely to benefit from the following methodological considerations. First, future research will benefit from the inclusion of clinical, as well as non-clinical populations. It will also be useful to investigate the specificity of cognitive factors to OCD subtypes (e.g., checking, contamination fears). Second, experimental analysis of the belief domains, particularly research that directly manipulates and/or isolates these domains, can enhance knowledge. Third, future research will be likely to benefit from consideration of the causal rules of these belief domains on OCD, including consideration of temporal precedence obtained through longitudinal investigations. Fourth, it seems important to examine the convergent and discriminant validity, as well as the predictive utility, of identifying and assessing six domains of cognition, particularly given the apparent overlap between some of these domains. Fifth, future research can benefit from an examination of how these belief domains interact and affect performance on cognitive and neuropsychological tasks, as well as general information processing. Related to this issue is the need to assess the extent to which beliefs relevant to the intended manipulations have been successful, and the extent to which beliefs hypothesized to be irrelevant to the manipulation were not affected. Finally, consideration of the affective and behavioral consequences or implications of these domains is also important.

As illustrated by the many chapters in the present volume, we are now entering an exciting phase in research on the cognitive basis of obsessions, but face difficult challenges as well. Advances in research will likely derive from the use of multiple tasks that permit testing the proposed domains of cognition at multiple levels of processing (e.g., attention, memory). In addition, it could prove fruitful to employ physiological methods that provide indirect indicators of predictions of cognitive theories. For example, researchers may be able to apply techniques such as facial electromyography, and evoked potentials to test predictions of current theories about the cognitive domains of OCD. The recent use of virtual reality techniques may likewise provide new methods for manipulating the cognitive phenomenology of individuals with OCD and testing theoretical predictions. Ultimately, the aim of such research is to facilitate refined clinical case conceptualizations and to suggest new and more effective cognitive–behavioral treatment strategies.

References

Amir, N., Cashman, L., & Foa, E. B. (1997). Strategies of thought control in obsessive–compulsive disorder. *Behaviour Research and Therapy, 35,* 775–777.

Antony, M. M., Purdon, C. L, Huta, V., & Swinson, R. P. (1998). Dimensions of perfectionism across the anxiety disorders. *Behaviour Research and Therapy, 36,* 1143–1154.

Beck, A. T. (1976). *Cognitive therapy and the emotional disorders.* New York: International Universities Press.

Beck, A. T., & Emery, G. (1985). *Anxiety disorders and phobias: A cognitive perspective.* New York: Basic Books.

Bhar, S. S., & Kyrios, M. (1999). Cognitive personality styles associated with depressive and obsessive compulsive phenomena in a non-clinical sample. *Behavioural and Cognitive Psychotherapy, 27,* 329–343.

Bhar, S. S., & Kyrios, M. (2000). *Ambivalent self-esteem as meta-vulnerability for obsessive compulsive disorder*. Paper presented at the International Conference in Self-Concept, Theory, Research and Practice: Advances for the New Millennium, Sydney, Australia.

Blatt, S. J. (1995). The destructiveness of perfectionism: Implications for the treatment of depression. *American Psychologist, 50*, 1003–1020.

Bolton, D., Raven, P., Madronal-Luque, R., & Marks, I. M. (2000). Neurological and neuro-psychological signs in obsessive compulsive disorder: Interaction with behavioural treatment. *Behaviour Research and Therapy, 38*, 695–708.

Bonninger, D. S., Krosnick, J. A., & Berent, M. K. (1995). Origins of attitude importance: Self-interest, social identification, and value relevance. *Journal of Personality and Social Psychology, 68*, 269–279.

Bouchard, C., Rhéaume, J., & Ladouceur, R. (1999). Responsibility and perfectionism in OCD: An experimental study. *Behaviour Research and Therapy, 37*, 239–248.

Bradley, B. P. Mogg, K., & Williams, R. (1994). Implicit and explicit memory for emotional information in non-clinical subjects. *Behaviour Research and Therapy, 32*, 65–78.

Burns, D. D. (1980). The perfectionist's script for self-defeat. *Psychology Today*, November, 34–51.

Cartwright-Hatton, S., & Wells, A. (1997). Beliefs about worry and intrusions: The meta-cognitions questionnaire and its correlates. *Journal of Anxiety Disorders, 11*, 279–296.

Chang, E. C., & Rand, K. L. (1999). Perfectionism as a predictor of subsequent adjustment: Evidence for a specific diathesis-stress mechanism among college students. *Journal of Counseling Psychology, 46*, 515–523.

Clark, D. A., & Purdon, C. (1993). New perspectives for a cognitive theory of obsessions. *Australian Psychologist, 28*, 161–167.

Clark, D. A., & Purdon, C. (1995). The assessment of unwanted intrusive thoughts: A review and critique of the literature. *Behaviour Research and Therapy, 33*, 967–976.

Clark, D. A., Ball, S., & Pape, D. (1991). An experimental investigation of thought suppression. *Behaviour Research and Therapy, 29*, 253–257.

Clark, D. A., Purdon, C., & Byers, E. S. (2000). Appraisal and control of sexual and non-sexual intrusive thoughts in university students. *Behaviour Research and Therapy, 38*, 439–455.

Clark, D. A., Winton, E., & Thynn, L. (1993). A further experimental investigation of thought suppression. *Behaviour Research and Therapy, 31*, 207–210.

Cloninger, C. R. (1987). A systematic method for clinical description and classification of personality variance: A proposal. *Archives of General Psychiatry, 44*, 573–588.

Deckersbach, T., Otto, M. W., Savage, C. R., Baer, L., & Jenike, M. A. (2000). The relationship between semantic organization and memory in obsessive–compulsive disorder. *Psychotherapy and Psychosomatics, 69*, 101–107.

Ehntholt, K. A., Salkovskis, P. M., & Rimes, K. A. (1999). Obsessive–compulsive disorder, anxiety disorders, and self-esteem: An exploratory study. *Behaviour Research and Therapy, 37*, 771–781.

Emmelkamp, P. M. G. (1987). Obsessive–compulsive disorders. In L. Michelson & L. M. Ascher (eds), *Anxiety and stress disorders, cognitive behavioral assessment and treatment*. New York: Guilford.

Foa, E. B. (1979). Failure in treating obsessive-compulsives. *Behaviour Research and Therapy, 17*, 169–176.

Foa, E. B., Ilai, D., McCarthy, P. R., Shoyer, B., & Murdock, R. (1993). Information processing in obsessive–compulsive disorder. *Cognitive Therapy and Research, 17*, 173–189.

Freeston, M., & Ladouceur, R. (1993). Appraisal of cognitive intrusions and response style: Replication and extension. *Behaviour Research and Therapy, 31*, 185–191.

Freeston, M., Ladouceur, R., Gagnon, F., & Thibodeau, N. (1993). Beliefs about obsessional thoughts. *Journal of Psychopathology and Behavioural Assessment, 15*, 1–21.

Freeston, M., Ladouceur, R., Thibodeau, N., & Gagnon, F. (1991). Cognitive intrusions in a non-clinical population. I. Response style, subjective experience, and appraisal. *Behaviour Research and Therapy, 29,* 585–597.

Freeston, M., Ladouceur, R., Thibodeau, N., & Gagnon, F. (1992). Cognitive intrusions in a non-clinical population. II. Associations with depressive, anxious, and compulsive symptoms. *Behaviour Research and Therapy, 30,* 263–271.

Freeston, M., Rhéaume, J., & Ladouceur, R. (1996). Correcting faulty appraisals of obsessional thoughts. *Behaviour Research and Therapy, 34,* 443–446.

Frost, R. O., & Marten, P. A. (1990). Perfectionism and evaluative threat. *Cognitive Therapy and Research, 14,* 559–572.

Frost, R. O., & Steketee, G. (1997). Perfectionism in obsessive–compulsive disorder patients. *Behaviour Research and Therapy, 35,* 291–296.

Frost, R. O., Lahart, C. M., Dugas, K. M., & Sher, K. J. (1988). Information processing among non-clinical compulsives. *Behaviour Research and Therapy, 26,* 275–277.

Frost, R. O., Marten, P., Lahart, C., & Rosenblate, R. (1990). The dimensions of perfectionism. *Cognitive Therapy and Research, 14,* 449–468.

Frost, R. O., Meagher, B., & Riskind, J. H. (2001). Obsessive–compulsive features in pathological lottery and scratch ticket gamblers. *Journal of Gambling Studies, 17,* 5–20.

Frost, R. O., Steketee, G., Cohen, L., & Griess, K. (1994). Personality traits in subclinical and non-obsessive-compulsive volunteers and their parents. *Behaviour Research and Therapy, 32,* 47–56.

Frost, R. O., Turcotte, T. A., Heimberg, R. G., Mattia, J. I., Holt, C. S., & Hope, D. A. (1995). Reactions to mistakes among subjects high and low in perfectionistic concern over mistakes. *Cognitive Therapy and Research, 19,* 195–205.

Garber, J., & Hollon, S. D. (1991). What can specificity designs say about causality in psychopathology research? *Psychological Bulletin, 110,* 129–136.

Goodwin, A. H., & Sher, K. J. (1992). Deficits in set-shifting ability in non-clinical compulsive checkers. *Journal of Psychopathology and Behavioral Assessment, 14,* 81–91.

Guidano, V., & Liotti, G. (1983). *Cognitive processes and emotional disorders.* New York: Guilford.

Hewitt, P. L., & Flett, G. L. (1991). Perfectionism in the self and social contexts: Conceptualization, assessment, and association with psychopathology. *Journal of Personality and Social Psychology, 143,* 177–182.

Horowitz, M. (1975. Intrusive and repetitive thoughts after experimental stress. *Archives of General Psychiatry, 32,* 1457–1463.

Janeck, A. S., & Calamari, J. E. (2000). Thought suppression in obsessive–compulsive disorder. *Cognitive Therapy and Research, 23,* 497–509.

Jones, M. K., & Menzies, R. G. (1997). The cognitive mediation of obsessive–compulsive handwashing. *Behaviour Research and Therapy, 35,* 843–850.

Jones, M. K., & Menzies, R. G. (1998a). The role of perceived danger in the mediation of obsessive–compulsive washing. *Depression and Anxiety, 8,* 121–125

Jones, M. K., & Menzies, R. G. (1998b). Danger ideation reduction therapy (DIRT) for obsessive–compulsive washers. A controlled trial. *Behaviour Research and Therapy, 36,* 959–970.

Krohne, H. W. (1989). The concept of coping modes: Relating cognitive person variables to actual coping behavior. *Advances in Behaviour Research and Therapy, 11,* 235–248.

Krohne, H. W. (1993). Vigilance and cognitive avoidance as concepts in coping research. In H. W. Krohne (ed.), *Attention and avoidance.* (pp. 19–50). Toronto: Gottingen, Hogrefe & Huber.

Krosnick, J. A. (1988). The role of attitude importance in social evaluation: A study of political preferences, presidential candidate evaluations, and voting behavior. *Journal of Personality and Social Psychology, 55,* 196–210.

Kyrios, M., & Bhar, S. (1995, July). *A questionnaire measure of inflated responsibility and its relationship to depressive and obsessive–compulsive phenomena.* Paper presented at the World Congress of Behavioural and Cognitive Therapies, Copenhagen.

Kyrios, M., & Bhar, S. (1997, September). *Experimental manipulation of inflated responsibility and obsessive–compulsive disorder.* Paper presented at the Congress of the European Association for Behavioural and Cognitive Therapies, Venice.

Kyrios, M., & Iob, M. (1998). Automatic and strategic processing in obsessive–compulsive disorder: Attentional bias, cognitive avoidance or more complex phenomena? *Journal of Anxiety Disorders, 12,* 271–292.

Kyrios, M., Wainwright, K., Purcell, R., Pantelis, C., & Maruff, P. (1999, November). *Neuropsychological predictos of outcome following cognitive–behavioral therapy for OCD. A pilot study.* Paper presented at the Association for the Advancement of Behavior Therapy, Toronto.

Ladouceur, R., Blais, F., Freeston, M. H., & Dugas, M. J. (1998). Problem solving and problem orientation in generalized anxiety disorder. *Journal of Anxiety Disorders, 12,* 139–152.

Ladouceur, R., Freeston, M. H., Gagnon, F., Thibodeau, N., & Durmont, J. (1994). Idiographic considerations in the cognitive–behavioral treatment of obsessional thoughts. *Journal of Behaviour Therapy and Experimental Psychiatry, 24,* 301–310.

Ladouceur, R., Gosselin, P., & Dugas, M. J. (2000). Experimental manipulation of intolerance of uncertainty: A study of a theoretical model of worry. *Behaviour Research and Therapy, 9,* 933–941.

Ladouceur, R., Leger, E., Rhéaume, J., & Dube, D. (1996). Correction of inflated responsibility in the treatment of obsessive–compulsive disorder. *Behaviour Research and Therapy, 34,* 767–774.

Ladouceur, R., Rhéaume, J., Freeston, M. H., Aublet, F., Jean, K., Lachance, S., Langlois, F., & DePokomandy-Morin, K. (1995). Experimental manipulations of responsibility: An analogue test for models of obsessive–compulsive disorder. *Behaviour Research and Therapy, 35,* 423–427.

Lopatka, C. (1994). *Responsibility in obsessive–compulsive disorder: Is it worth checking?* Unpublished doctoral dissertation, University of British Columbia.

Lopatka, C., & Rachman, S. (1995). Perceived responsibility and compulsive checking: An experimental analysis. *Behaviour Research and Therapy, 33,* 673–684.

MacDonald, P. A., Antony, M. M., MacLeod, C. M., & Richter, M. A. (1997). Memory and confidence in memory judgments among individuals with obsessive compulsive disorder and non-clinical controls. *Behaviour Research and Therapy, 35,* 497–505.

Milner, A. D., Beech, H. R., & Walker, V. J. (1971). Decision processes and obsessional behavior. *British Journal of Social and Clinical Psychology, 10,* 88–89.

Muris, P., Merckelbach, H., van den Hout, M., & de Jong, P. (1992). Suppression of emotional and neutral material. *Behaviour Research and Therapy, 30,* 639–642.

Niler, E. R., & Beck, S. J. (1989). The relationship among guilt, dysphoria, and anxiety and obsessions in normal population. *Behaviour Research and Therapy, 27,* 213–220.

Obsessive Compulsive Cognitions Working Group (1997). Cognitive assessment of obsessive–compulsive disorder. *Behaviour Research and Therapy, 35,* 667–681.

O'Connor, K., & Robillard, S. (1995). Interference processes in obsessive–compulsive disorder: Some clinical observations. *Behaviour Research and Therapy, 33,* 887–896.

Pacht, A. R. (1984). Reflections on perfection. *American Psychologist, 39,* 386–390.

Persons, J., & Foa, E. B. (1984). Processing of fearful and neutral information by obsessive-compulsives. *Behaviour Research and Therapy, 22,* 259–265.

Purcell, R., Maruff, P., Kyrios, M., & Pantelis, C. (1998). Neuropsychological deficits in obsessive–compulsive disorder: A comparison with unipolar depression, panic disorder, and normal controls. *Archives of General Psychiatry, 55,* 415–423.

Purdon, C. (1999). Thought suppression and psychopathology. *Behaviour Research and Therapy,* *37,* 1029–1054.

Purdon, C. (1998). *The role of thought suppression and meta-cognitive beliefs in the persistence of obsession-like intrusive thoughts.* Unpublished Doctoral Dissertation.

Purdon, C., & Clark, D. A. (1994a). Obsessive intrusive thoughts in nonclinical subjects. Part II. Cognitive appraisal, emotional response and thought control strategies. *Behaviour Research and Therapy, 32,* 403–410.

Purdon, C., & Clark, D. A. (1994b). Perceived control and appraisal of obsessional intrusive thoughts: A replication and extension. *Behavioural and Cognitive Psychotherapy, 22,* 269–285.

Rachman, S. (1997). A cognitive theory of obsessions. *Behaviour Research and Therapy, 35,* 793–802.

Rachman, S. (1998). A cognitive theory of obsessions: Elaborations. *Behaviour Research and Therapy, 36,* 793–802.

Rachman, S., Shafran, R., Mitchell, D., & Trant, J., & Teachman, B. (1996). How to remain neutral: An experimental analysis of neutralization. *Behaviour Research and Therapy, 34,* 889–898.

Rachman, S., Thordarson, D., Shafran, R., & Woody, S. (1995). Perceived responsibility: Structure and significance. *Behaviour Research and Therapy, 33,* 779–784.

Radomsky, A. S., & Rachman, S. (1999). Memory bias in obsessive–compulsive disorder (OCD). *Behaviour Research and Therapy, 37,* 605–618.

Rasmussen, S. A., & Eisen, J. L. (1992). Epidemiology and clinical features of obsessive compulsive disorder. In M. A. Jenike, L. Baer, & W. E. Minichiello (eds), *Obsessive compulsive disorders: Theory and management,* 2nd ed. (pp. 10–27). London: Year Book Medical.

Reed, G. F. (1969). "Under-inclusion" — a characteristic of obsessional personality disorder: I. *British Journal of Psychiatry, 115,* 781–785.

Reed, G. F. (1991). The cognitive characteristics of obsessional disorder. In P. A. Magaro (ed.), *Cognitive bases of mental disorders* (pp. 77–99). London: Sage.

Reiss, S., Peerson, R. A., Gursky, D. M., & McNally, R. J. (1986). Anxiety sensitivity, anxiety frequency, and the prediction of fearfulness. *Behaviour Research and Therapy, 24,* 1–8.

Reynolds, M., & Salkovskis, P. M. (1991). The relationship among guild, dysphoria, anxiety and obsessions in a normal population — an attempted replication. *Behaviour Research and Therapy, 29,* 259–265.

Rhéaume, J., Freeston, M. H., Dugas, M. J., Letarte, H., & Ladouceur, R. (1995). Perfectionism, responsibility, and obsessive–compulsive symptoms. *Behaviour Research and Therapy, 33,* 785–794.

Rhéaume, J., Ladouceur, R., Freeston, M. H., & Letarte, H. (1995). Inflated responsibility and its role in OCD-I. Validation of a theoretical definition of responsibility. *Behaviour Research and Therapy, 33,* 159–169.

Richards, H. C. (1997, September). *Memory and OCD: What is the nature of the relationship?* Paper presented at the Congress of the European Association for Behavioural and Cognitive Therapies, Venice.

Richter, M. A., Summerfeldt, L. J., Joffe, R. T., & Swinson, R. P. (1996). The Tridimensional Personality Questionnaire in obsessive–compulsive disorder. *Psychiatry Research, 65,* 185–188.

Riskind, J. H. (1989). The mediating mechanisms in mood and memory: A cognitive-priming formulation. *Journal of Social Behavior and Personality, 4,* 173–184.

Riskind, J. H. (1997). Looming vulnerability to threat: A cognitive paradigm for anxiety. *Behaviour Research and Therapy, 35,* 5, 386–404.

Riskind, J. H., & Williams, N. L. (1999a). Specific cognitive content of anxiety and catastrophizing: Looming vulnerability and the looming maladaptive style. *Journal of Cognitive Psychotherapy, 13,* 41–54.

Riskind, J. H., & Williams, N. L. (1999b). Cognitive case conceptualization and the treatment of anxiety disorders: Implications of the looming vulnerability model. *Journal of Cognitive Psychotherapy, 13*, 295–315.

Riskind, J. H., & Williams, N. L. (2000). *Cognitive vulnerability to obsessional thoughts: The effects of multiple forms of looming vulnerability on intrusive thought frequency.* Manuscript submitted for publication.

Riskind, J. H., & Williams, N. L. (In press). A unique vulnerability common to all the anxiety disorders: the looming maladaptive style. In L. Alloy & J. H. Riskind (eds), *Cognitive vulnerability to emotional disorders.* Erlbaum.

Riskind, J. H., Abreu, K., Strauss, M., & Holt, R. (1997). Looming vulnerability to spreading contamination in subclinical OCD. *Behaviour Research and Therapy, 35*, 405–414.

Riskind, J. H., Wheeler, D. J., & Picerno, M. R. (1997). Using mental imagery with subclinical OCD to "freeze" contamination in its place: Evidence for looming vulnerability theory. *Behaviour Research and Therapy, 35*, 757–768.

Riskind, J. H., Williams, N. L., Gessner, T. L., Chrosniak, L. D., & Cortina, J. M. (2000). The looming maladaptive style: Anxiety, danger, and schematic processing. *Journal of Personality and Social Psychology, 79*, 837–852.

Rode, C., Cosmides, L., Hell, W., & Tooby, J. (1999). When and why do people avoid unknown probabilities in decisions under uncertainty? Testing some predictions from optimal foraging theory. *Cognition, 72*, 269–304.

Ruthledge, P. C. (1996). Obsessionality and the attempted suppression of unpleasant persoanl intrusive thoughts. *Behaviour Research and Therapy, 36*, 403–416.

Salkovskis, P. M. (1985). Obsessional-compulsive problems: A cognitive–behavioural analysis. *Behaviour Research and Therapy, 23*, 571–583.

Salkovskis, P. M. (1989). Cognitive–behavioural factors and the persistence of intrusive thoughts in obsessional problems. *Behaviour Research and Therapy, 27*, 677–682.

Salkovskis, P. M. (1996). The cognitive approach to anxiety: threat beliefs, safety-seeking behaviour, and the special case of health anxiety and obsessions. In P. M. Salkovskis (ed.), *Frontiers of cognitive therapy* (pp. 48–74). New York: Guilford.

Salkovskis, P. M., & Campbell, P. (1994). Thought suppression in naturally occurring negative intrusive thoughts. *Behaviour Research and Therapy, 32*, 1–8.

Salkovskis, P. M., Rachman, S., Ladouceur, R., Freeston, M., Taylor, S., Kyrios, M., & Sica, C. (1996). Defining responsibility in obsessional problems. In Obsessive Compulsive Cognitions Working Group. Northampton: Smith College.

Salkovskis, P. M., Shafran, R., Rachman, S., & Freeston, M. H. (1999). Multiple pathways to inflated responsibility beliefs in obsessional problems: Possible origins and implications for therapy and research. *Behaviour Research and Therapy, 37*, 1055–1072.

Salkovskis, P. M., Westbrook, D., Davis, J., Jeavons, A., & Gledhill, A. (1997). Effect of neutralizing on intrusive thoughts: An experiment investigating the etiology of obsessive–compulsive disorder. *Behaviour Research and Therapy, 35*, 211–219.

Salkovskis, P. M., Wroe, A. L., Gledhill, A., Morrison, N., Forrester, E., Richards, C., Reynolds, M., & Thorpe, S. (2000). Responsibility attitudes and interpretations are characteristic of obsessive compulsive disorder. *Behaviour Research and Therapy, 38*, 347–372.

Savage, C. R., Deckersbach, T., Wilhelm, S., Rauch, S. L., Baer, L., Reid, T., & Jenike, M. A. (2000). Strategic processing and episodic memory impairment in Obsessive–Compulsive Disorder. *Neuropsychology, 14*, 141–151.

Schmidt, N. B., & Woolaway-Bickel, K. (In press). Cognitive vulnerability to panic disorder. In L. Alloy & J. H. Riskind (eds), *Cognitive vulnerability to emotional disorders.* Mahwah, NJ: Erlbaum.

Schmidt, N. B., Lerew, D. R., & Trakowski, J. H. (1995). Body vigilance in panic disorder. Evaluating attention to bodily perturbations. *Journal of Consulting and Clinical Psychology, 65*, 214–220.

Shafran, R. (1997). The manipulation of responsibility in obsessive–compulsive disorder. *British Journal of Clinical Psychology, 36*, 397–407.

Shafran, R., Thordarson, D., & Rachman, S. (1996). Thought–action fusion in obsessive–compulsive disorder. *Journal of Anxiety Disorders, 10*, 379–392.

Shafran, R., Watkins, E., & Charman, T. (1996). Guilt in obsessive–compulsive disorder. *Journal of Anxiety Disorders, 10*, 509–516.

Smari, J., Sigurjonsdottir, H., & Sacmundsdottir, I. (1994). Thought suppression and obsession–compulsion. *Psychological Reports, 75*, 227–235.

Steketee, G., Frost, R. O., & Cohen, I. (1998). Beliefs in obsessive–compulsive disorder. *Journal of Anxiety Disorders, 12*, 525–537.

Steketee, G., Frost, R. O., & Kyrios, M. (2001). *Beliefs and decision-making about possessions among compulsive hoarders*. Manuscript under review.

Summerfeldt, L. J., Huta, V., & Swinson, R. P. (1998). Personality and obsessive compulsive disorder. In R. P. Swinson, M. M. Antony, S. Rachman, & M. A. Richter (eds), *Obsessive–compulsive disorder: Theory, research, and treatment* (pp. 79–119). London: Guilford.

Tallis, F. (1994). Obsessions, responsibility, and guilt: Two case reports suggesting a common and specific aetiology. *Behaviour Research and Therapy, 32*, 143–145.

Tallis, F., Pratt, P., & Jamani, N. (1999). Obsessive compulsive disorder, checking and non-verbal memory: A neuropsychological investigation. *Behaviour Research and Therapy, 37*, 161–166.

Taylor, S., & Rachman, S. (1994). Stimulus estimation and the overprediction of fear. British *Journal of Clinical Psychology, 33*, 173–181.

Trinder, H., & Salkovskis, P. M. (1994). Personally relevant intrusions outside the laboratory: Long term suppression increases intrusions. *Behaviour Research and Therapy, 32*, 833–842.

van Oppen, P., & Arntz, A. (1994). Cognitive therapy for obsessive compulsive disorder. *Behaviour Research and Therapy, 32*, 79–87.

Wade, D., Kyrios, M., & Jackson, H. (1998). A model of obsessive–compulsive phenomena in a nonclinical sample. *Australian Journal of Psychology, 50*, 11–17.

Wegner, D. M. (1989). *White bears and other unwanted thoughts*. New York: Viking.

Wegner, D. M. (1994). Ironic processes of mental control. *Psychological Review, 101*, 34–52.

Wegner, D. M., Schneider, D. J., Carter, S., & White, T. (1987). Paradoxical effects of thought suppression. *Journal of Personality and Social Psychology, 53*, 5–13.

Wells, A., & Davies, M. (1994). The Thought Control Questionnaire: A measure of individual differences in the control of unwanted thoughts. *Behaviour Research and Therapy, 32*, 871–878.

Wells, A., & Papageorgiou, C. (1997). Relationship between worry, obsessive–compulsive symptoms and meta-cognitive beliefs. *Behaviour Research and Therapy, 36*, 899–913.

World Health Organization (1996). *The global burden of disease*. WHO.

Yaryura-Tobias, J. A., & Neziroglu, F. A. (1983). *Obsessive–compulsive disorders pathogenesis–diagnosis–treatment*. New York: Marcel Dekker.

Chapter 9

Information Processing in Obsessive Compulsive Disorder

Nader Amir and Michael J. Kozak

Introduction

Of what import is yet another chapter on information-processing approaches to anxiety? Information processing is quite psychological, and it has become popular to tout the promise of biological approaches to behavior, to the neglect of the psychological. Much contemporary thinking seems to deny a role for psychological events in the study of psychopathology. Have we not just recently witnessed the "decade of the brain", followed immediately by "the decade of behavior"? As noted by Miller and Keller (2000), a tilt away from psychological constructs is reflected in the National Institute of Mental Health's emphasis on bio-behavioral factors that might "underlie" mood states, and the National Institute of Health's efforts to reorganize peer-review of research on mental disorders in "the context of the biological question that is being investigated" (National Institute of Health, 1999, p. 2). The present chapter on information processing in obsessive compulsive disorder (OCD) takes a strikingly different view that understanding the meanings of events to an individual is essential to understanding that person's emotions, including anxiety. Further, identifying disordered mechanisms for such meanings is essential to understanding emotional disorders, including anxiety disorders, of which OCD is an exemplar. Is this view defensible?

Arguments that psychological theorizing is essential to understanding emotion, and that cognitive events are neither epiphenomenal nor simply unimportant are, of course, not new. Those who are unfamiliar with the arguments might refer to Fodor's (1968) and Dennett's (1978) writings on psychological explanation. A case for the necessity of such constructs in explaining anxiety in particular has been explicated by Kozak and Miller (1982) and Miller and Kozak, (1993). Additionally, Foa and Kozak (1993) have argued for the importance of meaning in understanding fear. These arguments will not be repeated in this chapter, but their conclusions constitute assumptions that underlie information processing approaches to psychopathology, including that of OCD.

In a recent review of findings on information processing in OCD, McNally (1999) outlined a number of assumptions that guide this approach. One fundamental assumption is that introspection is itself an insufficient tool to investigate cognition and emotion. Lang's (1968) classic consideration of the imperfect relationship between introspective observations and third-person observations of behavior and physiology highlighted the limitations of a strictly introspective approach. It is also assumed that cognitive biases are not simply epiphenomenal. Philosophical and theoretical arguments for this assumption are available from the authors cited above, but whether hypothesized cognitive biases are important causal mechanisms in OCD remains an empirical question. The present review considers this question.

A third assumption of information processing approaches is that cognition is subject to a separate level of analysis than are neurobiological phenomena (McNally, 1999). The relationship between psychological and neurobiological phenomena has been much debated, and no clear consensus has emerged regarding the merits of reductionism. The information processing approach rejects "naive" forms of reductionism, and proceeds as if the domain of cognitive function merits its own investigation, beyond any efforts devoted to biology, chemistry, and physics. However, the approach does not discount the goal of compatibility among the constructs of different sciences. Accordingly, psychological explanations should be informed by the findings of other sciences, and vice versa, with explanatory preeminence ceded to no single discipline. Another interesting assumption articulated by McNally (1999) is that cognitive processes hypothesized in anxiety can be either content-independent, or they can be specific to an individual's fear topography. Furthermore, some cognitive processes may be common to a diagnostic class, such as attentional bias to anxiety; others might be specific to a particular disorder.

In this chapter we review the available findings on cognition in OCD, discuss the extent to which they are particularly characteristic of anxiety, or specific to OCD, and consider their implications for understanding OCD. Information-processing biases researchers have investigated whether anxious individuals are characterized by attention, memory, or interpretation biases for threat-relevant information. Anxiety disordered individuals have consistently exhibited preferential attention to threat-relevant information (Williams, Mathews, & MacLeod, 1996) but preferential memory for threat-relevant information has received mixed support (e.g., Amir, McNally, Riemann, & Clements, 1996; Rapee, McCallum, Melville, Ravenscroft, & Rodney, 1994). Anxious individuals also tend to interpret ambiguous information as threatening (e.g., Amir, Foa, & Coles, 1997; McNally & Foa, 1987). We follow a similar strategy for examining information-processing bias in OCD, keeping in mind the guidelines proposed by McNally (1999).

Attentional Bias

Because of the limited capacity of the attentional system, humans are forced to prioritize sources of information using excitatory and inhibitory mechanisms. It is precisely this balance of the two processes (i.e., activation and inhibition) that may be faulty in individuals with OCD. To examine this hypothesis, researchers have examined both preferential attention to threat-relevant information and deficits in inhibiting distracting information. A promising method for examining attention is priming (Fox, 1994; Tipper, 1985). Priming is defined as the influence of prior presentation of a stimulus on later processing of that stimulus. Positive priming (or simply priming) refers to the decrease in the latency to identify a given item if that item has been previously encountered. Negative priming, on the other hand, refers to an increase in the latency to identify a given item if that item was previously ignored. This suggests that ignoring involves active inhibition. Thus, the presentation of a prime display may either facilitate or inhibit the later processing of a target, depending on the type of processing that is performed on the prime.

Researchers have used a negative priming paradigm to investigate whether individuals with OCD show inhibitory abnormalities. In a typical negative priming paradigm, subjects are simultaneously shown two stimuli (e.g., two words superimposed on one another one in red and one in green). Subjects are asked to read the word written in green and to ignore the word written in red. If the word written in red (ignored word) becomes the target on the next trial, participants exhibit delay in naming the target on the second trial (i.e. exhibit negative priming) because the active inhibition of the distractor on the first trial delays the naming of the word in the second trial. In a typical semantic negative priming task, the to-be-ignored word on the first trial and the to-be-attended word in the second trial are not identical but semantically related (e.g. doctor, nurse). Enright and Beech (1990, 1993a, 1993b) and Enright, Beech, and Claridge (1995) examined negative priming in individuals with OCD in a series of experiments. They found that individuals with OCD are characterized by deficits in the ability to inhibit processing of to-be-ignored information. No such inhibitory deficits were observed in other anxiety disorders. The inhibitory deficits in OCDs were observed in both standard negative priming tasks and semantic negative priming task. However, not all studies examining negative priming have replicated this finding (e.g., MacDonald, Antony, MacLeod, & Swinson, 1999). Thus, the bulk of the data suggests that OCD may involve inhibitory deficits of general information.

As stated earlier, however, information-processing bias may be content-independent or content-dependent. To examine content specific attentional bias for threat, researchers have used other paradigms. For example, Foa and McNally (1986) used a dichotic listening task to examine whether individuals with OCD would pay particular attention to words that related to their concern. Participants chose a word (e.g.,"cancer", "mouse feces") of particular significance to their OCD concerns. Their words were then embedded randomly in two prose passages, one presented to the right ear and one presented to the left ear. These researchers also created neutral passages by randomly embedding the word "pick" ten times in two prose passages. Participants were told to repeat aloud ("shadow") the passage presented to the right ear and to press a button whenever they heard the threat target ("cancer") or the non-threat target ("pick"). In this study, individuals with OCD detected threat targets more often than non-threat targets.

Researchers have also used the emotional Stroop paradigm to examine attentional bias for threat in individuals with OCD. The emotional Stroop paradigm is a popular measure of attentional bias in anxious patients (Williams, Mathews, & MacLeod, 1996). In this paradigm, participants are asked to name the colors in which emotional words are written while ignoring the meanings of the words. Anxious subjects are slower at naming the color of threat-related than non-threat-related words. This interference suggests that anxious individuals may be paying particular attention to threatening information relevant to their current concerns. Using this method, a number of researchers have shown that individuals with OCD are characterized by an attentional bias for OCD-relevant information (Foa, Ilai, McCarthy, Shoyer, & Murdock, 1993; Lavey, van Oppen, & van den Hout, 1994). This attentional bias in individuals with OCD does not seem to be present for general threat words as revealed by two studies (McNally, Riemann, & Kim, 1990; McNally *et al.*, 1994) showing that individuals with OCD do not show Stroop interference for panic-related (e.g., "suffocate") or PTSD-related (e.g., "bodybags") words. In summary, there is ample evidence, using diverse methods from different laboratories, that individuals with OCD show disorder-specific attentional bias for threat. However, whether this bias is disorder-specific or content-specific is not clear. That is, the bias observed in individuals with OCD may be related to their current concern (e.g., OCD-related material) and not specific to the disorder (Reimann & McNally, 1995).

Memory Bias

Clinical observation suggests that OCD patients often express doubt about their memory for their actions and surroundings (e.g., "Did I turn the oven off?", "Did I wash my hands completely?"). This doubt may reflect: (a) general memory deficits; (b) deficit in memory for OCD-relevant material; or (c) a lack of confidence in their memory.

Memory Deficits

Relevant to the first hypothesis, neuropsychological studies indicate that individuals with OCD show deficits in nonverbal memory, compared to non-anxious controls (Boone, Ananth, Philpott, Kaur, & Djenderjian, 1991; Christensen, Kim, Dyksen, & Hoover, 1992; Cohen *et al.*, 1996; Dirson, Bouvard, Cottraux, & Martin, 1995; Savage *et al.*, 1996; Zielinski, Taylor, & Juzwin, 1991). Furthermore, individuals with subclinical checking concerns have been found to show poorer recall for previously completed actions than do non-checkers (Rubenstein, Peynircioglu, Chambless, & Pigott, 1993). This pattern appears stronger for checkers than for washers (Sher, Frost, Kushner, Crews, & Alexander, 1989; Sher, Frost, & Otto, 1983). Contrary to the above results, other investigations have failed to find evidence of an overall memory deficit among people with OCD (Abbruzzese, Bellodi, Ferri, & Scarone, 1993; Brown, Kosslyn, Breiter, Baer, & Jenike, 1994; Foa, Amir, Gershuny, Molnar, & Kozak, 1997; MacDonald, Antony, MacLeod, & Richter, 1997; McNally & Kohlbeck, 1993).

Studies have also examined memory for OCD-relevant events in patients with OCD. For example, individuals with OCD sometimes report uncertainty about whether they performed an action or whether they simply imagined performing that action. Such uncertainty may motivate them to repeat the action. McNally and Kohlbeck (1993) examined possible deficits in memory for actions in patients with OCD compared to controls and found no group differences. Constans, Foa, Franklin and Mathews (1995) examined the hypothesis that OCD patients have a memory deficit for OCD-related material. OCD checkers and non-anxious controls were presented with a series of situations. Half of the situations involved objects that were likely to elicit an urge to check (e.g., candle, knife) and the other half involved neutral objects (e.g., chair, book). Contrary to the hypothesis, checkers were *more* accurate in remembering the position of objects that were left in an unsafe, than in a safe, position. No such differences emerged in the controls. Finally, Radomsky and Rachman (1999) found similar results using a different paradigm. OC washers and non-anxious controls were asked to look at everyday (neutral valence) objects, touched with either a clean cloth or one they were told was "probably dirty." In a subsequent recall test, OCD patients recalled more contaminated objects than clean objects, and recalled fewer clean objects than did non-anxious controls. Thus, these two studies suggest that people with OCD show a specific bias toward remembering threat material relevant to OCD.

Confidence in Memory

Studies have also examined level of confidence in memory in OCD subjects. For example, several studies have found that OCD checkers lack confidence in their memory (McNally & Kohlbeck, 1993; Sher, *et al.*, 1983) and are less satisfied with the vividness of their memories (Constans *et al.*, 1995). Also, non-patients with high MOCI checking scores reported less vivid memories than individuals with low MOCI scores (Sher *et al.*, 1989). Other researchers have also discovered that individuals with OCD experience lower confidence in memory (Constans *et al.*, 1995; Foa *et al.*, 1997; MacDonald, *et al.*, 1997). Thus, there is converging evidence that OCD is associated with low memory confidence. It is not clear whether checkers suffer more from such low confidence than do non-checkers, although a study with a non-clinical population of checkers suggests this may be the case (Sher *et al.*, 1983). It is also unclear whether confidence is lower for threat-relevant stimuli than for threat-irrelevant stimuli. For example, Foa *et al.* (1997) found lower confidence in memory for OCD-related stimuli, whereas Constans *et al.* (1995) did not.

To address some of these issues, Tolin *et al.* (2001) assessed memory and memory confidence over six presentations of objects designed to simulate a checking ritual. To maximize ecological validity and ensure that the stimuli were relevant for each OCD participant, OCD subjects selected safe, unsafe, and neutral objects from a pool of everyday objects. Tolin *et al.* examined learning and memory in individuals with OCD, anxious controls (AC), and non-anxious controls (NAC) by asking them to recall as many objects as possible and to rate their confidence in each memory. Learning was examined by repeating this process, using the same stimuli, six times. No group differences emerged in memory accuracy; however, in those with OCD, memory confidence for unsafe objects showed a progressive decline over repeated trials. NAC and AC groups did not show this decline in confidence. Furthermore, those with primarily checking rituals reported lower confidence in long-term memory than did OCD subjects without primarily checking rituals. Tolin *et al.* (2001) suggested that when individuals with OCD are repeatedly exposed to threat-related stimuli (such as repeated checking), their confidence in remembering these stimuli paradoxically decreases.

Mechanisms in Memory Differences

What would be the mechanism responsible for this difference in recollective experiences between individuals with and without OCD symptoms? Cognitive psychologists have developed a number of methods to delineate different characteristics of one's recollective experiences. For example, researchers have begun examining components of correct and false recognition. Recognition can take place in two distinct forms, that is, it can be accompanied by conscious recollection of some aspect of the experience or by a feeling of familiarity with the experience. These two forms of recognition are typically examined using Tulving's (1985) remember/know task, in which subjects are asked to classify recognition for previously presented items based on familiarity with the item (a know judgment) or a specific recollection of its presentation (a remember judgment). Studies employing this paradigm have found that remember and know judgments are differentially influenced by various factors (for a review see Knowlton, 1998), thereby suggesting that different memory systems may be involved in each type of recognition.

This distinction between systems is not simply due to a difference in level of confidence (Gardner, Gawlik, & Richardson-Klaven, 1994) or "trace strength" (e.g., Gardner & Java, 1991). The two subjective states have been shown to be differentially related to measures of frontal lobe functioning (Parkin & Walter, 1992), event-related potential (Smith, 1993), degree of sedation (Curran, Gardiner, Java, & Allen, 1993), and left versus right temporal lobe lesions (Blaxton & Theodore, 1997). Amir, Klumpp, Freshman, and Przeworski (2000) use a modified version of the false memory paradigm and Tulving's remember/know task to examine whether individuals with and without obsessive-compulsive symptoms differ in their source knowledge (remember vs. know) for recognition, as well as false recognition of OCD-relevant (e.g., germ), positive, or neutral information. These researchers constructed two matched sets of six OCD-relevant threat scenarios, six neutral scenarios, and six positive scenarios. They hypothesized that compared to individuals without OCD symptoms, those with OCD symptoms would rely more on feelings of familiarity (i.e., "know"), particularly when falsely recalling threat words. Results demonstrate that, although groups did not differ in correct or false memory of threat, neutral words, or positive words, individuals with OCD symptoms were more likely to use feelings of familiarity when making a false recognition. This enhanced reliance on feelings of familiarity in individuals with OCD symptoms may reflect ongoing activation of threatening cues and indicate that these individuals are less conservative about rating the quality of their memory, rating more recognized words as "know" than "remember" compared to those without OCD symptoms.

Directed forgetting.   Investigators have also examined the mechanisms of forgetting in individuals with OCD, using the directed forgetting paradigm. This paradigm has been used successfully to study memory processes in anxious populations (Cloitre, Cancienne, Brodsky, Dulit, & Perry, 1996; McNally, Metzger, Lasko, Clancy, & Pitman, 1998; Wilhelm, McNally, Baer, & Florin, 1996) and is uniquely suited to address the mechanisms of encoding and retrieval (Bjork, 1989; Johnson, 1994). In the directed-forgetting paradigm participants are presented with words, each followed by a cue either to remember the word or to forget it. On a later free recall test, participants are asked to remember all the words in the experiment, regardless of original instructions. Participants remember more of the to-be-remembered (TBR) words than the to-be-forgotten (TBF) words (e.g., Bjork, 1989; Zacks, Radvansky, & Hasher, 1996). The enhanced recall of TBR words compared to TBF words may involve: (a) diminished rehearsal of the TBF words; (b) retrieval inhibition of the TBF words; and/or (c) segregation of the TBR and TBF words into distinct memory sets (Zacks & Hasher, 1994). Various methods have been proposed for disentangling the role of encoding and retrieval inhibition (e.g., Basden, Basden, & Gargano, 1993). For example, performance on recall and recognition tests can be compared to assess the role of retrieval cues.

Researchers have used the directed forgetting paradigm to examine memory processes in various clinical and analogue samples. Wilhelm *et al.* (1996) found that individuals with OCD exhibited a deficit in their ability to forget threat-relevant material, but not positive or neutral material. Non-anxious controls did not show this bias. Furthermore, in this study the directed-forgetting effect was present on both recall and recognition tests. Wilhelm *et al.* (1996) suggested that the performance differences were best attributed to differential encoding of the TBR words rather than the differential retrieval inhibition of TBR words.

In summary, studies examining memory biases in individuals with OCD have produced inconsistent, if not contradictory, results. One implication of these findings is that faulty memory processes in OCD may be more specific (e.g., confidence in memory, or ability to forget) than generic (overall recall or recognition).

Interpretation Bias

Individuals with OCD may be characterized by an interpretation bias for threat. Unlike studies of attentional and memory biases, studies of interpretation bias have focused on various aspects of interpretation. For example, because of the prominent role of the construct of responsibility in some current cognitive models of OCD (e.g., Salkovskis, 1989) researchers have examined whether individuals with OCD show exaggerated perception of responsibility in ambiguous situations. Alternatively, individuals with OCD may assign exaggerated importance to negative thoughts or may equate them with actions (Thought–action fusion; see Chapter four).

Responsibility

Each of the above interpretations of ambiguous events had been studied experimentally. Clinical observations suggest that individuals with OCD suffer from excessive personal responsibility for harm to others. Foa, Steketee, and Young (1984) noted that individuals with agoraphobia generally fear harm that might come to themselves, whereas people with OCD are often preoccupied with harm that may come to others. Rachman (1993) suggested that many patients with OCD, especially those with checking compulsions, experience urges to ritualize only in those circumstances in which they assume personal responsibility for safety. Finally, Salkovskis (1985, 1989) proposed that an exaggerated sense of responsibility for negative thoughts (e.g., "I might stab my child") and anticipated negative events ("I will run over a pedestrian if I'm not careful") underlies the psychopathology of OCD. In order to reconcile the discrepancy between his proposition and the observation that some people with OCD are not concerned with others' safety, Salkovskis extended the customary use of the concept of responsibility to include feelings of liability for one's own harm. In a later exposition of this theory, Salkovskis, Richards, and Forrester (1995) suggested that OCD patients are characterized not only by a heightened sense of responsibility, but also by a lack of omission bias; that is, they believe that not acting in a situation which could potentially lead to harm is as bad as directly causing the harm.

To explore the relationship between responsibility and neutralizing, Freeston, Ladouceur, Thibodeau, and Gagnon (1992) administered the Cognitive Intrusions Questionnaire to college students. Factor analysis of responses on the questionnaire yielded five factors, only one of which was significantly related to questions of compulsive activity. This factor, the valence factor, represented the subject's evaluation of the intrusion and the degree to which the subject felt responsible and guilty. The highest loading item on this factor was, "To what extent would you feel responsible if the thought content were to happen?" The authors interpreted these results as demonstrating a link between responsibility and compulsive behavior. Rachman, Thordarson, Shafran, and Woody (1995) examined the relationship between responsibility and OCD symptoms in a sample of college students. To this end, they devised a questionnaire that measured four aspects of responsibility: responsibility for harm, responsibility in social contexts, a positive outlook towards responsibility, and thought–action fusion. Only the thought–action fusion aspect correlated with OC symptom severity as measured by the Maudsley Obsessive–Compulsive Inventory (MOCI; Hodgson & Rachman, 1977). The authors concluded that inflated responsibility is not a general characteristic of OCD, but rather, may be specific to personally relevant situations.

To explore the role of responsibility in the performance of compulsions, Ladouceur *et al.* (1995) carried out two experiments in which they manipulated degree of responsibility in college students. In the first experiment, participants were asked to determine whether they had heard a sound before. They were allowed to listen to the sound as many times as they wanted (i.e., check) before responding. Although the manipulation was successful in producing more feelings of responsibility in the High Responsibility (HR) group, participants in this group did not exhibit more checking behavior than those in the Low Responsibility (LR) group. The authors attributed the negative results to the absence of a relationship between the responsibility manipulation and the performed task. Therefore, in a second experiment, participants in the HR group were instructed to sort different kinds of pills presumably intended for public consumption. Participants in the LR group were told that the pill-sorting task was designed to inform the experimenter about color perception. Participants in the HR condition exhibited more preoccupation with making errors and were more anxious during the task compared to those in the LR condition. However, no group differences emerged on self-report of doubting, urges to check, and time required to complete the task.

To date two studies have examined responsibility experimentally in OCD (Lopatka & Rachman, 1995; Shafran, 1997). Both studies examined the hypotheses that inflating responsibility would increase the urge to check, the degree of discomfort experienced, and the estimated probabilities of bad outcomes. Deflating responsibility was hypothesized to decrease urge, discomfort, and estimated probabilities. In the Lopatka and Rachman (1995) study, participants were instructed to perform a task at home that usually evoked an urge to check under high responsibility instructions (HRI), low responsibility instructions (LRI), and controlled instructions (CI). Responsibility was manipulated using contracts in which the experimenter assumed complete responsibility for potential negative events following the task (LRI) or the participant assumed complete responsibility (HRI). Although the HRI condition produced a higher degree of responsibility compared with the CI condition, the HRI condition did not produce stronger urges to check, higher discomfort, or higher estimated probability of harm. In contrast, the low responsibility instructions reduced the subjects' discomfort, urges to check, and estimated probability of harm. Thus, the hypothesis that responsibility plays a role in OCD was partially supported.

Shafran (1997) replicated these results in a sample of OCs with varied phenomenology and added a measure estimating responsibility for thoughts and control over the thoughts. The results indicated that estimates of responsibility for thoughts and control over the threat did not differ when responsibility was manipulated. There was no significant interaction between the responsibility manipulation and the type of compulsion. It is important to note that in both the Lopatka and Rachman study and the Shafran study, perceived responsibility and degree of estimated probability of harm were similarly affected by the responsibility manipulation. Therefore, it is unclear whether responsibility or estimated probabilities was the crucial variable in determining the urge to check and its associated discomfort.

Foa, Amir, Bogert, Molnar, and Przeworski (2001) examined the proposition that inflated responsibility is implicated in OCD. To this end, the authors developed the Obsessive Compulsive Responsibility Scale (OCRS). The OCRS comprised 27 situations, nine low-risk, nine OCD-relevant, and nine high risk. Examples of low risk situations were: "You see some stuffing coming out of a prize stuffed animal at a carnival," and "You see a piece of string on the ground." Examples of OCD-relevant situations were: "You see some nails on a road," and "You see a box of stale crackers in an office cabinet." Examples of high-risk situations were "You see a person sitting alone in a diner is choking," and "You see a person faint in a supermarket." Subjects rated each situation on three ratings scales: (a) the urge to rectify the situation; (b) the degree of distress felt upon leaving the situation unrectified; and (c) the degree of personal responsibility felt if the unrectified situation later resulted in harm. Each rating was on an eight-point (zero–seven) Likert-type scale. Compared to anxious controls with social anxiety and non-anxious controls, individuals with OCD reported more urges to rectify situations involving potential risk, distress upon leaving such situations unrectified, and responsibility if the unrectified situations resulted in harm in low risk and OC-relevant situations. No group differences were detected in high-risk situations. These authors suggested that control subjects, relative to those with OCD, were better able to differentiate between situations that merit concern and ones that do not.

Thought–Action Fusion

In a further attempt to examine interpretation of ambiguity in their environment by those with OCD, researchers have examined the relationship between their thoughts and their actions. Rachman (1993) suggested that patients with OCD may fuse actions and thoughts. That is, these individuals may be more likely than non-anxious individuals to consider a thought about a negative event as synonymous with the occurrence of the actual negative event (See chapter two for a more thorough discussion). This concept may aid in explaining the maintenance, and possibly the etiology, of OCD for at least two reasons. First, if individuals with OCD believe that thinking about an unacceptable or disturbing event makes the event more likely to occur in reality, they may engage in rituals to prevent the negative consequence. Second, such individuals may believe that obsessional thoughts and negative acts are morally equivalent, thus feeling distress for having the negative thought. Research with clinical populations, as well as non-clinical populations with elevated scores on measures of OCD, supports the utility of the thought–action fusion (TAF) construct (Rachman, Thordarson, Shafran, & Woody, 1995). This research has used the Thought–Action Fusion Scale (TAFS), a psychometrically valid measure of the construct. The TAFS comprises three subscales: TAF-Moral (TAFM; 12 items) (e.g., "If I wish harm on someone, it is almost as bad as doing harm"), TAF-Likelihood-Self (TAFLS; three items), (e.g., "If I think of myself being injured in a fall, this increases the risk that I will have a fall and be injured"), and TAF-Likelihood-Other (TAFLO; four items), (e.g., "If I think of a friend or relative having a car accident, this increases the risk that he/she will have a car accident").

In two experiments, Shafran, Thordarson, and Rachman (1996) found that individuals with scores of 11 or higher on the MOCI (Hodgson & Rachman, 1977) had higher scores on the TAF-Likelihood than a sample of students and community volunteers. Furthermore, results of correlational analyses revealed that the TAF-Likelihood scores were positively correlated with severity of obsessive compulsive symptoms, as measured by the MOCI. Thus, there are both theoretical and empirical reasons to believe that the fusion of thoughts and actions, as measured by the TAFS, is an important construct in OCD. In addition, there is evidence that TAF can be experimentally induced (e.g., Rassin, Merckelbach, Muris, & Spaan, 1999). There are, however, a number questions that should be addressed to strengthen the case for a causal association between TAF and obsessive compulsive symptoms.

First, is the fusion of thoughts and actions in OCD confined to disastrous consequences of thoughts about negative events, or do individuals with obsessive compulsive symptoms believe that their thoughts about positive events are capable of producing positive outcomes, possibly preventing harm? Shafran *et al.* (1996) had people with OCD evaluate positive events (e.g., "If I think of winning the lottery, that will increase the chance that I will win the lottery"), but suggested that these items were of little relevance to OCD and therefore eliminated them from a revised version of the TAFS. However, clinical observation suggests that individuals with obsessive compulsive symptoms seem more concerned about preventing losses (i.e., about harm prevention) than about obtaining rewards from their thoughts.

Second, do individuals with obsessive compulsive symptoms rate negative events as more costly? If individuals with OCD rate negative events as more costly, then this exaggerated sensitivity to cost may explain their tendency to equate thoughts about negative events with the actual negative event. That is, the exaggerated cost associated with these negative events may be the cause of their fusion with actions. Alternatively, their tendency to equate thoughts and actions may explain their tendency to assign higher cost to negative thoughts than do non-anxious individuals. Because the TAFS does not inquire about the cost, or negative value, assigned to the negative events, it is not possible to examine these two alternative explanations.

Third, do individuals with obsessive compulsive symptoms believe that having negative thoughts implies something important about their self-worth? Perhaps they feel more responsible for having thoughts of negative events than do non-anxious individuals, thinking that these thoughts indicate that they are "a bad person." Because of the popularity of responsibility in some approaches to OCD (e.g., Salkovskis, 1989), it is likely that individuals with OCD take responsibility for having these negative thoughts and hence assign more importance to having them. This increased importance may explain the exaggerated tendency to fuse thoughts and actions.

To address some of the above concerns, Amir, Freshman, Ramsey, Neary, and Brigidi, (2001) modified the TAF questionnaire to address the questions raised above by expanding the "likelihood of events happening to others" subscale to include thoughts about positive events and thoughts involving prevention of harm (harm avoidance). They also added ratings of the cost of the negative and positive events and of the implication of the unwanted thought for self-perception. This last modification was designed to assess the extent of responsibility the individual felt for the thought. Replicating previous findings, they found that individuals with obsessive compulsive symptoms gave higher ratings to the likelihood of negative events happening as a result of their negative thoughts. Individuals with obsessive compulsive symptoms also rated the likelihood that they would prevent harm by their positive thoughts higher than did individuals without obsessive compulsive symptoms. These results suggest that the role of thought–action fusion in OCD may extend to exaggerated beliefs about thoughts regarding the reduction of harm. These results are reminiscent of findings on strength of belief in OCD (for review, see Kozak & Foa, 1994). Some individuals with OCD have fixed mistaken beliefs about harm related to their obsessive fears, for example, the belief that the number 666 on a license plate is an ill omen. Such ideas indicate that individuals with OCD can have magical beliefs about the properties of objects, as well as about thoughts. Research is needed to examine the link between these two varieties of belief, and to examine whether they are different aspects of the same cognitive phenomenon.

Efforts to Control Intrusive Thoughts

The tendency to fuse thoughts and actions in individuals with OCD may also lead to attempts to suppress these thoughts. Furthermore, intrusive distressing thoughts (obsessions) are one of the core features of OCD and are also common in the general population (Clark & de Silva, 1985; Rachman & de Silva, 1978; Salkovskis & Harrison, 1984). However, although these thoughts are similar in content to those experienced by individuals with OCD, they are associated with less distress than the obsessions of individuals with OCD (Rachman & de Silva, 1978; Salkovskis & Harrison, 1984). If both individuals with and without OCD experience intrusive, distressing thoughts why are they debilitating the former but not the latter?

One possible explanation is the use by individuals with OCD of problematic strategies to manage or control their intrusive thoughts. Wells and Davies (1994) proposed that strategies to cope with distressing intrusive thought can be categorized into five clusters: distraction (e.g., I do something that I enjoy), punishment (e.g., I get angry at myself for having the thought), worry (e.g., I dwell on other worries), re-appraisal (e.g., I analyze the thought rationally), and social (e.g., I ask my friends if they have similar thoughts). Wells and Davies found that the use of punishment and worry strategies to control intrusive thoughts was related to measures of anxiety and obsessive compulsive symptoms in a non-clinical sample.

Amir, Foa, and Cashman (1997) compared the control strategies employed by patients with OCD to those employed by non-patient controls. They also examined the relationship between control strategies and OCD symptom severity (obsessions and compulsions). They hypothesized that individuals with OCD would use punishment and worry strategies more often than non-patient controls to manage their intrusive thoughts. They further hypothesized that the degree of using punishment and worry would be related to OCD severity, especially severity of obsessions. Results revealed that OCD patients used punishment, worry, reappraisal, and social control more often than non-patients. Conversely, non-patients used distraction more often than OCDs. Interestingly, use of punishment strategy was the strongest discriminator of OCDs and non-patients, mostly because of the low frequency of its use by non-patients. Furthermore, punishment and worry were the only methods of thought control that correlated with OCD symptoms. These results suggest that OCD patients may use maladaptive methods of thought control when faced with obsessions. Ladouceur *et al.* (2000) compared strategies used by individuals with OCD, other anxiety, and healthy volunteers. These researchers concluded that people with OCD, those with other anxiety disorders, as well as non-anxious controls, draw on a similar pool of strategies to control unwanted thoughts.

Partially in an attempt to reconcile and combine the efforts of various investigations assessing cognitions in individual with OCD, in 1995 the Obsessive Compulsive Cognitions Working Group initiated a collective process to develop two measures of cognition relevant to current cognitive–behavioral models of OCD (OCCWG, 1997). This collaboration led to the development of a questionnaire (OCCWG, 1997). Future directions include the development and validation of a comprehensive assessment method using two scales: (a) The Obsessive Beliefs Questionnaire consisting of 87 items representing dysfunctional assumptions covering six domains: overestimation of threat, tolerance of uncertainty, importance of thoughts, control of thoughts, responsibility, and perfectionism; and (b) The Interpretation of Intrusions Inventory consisting of 31 items that refer to interpretations of intrusions that have occurred recently. Three of the above domains represent importance of thoughts, control of thoughts, and responsibility. Preliminary results on reliability and validity indicate excellent internal consistency, stability, convergent validity, and discriminant validity (OCCWG, 2001). However, high correlations between some of the scales indicate overlap, particularly among importance of thoughts, control of thoughts, and responsibility that should be addressed in subsequent empirical and theoretical investigations (OCCWG, in preparation).

Conclusions

Information processing models of psychopathology attempt to identify abnormalities in attention, memory, and interpretation among individuals with pathological anxiety. These abnormalities are thought to be causally involved in the pathogenesis of various emotional disorders and perhaps help explain the symptoms of these disorders. The research, reviewed above, is an initial attempt to identify such faulty mechanisms. For example, there is good evidence that individuals with OCD have attentional abnormalities. These abnormalities seem to involve both a general inability to inhibit processing of irrelevant information, as well as distraction by threat relevant cues. Studies of memory bias suggest that memory per se, might not be implicated in OCD. However, individuals with OCD might have lower confidence in their memories and this deficit in confidence may motivate checking. Finally, a host of studies demonstrate that individuals with OCD tend to assign different attributions to their thoughts and actions. For example, they might feel responsible for having certain thoughts and attempt to suppress these thoughts. In summary, the symptoms of OCD might be caused by biases in information processing. If so, the identification of such biases might aid in the identification of basic mechanism in OCD leading to better understanding and better treatment of its symptoms.

Acknowledgement

The authors would like to thank Fran Arnold and Jennifer Sullivan for their help in the preparation of this chapter. The preparation of this chapter was supported by a faculty development grant from the Institute for Behavioral Research (IBR) at University of Georgia awarded to the first author.

References

Abbruzzese, M., Bellodi, L., Ferri, S., & Scarone, S. (1993). Memory functioning in obsessive–compulsive disorder. *Behavioural Neurology, 6*, 119–122.

Amir, N., Foa, E. B., & Cashman, L. (1997). Strategies of thought control in obsessive–compulsive disorder. *Behaviour and Research Therapy, 35*, 775–777.

Amir, N., Foa, E. B., & Coles, M. (1997). Factor structure of the Yale–Brown Obsessive–Compulsive Scale. *Psychological Assessment, 9*, 312–316.

Amir, N., Freshman, M., Ramsey, B., Neary, E., & Brigidi, B. (2001). Thought–action Fusion in Individuals with OCD Symptoms. *Behaviour Research and Therapy, 37*, 765–776.

Amir, N., Klumpp, H., Freshman, M., & Przeworski, A. (2000). Memory bias in obsessive–compulsive disorder: The role of reconstruction of familiar threat-related items. Submitted for publication.

Amir, N., McNally, R. J., Riemann, B. C., & Clements, C. (1996). Implicit memory bias for threat in panic disorder: Application of the white noise paradigm. *Behaviour Research and Therapy, 34*, 157–162.

Basden, B. H., Basden, D. R., & Gargano, G. J. (1993). Directed forgetting in implicit and explicit memory tests: A comparison of methods. *Journal of Experimental Psychology: Learning, Memory, & Cognition, 19,* 603–616.

Beck, A. T., Epstein, N., Brown, G., & Steer, R. A. (1988). An inventory for measuring clinical anxiety: Psychometric properties. *Journal of Consulting and Clinical Psychology, 56,* 893–897.

Beck, A. T., Steer, R. A., & Garbin, M. G. (1988). Psychometric properties of the Beck Depression Inventory: Twenty-five years of evaluation. *Clinical Psychology Review, 8,* 77–100.

Bjork, R. A. (1989). Retrieval inhibition as an adaptive mechanism in human memory. In H. L. Roediger, III & F. I. M. Craik (eds), *Varieties of Memory and Consciousness: Essays in Honour of Endel Tulving* (pp. 309–330). Hillsdale, NJ: Erlbaum.

Blaxton, T., & Theodore, W. (1997). The role of the temporal lobes in recognizing visuo-spatial materials: Remembering versus knowing. *Brain and Cognition, 35,* 5–25.

Boone, K. B., Ananth, J., Philpott, L., Kaur, A., & Djenderjian, A. (1991). Neuropsychology and behavioral neuropsychological characteristics of nondepressed adults with obsessive–compulsive disorder. *Neurology, 4,* 96–109.

Brown, H. D., Kosslyn, S. M., Breiter, H. C., Baer, L., & Jenike, M. A. (1994). Can patients with obsessive–compulsive disorder discriminate between perceptions and mental images? A signal detection analysis. *Journal of Abnormal Psychology, 103,* 445–454.

Christensen, K. J., Kim, S. W., Dyksen, M. W., & Hoover, K. M. (1992). Neuropsychological performance in obsessive–compulsive disorder. *Biological Psychiatry, 31,* 4–18.

Clark, D. A., & de Silva, P. (1985). The nature of depressive and anxious intrusive thoughts: Distinct or uniform phenomena? *Behaviour Research and Therapy, 23,* 383–393.

Cloitre, M., Shear, K. M., Cancienne, J., & Zeitlin, S. B. (1994). Implicit and explicit memory for catastrophic associations for bodily sensations words in panic disorder. *Cognitive Therapy and Research, 18,* 225–240.

Cohen, L. J., Hollander, E., DeCaria, C. M., Stein, D. J., Simeon, D., Liebowitz, M. R., & Aronowitz, B. R. (1996). Specificity in neuropsychological impairment in obsessive–compulsive disorder: A comparison with social phobic and normal control subjects. *Journal of Neuropsychiatry, 8,* 82–85.

Constans, J. I., Foa, E. B., Franklin, M. E., & Mathews, A. (1995). Memory for actual and imagined events in OC checkers. *Behaviour Research and Therapy, 33,* 665–671.

Curran, H. V., Gardiner, J. M., Java, R. I., & Allen, D. (1993). Effects of lorazepam upon recollective experience in recognition memory. *Psychopharmacology, 119,* 374–378.

Dennett, D. (1978). *Brainstorms: Philosophical essays on mind and psychology.* Cambridge, MA: MIT Press.

Dirson, S., Bouvard, M., Cottraux, J., & Martin, R. (1995). Visual memory impairment in patients with obsessive–compulsive disorder: A controlled study. *Psychotherapy and Psychosomatics, 63,* 22–31.

Enright, S. J., & Beech, A. R. (1990). Obsessional states: Anxiety disorders or schizotypes? An information processing and personality assessment. *Psychological Medicine, 20,* 621–627.

Enright, S. J., & Beech, A. R. (1993a). Further evidence of reduced cognitive inhibition in obsessive–compulsive disorder. *Personality and Individual Differences, 14,* 387–395.

Enright, S. J., & Beech, A. R. (1993b). Reduced cognitive inhibition in obsessive–compulsive disorder. *British Journal of Clinical Psychology, 32,* 67–74.

Enright, S. J., Beech, A. R., & Claridge, G. S. (1995). A further investigation of cognitive inhibition in obsessive–compulsive disorder and other anxiety disorders. *Personality and Individual Differences, 19,* 535–542.

Foa, E. B., & Kozak, M. J. (1993). Pathological anxiety: Meaning and the structure of fear. In N. Birbaumer and A. Ohman (eds) *The structure of emotion: Physiological, cognitive, and clinical aspects* (pp. 110–121). Seattle WA: Hogrefe and Huber.

Foa, E. B., & McNally, R. J. (1986). Sensitivity to feared stimuli in obsessive–compulsives: a dichotic listening analysis. *Cognitive Therapy and Research, 10*, 477–485.

Foa, E. B., Amir, N., Bogert, K. V., Molnar, C., & Przeworski, A. (2001). Inflated perception of responsibility for harm in obsessive–compulsive disorder. *Journal of Anxiety Disorders*.

Foa, E. B., Amir, N., Gershuny, B., Molnar, C., & Kozak, M. J. (1997). Implicit and explicit memory in obsessive–compulsive disorder. *Journal of Anxiety Disorders, 11*, 119–129.

Foa, E. B., Iiai, D., McCarthy, P. R., Shoyer, B., & Murdock, T. B.. (1993). Information processing in obsessive–compulsive disorder. *Cognitive Therapy and Research, 17*, 173–189.

Fodor, J. A. (1968). *Psychological explanation*. New York: Random House.

Fox, E. (1994). Interference and negative priming from ignored distracters: The role of selection difficulty. *Perception and Psychophysics, 56*, 565–574.

Freeston, M. L., Ladoucear, R., Thibodeau, N., & Gagnon, F. (1992). Cognitive intrusions in a non-clinical population: II. Associations with depressive, anxious, and compulsive symptoms. *Behaviour Research and Therapy, 30*, 263–271.

Gardiner, J. M., Gawlick, B., & Richardson-Klavehn, A. (1994). Maintenance rehearsal affects of knowing, not remembering: Elaborative rehearsal affects remembering, not knowing. *Psychonomic Bulletin and Review, 1*, 107–110.

Gardner, J. M., & Java, R. I. (1991). Forgetting in recognition memory with and without recollective experience. *Memory and Cognition, 19*, 617–623.

Hodgson R. J., & Rachman, S. (1977). Obsessional–compulsive complaints. *Behaviour Research and Therapy, 15*, 389–395.

Johnson, H. M. (1994). Processes of successful intentional forgetting. *Psychological Bulletin, 116*, 274–292.

Knowlton, B. J. (1998). The relationship between remembering and knowing: A cognitive neuroscience perspective. *Acta Psychologica, 98*, 253–265.

Kozak, M., J., & Foa, E. B. (1994). Obsessions, overvalued ideas, and delusions in obsessive–compulsive disorder. *Behaviour Research and Therapy, 32*, 343–353.

Kozak, M. J., & Miller G. A. (1982). Hypothetical constructs versus intervening variables: A reappraisal of the three-systems model of anxiety assessment. *Behavioral Assessment, 4*, 347–358.

Ladouceur R., Freestone M. H., Rhéaume J., Dugas, M. J., Gagmon, F., Thibodeau, N., & Fournier, S. (2000). Strategies used with intrusive thoughts: A comparison of OCD patients with anxious and community controls. *Journal of Abnormal Psychology, 109*, 179–187.

Ladouceur, R., Rhéaume, J., Freeston, M. H., Aublet, F., Jean, K., Lachance, S., Langlois, F., & De Pokomandy-Morin, K. (1995). Experimental manipulations of responsibility: An analogue test for models of obsessive–compulsive disorder. *Behaviour Research and Therapy, 33*, 937–946.

Lang, P. J. (1968). Fear reduction and fear behavior: Problems in treating aconstruct. In J. M. Schlien (ed.), *Research in Psychotherapy, III* (pp. 90–102). Washington, D.C.: American Psychological Association.

Lavey, E. H., van Oppen, P., & van den Hout, M. A. (1994). Selective processing of emotional information in obsessive–compulsive disorder. *Behaviour Research and Therapy, 32*, 243–246.

Lopatka, C., & Rachman, S. (1995). Perceived responsibility and compulsive checking: An experimental analysis. *Behaviour Research and Therapy, 33*, 673–684.

MacDonald, P. A., Antony, M. M., MacLeod, C. M., & Richter, M. A. (1997). Memory and confidence in memory judgments among individuals with obsessive–compulsive disorder and non-clinical controls. *Behaviour Research and Therapy, 35*, 497–505.

MacDonald, P. A., Antony, M. M., MacLeod, C. M., & Swinson, R. P. (1999). Negative priming for obsessive–compulsive checkers and noncheckers. *Journal of Abnormal Psychology, 108*, 679–686.

McNally, R. J. (1999). Information-processing abnormalities in obsessive–compulsive disorder. In W. Goodman, M. Rudorfer, & J. Maser (eds) *Obsessive–compulsive disorder: contemporary issues in treatment*. Mahwah, NJ: Lawrence Erlbaum.

McNally, R. J., & Foa, E. B. (1987). Cognition and agoraphobia: Bias in the interpretation of threat. *Cognitive Therapy and Research, 11*, 567–581.

McNally, R. J., & Kohlbeck, P. A. (1993). Reality monitoring in obsessive–compulsive disorder. *Behaviour Research and Therapy, 31*, 249–253.

McNally, R. J., Amir, N., Louro, C. E., Lukach, B. M., Riemann, B. C., & Calamari, J. E. (1994). Cognitive processing of idiographic emotional information in panic disorder. *Behaviour Research and Therapy, 22*, 119–122.

McNally, R. J., Metzger, L. J., Lasko, L. J., Clancy, S. A., & Pitman, R. K. (1998). Directed forgetting of trauma cues in women with histories of childhood sexual abuse. *Journal of Abnormal Psychology, 107*, 596–601.

McNally, R. J., Riemann, B. C., & Kim, E. (1990). Selective processing of threat cues in panic disorder. *Behaviour Research and Therapy, 28*, 407–412.

Miller, G. A., & Keller, J. (2000). Psychology and neuroscience: Making peace. *Current Directions in Psychological Science, 9*, 30–33.

Miller, G. A., and Kozak, M. J. (1993). A philosophy for the study of emotion: Three systems theory. In N. Birbaumer & A. Ohman (eds) *The structure of emotion: physiological, cognitive, and clinical aspects* (pp. 31–47). Seattle WA: Hogrefe and Huber.

Mogg, K., Mathews, A., & Weinman, J. (1987). Memory bias in clinical anxiety. *Journal of Abnormal Psychology, 96*, 94–98.

National Institute of Mental Health. (1999, February). Peer review notes. Washington, D.C.

Neill, W. T., Beck, J. L., Bottalico, K. S., & Molloy, R. D. (1990). Effects of intentional versus incidental learning on explicit and implicit tests of memory. *Journal of Experimental Psychology: Learning, Memory, and Cognition, 16*, 457–463.

Obsessive Compulsive Cognitions Working Group. (1997). Cognitive assessment of obsessive–compulsive disorder. *Behaviour Research and Therapy, 35*, 667–681.

Obsessive Compulsive Cognitions Working Group. (2001). Development and initial validation of the Obsessive–Beliefs Questionnaire and the Interpretation of Intrusions Inventory. *Behaviour Research and Therapy, 39*, 987–1006.

Parkin, A. J., & Walter, B. M. (1992). Recollective experience, aging, and frontal dysfunction. *Psychology and Aging, 7*, 290–298.

Rachman, S. (1993). Obsessions, responsibility, and guilt. *Behaviour Research and Therapy, 31*, 149–154.

Rachman, S., & de Silva, P. (1978). Abnormal and normal obsessions. *Behaviour Research and Therapy, 16*, 233–248.

Rachman, S., Thordarson, D. S., Shafran, R., & Woody, S. (1995). Perceived responsibility: Structure and significance. *Behaviour Research and Therapy, 33*, 779–784.

Radomsky, A. S., & Rachman, S. (1999). Memory bias in obsessive–compulsive disorder (OCD). *Behaviour Research and Therapy, 37*, 605–618.

Rapee, R. M., McCallum, S. L., Melville, L. F., Ravenscroft, H., & Rodney, J. M. (1994). Memory bias in social phobia. *Behaviour Research and Therapy, 32*, 89–99.

Rassin, E., Merckelbach, H., Muris, P., & Spaan, V. (1999). Thought–action fusion as a causal factor in the development of intrusions. *Behaviour Research and Therapy, 37*, 231–237.

Riemann, B. C, & McNally, R. J. (1995). Cognitive processing of personally relevant information. *Cognition and Emotion, 9*, 325–340.

Rubenstein, C. S., Peynircioglu, Z. F., Chambless, D. L., & Pigott, T. A. (1993). Memory in subclinical obsessive–compulsive checkers. *Behaviour Research and Therapy, 31*, 759–765.

Salkovskis, P. M. (1985). Obsessional–compulsive problems: A cognitive–behavioural analysis. *Behaviour Research and Therapy, 23*, 571–583.

Salkovskis, P. M. (1998, July). *Cognitive, behavioural and biological interactions in psychological problems: Why OCD is not a neurological disorder and other controversies.* Presented to the World Congress of Behavioural and Cognitive Therapies, Acapulco.

Salkovskis, P. M., & Harrison, J. (1984). Abnormal and normal obsessions: A replication. *Behaviour Research and Therapy, 22*, 549–552.

Salkovskis, P. M., Richards, H. C., & Forrester, E. (1995). The relationship between obsessional problems and intrusive thoughts. *Behavioural and Cognitive Psychotherapy, 23*, 281–299.

Savage, C. R., Keuthen, N. J., Jenike, M. A., Brown, H. D., Baer, L., Kendrick, A. D., Miguel, E. C., Rauch, S. L., & Albert, M. S. (1996). Recall and recognition memory in obsessive–compulsive disorder. *Journal of Neuropsychiatry, 8*, 99–103.

Shafran, R. (1997). The manipulation of responsibility in obsessive–compulsive disorder. *British Journal of Clinical Psychology, 36*, 397–407.

Shafran, R., Thordarson, D. S., & Rachman, S. (1996). Thought–action fusion in obsessive–compulsive disorder. *Journal of Anxiety Disorders, 10*, 379–391.

Sher, K. J., Frost, R. O., & Otto, R. (1983). Cognitive deficits in compulsive checkers: An exploratory study. *Behaviour Research and Therapy, 21*, 357–363.

Sher, K. J., Frost, R. O., Kushner, M., Crews, T. M., & Alexander, J. E. (1989). Memory deficits in compulsive checkers: Replication and extension in a nonclinical sample. *Behaviour Research and Therapy, 27*, 65–69.

Smith, M. E. (1993). Neuropsychological manifestations of recollective experience during recognition memory judgments. *Journal of Cognitive Neuroscience, 5*, 1–13.

Tipper, S. P. (1985). The negative priming effect: Inhibitory effects of ignored primes. *Quarterly Journal of Experimental Psychology, 37A*, 571–590.

Tolin, D. F., Abramowitz, J. S., Brigidi, B. D., Amir, N., Street, G. P., & Foa, E. B. (2001). Memory and confidence biases in obsessive–compulsive disorder. *Behaviour Research and Therapy, 39*, 913–927.

Tulving, E. (1985). Memory and consciousness. *Canadian Psychologist, 26*, 1–12.

Wells, A., & Davies, M. I. (1994). The thought control questionnaire: A measure of individual differences in the control of unwanted thoughts. *Behaviour Research and Therapy, 32*, 871–878.

Wilhelm, S., McNally, R. J., Baer, L., & Florin, I. (1996). Directed forgetting in obsessive–compulsive disorder. *Behaviour Research and Therapy, 34*, 633–641.

Williams, J. M. G., Mathews, A., & MacLeod, C. (1996). The emotional Stroop task and psychopathology. *Psychological Bulletin, 120*, 3–24.

Zacks, R. T., & Hasher, L. (1994). Directed ignoring: inhibitory regulation of working memory. In D. Dagenbach, & T. H. Carr (eds) *Inhibitory processes in attention, memory, and language.* San Diego: Academic Press.

Zacks, R. T., Radvansky, G. A., & Hasher, L. (1996). Studies of directed forgetting in older adults. *Journal of Experimental Psychology: Learning, Memory, and Cognition, 22*, 143–156.

Zielinski, C. M., Taylor, M. A., & Juzwin, K. R. (1991). Neuropsychological deficits in obsessive–compulsive disorder. *Neuropsychiatry, Neuropsychology, and Behavioral Neurology, 4*, 110–126.

Chapter 10

Insight: Its Conceptualization and Assessment

Fugen Neziroglu and Kevin P. Stevens

Introduction

Insight as a term has been used to describe and define various cognitive functions and mental phenomena. Insight has been a central topic of discussion for many philosophers as well. This chapter seeks to examine the concept of insight at its interface between mental health professions and the cognitive sciences and will attempt to define its place in reference to other similar concepts such as judgment and metacognition. We will also review methods and measures for the assessment of insight and their import as a prognostic variable in treatment protocols. Finally, we will examine the role of insight with respect to the cognitive domains identified by the OCCWG (1997, 2001).

Definitions

Insight can be defined as an understanding of the motivations behind one's thoughts or behaviors. Insight may also be defined as a recognition of the sources of one's emotional or mental problems. Outside of a psychotherapeutic context, insight may connote a sudden understanding of a problem following a period of time in which the brain is organizing seemingly unrelated material in accordance with various organizational strategies (Halpern, 1984). In a somewhat narrow application, Bastick (1982) defined insight operationally as a sudden increase in the number of correct responses on a learning task. Psychiatrically, insight is seen as an ability on the part of a person to understand and comprehend causes and meanings of a situation (Kaplan & Saddock, 1993).

Differentiation of Insight from Judgment, Knowledge, and Metacognition

Terms such as insight, judgment, knowledge, and metacognition are often used interchangeably in both academic and clinical settings. Differences between the terms do exist, however. A broad analogy may provide a summary understanding of the relatedness of these terms: judgment is to insight as knowledge is to metacognition. Whereas judgment may be defined as an ability to correctly assess and consequently operate adaptively within the parameters of an assessment (Kaplan & Saddock, 1993), insight refers to a *sudden* gain in the understanding of a mental set, whether in a learning task or, more generally, in how one operates on his/her environment. Judgment therefore imbues a sense of discernment and choice of actions among various conceived options of which one is aware. Perhaps a major distinction between insight and judgment concerns the apparent passivity and the receptive quality of the latter, whereas the former is marked by an active and an expressive mental and behavioral undertaking.

Knowledge, on the other hand, refers to a "store" or "node network" of learned or encoded information that may be available for retrieval and further processing to either solve a problem or to generate new knowledge or node connections (Matlin, 1989). Knowledge, appears to envelope the concepts of judgment and insight in that sound judgment may be exercised given true insight. The cognitive, affective, and behavioral responses and operations that follow can then be abstracted and encoded as experiential knowledge.

Just as judgment may be affected by the extent of insight one has regarding particular matters, so is knowledge relatively limited by the extent of one's metacognition. Metacognition is more broadly akin to insight in that both entail knowledge about and, more importantly, awareness of one's cognitive processes. Metacognition is, however, a general cognitive process used to analyze specific and different cognitions, stores, and mental processes. It can be used as a guide in the generation of new knowledge and in the selection of mental sets to solve familiar and new problems (Cavanaugh & Perlmutter, 1982). Whereas metacognition may be conceived of as superintendent of cognition, insight appears to represent more the process in which one gathers understanding.

Terms such as insight, judgment, knowledge, cognition, awareness, and metacognition appear related in meaning, so that generating separate definitions may appear moot or pedantically academic in character. The phenomena of blindsight and the phantom limb may highlight the differences when these concepts operate relatively independently.

The phenomenon of blindsight (Weiskrantz, 1986; Weiskrantz, Warrington, Sanders, & Marshall, 1974) is the condition in which persons and animals without vision begin to identify visual stimuli without being aware of them. In this condition, the normally used visual cortices and pathways do not process visual information and yet over time, persons begin to respond to visual sensation. Blindsight has been demonstrated in monkeys where the entire primary visual cortex has been removed experimentally. Blindsighted individuals learn over time to orient toward light, identify the presence and absence of stimuli, discriminate shapes and edges, and can avoid obstacles while walking or running. Particularly in the case of avoiding obstacles, ones sees clearly the execution of sound judgment without apparent insight.

It appears that blindsight, or unconscious vision, is made possible as the brain recruits intact pathways of the primitive subcortical mammalian visual pathway that are not normally used in humans and monkeys. These pathways are also not routed through sections of the brain that produce awareness that can be verbalized. While persons improve their blindsight abilities with training, they never gain verbal consciousness of this. While blindsight improves, no research that we are aware of has demonstrated that humans have utilized metacognitive processes to evaluate and select this new modality in decision making or concept formation. Blindsighted individuals remain unaware of their improved "visual skills".

Thus, in the phenomenon of blindsight we see judgment (e.g., to act, to avoid obstacles, to determine the presence or absence of an object) occurring without insight and knowledge that comes to exist presumably independently of the auspices of one's metacognition. While their abilities improve, they remain unaware of this. What appears to have parsed these concepts is consciousness; in particular, verbal consciousness. For it remains difficult to conceive of an individual who can run and actively avoid obstacles without truly being aware of them at some level. Rather, it seems that the various concepts such as knowledge, insight, awareness, judgment, and understanding are present and operative but not with their usual verbal overlays. This conceptualization brings blindsight closer to a pure but limited stimulus–response (S–R) model. S–R models are particularly good at explaining behavior emitted without apparent awareness (Bruner, 1992; Greenwald, 1992; Kilstrohm, 1987). Examples of such behaviors include automatic behaviors, where verbal stimuli have dropped out of response chains; not being aware of shifting gears while driving, subtle mood changes following changes in weather and lighting; particular food cravings; or possibly certain compulsive behaviors.

It appears, then, that language and verbal abilities provide the means to link judgment to insight and knowledge to metacognition. This can also be observed in the phantom limb phenomenon. In this phenomenon, amputees experience tactile sensations such as pain, itching, touch, and tension in appendages and limbs that have been amputated and now no longer exist. The reason for the phantom limb phenomenon lies in the neural reorganization and mapping in the brain of adjacent areas that take over the areas that once controlled the amputated body parts. These latent circuits allow for the expansion of an adjacent cortical area. For example, tactile stimulation to the index finger of a monkey would produce the perception of touch to an actually amputated adjacent finger. The brain itself is unaware of the origination of impulses and falsely registers these as originating from non-existing bodily areas. In cases of phantom limb, the person is certainly aware of a missing limb or appendage. That is, they have access to visually based knowledge of this. During the course of rehabilitation and adaptation, a person's judgment and metacognition is at least partially altered as far as the amputation has altered gait, mobility, balance, writing skills, daily living skills, interpersonal interactions, and even self-perceptions. Phantom limb pain and general stimulation often persists and cannot be treated by opiates or even further surgery to the neuromas at the point of entry into the spinal column. The sensory and perceptual mechanism persists in the brain and there is no personal insight that the brain is being remapped, despite having intellectual knowledge of this.

While verbal knowledge and analysis can bridge the gap between altered knowledge and metacognition, the altered judgment does not occur because of altered insight concerning the origination of neural impulses in the brain. Language is critically missing in this instance. While language and insight regarding neural mapping is not available, one sees more clearly in the case of the phantom limb phenomenon than in unconscious vision that different levels of insight do exist.

Different Levels of Insight

Differentiating between varying levels of insight begins to make more sense in clinical and applied settings, particularly as this may provide a qualitative prognostic indication of treatment outcome. This has traditionally been done by psychiatrists as part of a mental status examination (see Kaplan & Saddock, 1993). Levels of insight range from complete denial to partial insight to full insight.

True emotional insight is said to exist when the patient's awareness and understanding of his or her thoughts, feelings, and motives can be used to exert a change in their behavior. This is the highest degree of insight possible, characterized by sound judgment and knowledge that is utilized appropriately by metacognitive processes.

Intellectual insight is more commonly seen in psychotherapeutic contexts and occurs when patients understand that their degree of maladaptation is due to their own thoughts, feelings, and behaviors. The characteristic of intellectual insight is that patients cannot or do not apply this metacognitive knowledge to alter behavior patterns and interpersonal tendencies. In this level of insight, sound judgment is not exercised, and insight and metacognitive processes fail to generate appropriate strategies to solve the problems. Patients in this category are often seen to repeat the same mistakes over and over again. They fail to learn from previous mistakes and prior experiences.

Partial internally based and externally based insights occur when there is an awareness of a disorder that is falsely attributed to either unknown factors within the person or external factors such as other's behaviors or organic factors. These levels of insight are characterized by persons not being attuned to their own emotional states. In our experience, we see this level of insight predominantly in persons with character disorders, anger management issues, as well as in drug and alcohol abusers. Level of insight varies to the extent that persons may only exhibit a slight awareness of being maladapted and needing help, while at the same time denying this and actively sabotaging treatment gains.

Denial of illness is the lowest level of insight possible and likely only occurs in people with severe mental illnesses characterized by predominant chemical and/or anatomical organic deficits as is seen in people during a full blown manic phase, and persons with psychotic and dementing disorders.

Overvalued Ideas and their Relationship to Insight and Judgment

We have already stated that level of insight varies from total awareness to denial of illness. This means that judgment is either very good or completely lacking depending on the level of insight. Overvalued ideas are pathological thought processes with poor insight. Kozak and Foa (1994) have suggested that overvalued ideas are on a continuum between rational thought and delusions. We propose that overvalued ideas do not fluctuate spontaneously, but are fixed and possibly modifiable only if challenged.

Several types of abnormal thought processes exit, one of which is overvalued ideas. Others include delusional, fixed, and obsessional ideas. The level of insight and judgment distinguishes one from the other. Delusions refer to ideas that are a result of a primary pathological experience or sensory/perceptual misinterpretation. This is then further elaborated with circumstantial verbal reasoning that inevitably draws on external events, episodes, and conditions that serve to validate the original delusional belief. There is clearly an absence of insight in such cases. Fixed ideas are unchangeable thoughts that do not affect the persons' everyday life. The individual's judgment is impaired in one area, but the person has good insight in the unaffected areas. Obsessions are parasitic ideas within an intact intellect, intruding into the normal thought process or ideation, against the will (Westphal, 1872). These ideas are intrusive, forceful and, to varying degrees, ego dystonic. A similar definition was accepted many years later in the Diagnostic and Statistical Manual (American Psychiatric Association, 1994). Within obsessions, a continuum of insight ranges from very good to very poor. Taken together, these forms of pathology are part of formal thought disorder. Some discussion in the literature has focused on the form and function of thought disorders and whether they should be properly referred to as a language disturbance (Thomas, 1995).

As for overvalued ideas present in obsessive–compulsive spectrum disorders (Yaryura-Tobias & Neziroglu, 1997a, b), judgment is impaired and the thought process is considered abnormal. An overvalued idea is a strong belief with an underlying affective component. Wernicke (1906) stated that overvalued ideas are elaborated mental observations or perceptions that are accepted in exaggerated and bizarre ways to the exclusion of other observations. It is, however, the affective component of the mental perceptions that leads to overvaluation of ideas. Judgment is clouded by affect, whether based in fear or anxiety.

Wernicke questions how affect can influence the property of ideas whereby normal valuation of ideas are changed and become either overvalued or undervalued in relation to affect. Overvalued ideas have the attribute, as opposed to undervalued ideas, to be easily drawn from the periphery and are resistant to modification. Wernicke also suggested that, similar to hallucinations, overvalued ideas strongly involve the process of misattribution. This misattribution is due to the lack of clear perceptions that give rise to illusions. The illusions appear to be hallucination-like and take on extraordinary meaning, much like random association of events leading to bizarre or eccentric beliefs and suspicions. The overvalued ideas are governed by language and affect, which are derived from mental illusions or misattributions. These misattributions are due to poor insight, which is governed by affect. According to Wernicke, anxious affect leads to anxious ideas that can be differentiated into autopsychic, allopsychic, or somatopsychic events. Autopsychic ideas refer to feelings of inferiority and self-blame. Allopsychic anxious ideas comprise menace and adversity (predicting doom) such that the environment is perceived as dangerous. Somatopsychic ideas are based on the idea that physical symptoms are indicative of horrible illness and death. All these ideas have varying degrees of insight depending on the intensity of the anxiety.

This differentiation of anxious ideas possibly sheds some light on different major themes in obsessive–compulsive disorder (OCD). For example, allopsychic ideas could segue into feared consequences involving harm to self or others. Somatopsychic ideas are related to contamination and health obsessions such as AIDS. If there is considerable anxious or general affective activation along with a tendency to misattribute perceptions (such as via doubting, for example), then the person with OCD will also likely experience a heightening of overvalued ideas. Autopsychic ideas, or the belief in one's inferiority and tendency to self-blame, may be more closely linked to a particular cognitive distortion seen in OCD, namely, the tendency to experience an overinflated sense of responsibility. This faulty idea, which may be in part maintained by the process in which overvalued ideas are solidified, also seems to be functionally related to checking compulsions. The question as to why checking compulsions are maintained may partly be answered by considering the neuropsychological circuits involved in visual–spatial tasks, as well as brain centers that signal completion and closure. Perhaps if these latter sites do not function properly, there is no perception of closure, leaving the person compelled to repeat the check. Perhaps a subjective sense of confidence in having completed a check or a poor memory trace leads to doubt surrounding the completion of the check. In either case, as the sense of incompletion (i.e., lack of awareness or memory trace) is pitted against an idea of pathological responsibility, one would expect an increase of cognitive–affective arousal. This process is likely to perpetuate itself in a vicious cycle.

For comparative purposes, others, such as Jaspers (1913), viewed overvalued ideas as they are seen in social reformers, inventors, or any individual of strong conviction, whereas delusions are strictly seen in patients. Overvalued ideas, according to Jaspers (1913) are challengeable, transient, isolated, and bound to personality and situation, whereas delusions are unchangeable and fixed, and not necessarily bound to personality or situation. The first two symptoms, delusional and fixed ideas, are unchangeable and overlap in qualities with paranoid reactions or states. These conditions have unclear boundaries and are weakly differentiated from paranoid schizophrenia (Carpenter & Stevens, 1994). Once again insight is somewhat better in overvalued ideas compared to delusions.

The obsessive compulsive belief domains identified by the OCCWG (1997, 2001) can be viewed as beliefs that may become overvalued. For instance, an OCD client's belief that exposure to everyday adhesive material will cause serious health problems is an over-estimation of the probability of negative events. This belief may lead the individual to avoid all forms of tape, stickers, and any adhesive material. The belief may constitute an overvalued idea to the extent that the client is convinced the belief is reasonable and accurate, and to the extent he/she fails to doubt the belief over a period of time. If this person had an obsession with relatively good insight and not an overvalued idea, then he/she would begin to take steps to alter the belief and the resulting behavior (i.e., they would stop avoiding adhesives and challenge their estimation of the probability of something bad happening after contact). If this person had an obsession with intellectual insight only, he/she would understand that his/her belief about harm is exaggerated and is causing him/her serious distress and interference, but he/she would not be able to use this information to solve the problem.

The cognitive theory on which the OCCWG belief domains are based suggests that the general beliefs about importance of thoughts, control of thoughts, overestimation of responsibility, overestimation for negative events, tolerance for uncertainty, and perfectionism form the backdrop for the interpretation of intrusive thoughts (Rachman, 1997; Salkovskis, 1985). The interpretations of intrusive thoughts have to do with the conclusions about the importance of an intrusive thought, their responsibility for harm caused by the thought, and the necessity for controlling the thought. The extent to which these beliefs and interpretations are overvalued, that is, the magnitude of conviction in these beliefs, will determine the degree of emotional distress and interference created by the disorder.

The degree of insight, that is, the extent to which the patient understands that these beliefs lead to their symptoms, will determine their willingness to examine and challenge these beliefs.

Assessment of Insight

The mental status examination provides a means of assessing judgment and insight. The assessment of judgment entails asking patients questions that tap into their knowledge of conventional standards of behavior, their ability for social judgment, and their level of social maturity. The format for assessing insight is less structured and entails asking patients directly whether they believe they are ill, what possibly caused this, and whether or not they feel that treatment is necessary. Depending on answers to these questions, the clinician can then probe further to make a determination as to the patient's level of insight.

A more quantitative approach involves an examination of selected MMPI-2 scales when this is feasible. For example, scale three (Hy) may be interpreted as a threshold, where patients are aware of the symptoms associated with scales that are more elevated than Hy and not aware of symptoms that are associated with scales that are less elevated than Hy (Schare, 1993, personal communication). In our experience, we tend to find that low scores on scales five and nine of the MMPI-2 correlate roughly with intellectual insight. That is, patients with this pattern become more aware of their condition, behavioral patterns, and symptoms over the course of therapy, but tend not to maintain treatment gains. Finally, the validity scales F and K tend to indicate naive and poorly defined self concept, along with diminished insight and awareness for treatment interventions (Butcher, 1990).

Few scales assess insight directly. Only recently has there been an attempt to assess insight more systematically. Two reliable and valid clinically administered scales are the Brown Assessment of Beliefs Scale (BABS; Eisen *et al.*, 1998) and the Overvalued Ideas Scale (Neziroglu, McKay, Yaryura-Tobias, Stevens, & Todaro, 1999). The BABS was developed to "assess delusions across a wide range of psychiatric disorders" (p. 102). It is a seven-item scale that is not specific to OCD but does measure insight of patients diagnosed with OCD, body dysmorphic disorder, and mood disorders with psychotic features. The seven items comprise conviction, perception of other's view of beliefs, explanation of differing views, fixity of ideas, attempts to disprove beliefs, insight, and ideas/delusions of reference. The last item is not included in the total score. The BABS has specific probes and five anchors for each item. The scores for each item range from zero (nondelusional) to four (delusional). The authors of the scale concluded that the scale is a valid measure of delusionality. According to Kozak and Foa (1994) overvalued ideas are different from delusions. For them patients with delusions accept and are less bothered by their behaviors performed as a response to the thought than patients with overvalued ideas who are highly bothered by the behavioral response to the thought. However, the latter group still has a high degree of conviction that the feared outcome has a high probability of occurring. Regardless of whether the BABS measures delusionality or overvalued ideas, it assesses insight. It is inferred that in delusions there is less insight as compared to overvalued ideas.

The Overvalued Ideas Scale (OVIS; Neziroglu *et al.*, 1999) is a ten-item clinician administered scale that assesses the extent of a patient's obsessions and associated compulsions on several different continua, each rated from one to ten. Item content reflects strength, reasonableness, and accuracy of the belief, as well as strength of the belief over the past week; the extent to which others share the same beliefs; how the patient attributes similar or differing beliefs; how effective the compulsions are; the extent to which their disorder has caused their obsessive belief; and their degree of resistance to the belief. The average of the items provides an estimate of overvalued ideation OVI, where higher scores represent greater levels of OVI. The OVIS has numerous anchor points and probe questions to aid the clinician in quantifying OVI.

Besides these two scales with established reliability and validity measurements, there have been other attempts at measuring overvalued ideas in OCD. One is in the form of a single item assessment (item 11 of the Yale Brown Obsessiven Compulsive Scale; Goodman *et al.*, 1989a). Another involves clinician-based ratings of bizarreness and fixidity (Lelliot, Noshirvani, Basoglu, Marks, & Monteiro, 1988). Both of these assessments lack reliability and validity data, however, in addition, another instrument was designed for the American Psychiatric Association field trial (Eisen *et al.*, 1995). This scale measured patients' confidence that the harmful consequence will happen; patients' recognition of the disparity of their beliefs from conventional beliefs; patients' understanding of why they have unrealistic beliefs; flexibility in changing mistaken beliefs; and bizarreness of obsessive ideas. Internal item consistency was very low, and therefore the single item, "belief in consequence" was used to address whether the individual believes that his or her feared consequences are reasonable. Again, the psychometric properties of this scale or item have not been reported.

Factors that Influence and Limit Insight

Besides attempting to clarify the nature and scope of insight, there are likely many factors that may limit insight. These thoughts may include, for example, limited cognitive abilities such as low general intelligence, as well as poorly developed specific skills such as memory encoding and retrieval. Certainly pre-cognitive operations involving sensory processing and perceptual abstraction that influence and form a basis of insight, may affect insight if those pathways are damaged or deficient, as in the case with faulty proprioceptive feedback loops in schizophrenics. Other factors influencing insight undoubtedly include affect and affective regulation skills and general organic conditions and illnesses. These factors, singularly and probably in combination, likely underlie attentional biases seen in OCD. The main affective component of OCD, anxiety, is likely to act as a conditioning force to stimuli that become value laden. That is, once neutral stimuli are likely to signal danger and draw attentional resources to a disproportionate degree. Attentional biases are clearly evident in OCD and can readily be seen as patients become fixated on red colored specs, which are misperceived as contaminated blood drops.

Besides internal operations, one may also speculate on the influences of socio-economic contingencies. Social and economic parameters often subtly influence judgment and perception. Indeed, awareness — raising campaigns are often initially needed to direct people's attention toward specific issues before behavioral changes are even possible. For example, how many of us are aware that poverty is functional in that it allows people to consume new products while poorer persons buy second hand and no-frills products that are otherwise slated for waste? Are we aware of the possibility that recent explosions in the amount of overt sexuality and pornography may actually represent very primitive simian responses to quell rising levels of aggression and violence (Chance, 1988)? We know intellectually that families are among the most violent and discordant of institutions and yet rarely is there mention of biologically based mechanisms of aggression triggered in response to "colonies" being at their "carrying capacity" in relation to the amount of physical space in crowded cities and apartment dwellings. These examples are perhaps beyond the scope of the chapter's emphasis on insight, OVI, and OCD; however, their mention serves to re-iterate both the importance and at times lack of insight in relation to behavior and learning.

Cognitive therapy for OCD has focused on two features central to the concept of insight. First, cognitive therapy typically begins with an attempt to educate the client about the nature of OCD symptoms and the cognitive-behavioral model of OCD. It is assumed that individuals need to understand (or be convinced) that there is a relationship between the interpretation of their intrusive thoughts and their OCD symptoms. Seen in this way, the initial step in cognitive therapy for OCD is to build insight. People with OCD must understand exactly how their thinking leads to emotional distress, avoidance and ritualizing before they can undertake the task of challenging their beliefs. The second and related feature of cognitive therapy involves challenging the overvalued ideas related to probability overestimation, responsibility, importance of thoughts, etc. Much of the process of cognitive therapy is devoted to challenging these beliefs and entertaining alternative ones (Freeston, Rhéaume, & Ladouceur, 1996; Van Oppen & Arntz, 1994).

In summary, we have attempted to delineate and define insight as a concept and particularly how it is influenced and expressed via related concepts. Insight remains a somewhat vague and certainly complex construct that appears multi-determined and, likewise, influenced by many more internal and external factors. Following adequate observation and assessment, we look forward to the development of effective interventions (cognitive, behavioral, nutritional, and pharmacological) that might increase insight and general treatment gains.

References

American Psychiatric Association (1994). *Diagnostic and statistical manual of mental disorders* (4th ed.). Washington, DC: Author

Bastick, J. (1982). *Intuition: How we think and act*. Chichester, UK: Wiley.

Bruner, J. (1992). Another look at New Look I. *American Psychologist, 47*, 780–783.

Butcher, J. N. (1990). *MMPI-2 in psychological treatment*. New York: Oxford University Press.

Carpenter, W. T., & Stephens J. H. (1979). An attempted integration of information relevant to schizophrenic subtypes. *Schizophrenica Bulletin, 5*, 490–506.

Cavanaugh, J. C., & Perlmutter, M. (1982). Metamemory: A critical examination. *Child Development, 53*, 11–28.

Chance, M. (1988). *Social fabrics of the mind* (pp. 1–29). London: LE & A Publishers.

Eisen, J. L., Phillips, K. A., Baer, L., Beer, D. A., Foa, E. B., Kozak, M. J., Goodman, W. K., Hollander, E., Jenike, M. A., & Rasmussen, S. A. (1995). DSM-IV field trial: Obsessive–compulsive disorder. *American Journal of Psychiatry, 152*, 90–96.

Freeston, M. H., Rhéaume, J., & Ladouceur, R. (1996). Correcting faulty appraisals of obsessional thought. *Behaviour Research and Therapy, 34*, 443–446.

Goodman, W. K., Price, L. H., Rasmussen, S. A., Mazure, C., Delgado, P., Geiniger, G. R., & Charney, D. S. (1989a). The Yale Brown Obsessive–Compulsive Scale: II. validity. *Archives of General Psychiatry, 46*, 1012–1016.

Goodman, W. K., Price, L. H., Rasmussen, S. A., Mazure, C., Fleischman, R. L., Hill, D. L., Heninniger, G. R., & Charney, D. S. (1989). The Yale Brown Obsessive–Compulsive Scale: I. Development, use and reliability. *Archives of General Psychiatry, 46*, 1006–1011.

Greenwald, A. G. (1992). New Look 3: Unconscious cognition reclaimed. *American Psychologist, 47*, 766–779.

Halpern, D. F. (1984). *Thought and knowledge: An introduction to critical thinking.* Hillsdale, NJ: Erlbaum.

Jaspers, K. (1913). *Psicopatologia general (allgemeine psychopatologie)* (R.O. Saubidet, Trans.). Buenos Aires: Beta Publishers. (Original work published 1955).

Kaplan, H. I., & Saddock, B. J. (1993). *Synopsis of psychiatry (6th edition-revised).* Baltimore: Williams & Wilkins.

Kilhstrom, J. F. (1987). The cognitive unconscious. *Science, 237*, 1445–1452.

Kozak, M. J., & Foa, E. B. (1994). Obsessions, overvalued ideas, and delusions in obsessive–compulsive disorder. *Behaviour Research and Therapy, 32*, 343–353.

Lelliot, P. T., Noshirvani, H. F., Basoglu, M., Marks, I. M., & Monteiro, W. O. (1988). Obsessive–compulsive beliefs and treatment outcome. *Psychological Medicine, 18*, 697–702.

Matlin, M. W. (1989). *Cognition* (2nd ed.). New York: Holt, Rinehart & Winston.

Neziroglu, F., McKay, D., Yaryura-Tobias, J. A., Stevens, K. P., & Todaro, J. (1999). The Overvalued Ideas Scale: Development, reliability and validity in obsessive–compulsive disorder. *Behaviour Research and Therapy, 37*, 881–902.

Obsessive Compulsive Cognitions Working Group (2000). Development and initial validation of the Obsessive Beliefs Questionnaire and the Interpretation of Intrusions Inventory. *Behaviour Research and Therapy, 39*, 987–1006.

Obsessive Compulsive Working Group (1997). Cognitive assessment of obsessive compulsive disorder. *Behaviour Research and Therapy 35(&)*, 667–687.

Rachman, S. (1997). A cognitive theory of obsessions. *Behaviour Research and Therapy, 35*, 793–802.

Salkovkis, P. M., & Warwick H. M. (1985). Cognitive therapy of obsessive compulsive disorder: Treating treatment failures. *Behavioural Psychotherapy, 13*, 243–255.

Schare, M. (1993). Personal Communication.

Thomas, P. (1995). Thought disorder or communication disorder: Linguistic science provides a new approach. *British Journal of Psychiatry, 166*, 287–290.

van Oppen, P., & Arntz, A. (1994). Cognitive therapy for obsessive compulsive disorder. *Behaviour Research and Therapy, 32*, 79–87.

Weiskrantz, L. (1986). *Blindsight: A case study and implications.* New York: Oxford University Press.

Weiskrantz, L., Warrington, E. K., Sanders, M. D., & Marshall, J. (1974). Visual capacity in the hemianopic field following a restricted occipital ablation. *Brain, 97*, 709–728.

Wernicke, C. (1906). *Grundrisse der psychiatrie* (Foundations of psychiatry). Leipzig: Verlag.

Westphal, C. (1872). *Ueber zwangsvorstell* (On compulsions) (pp. 390–397). Berliner Klinischen: Wochenschrift.

Yaryura-Tobias, J. A., & Neziroglu, F. A. (1997a). *Biobehavioral treatment of obsessive–compulsive spectrum disorders.* New York: W.W. Norton.

Yaryura-Tobias, J. A., & Neziroglu, F. A. (1997b). *Obsessive–compulsive disorder spectrum: pathogenesis, diagnosis, and treatment.* Washington D.C.: American Psychiatric Press.

Commentary on Cognitive Approaches to Obsessive Compulsive Disorder: Critical Issues and Future Directions in Measurement

Steven Taylor

The four chapters in this section consider the major approaches to investigating cognition in obsessive compulsive disorder (OCD): (1) self-report measures, such as the Obsessional Beliefs Questionnaire; (2) interview measures, such as the Overvalued Ideas Scale; (3) measures of information processing biases, such as the modified Stroop test; and (4) experimental designs that explore the effects of cognitive variables by systematically manipulating them. While these chapters address many important issues, they raise some essential questions that need to be further investigated. In this commentary I will address the following questions, which are essential to the task of evaluating the role of cognition in OCD:

- What are the fundamental constructs?
- What causes cognitions?
- What are the most promising methods for investigating cognition in OCD?

What are the Fundamental Constructs?

Several years of research have been devoted to the development and refinement of self-report measures of beliefs and appraisals thought to be important in OCD (see Taylor, Kyrios, Thordarson, Steketee, & Frost, 2002). The Obsessive Compulsive Cognitions Working Group (OCCWG, 1997) proposed, for example, that there are several different domains of beliefs, each purportedly playing a role in producing obsessions and compulsions. These domains, such as inflated responsibility and perfectionism, are described in detail in other chapters in this volume.

The OCCWG has devoted much of its efforts to developing self-report measures of these domains. Has this time been well spent? The Obsessional Beliefs Questionnaire (OBQ) and the Interpretation of Intrusions Inventory (III) have been found to perform satisfactorily on various indices of reliability. The validity of these measures requires further study, particularly with regard to discriminative validity and factorial validity. The subscales of the OBQ, for example, are highly correlated with one another. They also are

Cognitive Approaches to Obsessions and Compulsions – Theory, Assessment, and Treatment
Copyright © 2002 by Elsevier Science Ltd.
ISBN: 0-08-043410-X

highly correlated with measures of depression and general anxiety, with these correlations being about as large as those with measures of OCD symptoms (see OCCWG, 2001, in preparation).

These findings raise an important question: Do the subscales assess distinct constructs or do they simply assess a general tendency to hold irrational beliefs? If subsequent research supports the latter, then the credibility of the cognitive models of OCD would be in jeopardy, because the models would lose their explanatory specificity. That is, their key cognitive constructs would not distinguish OCD from other disorders. The models would fail to explain, for example, why a person with extreme perfectionism develops obsessions and compulsions instead of some other problem, such as severe depression.

A critical issue for future research is to identify two sorts of cognitive factors: Those that lead a person to specifically develop obsessions and compulsions, and nonspecific factors that predispose a person to develop anxiety or mood disorders in general. Although this was a goal in developing the OBQ and III, it has not been satisfactorily achieved. The OBQ and III appear to be, to a large extent, measures of nonspecific factors. We need to identify specific factors to understand what causes people to develop obsessions and compulsions, as opposed to other clinical problems.

It may be that specific factors can be identified if the cognitive constructs (belief domains) are further refined or narrowed in their definitions. For example, it may be possible to define various subtypes of inflated responsibility, such as responsibility for thoughts, responsibility for actions committed, and responsibility for actions omitted. Some subtypes of responsibility might be specifically related to OCD, whereas other subtypes might be nonspecific. People with OCD are often concerned about omitting certain acts; e.g., failing to pick up a shard of glass on the pavement, which conceivably could injure someone. This form of responsibility might distinguish OCD from other clinical problems.

Once we are able to identify the cognitive domains that are specifically correlated with obsessions and compulsions, then these findings can guide experimental research to see if these variables play a central causal role in OCD. Although experimental research to date has been useful in furthering our understanding of OCD (Riskind, Williams, & Kyrios, 2002), it is currently unclear whether these experiments investigated cognitive constructs that are specific to OCD, or whether they have examined nonspecific constructs.

What Causes Cognitions?

Cognitive models of OCD assume that cognitive factors play several important causal roles in OCD. They are thought to be predisposing factors, for example, certain beliefs, such as inflated beliefs in personal responsibility are thought to make a person vulnerable to developing OCD. Particular types of beliefs and appraisals are also thought to maintain OCD (see, for example, Salkovskis, 1996).

Correlational studies have repeatedly shown that OCD-related beliefs and appraisals have moderate-to-large correlations with measures of OCD symptoms (e.g., OCCWG, 2001, in preparation). A small but steadily growing number of experimental studies also suggest that experimentally-manipulated changes in particular beliefs and appraisals (e.g., responsibility beliefs) leads to changes in particular OCD symptoms (e.g., compulsive checking; see Chapter eight). Taken together, the correlational and experimental findings suggest that beliefs and appraisals play some role in causing OCD (but possibly also in causing other clinical problems, such as depression and generalized anxiety). To understand better the causes of OCD it is important to identify the causes of cognitions.

The research on cognitive factors in panic disorder provides an instructive parallel. Here, a central cognitive variable is anxiety sensitivity (AS). This is the fear of arousal-related sensations (ARS), arising from beliefs that these sensations have harmful consequences. Palpitations, for example, are feared in people with high AS because they believe that rapid heartbeat leads to cardiac arrest. People with low AS, by comparison, believe that rapid heartbeat is harmless (for extended discussions of AS, see Taylor, 1999, 2000). A number of longitudinal studies have shown that the severity of AS is one of the best known predictors of a person's risk for experiencing future panic attacks (Taylor, 1999). A good deal of experimental evidence also suggests that AS is an important causal variable in panic disorder (Taylor, 2000). Yet, AS is not sufficient to explain panic disorder; it is important to understand what causes AS to become elevated in the first place. Our recent research suggest that a combination of genetic factors and early learning experiences influences a person's level of AS, which in turn influences the propensity to develop panic attacks (Jang, Stein, Taylor, & Livesley, 1999; Stewart *et al.*, 2001).

Similarly, some constellation of environmental and genetic factors may play a role in producing OCD-related beliefs, which in turn give rise to obsessions and compulsions. An important direction for future research is to investigate the nature and strength of these environmental and genetic influences. If beliefs and appraisals are important causal factors in OCD, then it should be possible to demonstrate that these variables influence OCD symptoms, even if one controls for the direct effects of early learning experiences. We conducted an analogous test in our study of AS (Stewart *et al.*, 2001). Using structural equation modeling, we tested a model that specified three causal pathways: (a) particular types of early learning experiences cause AS, (b) these learning experiences directly cause panic attacks, and (c) AS causes panic attacks. The results supported paths one and three but not two. The findings suggest that early learning does not directly cause panic attacks. Instead, early learning influences AS, which in turn influences the risk of having panic attacks. The same sort of test could be used to assess the role of beliefs and appraisals in OCD; i.e., to see whether early learning experiences directly account for OCD symptoms, or whether these early experiences are mediated through their effects on beliefs and appraisals, which then influenced OCD symptoms.

To further understand OCD, it also would be important to better integrate biological findings with cognitive research. Neuroimaging studies have shown that OCD is characterized by increased activity in the orbital–frontal cortex and in some structures of the basal ganglia (Swinson, Antony, Rachman, & Richter, 1998). How does activity in these areas relate to cognitive variables? For example, are increases in personal responsibility associated with increases in activation in the orbital–frontal cortex? A better understanding of these brain-cognition relations is likely to improve our understanding of where cognitive variables lie in the causal chain of events. And, more importantly, such studies will advance our understanding of the basic mechanisms of OCD.

What are the Most Promising Methods for Investigating Cognition in OCD?

Researchers have relied heavily on self-report measures to study cognitive factors in OCD. As noted by Amir and Kozak (2002) in Chapter nine, self-report methods have their limitations. Many aspects of cognition, for example, are not available to introspection. Amir and Kozak (2002) advocate the use of information–processing strategies. As these authors show, such approaches have produced evidence of various information-processing biases in OCD. Concern-relevant biases in selective attention are among the most robust findings. Memory biases are among the most fragile phenomena, identified using some experimental paradigms but not others.

Despite the many intriguing findings obtained from information-processing studies, this program of research has so far told us little about the causes of obsessions and compulsions. The processing biases may be largely — or perhaps entirely — consequences of OCD rather than causes. Much also needs to be learned about the biological correlates of these biases. Thus, there are two important avenues for future information-processing research. One avenue could look at the causal role of processing biases. This could be done in several ways. Biases could be experimentally manipulated in order to explore their effects on OCD symptoms. Longitudinal studies could be conducted to determine whether these biases predict important phenomena, such as the later development of OCD. Biological studies, such as neuroimaging research, could be conducted to better understand the way that the biases are instantiated in the brain. What we don't need, in my opinion, are more Stroop studies or related investigations that merely demonstrate information-processing biases in OCD.

It is important that researchers and clinicians not lose sight of the importance of self-report methods in understanding OCD. In clinical practice, self-report measures such as the OBQ are useful in treatment planning (Taylor, Thordarson, & Söchting, 2001). Information-processing approaches are less informative in this regard. Self-report measures also might prove to be most important in understanding the mechanisms of OCD, especially if information-processing biases turn out to be merely consequences (rather than causes) of OCD. Research into the causes of panic disorder again provides an instructive parallel. Recall that AS is one of the best-known indicators of a person's risk for developing panic attacks. AS is measured by a simple 16-item self-report questionnaire. In the study of panic disorder, we have yet to find an information-processing paradigm with such power in predicting panic. If a goal of science is the prediction of important phenomena, then self-report methods in panic research have proved themselves to be more powerful than information-processing paradigms. The same might be the case in the study of OCD. Longitudinal studies will eventually answer this important question.

It remains to be seen whether interview-based measures are as useful as self-report questionnaires. Interviews enable researchers and clinicians to explore a patient's beliefs and appraisals in great depth and detail, and therefore furnish more information than self-report questionnaires. Recently developed interview measures of overvalued ideation have proved useful, for example, for predicting treatment outcome (Neziroglu & Stevens, 2002). This suggests that our understanding of OCD may be advanced by developing interview measures of other cognitive constructs, such as responsibility beliefs.

Other approaches also seem promising to some extent. Several studies have documented neuropsychological abnormalities and neurological soft signs in OCD (Riskind *et al.*, 2002). The specificity of these results remains in question, because similar findings have been reported for other disorders (Stowe & Taylor, 2001). Further studies using neuropsychological or neurological tests can address two important issues. The first is whether the neuropsychological abnormalities and neurological soft signs are markers for some nonspecific vulnerability factor; i.e., a factor that make a person vulnerable to develop any of a number of mental disorders. The second is whether the neuropsychological abnormalities and neurological soft signs are simply consequences of mental disorders, rather than causes.

Summary and Conclusion

To better understand the causes of obsessions and compulsions, further work needs to be done to identify cognitive domains (beliefs and appraisals) that are specific to OCD. Some of the beliefs and appraisals identified so far may be nonspecific, playing a role in obsessions, compulsions, and in many other clinical problems such as depression and generalized anxiety. Further work also needs to be done to identify the causes of important beliefs and appraisals. Advances in understanding OCD are most likely to occur if we can integrate the various methods of assessment. For example, integrating neuroimaging methods with findings from self-report methods and with results from information-processing studies. To date, information-processing studies have been insufficient for understanding the causes of OCD. Self-report methods should not be under-valued. These methods can help us identify central cognitive domains, and thereby guide the focus of experimental research. Self-report methods also have great clinical value and much promise in predicting important phenomena, such as the development of obsessions and compulsions. Interview methods are also promising. Useful information may also be gleaned from neuropsychological and neurological tests. However, these methods may be best suited for understanding nonspecific cognitive factors. That is, nonspecific causes (or perhaps consequences) OCD and other disorders.

References

Amir, N., & Kozak, M. J. (2002). Information processing in OCD. In R.O. Frost & G. Steketee (eds), *Cognitive approaches to obsessions and compulsions: Theory, assessment and treatment.* (pp. 165–181). Oxford: Elsevier.

Jang, K. L., Stein, M. B., Taylor, S., & Livesley, W. J. (1999). Gender differences in the aetiology of anxiety sensitivity: A twin study. *Journal of Gender Specific Medicine, 2*, 39–44.

Neziroglu, F., & Stevens, K. (2002). Insight: Its conceptualization and measurement. In R.O. Frost & G. Steketee (eds), *Cognitive approaches to obsessions and compulsions: Theory, assessment and treatment.* (pp. 183–193). Oxford: Elsevier.

Obsessive Compulsive Cognitions Working Group. (1997). Cognitive assessment of obsessive–compulsive disorder. *Behaviour Research and Therapy, 35*, 667–681.

Obsessive Compulsive Cognitions Working Group. (2001). Development and initial validation of the Obsessive–Beliefs Questionnaire and the Interpretation of Intrusions Inventory. *Behaviour Research and Therapy, 39*, 987–1006.

Obsessive Compulsive Cognitions Working Group. (in preparation). *The Obsessive Beliefs Questionnaire and the Interpretation of Intrusions Inventory: Findings of Stage III*. Manuscript in preparation.

Riskind, J. H., Williams, N. L., & Kyrios, M. (2002). Experimental methods for studying cognition. In R.O. Frost & G. Steketee (eds), *Cognitive approaches to obsessions and compulsions: Theory, assessment and treatment*. (pp. 139–164). Oxford: Elsevier.

Salkovskis, P. M. (1996). Cognitive–behavioural approaches to the understanding of obsessional problems. In R.M. Rapee (ed.), *Current controversies in the anxiety disorders* (pp. 103–134). New York: Guilford.

Stewart, S. H., Taylor, S., Jang, K. L., Cox, B. J., Watt, M. C., Fedoroff, I. C., & Borger, S. C. (2001). Causal modeling of relations among learning history, anxiety sensitivity, and panic attacks. *Behaviour Research and Therapy, 39*, 443–456.

Stowe, R., & Taylor, S. (2001). Posttraumatic stress disorder. *Encyclopedia of life sciences*. London: Nature Publishing Group.

Swinson, R. P., Antony, M. M., Rachman, S., & Richter, M. A. (1998). *Obsessive–compulsive disorder: Theory, research, and treatment*. New York: Guilford.

Taylor, S. (1999). *Anxiety sensitivity: Theory, research, and treatment of the fear of anxiety*. Mahwah, NJ: Erlbaum.

Taylor, S. (2000). *Understanding and treating panic disorder: Cognitive–behavioral approaches*. New York: Wiley.

Taylor, S., Kyrios, M., Thordarson, D. S., Steketee, G., & Frost, R. O. (2002). Development and validation of instruments for measuring intrusions and beliefs in OCD. In R.O. Frost & G. Steketee (eds), *Cognitive approaches to obsessions and compulsions: Theory, assessment and treatment*. (pp. 117–137). Oxford: Elsevier.

Taylor, S., Thordarson, D., & Söchting, I. (2001). Assessment, treatment planning, and outcome evaluation for obsessive–compulsive disorder. In M.M. Antony, & D.H. Barlow (eds), *Handbook of assessment, treatment planning, and outcome evaluation: Empirically supported strategies for psychological disorders*. New York: Guilford.

Section C

Cognition in Disorders Related to Obsessive Compulsive Disorder

Chapter 11

Cognitive Theory of Body Dysmorphic Disorder

Sabine Wilhelm and Fugen Neziroglu

The Clinical Picture of Body Dysmorphic Disorder

Body dysmorphic disorder (BDD), a preoccupation with an imagined or slight defect in appearance, has only recently received empirical attention (e.g., Neziroglu & Yaryura-Tobias, 1993a, b; Phillips, 1991; Phillips, McElroy, Keck, Pope, & Hudson, 1993). Preliminary estimates suggest that BDD may be common, with a rate of 1.9 percent in the general population (Rich, Rosen, Orosan, & Reiter, 1992). Common complaints involve imagined or minor flaws of the head and face, but any body part can be the focus of concern. Individuals with BDD often complain about acne, scarring, wrinkles, paleness, excessive facial hair, hair thinning, or the shape or size of body parts such as the nose, lips or teeth. Some people with BDD have concerns focusing on bodily asymmetry. Muscle dysmorphia is a variant of BDD in which individuals consider themselves small and weak when, in fact, they are quite muscular and large (Pope, Gruber, Choi, Olivardia, & Phillips, 1997).

Most people suffering from BDD are severely distressed by their supposed flaws and describe their preoccupations as painful and tormenting (American Psychiatric Association, 1994). The preoccupations are difficult to control and very time consuming; some individuals spend several hours per day thinking about their defect. About 90 percent of the individuals suffering from BDD perform repetitive behaviors intended to check, improve, or hide the supposed defect (Neziroglu, Anderson, & Yaryura-Tobias, 1999). These behaviors include checking the perceived flaw in mirrors or other reflecting surfaces, such as store windows or car bumpers. Many individuals camouflage the perceived flaw with make-up, hair, body position, or clothing (e.g., wearing a hat to hide protruding ears or balding). Other patients engage in excessive grooming behaviors, such as combing, cutting, or styling their hair. Some patients pick at their skin for several hours per day, trying to remove blemishes. Indeed, they may pick their skin so deeply that they require emergency surgery (O'Sullivan, Phillips, Keuthen, & Wilhelm, 1999; Phillips & Taub, 1995). Many individuals with BDD ask for reassurance related to the imagined defect. BDD patients may also frequently compare their appearance with that of other people. The repetitive behaviors can consume several hours per day and usually only provide temporary relief. In addition, BDD patients frequently seek medical care and plastic surgery (Hollander, Cohen, & Simeon, 1993; Neziroglu & Yaryura-Tobias, 1997; Phillips *et al.*, 1993). Avoidance of social situations or bright lights, for example, is common. Individuals with BDD usually have a difficult approach-avoidance relationship with mirrors; caught between wanting to avoid their reflection and wanting to fix it. They often alternate between episodes of mirror avoidance and mirror checking.

BDD is also associated with high levels of occupational and social disability, including unemployment, absenteeism, lost productivity, and marital dysfunction. In its most severe form, it incapacitates its sufferers and keeps them housebound for many years. In one study, rates of suicide attempts related to appearance concerns were 17 percent (Phillips *et al.*, 1993).

Available data suggest that BDD usually begins during adolescence (e.g., Phillips, Atala, & Albertini, 1995). It tends to be chronic, often enduring for decades without remission (Phillips, 1991; Phillips *et al.*, 1993). The sex ratio is approximately 1:1 (Phillips & Diaz, 1997).

Insight in BDD is frequently poor and approximately 50 percent of patients are delusional (Phillips, 1991; Phillips *et al.*, 1993). Ideas or delusions of reference occur in two-thirds of cases, involving the belief that others take special notice of the perceived defect, for example, staring at it or mocking it (Phillips, McElroy, Keck, Pope, & Hudson, 1994). If the preoccupation with the appearance flaw takes on delusional intensity, sufferers are unable to consider that they may be incorrect with respect to perception of their own appearance. In those cases the diagnosis of delusional disorder, somatic type, should be considered. Phillips (1998) recommends that individuals with delusional BDD should be double classified as both, delusional disorder and BDD. This suggests that the delusional and non-delusional forms of BDD may actually be a single disorder, varying only in the degree of insight (Phillips *et al.*, 1994). Thus, delusionality may be a dimensional construct, with insight occurring on a continuum and occasionally changing over time (Phillips & McElroy, 1993).

Comparison with Obsessive Compulsive Disorder (OCD)

Similarities between OCD and BDD

BDD is classified as a somatoform disorder in the Diagnostic and Statistical Manual of Mental Disorders (DSM-IV, American Psychiatric Association, 1994). However, due to the many similarities with OCD, psychopathologists often categorize it as an OCD spectrum disorder (for a review see Yaryura-Tobias & Neziroglu, 1997a, b). Indeed, the symptoms of BDD are similar to those of OCD, including recurrent persistent thoughts and compulsive behaviors, such as mirror checking. When compared to OCD patients, BDD patients are similar on measures of depression, state, and trait anxiety, but OCD patients have higher levels of physical symptoms of anxiety (McKay, Neziroglu, & Yaryura-Tobias, 1997). Some reports suggest that BDD occurs at high rates in patients with OCD (Brawman-Mintzer *et al.*, 1995; Hollander & Phillips, 1992; Neziroglu & Yaryura-Tobias, 1997; Phillips *et al.*, 1993; Wilhelm, Otto, Zucker, & Pollack, 1997). In a recent study comparing individuals with BDD to those with OCD, no significant differences were found in sex ratio, employment status, most course and impairment variables, or comorbidity (Phillips, Gunderson, Mallya, McElroy, & Carter, 1998).

Differences between OCD and BDD

Although BDD may be related to OCD, there are some important differences. For example, the thoughts of the individuals with BDD are often not experienced as intrusive or senseless as obsessions in people with OCD. Those with BDD have much higher levels of overvalued ideas (McKay, Neziroglu, & Yaryura-Tobias, 1997). Moreover, in BDD the thoughts are limited to imagined physical flaws, and individuals with BDD are less likely to resist the thoughts. In contrast to OCD, insight is often limited or absent in BDD (Eisen, Philips, & Rasmussen, 1996; McKay, Neziroglu, & Yaryura-Tobias, 1997; Neziroglu, Stevens, Liquori, & Yaryura-Tobias, 2000). Indeed, Phillips *et al.* (1994) found that BDD patients are delusional a substantial part of the time, which is not the case for OCD patients. Another dissimilarity is that BDD preoccupations more often appear to be associated with shame, rejection sensitivity, and low self-esteem, and checking behaviors seem to increase rather than decrease anxiety (Phillips, 2000). However, not all compulsive behaviors in BDD patients are anxiety increasing; for example, reassurance seeking is anxiety decreasing. Mirror checking tends to increase depression rather than anxiety, an aspect of BDD that requires further investigation. A recent study also showed that individuals with BDD were significantly less likely to be married than individuals with OCD, and were significantly more likely to have suicidal ideation or have made a suicide attempt because of their illness. They also had an earlier onset of major depression and a higher lifetime prevalence of major depression, social phobia, and psychotic disorders (Phillips *et al.*, 1998).

Unlike OCD, BDD shares many features with social phobia. A recent study investigating the prevalence of BDD in anxiety disorders showed that social phobia preceded the onset of BDD in all individuals who suffered from both disorders (Wilhelm *et al.*, 1997). This suggests that BDD develops in individuals with early onset and chronic social phobia. Because of the similarities with OCD and social phobia, psychopathologists recently discussed whether BDD should be classified as an anxiety disorder rather than a somatoform disorder (see Phillips, 1998).

Beliefs and Attitudes in BDD

Individuals with BDD usually think that others share their view of the perceived defect. They assume that others take notice and are disgusted by it. Attention by others often makes the BDD sufferer feel ashamed, because they believe that the perceived defect reveals some personal flaw and is indicative of their self-worth. Personal and physical appearance values have become interwoven. Indeed, in a recent questionnaire study to elicit attitudes from BDD patients, Veale and colleagues found that a large number of individuals endorsed beliefs such as "if my appearance is defective, I am inadequate" or "if my appearance is defective then I am worthless" and "If I am unattractive, I will be alone and isolated all my life" (Veale, Boockock *et al.*, 1996). Geremia and Neziroglu (2000) found the following beliefs in individuals with BDD: "If I looked better, my whole life would be better." "Happiness comes from looking good." "If there is one flaw in my overall appearance, then I feel unattractive." "How I feel about myself as a person is usually related to how I feel about the way I look." "If my (body part of concern) is not beautiful, then it must be ugly." "I feel that my (body part of concern) is unattractive/ugly, it means that it looks unattractive/ugly."

On the basis of his clinical work and research, Cash (1997) has identified certain beliefs or assumptions typical for a wide range of individuals who are distressed about their appearance (e.g., acne sufferers, patients with eating disorders, people with subclinical appearance concerns). These assumptions are similar to those described above, including, for example, "One's outward physical appearance is a sign of the inner person". In addition, Cash lists other assumptions such as, "The first thing that people will notice about me is what is wrong with my appearance." "If I could look as I wish, my life would be so much happier." Although, to our knowledge, Cash never verified these beliefs in research studies specifically investigating individuals with BDD, clinical observations of the authors suggest that they may be relevant for this group.

Perfectionism may also play a major role in BDD (Neziroglu *et al.*, 1999; Pacht, 1984). In the survey of BDD patients mentioned above, 69 percent affirmed the belief, "I have to have perfection in my appearance" (Veale, Boockock *et al.*, 1996). From an evolutionary perspective, trying to look as perfect and symmetrical as possible has adaptive significance as flaws and asymmetries in appearance may interfere with mating success in animals and humans (for detailed reviews see, Ectoff, 1999; Veale, Gournay *et al.*, 1996). For example, Moller and Thornhill (1998) found that symmetry is clearly related to sexual attraction in most species, including humans. Symmetry may be favored by animals and humans because it is a measure of overall fitness and might indicate for example, absence of parasites, infections, or exposure to radiation (see Gangestad, Thornhill, & Yeo, 1994).

Because good looks increase the chances to find a biologically fit partner, it makes sense that humans as well as animals are concerned about it. However, in BDD beliefs about symmetry or wanting to look good are held very rigidly. These perfectionistic beliefs or assumptions might contribute to negative evaluation of and increased attention to minor flaws in appearance (Neziroglu, Anderson, & Yaryura-Tobias, 1999; Veale, Gournay *et al.*, 1996). Indeed, the greater demand for symmetry and perfection might lead to selective attention to asymmetries and minor appearance defects (see below). So far, evidence likening perfectionism and BDD merely comes from anecdotal reports or descriptive studies that assessed beliefs. Future studies will have to investigate whether BDD patients have higher levels of perfectionism than non-BDD individuals using validated measures.

Perfectionism has also been reported in a number of other disorders. High levels of perfectionism have been reported for individuals with OCD (Frost & Steketee, 1997), panic disorder (Frost & Steketee, 1997), social phobia (Juster, Heimberg, Frost, Holt, & Mattia, 1996), eating disorders (Bastani, Rao, Weltzin, & Kaye, 1995), and depression (Hewitt & Flett, 1991). Thus, perfectionism is not exclusive to BDD and may be associated with a number of different illnesses. (See Chapter six in this volume.) Nevertheless, it may be an important factor in the development and maintenance of BDD.

Similarities between OCD and BDD Beliefs

An international group of researchers has recently attempted to determine the most relevant domains of OCD-related beliefs and appraisals [Obsessive Compulsive Cognitions Working Group (OCCWG), 1997]. This group identified six general domains of belief relevant to OCD, including inflated responsibility, overestimation of threat, intolerance of uncertainty, importance of thoughts, the need to control thoughts, and perfectionism. The OCCWG is currently engaged in psychometric testing of a self-report measure that assesses beliefs hypothesized to be characteristic of individuals with OCD, the Obsessive Beliefs Question-naire (OBQ). When the questionnaire was administered to 12 patients with BDD and 15 OCD patients, the only difference between the two groups was that the OCD patients scored higher with respect to overinflated sense of responsibility (Neziroglu, Wilhelm, & Knauz, 2001, unpublished data). These findings have to be interpreted with caution given the small number of patients; however, they might shed light on cognitive similarities and differences between OCD and BDD patients.

Cognitive theorists have suggested that perfectionistic beliefs or assumptions may play an important role in the development and maintenance of OCD (Guidano & Liotti, 1983; McFall & Wollersheim, 1979). Evidence associating perfectionism and OCD stems from studies of nonclinical populations (e.g., Frost, Marten, Lahart, & Rosenblate, 1990; Frost, Steketee, Cohn, & Greiss, 1994) and of OCD patients (e.g., Ferrari, 1995; Frost & Steketee, 1997). Various kinds of perfectionism in OCD have been postulated, including the need for things to be "just right," and the need for perfect symmetry (Freeston, Léger, Rhéaume, & Ladouceur, 1996; for a review see Steketee, Frost, Rheaume, & Wilhelm, 1998). In OCD, concern about symmetry and perfection has been associated with hoarding, ordering, repeating, and counting compulsions (Baer, 1994). Although both BDD and OCD sufferers report demands for symmetry and perfection, only minor differences seem to distinguish the two groups. In BDD patients the need for symmetry focuses on their own appearance in OCD symmetry demands focus on objects and activities (Veale, Gournay *et al.*, 1996). Whereas in OCD the tolerance for making mistakes may be small (see also Pitman, 1987), in BDD the tolerance for having flaws in appearance may be very limited. Doubts about actions may be characteristic of certain subtypes of OCD, but it may be less typical for those with BDD (e.g., Frost & Steketee, 1997). Individuals suffering from BDD might check their appearance because of doubts of severity of the defect (Veale, Gournay *et al.*, 1996). They appear to be uncertain whether the defect is still present to the same extent and doubt their own perception. Similar to OCD patients they may be unable to tolerate uncertainty. Checking behavior is also related to magical thinking, with sufferers hoping that the defect has magically disappeared since the last time it was checked (Neziroglu *et al.*, 1999, 2000).

Cognitive Processes in BDD

Since the 1980s researchers have begun to stress the role of cognitive factors in the etiology and maintenance of psychological disorders. Their research employs concepts and methods of cognitive psychology to show information processing biases in these disorders (e.g.,

Beck & Emery, 1985; Williams, Watts, MacLeod, & Mathews, 1997). Information processing pertains to the way in which individuals perceive, attend to, and retrieve information (Hollon & Kriss, 1984; Ingram & Kendall, 1986). The beliefs and assumptions described in the previous section likely influence the processing of information. The quantity of all stimuli available at a particular time is too much to process. Therefore, information processing is selective. Selection is not random, but is based on underlying beliefs that guide the screening, encoding, managing, storing, and recall of information (Beck & Clark, 1988). This leads to the elaboration and encoding of information consistent with existing beliefs, whereas inconsistent or irrelevant information is ignored, forgotten, or distorted until it fits the belief (Beck & Clark, 1988; see also Alba & Hasher, 1983). Individuals may also be more likely to retrieve information consistent with their beliefs. Thus, maladaptive beliefs may play a major role in the etiology and maintenance of BDD. The negative beliefs described in the previous section systematically affect information processing, and therefore are consistently reinforced.

Psychopathlologists have not only adopted information processing theories, but also experimental paradigms of cognitive psychology to determine where in the system the dysfunctions are located (for reviews see, for example, Dalgleish & Watts, 1990; Eysenck, 1992; Logan & Goetsch, 1993; Williams *et al.*, 1997). These rigorous methods are mainly applied to investigate attentional and memory biases. Surprisingly, little research has been done concerning attentional biases in BDD. Recently, Buhlmann, McNally, Wilhelm, and Florin (2000) found empirical support for the contention that attentional resources are drawn toward body image themed words in BDD. They conducted a modified Stroop (1935) experiment. In Stroop experiments, subjects are presented words of varying emotional significance and asked to name the color in which the word is printed while ignoring its meaning. Delays in the naming of the color, or "Stroop interference," occur whenever the subjects attend to the meaning of the word, despite their attempt to attend only to its color. If an attentional bias for body image-related information exists in BDD patients, they ought to take longer to color-name body image-related words than words unrelated to body image. Indeed, Buhlmann *et al.* (2000) found delayed color-naming latencies for emotional material unrelated to body image (e.g., kindness, peril) and for body image related information (e.g., attractive, disfigured), in comparison with neutral material (e.g., carpet). In other words, BDD patients experienced difficulty maintaining attentional focus in the presence of cues with emotional significance, and especially those related to their current appearance concerns.

Hanes (1998) found that both BDD and OCD subjects showed deficits in maintaining attentional focus (Stroop) and planning abilities (Tower of London). A recent neuropsychological study investigated memory in BDD (Deckersbach *et al.*, 2000). Results showed that BDD subjects differed significantly from healthy control subjects on verbal and nonverbal memory tasks. The study also revealed that group differences were mediated by deficits in organizational strategies in the BDD group. BDD subjects seemed to have difficulty appreciating the overall perceptual and semantic attributes present in complex tests. For example, they approached a complex figure (i.e., the Rey-Osterrieth Complex Figure Test) by focusing on unimportant details, instead of trying to identify more global organizational features. Deficits in immediate and delayed recall were associated with these impairments in organization. Very similar findings have been reported for OCD patients (Savage *et al.*, 2000).

Thus, BDD patients, like those with OCD, may focus overly on certain details of their environment or themselves, while ignoring other potentially more important ones. BDD patients may overfocus on a small defect in appearance that other people would consider minimal or would not notice. At the same time, BDD patients might ignore the rest of the face. This could lead to a perceptual distortion that makes the defect appear very prominent so that a minor scar might be perceived as huge and obvious. Thus, selective attention to visual input others would ignore might contribute to, create, or maintain the defect in BDD sufferers. We have already noted that BDD patients tend to compare themselves with others in a ritualistic way. They are likely to try measuring up against others who have "better skin," a "shorter nose," etc. Again, selective attention might be at work, as patients usually do not compare themselves with someone with appearance problems worse than their own. Of course, selective attention to appearance-related themes may also lead to a large number of thoughts regarding the defect.

Selective attention may be a critical factor in the development and maintenance of many emotional disorders (Wells & Matthews, 1994). Negative beliefs and assumptions may not only lead to and be supported by selective attention, but also by social information processing biases. Recently, one of our patients encountered an unfriendly clerk in a store, although most people would attribute the unfriendly behavior to difficulty communicating or to a personality flaw in the clerk, our BDD patient blamed the clerk's behavior on his appearance. He was convinced that the clerk was unfriendly because he was so disgusted with the way the patient looked. Thus, a BDD sufferer is likely to interpret a general social situation as appearance-related. Their preoccupation in social situations is very intense, and they often expect to be stared at by other people (Rosen, 1995). They can be so convinced of their ugliness that they interpret any interaction with others as a response to the defect.

Cognitive Processing Similarities and Differences between OCD and BDD

We have already described similarities in the clinical picture of OCD and BDD patients: BDD sufferers have recurrent thoughts about appearance and engage in appearance related compulsions. Information processing studies in OCD and BDD lead to similar results, both groups are characterized by deficits in inhibition or selective attention (Buhlmann *et al.*, 2000; Foa, Ilai, McCarthy, Shoyer, & Murdock, 1993). Recent studies showed that the neuropsychological profile may be similar in OCD and BDD, and both groups may be characterized by executive dysfunction (Deckersbach *et al.*, 2000). Thus, on the basis of these phenomenological and cognitive similarities, it is possible that the cognitive models, which have been proposed for OCD, may also be relevant for BDD.

Salkovskis (1985, 1989) has suggested a cognitive model of OCD that describes intrusive thoughts as part of normal experiences. What differentiates individuals with OCD is not that they have intrusive thoughts, but how they react to them. Although most people disregard intrusions, people with OCD pay attention to them and think that they are especially important. The interpretation of intrusions might be influenced by beliefs or other factors, such as stress and moodstate. Processing of intrusions can produce either neutral or negative emotions. Neutral emotions do not lead to actions, whereas negative emotions provoke the desire to either avoid situations that trigger intrusions or attempts to neutralize them with compulsions or other discomfort reducing activities. In sum, the cognitive model for OCD proposes that people interpret day to day events (intrusions) in a maladaptive way that leads to further negative mental processing and emotional, as well as behavioral, consequences.

The application of cognitive paradigms for body image disturbance is relatively new and has mostly been narrowly confined within the field of body shape and eating disorders (for an overview see Thompson, Heinberg, Altabe, & Tantleff-Dunn, 1999). Nevertheless, cognitive models for BDD may be similar to those proposed for OCD (Geremia & Neziroglu, 2000; Veale, Gournay *et al.*, 1996).

Cognitive Model for BDD

Obsessive thinking in BDD involves recurrent, intrusive thoughts about appearance (Neziroglu & Yaryuara-Tobias, 1993a, b; Yaryura-Tobias & Neziroglu, 1997a, b). Almost everyone has some minor flaws in appearance and occasionally thinks about them. What separates individuals with BDD is not that they have minor defects in appearance, but how they react to them. Although many people can just disregard their minor appearance flaws, people with BDD focus on them and attach special significance to them. The negative evaluation of flaws might be influenced by perfectionistic beliefs about appearance or by assumptions that these flaws reveal something negative about the person's character. Fear of negative evaluation might also predispose individuals to develop BDD (Wilhelm *et al.*, 1997). These beliefs might have evolved because of a biological predisposition, family, and cultural values and childhood experiences (Veale, Gournay *et al.*, 1996; Yaryura-Tobias & Neziroglu, 1997a). Other factors, such as stress and current mood, may also play a role in the BDD sufferer's reaction to the flaw. Processing of perceived appearance flaws leads to negative feelings that cause the sufferer to either avoid situations that trigger the unpleasant feelings or to neutralize them with appearance related rituals or other activities (e.g., reassurance seeking). Avoidance behavior, hiding of the defect and checking, are reinforcing because they provide a short term relief of discomfort. Thus, the rituals and avoidance are the engine that maintains the dysfunctional beliefs in people with BDD, just like in individuals suffering from OCD.

In sum, the cognitive model for BDD may be very similar to the model for OCD. It proposes that people interpret normal visual input, such as minor flaws, in a biased way that results in further negative mental, emotional, and behavioral consequences.

Summary and Comment

Body dysmorphic disorder is a preoccupation with an imagined defect in appearance. In the past few years it has developed from being a neglected psychiatric illness to one that is becoming better understood and more frequently studied. Just like patients with OCD, individuals with BDD suffer from recurrent persistent thoughts, and often engage in compulsive behaviors. Because of the striking phenomenological and cognitive analogies of BDD and OCD, it might be useful to categorize BDD as an anxiety disorder (see Phillips, 1998). On the basis of cognitive models for OCD, we developed a model for BDD that emphasizes problems with appearance appraisal and cognitive processing. We hypothesize that body image disturbance is associated with maladaptive beliefs and altered interpretations of appearance-related information. So far, few researchers have identified beliefs that may be important for the development and maintenance of BDD. Research on cognitive processes has suggested some biases or deficits with respect to attention and memory. To date, the research efforts on BDD in general have been very limited, and particularly research on cognition in BDD is needed. An important question to be examined in future studies is whether BDD patients actually see a physical anomaly (such as an unusually long nose) that cannot be detected by others. Alternatively, they might overreact and selectively attend to minor flaws that other people consider unimportant. Thus, there might just be a difference in the interpretation of appearance by individuals with BDD.

Further study of cognition in BDD will also have to determine which beliefs and specific belief domains (e.g., perfectionism) are important for the etiology and maintenance of BDD. We summarized some evidence that BDD sufferers may have maladaptive assumptions with respect to the meaning of their defect. So far, research on cognitive processes, cognitive content, and treatment has developed independently. However, an integration of these various cognitive approaches may be very fruitful. Indeed, cognitive interventions that focus on maladaptive beliefs seem to be very useful. Cognitive interventions may be particularly beneficial if they focus on the basic assumptions about the self, the world, and the future. Our clinical experience suggests that BDD patients may relapse if these assumptions are not addressed during treatment.

References

Alba, J. W., & Hasher, L. (1983). Is memory schematic? *Psychological Bulletin, 93*, 203–231.

American Psychiatric Association (1994). *Diagnostic and statistical manual of mental disorders* (4th ed.). Washington, DC: American Psychiatric Press.

Baer, L. (1994). Factor analysis of symptom subtypes of obsessive compulsive disorder and their relation to personality and tic disorders. *Journal of Clinical Psychiatry, 55*, 18–23.

Bastani, A. M., Rao, R., Weltzing, T., & Kaye, W. H. (1995). Perfectionism in anorexia nervosa. *International Journal of Eating Disorders, 17*, 147–152.

Beck, A. T., & Clark, D. A. (1988). Anxiety and depression: An information processing perspective. *Anxiety Research, 1*, 23–36.

Beck, A. T., & Emery, G. (1985). *Anxiety disorders and phobias: A cognitive perspective*. New York: Basic Books.

Brawman-Mintzer O., Lydiard, B. L., Phillips, K. A., Morton, A., Czepowicz, V., Emmanuel, N., Villareal, G., Johnson, M., & Ballenger, J. C. (1995). Body dysmorphic disorder in patients with anxiety disorders and major depression: A comorbidity study. *American Journal of Psychiatry, 152*, 1665–1667.

Buhlmann, U., McNally, R., Wilhelm, S., & Florin I. (2000). Selective processing of emotional information in body dysmorphic disorder. Submitted for publication.

Cash, T. F. (1997). *The body image workbook: An eight step program for learning to like your looks*. Oakland, CA: New Harbinger.

Dalgleish, T., & Watts, F. N. (1990). Biases of attention and memory in disorders of anxiety and depression. *Clinical Psychology Review, 10*, 589–604.

Deckersbach, T., Savage, C. R., Phillips, K. A., Wilhelm, S., Buhlmann, U., Rauch, S. L., Baer, L., & Jenike, M. A. (2000). Characteristics of memory dysfunction in body dysmorphic disorder. *Journal of the International Neuropsychological Society* (in press).

Ectoff, N. (1999). *Survival of the prettiest*. New York: Doubleday

Eisen, J. L., Philips, K. A., & Rasmussen, S. A. (1996). *Delusionality in OCD, body dysmorphic disorder and mood disorders*. Syllabus and Proceedings Summary of the annual meeting of the American Psychiatric Association (p. 165). New York: American Psychiatric Association.

Eysenck, M. W. (1992). *Anxiety: The cognitive perspective*. Hove, UK: Erlbaum.

Ferrari, J. R. (1995). Perfectionism cognitions with nonclinical and clinical samples. *Journal of Social Behavior and Personality, 10*, 143–156.

Foa, E. B., Ilai, D., McCarthy, P. R., Shoyer, B., & Murdock, T. (1993). Information processing in obsessive–compulsive disorder. *Cognitive Therapy and Research, 17*, 173–189.

Freeston, M. H., Léger, E., Rhéaume, J., & Ladouceur, R. (1996). *The treatment utility of cognitive assessment in obsessive compulsive disorder*. Poster presented at the annual meeting of the Association for Advancement of Behavior Therapy, New York.

Frost, R. O., Marten, P., Lahart, C., & Rosenblate, R. (1990). The dimensions of perfectionism. *Cognitive Therapy and Research, 14*, 449–468.

Frost, R. O., & Steketee, G. (1997). Perfectionism in obsessive compulsive disorder. *Behaviour Research and Therapy, 35*, 291–296.

Frost, R. O., Steketee, G., Cohn, L., & Greiss, K. (1994). Personality traits in subclinical and non-obsessive compulsive volunteers and their parents. *Behaviour, Research and Therapy, 32*, 47–56.

Gangestad, R., Thornhill, R., & Yeo, R. A. (1994). Facial attractiveness, developmental stability, and fluctuating asymmetry. *Ethology and Sociobiology, 15*, 73–85.

Geremia, G., & Neziroglu, F. (2000). Cognitive therapy for body dysmorphic disorder. Submitted for publication.

Guidano, V. F., & Liotti, G. (1983). *Cognitive processes and emotional disorders*. New York: Guilford.

Hanes, K. (1988). Neuropsychological performance in body dysmorphic disorder. *Journal of the International Neuropsychological Society, 4*, 167–171.

Hewitt, P. L., & Flett, G. L. (1991). Perfectionism and depression: A multidimensioanl analysis. *Journal of Social Behavior and Personality, 5*, 423–438.

Hollander, E., Cohen, L. J., & Simeon, D. (1993). Body dysmorphic disorder. *Psychiatric Annuals, 23*, 359–364.

Hollander, E., & Phillips, K. A. (1992). Body image and experience disorders. In E. Hollander (ed.), *Obsessive–compulsive related disorders* (pp. 17–48). Washington, DC: American Psychiatric Press.

Hollon, S. D., & Kriss, M. R. (1984). Cognitive factors in clinical research and practice. *Clinical Psychology Review, 4*, 35–76.

Ingram, R. E., & Kendall, P. C. (1986). Cognitive clinical psychology: Implications of an information processing perspective. In R. E. Ingram (ed.), *Information processing approaches to clinical psychology* (pp. 3–21). Orlando, FL: Academic Press.

Juster, H. R., Heimberg, R. G., Frost, R. O., Holt, C. S., & Mattia, J. I. (1996). Social phobia and perfectionism, *Personality and Individual Differences, 21*, 403–410.

Logan, A. C., & Goetsch, V. L. (1993). Attention to external threat cues in anxiety states. *Clinical Psychology Review, 13*, 541–559.

McFall, M. E., & Wollersheim, J. P. (1979). Obsessive–compulsive neurosis: A cognitive–behavioral formulation and approach to treatment. *Cognitive Therapy and Research, 3*, 333–348.

McKay, D., Neziroglu, F., & Yaryura-Tobias, J. A. (1997). Comparison of clinical characteristics in obsessive compulsive disorder and body dysmorphic disorder. *Journal of Anxiety Disorders, 11*, 447–454.

Moller, A. P., & Thornhill, R. (1998) Bilateral symmetry and sexual selection: A meta analysis. *American Naturalist, 151*, 174–192.

Neziroglu, F., Anderson, M., & Yaryura-Tobias, J. A. (1999). An in-depth review of obsessive compulsive disorder, body dysmorphic disorder, hypochondriasis, and trichotillomania: Therapeutic issues and current research. *Crisis Intervention, 5*, 59–94.

Neziroglu, F., Stevens, K., Liquori, B., & Yaryura-Tobias, J. A. (2000). Cognitive and behavioral treatment of obsessive compulsive disorders. In W. K. Goodman, M. V. Rudorfer, & J. D. Maser (eds) *Obsessive–compulsive disorder: contemporary issues in treatment* (pp. 233–250). Englewood Cliffs, NJ: Lawrence Erlbaum.

Neziroglu, F., Wilhelm, S., & Knauz, R. (2001). Available from Fugen Neziroglu, Institute for Bio-Behavioral Therapy and Research, Department of Psychology, Suite 102, 935 Northern Blvd., Great Neck, NY 112021 5034, USA. Unpublished data.

Neziroglu, F., & Yaryura-Tobias, J. A. (1993a). Exposure, response prevention, and cognitive therapy in the treatment of body dysmorphic disorder. *Behavior Therapy, 24*, 431–438.

Neziroglu, F., & Yaryura-Tobias, J. A. (1993b). Body dysmorphic disorder: Phenomenology and case descriptions. *Behavioural Psychotherapy, 21*, 27–36.

Neziroglu, F., & Yaryura-Tobias, J. A. (1997). A review of cognitive behavioral and pharmacological treatment of body dysmorphic disorder. *Behavior Modification, 21*, 324–340.

Obsessive Compulsive Cognitions Working Group (1997). Cognitive assessment of obsessive–compulsive disorder. *Behaviour Research and Therapy, 35*, 667–681.

O'Sullivan R. L., Philips K. A., Keuthen, N. J., & Wilhelm, S. (1999). Near fatal skin picking from delusional body dysmorphic disorder responsive to fluvoxamine. *Psychosomatics, 40*, 79–81.

Pacht, A. R. (1984). Reflections on perfection. *American Psychologist, 39*, 386–390.

Phillips, K. A. (1991). Body dysmorphic disorder: The distress of imagined ugliness. *American Journal of Psychiatry, 148*, 1138–1149.

Phillips, K. A. (1998). Body dysmorphic disorder: Clinical aspects and treatment strategies. In M. A. Jenike, L. Baer, W. E. Minichiello (eds), *Obsessive–compulsive disorder: Theory and management* (3rd ed.) (pp. 187–199). Chicago, IL: Mosby.

Phillips, K. A. (2000). Connection between obsessive compulsive disorder and body dysmorphic disorder. In W. K. Goodman, M. V. Rudorfer, & J. D. Maser (eds) *Obsessive compulsive disorder: Contemporary issues in treatment* (pp. 23–42). Englewood Cliffs, NJ: Lawrence Erlbaum.

Phillips, K. A., Atala, K. D., & Albertini, R. S. (1995). Case study: Body dysmorphic disorder in adolescents. *Journal of the American Academy of Child and Adolescent Psychiatry, 34*, 1216–1222.

Phillips, K. A., & Diaz, S. (1997). Gender differences in body dysmorphic disorder. *Journal of Nervous and Mental Disease, 185*, 570–577.

Phillips, K. A., Gunderson, C. G., Mallya, G., McElroy, S. L., & Carter, W. (1998). A comparison study of body dysmorphic disorder and obsessive–compulsive disorder. *Journal of Clinical Psychiatry, 59*, 568–575.

Phillips K. A., & McElroy, S. L. (1993). Insight, overvalued ideation, and delusional thinking in body dysmorphic disorder: Theoretical and treatment implications. *Journal of Nervous and Mental Disease, 181*, 699–702.

Phillips, K. A., McElroy, S. L., Keck, P.E, Hudson, J. I., & Pope, H. G. (1994). A comparison of delusional and non delusional body dysmorphic disorder in 100 cases. *Psychopharmacological Bulletin, 30,* 179–186.

Phillips, K. A., McElroy, S. L., Keck, P. E., Pope, H. G., & Hudson, J. I. (1993). Body dysmorphic disorder: 30 cases of imagined ugliness. *American Journal of Psychiatry, 150,* 302–308.

Phillips, K. A., & Taub, S. L. (1995). Skin picking as a symptom of body dysmorphic disorder. *Psychopharmacology Bulletin, 31,* 279–288.

Pitman, R. K. (1987). A cybernetic model of obsessive compulsive psychopathology. *Comprehensive Psychiatry, 44,* 226–232.

Pope, H. G. Jr., Gruber, A. J., Choi, P., Olivardia, R., & Phillips, K. A. (1997). Muscle dysmorphia. An unrecognized form of body dysmorphic disorder, *Psychosomatics, 38,* 548–557.

Rich, N., Rosen, J. C., Orosan, T., & Reiter, J. (1992). *Prevalence of body dysmorphic disorder in nonclinical populations.* Paper presented at the annual convention of the Association for Advancement of Behavior Therapy, Boston.

Rosen, J. C. (1995). The nature of body dysmorphic disorder and treatment with cognitive behavior therapy. *Cognitive and Behavioral Practice, 2,* 143–166.

Salkovskis, P. M. (1985). Obsessional-compulsive problems: A cognitive-behavioral analysis. *Behaviour Research and Therapy, 23,* 571–584.

Salkovskis, P. M. (1989). Cognitive behavioral factors and the persistence of intrusive thoughts in obsessional problems. *Behaviour Research and Therapy, 27,* 677–682.

Savage, C. R., Deckersbach, T., Wilhelm, S., Rauch, S. L., Baer, L., Reid, T., & Jenike, M. A. (2000). Strategic processing and episodic memory impairment in obsessive–compulsive disorder. *Neuropsychology, 14,* 141–151.

Steketee, G., Frost, R. O., Rhéaume, J., & Wilhelm, S. (1998). Cognitive theory and treatment of obsessive-compulsive disorder. In M. A. Jenike, L. Baer, & W. E. Minichello (eds), *Obsessive–compulsive disorder: Theory and management* (3rd ed.) (pp. 368–399). Chicago: Mosby.

Stroop, J. R. (1935). Studies of interference in serial verbal reactions. *Journal of Experimental Psychology, 18,* 643–662.

Thompson, K. J., Heinberg L. J., Altabe, M., & Tantleff-Dunn, S. (1999). *Exacting beauty: Theory, assessment and treatment of body image disturbance.* Washington, DC: American Psychological Association.

Veale, D., Boockock, A., Gournay, K, Dryden, W., Shah, F., Wilson, R., & Walbrun J. (1996). Body dysmorphic disorder — A survey of 50 cases. *British Journal of Psychiatry, 169,* 196–201.

Veale, D., Gournay, K., Dryden, W., Boocock, A., Shah, F., Wilson, R., & Walburn, J. (1996). Body dysmorphic disorder: A cognitive behavioral model and pilot. *Behaviour Research and Therapy, 34,* 717–729.

Wells, A., & Matthews, G. (1994). *Attention and emotion.* Hillsdale, NJ: Lawrence Erlbaum.

Wilhelm, S., Otto, M. W., Zucker, B. G., & Pollack, M. H. (1997). Prevalence of body dysmorphic disorder in patients with anxiety disorders. *Journal of Anxiety Disorders, 11,* 499–502.

Williams, J. M. G., Watts, F. N., MacLeod, C., & Mathews, A. (1997). *Cognitive psychology and emotional disorders.* (2nd ed.) New York: Wiley.

Yaryura-Tobias, J. A., & Neziroglu, F. (1997a). *Obsessive-compulsive disorders spectrum: Pathogenesis, diagnosis and treatment.* Washington, DC: American Psychiatric Press.

Yaryura-Tobias, J. A., & Neziroglu, F. (1997b). *Bio-behavioral treatment of obsessive compulsive spectrum disorders.* Boston: Norton.

Chapter 12

Eating Disorders and Obsessive Compulsive Disorder

Roz Shafran

Introduction

This chapter begins by describing the main types of eating disorders and examining their phenomenological and cognitive overlap with obsessive compulsive disorder (OCD). Empirical studies looking at the statistical comorbidity between eating disorders and OCD (for example, how many patients with anorexia nervosa also have OCD; how many patients with OCD have anorexia nervosa) are reviewed. The need for a psychological, rather than statistical, analysis of the comorbidity between eating disorders and OCD is expressed, and it is argued that progress could be made in this task by examining shared beliefs between eating disorders and OCD. Six domains of belief have been identified by the OCCWG (1997) as important in OCD (responsibility, importance of thoughts, control over thoughts, overestimation of threat, intolerance of uncertainty and perfectionism). Each of these domains is explored in relation to eating disorders with the aim of better understanding the psychological relationship between OCD and eating disorders. It is hoped that such an improved understanding could facilitate the treatment of patients with comorbid disorders, although it should be noted that comorbid OCD does not necessarily indicate a significantly poorer prognosis for patients with anorexia nervosa or bulimia nervosa (Thiel, Zuger, Jacoby, & Schussler, 1998). The chapter concludes with clinical implications of this psychological analysis and suggestions for future research.

Types of Eating Disorder

Three types of eating disorders are currently recognized by the fourth edition of the Diagnostic and Statistical Manual (DSM-IV; APA, 1994). These are anorexia nervosa, bulimia nervosa and eating disorder not otherwise specified (EDNOS) or atypical eating disorder. In addition, binge eating disorder is identified as a diagnostic category for research purposes. A brief description of these disorders is given below for readers unfamiliar with their characteristics.

Anorexia Nervosa

Anorexia nervosa has distinct behavioral, cognitive and physical characteristics. Behaviorally, patients refuse to maintain normal body weight and restrict their eating. Sometimes, this extreme dietary restriction is punctuated by episodes of binge eating and purging, much like bulimia nervosa (see later). Patients sometimes exercise excessively in a compulsive manner; that is, they feel that exercise is something that they must do, rather than exercising for pleasure. Cognitively, the disorder is characterized by an intense fear of weight gain or becoming fat. Such patients often have a disturbance in their body image (see Thompson, Heinberg, Altabe, & Tanleff, 1999). This may be perceptual (the person perceives herself as larger than she is in reality), affective (the person feels fat), evaluative (the persons' self-evaluation is dependent on their body size) and/or cognitive (the person thinks she is fat). Such patients repeatedly check their weight and body shape. Even though the patients are physically underweight as indicated by a body mass index (weight in kg/height in m^2) less than 17.5, they often deny the seriousness of their situation. The physical impairment is evidenced in an absence of menstruation in post-menarchal females. Females with anorexia nervosa outnumber males approximately ten to one.

Bulimia Nervosa

First described as "an ominous variant of anorexia nervosa" (Russell, 1979, p. 429), the primary behavior that characterizes bulimia nervosa is the consumption of large quantities of food (approximately twice the amount that other people may eat under similar circumstances). This must occur in a discrete period of time and be accompanied by a sense of loss of control over eating; patients cannot stop themselves from eating. There is recurrent inappropriate compensatory behavior to prevent weight gain, some of which involve purging such as vomiting, using laxatives/diuretics, and others which do not (i.e., fasting, excessive exercise). For diagnostic purposes, the binge eating and compensatory behavior must occur at least twice weekly for at least three months. Despite the strong behavioral component of bulimia nervosa, the core psychopathology is cognitive; the self-evaluation of people with this disorder is dependent largely, or even exclusively, on shape and weight (Fairburn, 1997). Given the importance of shape and weight, it is not surprising that such patients weigh themselves repeatedly (up to 20 times daily) and check their shape. People with bulimia nervosa are of normal weight since the excess food ingested in a binge is balanced by the compensatory behavior. Over 90 percent of patients with bulimia nervosa are female.

Eating Disorders Not Otherwise Specified

Approximately 50 percent of patients attending an outpatient clinic present with a serious clinical eating disorder but do not meet diagnostic criteria for either anorexia nervosa or bulimia nervosa. This situation could be explained by many factors. For example, the patient may be menstruating despite having low body weight and all the other characteristics of anorexia nervosa. Alternatively, the patient may not express a fear of weight gain or becoming fat but may be restricting owing to a need for self-control (see Fairburn, Shafran, & Cooper, 1999), or the patient may be purging for shape and weight reasons but may not be experiencing frequent episodes of binge eating. For patients who experience binge eating in the absence of compensatory behavior, a new category of eating disorder called binge eating disorder has been proposed and has been the subject of research studies (Castonguay, Eldredge, & Agras, 1995; Fairburn, Cooper, Doll, Norman, & O'Connor, 2000; Peterson *et al.*, 2000).

Phenomenological Comparison with OCD

Similarities

Descriptions of the phenomenological overlap between OCD and eating disorders have been reported for over 50 years, with anorexia nervosa being viewed as a compulsive neurosis (DuBois, 1949; Palmer & Jones, 1939). It has even been argued that the overlap in phenomenology between eating disorders and OCD is so strong that eating disorders are a modern expression of OCD (e.g., Rothenberg, 1986). Bruch (1976) described "obsessive hyperactivity" as one of the four cardinal features of anorexia nervosa, demonstrating an apparent phenomenological overlap between obsessions, compulsions and anorexia nervosa. The repeated checking of shape and weight (Rosen, 1997) can be viewed as analogous to checking windows, doors etc., and repeatedly seeking reassurance about one's body shape (Rosen, 1997) is akin to repeated reassurance seeking in OCD (Rachman & Hodgson, 1980). The ritualistic behavior that accompanies eating in patients with anorexia nervosa in particular (for example, eating food in a particular order, only using certain utensils, only eating after a certain time of day, magical rituals to prevent weight gain or to lose weight; see Garner, Vitousek, & Pike, 1997) can be viewed as similar to the ordering compulsions that occur in the context of OCD (Rachman & Hodgson, 1980). Sometimes, fears of contamination can lead to a reduction in food intake and significant weight loss. In these circumstances, patients may be referred for the treatment of an eating disorder such as anorexia nervosa, but the psychopathology is that of OCD.

Of interest, the most common symptoms of OCD in patients with eating disorders are those of symmetry, order and arranging (Bastiani *et al.*, 1996; Matsunaga *et al.*, 1999). It appears that many patients with both bulimia nervosa and anorexia nervosa have an elevated need for symmetry and exactness compared to normal controls and this does not change with recovery from the eating disorder (Kaye, 1997; von Ranson, Kaye, Weltzin, Rao, & Matsunaga, 1999).

Differences

Compulsions in OCD are purposeful behaviors that most frequently arise in response to an obsession (Rachman & Hodgson, 1980). One of the fundamental characteristics of obsessions is that they are ego-dystonic and the person resists them (Lewis, 1936). In eating disorders, the checking of shape and weight, and compulsive exercise occur in response to the patient's preoccupation with eating, shape or weight (or their control). This preoccupation may be described by patients as an "obsession", but the thoughts rarely have the intrusive quality of obsessions. They are not ego-dystonic but are in keeping with the person's belief system regarding the importance of shape and weight (Vitousek, 1996), they are not viewed as repugnant and subsequently they are not resisted. In summary, there is a superficial overlap in some of the phenomenological features of the disorders but they remain distinct.

Statistical Comorbidity between OCD and Eating Disorders

Given the phenomenological overlap between OCD and eating disorders, it has been hypothesized that the two disorders have a special relationship and that they will co-occur more commonly than expected by chance. Using a variety of retrospective methodologies, between two and 48 percent of patients with eating disorders also have significant symptoms of OCD (Ben-Tovim, Marilov, & Crisp, 1979; Braun, Sunday, & Halmi, 1994; Halmi *et al.*, 1991; Herzog, Keller, Sacks, Yeh, & Lavori 1992; Thiel, Brooks, Ohlmeier, Jacoby, & Schussler, 1995; Thornton & Russell, 1997). The wide range in estimates of statistical comorbidity is likely to be a result of varied methodologies and use of different criteria for recording of clinically significant symptoms. One study also found some indication that OCD is elevated in relatives of probands with anorexia nervosa (Halmi *et al.*, 1991). More recently a controlled family genetics study found that obsessive compulsive personality disorder is elevated amongst relatives of patients with eating disorders (Lilenfeld *et al.*, 1998; see later).

Other studies have examined the scores of patients with eating disorders on measures of OCD such as the Yale–Brown Obsessive Compulsive Scale (YBOCS: Goodman *et al.*, 1989). The majority of these studies report that patients with eating disorders score higher on these measures than normal controls and sometimes as high as patients with OCD (e.g., Bastiani *et al.*, 1996). Importantly, patients with eating disorders often have a different symptom profile with most common symptoms being symmetry, order and arranging (Bastiani *et al.*, 1996; Matsunaga *et al.*, 1999). Some of these studies can be difficult to interpret since they confound the symptoms of the eating disorder with symptoms of OCD. For example, a patient might score higher on the YBOCS due to the symptoms of her eating disorder (e.g., she may have a need for symmetry and exactness in relation to the utensils used to eat her food out of fear that otherwise she would gain weight). Nevertheless, an elevation in scores on these measures remains even after removing items that could be due to the symptoms of the eating disorder (see Kaye, Weltzin, & Hsu, 1993). Furthermore, an elevation in obsessional symptoms (notably symmetry, order and exactness) can remain even after the eating disorder has been treated successfully (Bastiani *et al.*, 1996; von Ranson *et al.*, 1999).

It is estimated that between eight and 12 percent of patients with OCD also have an eating disorder (Kasvikis, Sakiris, Marks, Basogle, & Noshirvani, 1986; Rubenstein, Pigott, L'Heureux, Hill, & Murhy, 1992; Zribi, Chambon, & Cottraux, 1989) and that the rates are higher than expected by chance. However, the prevalence of eating disorders among people with OCD is lower than the prevalence of OCD in patients with anorexia nerovsa or bulimia nervosa. The finding that the incidence of OCD is higher in eating disorders than vice versa is intriguing, and is similar to the pattern of comorbidity between OCD and Tourettes Syndrome (TS) in which more patients with TS have comorbid OCD than patients with OCD have comorbid TS (e.g., Chee & Sachdev, 1997). Why this should be so is unclear.

A Psychological Approach to Comorbidity

The limitations of simply examining the frequency with which two disorders co-occur was pointed out by Rachman (1991). In a succinct paper, he argued that the "conventional studies of psychiatric comorbidity deal with co-occurrences of two or more psychiatric problems and are, in essence, statistical associations" (Rachman, 1991, p. 461). He suggested that introducing psychological analyses of comorbidity would improve the understanding of the disorders concerned and alert therapists to possible complications. It would also provide indications for treatment and prognosis, facilitate a better understanding of the relationship between the problems, and provide a means of determining whether the connection is static or dynamic. In this paper, he suggested that analyses of comorbidity should assess the connectedness between two disorders in a variety of ways. This might include the behavioral analysis of the functional interdependence of the disorders, assessing the patient's view of the connectedness of the two problems (although this is often inaccurate; Rachman & Lopatka, 1988) and "cognitive analyses". For example, it was suggested that the connecting cognitive link between claustrophobia and agoraphobia was the occurrence of alarming misinterpretations of certain bodily sensations.

This refreshing approach to comorbidity has not been used to illuminate the relationship between eating disorders and OCD. However, given the statistical co-occurrence and superficial overlap in phenomenology, a cognitive analysis of the links between the two disorders may facilitate an improved understanding of each of them and their treatment in patients who have both disorders. The work described in this volume (Chapters one–seven) has identified six domains of beliefs that are relevant to OCD. It is hoped that examining these beliefs in eating disorders will help improve understanding of the psychological connectedness of the two disorders. Also worthwhile is a converse analysis investigating how the cognitions identified as relevant to eating disorders apply to OCD.

Domains of OCD Beliefs in Eating Disorders

It is argued above that examining the beliefs identified as important in OCD will help improve understanding of the psychological connectedness of eating disorders and OCD, and this will be particularly worthwhile in order to improve treatments for patients who have both disorders. To date, there has been no direct investigation in eating disorders of responsibility, importance of thoughts, control over thoughts, intolerance of uncertainty and overestimation of threat. There has, however, been substantial interest in perfectionism in eating disorders. The aim of the subsequent sections is to examine these specific domains in eating disorders with the goal of improving our understanding of the psychological connectedness between them and OCD.

Perfectionism in Eating Disorders

Of all the domains identified by the OCCWG, the relationship between perfectionism and eating disorders has been most widely studied. This is because eating disorders have long been associated with perfectionism from theoretical, phenomenological and empirical perspectives (Casper, 1983; Halmi *et al.*, 2000; Vitousek & Manke, 1994).

Perfectionism has been incorporated into cognitive theories of the maintenance of both anorexia nervosa and bulimia nervosa (Slade, 1982; Fairburn, 1997; Fairburn, Shafran, & Cooper, 1999). For example, perfectionism and dichotomous thinking has been suggested to mediate the relationship between extreme concerns about shape and weight, and rigid and intense dieting (Fairburn, 1997). Moreover, such perfectionistic dieting is brittle and easily ruptured in certain circumstances such as low mood. Consistent with the all-or-nothing thinking that characterizes perfectionism, the breaking of dietary restraint can lead to a total loss of control over food intake and an episode of binge eating. In anorexia nervosa, it has been suggested that perfectionism leads the patient to view adherence to food restriction as success in the context of perceived failure (Slade, 1982). Most recently it has been argued that eating disorders are the expression of perfectionism in the domain of eating, shape and weight, and their control (Shafran, Cooper, & Fairburn, in press).

From a phenomenological perspective, people with anorexia nervosa have been described as "perfectionistic, compliant and isolated girls" (Vitousek & Manke, 1994, p. 139). Such is the phenomenological overlap that many people consider perfectionism part of anorexia nervosa, and some questionnaires to assess eating disorders have subscales to assess perfectionism, such as the Eating Disorders Inventory (Garner, Olmsted, & Polivy, 1983) and the Setting Conditions for Anorexia Nervosa Scale (SCANS; Slade & Dewey, 1986). The SCANS was a precursor of later attempts to measure perfectionism in people with eating disorders ((Mitzman, Slade, & Dewey, 1994; Waller, Wood, Miller, & Slade, 1992) and led to the development of the Positive and Negative Perfectionism Scale (PANPS; Terry-Short, Owens, Slade, & Dewey, 1995; see below).

There has been widespread investigation into the association between perfectionism and symptoms of eating disorders, most commonly using one of two multidimensional scales. The multidimensional perfectionism scale developed by Frost, Marten, Lahart, and Rosenblate (1990) and by Hewitt and Flett (1991) are described in Chapter six. In undergraduate students, eating disorder symptoms are associated with two of these subscales termed Concern over Mistakes and Doubts about Actions (Minarik & Ahrens, 1996), and with self-oriented and socially prescribed perfectionism (Hewitt, Flett, & Ediger, 1995). In this latter study, self-oriented perfectionism was related only to anorexic symptoms, whereas socially prescribed perfectionism was related to dieting, concerns with being thinner, disordered eating patterns, body image avoidance and self-esteem. Comparable findings have been obtained in a sample of adolescents (Davidson, 1989).

Findings from a recent experiment also indicate that eating difficulties are associated with conforming to the unrealistically high performance expectations of others (Pliner & Haddock, 1996). In this study, 100 extremely weight-concerned college students were assigned high or low goals or they selected their own goals in a performance situation. Subjects in the high and low goal group received false feedback indicating success or failure; it was found that individuals who were most weight concerned persisted in accepting an unrealistically high imposed goals and were most affected by the feedback. This study indicates that people with eating concerns conformed to the unrealistically high performance expectations of others more than their weight unconcerned peers (Pliner & Haddock, 1996).

Similar studies have been conducted in patients with eating disorders. Patients with anorexia nervosa scored higher on most measures of perfectionism than normal controls (Bastiani, Rao, Weltzin, & Kaye, 1995; Slade & Dewey, 1986), regardless of the particular subtype of anorexia nervosa (Halmi *et al.*, 2000). Elevated perfectionism has been found both in underweight patients (n=11) and in weight restored patients with anorexia nervosa (n=8). These sample sizes are small but provisionally suggest that perfectionism is not a function of low weight. Consistent with this, Srinivasagam *et al.* (1995) found that high levels of perfectionism persisted after long-term recovery from anorexia nervosa (n=20) and the majority of mean scores on Frost's subscales were higher than those for patients with anxiety disorders (Antony, Purdon, Huta, & Swinson, 1998).

Perfectionism has been identified as a specific risk factor for the development of eating disorders in large-scale community studies that examined risk factors for patients with bulimia nervosa, anorexia nervosa and binge eating disorders (Fairburn *et al.*, 1998; Fairburn, Cooper, Doll, & Welch, 1999). There was a trend for perfectionism to be higher in people with anorexia nervosa compared to patients with bulimia nervosa although perfectionism in bulimia nervosa, was still high. Comparable findings were evident among 890 female undergraduates, and perfectionism was identified as a risk factor for bulimic symptoms for women who perceived themselves as overweight (Joiner, Heatherington, Rudd, & Schmidt, 1997). A similarly large, well-controlled study recently found that relatives of anorexic and bulimic probands had increased risk of subclinical forms of an eating disorder, major depressive disorder, and OCD (Lilenfeld *et al.*, 1998). Perfectionism has been found to be elevated in all of these disorders (see above) but Lilenfeld *et al.* also found that the risk of obsessive compulsive personality disorder (in which perfectionism is a diagnostic feature) was elevated only among relatives of anorexic probands. The authors concluded there was evidence that anorexia nervosa and obsessive compulsive personality disorder may have shared familial risk factors.

The PANPS was devised to assess both the positive and negative aspects of perfectionism since it was hypothesized that positive perfectionism may be associated with anorexia nervosa (Mitzman *et al.*, 1994; Terry-Short *et al.*, 1995). The hypothesis was based upon clinical observations that such patients feel morally superior due to their food restriction, and that successful restriction made them feel triumphant, powerful and proud (Vitousek & Manke, 1994). This division of positive and negative corresponds to previous categories of healthy/unhealthy (Terry-Short *et al.*, 1995), normal/neurotic (Hamenchek, 1978), satisfied/dissatisfied (Slade & Dewey, 1996) and maladaptive evaluation concerns/positive achievement strivings (Frost, Heimberg, Holt, Mattia, & Neubauer, 1993; See also Chapter six in this volume). The PANPS has two factors: negative perfectionism that is a function of avoidance of negative consequences, and positive perfectionism that is a function of achievement of positive consequences. Personal standards, organization, self-oriented perfectionism and other oriented perfectionism were associated with positive perfectionism. Concern over mistakes, parental criticism, parental expectations, doubts about actions and socially prescribed perfectionism were associated with negative perfectionism (Terry-Short *et al.*, 1995). Patients with eating disorders scored higher than depressed patients, athletes and normal controls on negative perfectionism, but they also tended to score higher on positive perfectionism than either the controls or depressed patients but not athletes (Terry-Short *et al.*, 1995).

The relationship between positive perfectionism and body image has also been explored in a large study of 123 patients with anorexia and bulimia (Davis, 1997) and was found to be complex. Body image disparagement was most pronounced when positive and negative perfectionism were both elevated, and body esteem was positively associated with positive perfectionism only when levels of negative perfectionism were low (Davis, 1997). The author concluded that relationships between perfectionism and eating disorder symptoms are complex and that simple interpretations may be misleading.

In summary, there has been a great deal of research examining perfectionism in eating disorders. Perfectionism appears to be an important factor in the development and maintenance of eating disorders, and it is often a long-standing personality trait of patients with anorexia nervosa. Might it be the link between the elevated comorbidity between OCD and eating disorders? Is it possible that people with high levels of perfectionism are more at risk of developing both eating disorders and OCD than people with lower levels of perfectionism? This is an empirical question but the answer may depend on the domains that are salient and important to the individual. It may be that people with high levels of perfectionism whose salient domains are eating and cleanliness are at risk for an eating disorder and OCD with washing compulsions. For other individuals with high levels of perfectionism whose salient domains are eating and ensuring the safety of others, perhaps an eating disorder and OCD with checking compulsions might emerge. For those with high levels of perfectionism whose salient domain is only eating, OCD may be less likely to develop. In conclusion, if perfectionism is the psychological variable that connects eating disorders and OCD, then this connection may be affected by other factors such as the salience of the domain. Such a connection is also likely to be affected by the other cognitions that have been shown to be related to OCD.

Responsibility in Eating Disorders

Although patients with eating disorders are not considered to interpret their intrusions as indicating responsibility for harm, as in OCD, (see Chapter four), patients with anorexia nervosa are described as overconscientious and have a strong adherence to moral values (Casper, Hedeker, & McClough, 1992; Vitousek & Manke, 1994). There is some evidence that they avoid harm (e.g., Berg, Crosby, Wonderlich, & Hawley, 2000) and that this is genetically determined (Lilenfeld *et al.*, 2000, in press). Whether harm-avoidance operates through a mechanism of responsibility has yet to be tested, although it is not implausible. In summary, there are no data assessing responsibility in patients with eating disorders but descriptions of their personality characteristics and data regarding avoidance of harm are consistent with a patient group that has high levels of responsibility.

Importance of Thoughts: Thought–Shape Fusion

It has been suggested that patients with OCD place undue importance on their thoughts, perhaps because of the cognitive bias of thought–action fusion (TAF, Shafran, Thordarson, & Rachman, 1996, see Chapter two). Thought–action fusion has two components: moral TAF and likelihood TAF (Rachman, Thordarson, Shafran, & Woody, 1995; Shafran, Thordarson, & Rachman, 1996). Moral TAF refers to beliefs that thoughts are morally equivalent to actions; likelihood TAF refers to beliefs that thoughts can increase the probability of bad events actually occurring. A similar cognitive bias has been found to be associated with symptoms of eating disorders (Shafran, Teachman, Kerry, & Rachman, 1999). Thought–shape fusion (TSF) has three components. Moral TSF refers to beliefs that thinking about eating a forbidden food is almost as morally wrong as eating a forbidden food. Likelihood TSF refers to beliefs that thinking about eating a forbidden food is likely to make the person gain weight in reality. Feeling TSF, the third component, refers to beliefs that thinking about eating a forbidden food is likely to make the person feel as though he/she has gained weight or changed shape.

In a recent study, TSF in 119 students was found to be significantly associated with measures of eating disorder psychopathology ($r=0.61$). This association was not mediated by depression or scores on the Maudsley Obessional Compulsive Inventory (MOCI; Hodgson & Rachman, 1977).

In addition, thirty students with TSF participated in a behavioral experiment that elicited the distortion. This experimental study was based on a previous investigation of thought–action fusion (Rachman, Shafran, Mitchell, Trant, & Teachman, 1996). The results showed that, as with TAF, it was possible to elicit the distortion under laboratory conditions and that just thinking about eating fattening food elicited a feeling that it was likely that they had gained weight/changed shape, feelings of moral wrong doing and feelings of fatness. Their anxiety also increased, as did feelings of guilt. The procedure elicited the urge to check and to neutralize, and performance of such behaviors reduced anxiety, just as with the previous study on TAF. These findings have been replicated in a sample of patients with anorexia nervosa (Radomsky & de Silva, in preparation) with similar and equally strong findings.

How TSF may operate in eating disorders is uncertain. One suggestion (Whittal, personal communication) is that this cognitive bias operates on the preoccupation with eating that is common among patients with eating disorders who are attempting to restrict their food intake. Such patients are likely to experience unwanted intrusive thoughts of forbidden foods. Patients with thought–shape fusion will be likely to feel immoral and 'fat' after such intrusions. Simply placing such an interpretation on their thoughts is likely to increase the significance and persistence of the thoughts. In turn, this may result in an interpretation by the patient that she has lost control of her thoughts and is going crazy. In this way the domain of importance of thoughts in eating disorders may be closely linked to the domain regarding control over thoughts, as is the case in OCD.

Control over Thoughts in Eating Disorders

If patients with eating disorders have TSF, they may be attempting to suppress thoughts related to eating and food in the same way as patients with OCD attempt to suppress their unwanted thoughts (see Chapter three). In eating disorders, the need for control has been emphasized, particularly for patients with anorexia nervosa (see Fairburn *et al.*, 1999), but the control desired is in the domain of eating, shape and weight and the self as opposed to control over thoughts. Nevertheless, some research exists regarding thought suppression and weight preoccupations (Harnden, McNally, & Jimmerson, 1997). In this study, results suggested that thought suppression may foster the development of weight-related preoccupations, although the role of thought suppression in the maintenance of these preoccupations was unclear.

As with patients with OCD who experience intrusive thoughts, patients with eating disorders can interpret their preoccupations with eating, shape and weight as an indication that they are going crazy and losing control of their mind. For example, one patient with anorexia nervosa spent the majority of her day deciding what she would allow herself to eat that night. Her preoccupation interferred with her studies and she was intensely frustrated by her inability to concentrate on her work. As is common with patients with OCD, she interpreted this as a sign that she had lost mental control.

Intolerance of Uncertainty

It has been suggested that the need for certainty is an important factor in the maintenance of anorexia nervosa (Vitousek & Manke, 1994; Vitousek, 1996). People with AN are described as having a need for order and routine, and finding decision-making and choices aversive. Having a disorder such as anorexia nervosa is so restrictive that the structure of life becomes simpler and this is hypothesized to maintain the disorder (Vitousek & Orimoto, 1993). Such patients typically eat the same restricted range of foods day after day since they cannot tolerate the uncertainty of the impact of a new food with an unknown calorie content. It may be the case that the domain in which the patient has an intolerance for uncertainty differs. In patients with eating disorders it is likely to concern calorie-content, weight change and shape change rather than whether an action has been completed or not. The intolerance for uncertainty in the domain of eating, shape and weight may account for the clinical phenomena whereby some patients have a strong need to always know the calorie content of food items, weigh themselves frequently and check their shape excessively.

Overestimation of Threat

Astonishingly, to the best of the author's knowledge, there has been no study investigating threat estimation in general in patients with eating disorders. This is particularly surprising given the statistical comorbidity between anxiety disorders and eating disorders. There is some evidence that patients with eating disorders overestimate threat but in the area of eating, shape and weight, and self concept (Meyer, Waller, & Watson, 2000). For example, such patients overestimate the threat of weight gain from eating one biscuit (see Cooper & Hunt, 1998; Cooper & Turner, 2000) or overestimate the effects of weight gain (e.g., "I won't be able to cope and will collapse"). The data on harm avoidance (see section on responsibility above) suggest that such patients may indeed have an elevation in their estimates of threat in general, although this elevation may be lower than that of patients with OCD and other anxiety disorders. However, as argued with perfectionism, it is the domain in which their belief is expressed that is likely to be critical in understanding the impact of the cognition. If the patient does overestimate weight gain (i.e., the threat in the domain that is salient to her), then such an overestimate is likely to maintain her restraint. The relationship between the expression of the domain of the threat and general elevations in threat estimation remains to be elucidated.

Beliefs in Eating Disorder

It is important to mention some of the beliefs that have been identified as relevant for patients with eating disorders (see Vitousek, 1996 for a review). These beliefs are described as negative beliefs about the self (e.g., "I am stupid"), beliefs that weight and shape are a means to acceptance by others, beliefs that weight and shape are necessary for self-acceptance, and beliefs about control over eating (Cooper & Hunt, 1998; Cooper & Turner, 2000). Other researchers have identified beliefs that may be important including rigid weight regulation, weight and approval, and excessive self-control as a component of self-esteem (see Mizes & Christiano, 1995). None of these beliefs have been examined in patients with OCD.

Psychological Approach to Comorbidity: the Role of Cognitions

The aim of the above analysis was to examine the OCD-relevant domains in eating disorders with the goal of improving our understanding of the psychological connectedness between eating disorders and OCD. As suggested previously (OCCWG, 1997), high levels of these cognitions may not be unique to obsessive compulsive disorder, and the above review indicates that they are not. There is evidence that responsibility (harm-avoidance), overimportance of thoughts, need for control (though not of thoughts in the domains of aggression, blasphemy and sex), overestimation of threat (related to shape and weight), intolerance of uncertainty, and particularly perfectionism are also characteristic of eating disorders.

According to cognitive theory described in Chapter one, the six domains of appraisal make a person vulnerable to developing OCD and/or contribute to its maintenance. It may also be the case that they make a person vulnerable to developing an eating disorder. Two questions immediately arise from this hypothesis. First, how do they make a person vulnerable to developing either of these psychiatric disorders, and second, what characteristics would lead a person to develop OCD rather than an eating disorder (and vice versa). The answers to both of these questions are entirely speculative.

How these beliefs may operate to make one vulnerable to developing a psychiatric disorder is not known but a detailed cognitive–behavioral analysis of clinically-relevant perfectionism has led to some suggestions (Shafran *et al.*, 2000). In this analysis, it is proposed that the self-worth of patients with perfectionism is dependent on the pursuit and attainment of personally demanding standards in at least one salient domain (Shafran, Cooper, & Fairburn, in press). If the domain is eating, shape and weight (or their control), then perfectionism is likely to be an important factor that transforms normal dieting into a clinical eating problem. If the domain relates to intrusive thoughts (i.e., having perfect control over thoughts), then perfectionism may contribute to the transformation of normal unwanted intrusive thoughts into abnormal obsessions (see Chapters one and two in this volume).

A similar process may operate for threat estimation. In OCD, if a person overestimates the likelihood or consequences of threat occurring to a loved one, then this is likely to contribute to efforts to protect their loved one in any way possible. Such behavior may turn normal compulsions into abnormal ones (Muris, Merckelbach, & Clavan, 1997). In eating disorders, if a person overestimates the likelihood of gaining a large amount of weight, or the negative consequences of that weight gain (e.g., "nobody will ever find me attractive"), then this may act as a factor in the transformation from normal dieting into abnormal, extreme dieting to obtain a margin of safety from fatness (Vitousek & Orimoto, 1993). The same principle can be applied to the other beliefs, that is, having the belief will render the person vulnerable to developing a psychiatric disorder by turning a normal process (intrusive thoughts, dieting) into an abnormal one (obsessions, extreme dietary restriction). It is likely that the precise mechanisms that contribute to this transformation are common to both OCD and eating disorders, and include thought-suppression and information processing biases such as hypervigilance and avoidance behaviour.

What determines the domain to which the beliefs are applied is an empirical question. It may be dependent on early experiences, or else there may be a genetic contribution (Lilenfeld *et al.*, 1998). It may also sometimes be dependent on the particular environmental circumstances. For example, one patient with perfectionism was functioning well at school, and her self-worth was dependent on her doing well academically. In her second year at University, she obtained little feedback and her self-worth began to decrease. Coincidentally, she had gained a small amount of weight due to eating larger portions than she was accustomed to, while on holiday in the United States. Consequently, she began to diet. Her need to achieve goals transferred from her work (because of the absence of feedback) to her diet (the feedback was immediate). It is possible that if someone in her family had been ill at this time, or if there was an increase in her responsibility at work, then OCD may have developed.

Clinical and Research Implications of Psychological Analysis

Clinically it is important to identify the nature of beliefs that may have contributed to the development and maintenance of the problem. This is true both for OCD and for eating disorders. The two fields can inform each other. For the treatment of eating disorders, it may be appropriate to ask questions that elicit beliefs in each of the six domains identified for OCD. They may be playing an important role in the maintenance of the problem (especially perfectionism). For the treatment of OCD, it may be equally informative to identify beliefs that characterize eating disorders. For patients with both OCD and an eating disorder, examining these beliefs and their applicability to different domains (eating, shape and weight vs. intrusive thoughts) may be particularly illuminating.

From a research perspective, the hypothesis that the beliefs identified by OCCWG in the domain of eating, shape and weight (as opposed to intrusive thoughts) may be important in the maintenance of eating disorders should be tested. Such an investigation may necessitate the adaptation of the OBQ and III. Investigation of these domains in patients with comorbid eating disorders and OCD, compared with patients with eating disorder only or OCD only would also be illuminating. It might be hypothesized that patients with comorbid eating disorder and OCD may not necessarily have stronger beliefs in the six areas, but that these beliefs would be applied both to the domain of intrusive thoughts and to eating, shape and weight. The role of cognitions in the relationship between eating disorders and OCD would also be informed by the experimental manipulation of the beliefs to see the impact on each of the disorders. Such research would undoubtedly be challenging but would likely benefit patients who are experiencing two disabling and distressing disorders.

References

American Psychiatric Association. (1994). *Diagnostic and Statistical Manual of Mental Disorders*, (4th ed.), Washington, DC: Author.

Antony, M. M., Purdon, C. L., Huta, V., & Swinson, R. P. (1998). Dimensions of perfectionism across the anxiety disorders. *Behaviour Research and Therapy, 36*, 1143–1154.

Bastiani, A. M., Altemus, M., Pigott, T. A., Rubenstein, C., Weltzin, T. E., & Kaye, W. H. (1996). Comparison of obsessions and compulsions in patients with anorexia nervosa and obsessive–compulsive disorder. *Biological Psychiatry, 39*, 966–969.

Bastiani, A. M., Rao, R., Weltzin, T. E., & Kaye, W. H. (1995). Perfectionism in anorexia nervosa. *International Journal of Eating Disorders, 17*, 147–152.

Ben-Tovim, D. I., Marilov, V., & Crisp, A. H. (1979). Personality and mental state (PSE) within anorexia nervosa. *Journal of Psychosomatic Research, 23*, 321–325.

Berg, M. L., Crosby, R. D., Wonderlich, S. A., & Hawley, D. (2000). Relationship of temperament and perceptions of nonshared environment in bulimia nervosa. *International Journal of Eating Disorders, 28*, 148–154.

Braun, D. L., Sunday, S. R., & Halmi, K. A. (1994). Psychiatric comorbidity in patients with eating disorders. *Psychological Medicine, 24*, 859–867.

Bruch, H. (1976). The treatment of eating disorders. *Mayo Clinic Proceedings, 51*, 266–272.

Bulik, C. M. (1995). Anxiety disorders and eating disorders: a review of their relationship. *New Zealand Journal of Psychiatry, 24*, 51–62.

Casper, R. C., Hedeker, D., & McClough, J. F. (1992). Personality dimensions in eating disorders and their relevance for subtyping. *Journal of the American Academy of Child and Adolescent Psychiatry, 31*, 830–840.

Castonguay, L. G., Eldredge, K. L., & Agras, W. S. (1995). Binge eating disorder: Current state and future directions. *Clinical Psychology Review, 15*, 865–890.

Chee, K. Y., & Sachdev, P. (1997). A controlled study of sensory tics in Gilles de la Tourette syndrome and obsessive–compulsive disorder using a structured interview. *Journal of Neurology, Neurosurgery and Psychiatry, 62*, 188–192.

Cooper, M., & Hunt, J. (1998). Core beliefs and underlying assumptions in bulimia nervosa and depression. *Behaviour Research and Therapy, 36,* 895–898.

Cooper, M., & Turner, H. (2000). Underlying assumptions and core beliefs in anorexia nervosa and dieting. *British Journal of Clinical Psychology, 39,* 215–218.

Davis, C. (1997). Normal and neurotic perfectionism in eating disorders: an interactive model. *International Journal of Eating Disorders, 22,* 421–426.

Du Bois, F. (1949). Compulsion neurosis with cachexia (anorexia nervosa) *American Journal of Psychiatry, 20,* 106–107.

Fairburn, C. G. (1997). Eating disorders. In D.M. Clark & C.G. Fairburn (eds). *Science and practice of cognitive–behaviour therapy.* Oxford medical publications. Oxford, UK: Oxford University Press.

Fairburn, C. G., Cooper, Z., Doll, H. A., Norman, P., & O'Connor, M. (2000). The natural course of bulimia nervosa and binge eating disorder in young women. *Archives of General Psychiatry, 57,* 659–665.

Fairburn, C. G., Cooper, Z., Doll, H. A., & Welch, S. L. (1999). Risk factors for anorexia nervosa: Three integrated case control comparisons. *Archives of General Psychiatry, 56,* 468–476.

Fairburn, C. G., Doll, H. A., Welch, S. L., Hay, P. J., Davies, B. A., & O'Connor, M. E. (1998). Risk factors for binge eating disorder: a community based, case control study. *Archives of General Psychiatry, 55,* 425–432.

Fairburn, C. G., Shafran, R., & Cooper, Z. (1999). A cognitive–behavioral theory of anorexia nervosa. *Behaviour Research and Therapy, 37,* 1–13.

Frost, R. O., Heimberg, R. G., Holt, C. S., Mattia, J. I., & Neubauer, A. L. (1993). A comparison of two measures of perfectionism. *Personality and Individual Differences, 14,* 119–126.

Frost, R. O., Marten, P., Lahart, C. M., & Rosenblate, R. (1990). The dimensions of perfectionism. *Cognitive Therapy and Research, 14,* 449–468.

Garner, D. M., Olmsted, M. P., & Polivy, J. (1983). Development and validation of a multidimensional eating disorder inventory for anorexia nervosa and bulimia. *International Journal of Eating Disorders, 2,* 15–34.

Garner, D. M., Vitousek, K. M., & Pike, K. M. (1997). Cognitive–behavioral therapy for anorexia nervosa. In D.M. Garner & P.E. Garfinkel (eds). *Handbook of treatment for eating disorders* (2nd ed, pp. 94–144). New York: Guilford.

Goodman, W. K., Price, L. H., Rasmussen, S. A., Mazure, C., Fleischmann, R. L., Hill, C. L., Heninger, G. R., & Charney, D. S. (1989). The Yale–Brown Obsessive–Compulsive Scale (Y-BOCS): II. Validity. *Archives of General Psychiatry, 46,* 1012–1016.

Halmi, K. A., Eckert, E., Marchi, P., Sampugnaro, V., Apple R., & Cohen, J. (1991). Comorbidity of psychiatric diagnoses in anorexia nervosa. *Archives of General Psychiatry, 48,* 712–718.

Halmi, K. A., Sunday, S. R., Stober, M., Kaplan, A., Woodside, D. B., Fichter, M., Treasure, J., Berrettini, W. H., & Kaye, W. H. (2000). Perfectionism in anorexia nervosa: variation by clinical subtype, obsessionality and pathological eating behavior. *American Journal of Psychiatry, 157,* 1799–1805.

Hamachek, D. E. (1978). Psychodynamics of normal and neurotic perfectionism. *Psychology: A Journal of Human Behavior, 15,* 27–33.

Harnden, J. L., McNally, R. J., & Jimmerson, D. C. (1997). Effects of suppressing thoughts about body weight: A comparison of dieters and nondieters. *International Journal of Eating Disorders, 22,* 285–290.

Herzog, D. B., Keller, M. B., Sacks, N. R., Yeh, C. J., & Lavori, P. W. (1992). Psychiatric comorbidity in treatment-seeking anorexics and bulimics. *Journal of the American Academy of Child and Adolescent Psychiatry, 31,* 810–818.

Hewitt, P. L., & Flett, G. L. (1991). Perfectionism in the self and social contexts: conceptualization, assessment, and association with psychopathology. *Journal of Personality and Social Psychology,* *60*, 456–470.

Hewitt, P. L., Flett, G. L., & Ediger, E. (1995). Perfectionism traits and perfectionistic self presentation in eating disorder attitudes, characteristics, and symptoms. *International Journal of Eating Disorders, 18*, 317–26.

Hodgson, R. J., & Rachman, S. (1977). Obsessional-compulsive complaints. *Behaviour Research and Therapy, 15*, 389–395.

Joiner, T. E. Jr., Heatherton, T. F., Rudd, M. D., & Schmidt, N. B. (1997). Perfectionism, perceived weight status, and bulimic symptoms: two studies testing a diathesis stress model. *Journal of Abnormal Psychology, 106*, 145–153.

Kasvikis Y. G., Sakiris, F., Marks I. M., Basoglu, M., & Noshirvani, H. (1986). Past history of anorexia nervosa in women with obsessive–compulsive disorder. *International Journal of Eating Disorders, 5*, 1069–1075.

Kaye, W. H. (1997). Anorexia nervosa, obsessional behavior, and serotonin. *Psychopharmacology Bulletin, 33*, 335–344.

Kaye, W. H., Weltzin, T. E., & Hsu, L. G. (1993). Anorexia nervosa. In E. Hollander (ed.). *Obsessive–compulsive related disorders*. Washington DC: American Psychiatric Press.

Kaye, W. H., Weltzin, T. E., Hsu, L. G., Bulik, C., McConaha, C., & Sobkiewicz, T. (1992). Patients with anorexia nervosa have elevated scores on the Yale–Brown Osessive–Compulsive Scale. *International Journal of Eating Disorders, 12*, 57–62.

Lewis, A. J. (1936). Problems of obsessional illness. *Proceedings of the Royal Society of Medicine, 29*, 325–336.

Lilenfeld, L. R., Devlin, B., Bulik, C. M., Strober, M., Berrettini, W. H., Bacanu, S., Fichter, M. M., Goldman, D., Halmi, K. A., Kaplan, A., Woodside, D. B., Treasure, J., & Kaye, W. H. (in press). Deriving behavioral phenotypes in an International Multicenter Study of Eating Disorders. *Psychological Medicine*.

Lilenfield L. R., Kaye, W. H., Greeno, C. G., Merikangas K. R., Plotnicov, K., Pollice, C., Rao, R., Strober, M., Bulik, C. M., & Nagy, L. (1998). A controlled family study of anorexia nervosa and bulimia nervosa: Psychiatric disorders in first degree relatives and effects of proband comorbidity. *Archives of General Psychiatry, 55*, 603–610.

Lilenfeld, L. R., Stein, D., Bulik, C. M., Strober, M., Plotnicov, K. H., Pollice, C., Rao, R., Nagy, L., &. Kaye, W. H. (2000). Personality traits among currently eating disordered, recovered, and never ill first-degree female relatives of bulimic and control women. *Psychological Medicine, 30*, 1399–1410.

Matsunaga, H., Kirjike, N., Iwasaki, Y., Miyata, A., Yamagami, S., & Kaye, W. H. (1999). Clinical characteristics in patients with anorexia nervosa and obsessive–compulsive disorder. *Psychological Medicine, 29*, 407–414.

Meyer, C., Waller, G., & Watson, D. (2000). Cognitive avoidance and bulimic psychopathology: the relevance of temporal factors in a nonclinical population. *International Journal of Eating Disorders, 27*, 405–410.

Minarik, M. L., & Ahrens, A. H. (1996). Relations of eating and symptoms of depression and anxiety to the dimensions of perfectionism among undergraduate women. *Cognitive Therapy and Research, 20*, 155–169.

Mitzman, S. F., Slade, P., & Dewey M. E. (1994). Preliminary development of a questionnaire designed to measure neurotic perfectionism in the eating disorders. *Journal of Clinical Psychology, 50*, 516–22.

Mizes, J. S., & Christiano, B. A. (1995). Assessment of cognitive variable relevant to cognitive–behavioral perspectives on anorexia nervosa and bulimia nervosa. *Behaviour Research and Therapy, 33*, 95–105.

Muris, P., Merckelbach, H., & Clavan, M. (1997). Abnormal and normal compulsions. *Behaviour Research and Therapy, 35*, 249–252.

Obsessive–Compulsive Cognitions Working Group (1997). Cognitive assessment of obsessive–compulsive disorder. *Behaviour Research and Therapy, 35*, 667–681.

Palmer, H. D., & Jones, M. (1939). Anorexia nervosa as a manifestation of compulsive neurosis. *Archives of Neurology and Psychiatry, 41*, 856–860.

Peterson, C. B., Crow, S. J., Nugent, S., Mitchell, J. E., Engbloom, S., & Mussell, M. P. (2000). Predictors of treatment outcome for binge eating disorder. *International Journal of Eating Disorders, 28*, 131–138.

Pliner, P., & Haddock. G. (1996). Perfectionism in weight concerned and unconcerned women: an experimental approach. *International Journal of Eating Disorders, 19*, 381–389.

Rachman, S. (1991). A psychological approach to the study of comorbidity. *Clinical Psychology Review, 11*, 461–464.

Rachman, S., & Hodgson, R. (1980). *Obsessions and compulsions*. Englewood Cliffs, NJ: Prentice-Hall.

Rachman, S., & Lopatka, C. (1988). Accurate and inaccurate predictions of pain. *Behaviour Research and Therapy, 26*, 291–296.

Rachman, S., Shafran, R., Mitchell, D., Trant, J., & Teachman, B. (1996). How to remain neutral: an experimental analysis of neutralization. *Behaviour Research and Therapy, 34*, 889–898.

Rachman, S., Thordarson, D. S., Shafran, R., & Woody, S. R. (1995). Perceived responsibility: Structure and significance. *Behaviour Research and Therapy, 33*, 779–784.

Von Ranson, K. M., Kaye, W. H., Weltzin, T. E., Rao, R., & Matsunaga, H. (1999). Obsessive–compulsive disorder symptoms before and after recovery from bulimia nervosa. *American Journal of Psychiatry, 156*, 1703–1708.

Rosen, J. C. (1997). Cognitive–behavioral body image therapy. In D.M. Garner & P.E. Garfinkel (eds), *Handbook of treatment for eating disorders*, 2nd ed. (pp. 188–201). New York: Guilford.

Rothenberg, A. (1986). Eating disorder as a modern obsessive–compulsive syndrome, *Psychiatry, 153*, 6–15.

Rubenstein, C. S., Pigott T. A., L'Heureux, F., Hill, J. L., Murhy, D. L. (1992). A preliminary investigation of the lifetime prevalence of anorexia and bulimia nervosa in patients with obsessive–compulsive disorder. *Journal of Clinical Psychiatry, 53*, 309–314.

Russell, G. (1979). Bulimia nervosa: An ominous variant of anorexia nervosa. *Psychological Medicine, 9*, 429–448.

Shafran, R., Cooper, Z., & Fairburn, C. G. (in press). Perfectionism. A cognitive–behavioural analysis. *Behaviour Research and Therapy*.

Shafran, R., Teachman, B. A., Kerry, S., & Rachman, S. (1999). A cognitive distortion associated with eating disorders: thought–shape fusion. *British Journal of Clinical Psychology, 38*, 167–179.

Shafran, R., Thordarson, D. S., & Rachman, S. (1996). Thought–action fusion in obsessive–compulsive disorder. *Journal of Anxiety Disorders, 10*, 379–391.

Slade, P. D. (1982). Towards a functional analysis of anorexia nervosa and bulimia nervosa. *British Journal of Clinical Psychology, 21*, 167–179.

Slade, P. D., & Dewey, M. E. (1986). Development and preliminary validation of SCANS: A screening instrument for identifying people at risk of developing anorexia nervosa and bulimia nervosa. *International Journal of Eating Disorders, 5*, 517–538.

Srinivasagam, N. M., Kaye, W. H., Plotnicov, K. H., Greeno, C., Welzin, T. E., & Rao, R. (1995). Persistent perfectionism, symmetry, and exactness after long-term recovery from anorexia nervosa. *American Journal of Psychiatry, 152*, 1630–1634.

Terry-Short, L. A., Owens, G. R., Slade, P. D., & Dewey, M. E. (1995). Positive and negative perfectionism. *Personality and Individual Differences, 18*, 663–668.

Thiel., A., Brooks, A., Ohlmeier, M., Jacoby, G. E., & Schussler, G. (1995). Obsessive–Compulsive disease in patients with anorexia and bulimia nervosa. *American Journal of Psychiatry, 152*, 72–77.

Thiel, A., Zuger, M., Jacoby, G. E., & Schussler, G. (1998). Thirty-month outcome in patients with anorexia or bulimia nervosa and concomitant obsessive–compulsive disorder. *American Journal of Psychiatry, 155*, 244–249.

Thompson, J. K., Heinberg, L. J., Altabe, M., & Tantleff, D. S. (1999). *Exacting beauty: Theory, assessment, and treatment of body image disturbance.* Washington, DC: American Psychological Association.

Thornton, C., & Russell J. (1997). Obsessive–compulsive comorbidity in the dieting disorders. *International Journal of Eating Disorders, 21*, 83–87.

Vitousek, K. M. (1996). The current status of cognitive–behavioral models of anorexia nervosa and bulimia nervosa. In P.M. Salkovskis (ed.) *Frontiers of cognitive therapy* (pp. 383–418). New York: Guilford.

Vitousek, K. M., & Orimoto, L. (1993). Cognitive–behavioral models of anorexia nervosa, bulimia nervosa, and obesity. In P.C. Kendall & K.S. Dobson (eds), *Psychopathology and cognition* (pp. 191–242). New York: Academic Press.

Vitousek, K., & Manke, F. (1994). Personality variables and disorders in anorexia nervosa and bulimia nervosa. *Journal of Abnormal Psychology, 103*, 137–147.

Waller, G., Wood, A., Miller, J., & Slade, P. (1992). The development of neurotic perfectionism: A risk factor for unhealthy eating attitudes. *British Review of Bulimia and Anorexia Nervosa, 6*, 57–62.

Zribi, S., Chambon, O., & Cottraux, J. (1989). Anorexia nervosa: A frequent antecedent of obsessive–compulsive disorder. *Encephale, 15*, 355–358.

Chapter 13

A Cognitive Perspective on Obsessive Compulsive Disorder and Depression: Distinct and Related Features

David A. Clark

Introduction

Since the dawn of modern psychiatry, researchers and clinicians have recognized a close relationship between obsessions, compulsions and mood disturbance, especially depression. Rachman and Hodgson (1980) noted that Henry Maudsley made no distinction between obsessions and depression in his 1895 publication of *The Pathology of Mind*. By the mid-point of the 20th century, early psychiatric literature began to distinguish obsessive compulsive disorder as a neurotic illness (Rachman & Hodgson, 1980). In DSM-I (American Psychiatric Association [APA], 1952) depression and OCD were categorized under psychoneurotic disorders with a common root in anxiety. By the third edition and its revision (APA, 1987), the DSM recognized a clear distinction between major depression as a disturbance of mood and obsessive compulsive disorder (OCD) as a subtype of anxiety disorder with a characteristic subjective state of anxiousness and avoidant behavior.

The relationship between OCD and depression can be understood at a number of levels. Diagnostically OCD and major depressive disorder (MDD) have a high comorbidity rate. Temporally the two disorders are linked, with OCD more often leading to secondary depression than vice versa. OCD and MDD share certain common symptoms such as worry, doubt, indecisiveness, guilt, social withdrawal and isolation. There may be a common genetic diathesis to OCD and major depression (Billett, Richter, & Kennedy, 1998), and personality features like perfectionism, conscientiousness and low self-esteem have been implicated in both disorders. Commonalties are even apparent in pharmacotherapy and psychological interventions, with the pervasive use of serotonin reuptake inhibitors (SRIs) as first-line medication for both disorders and the more recent introduction of cognitive interventions, initially developed for depression, in the treatment of obsessions.

In keeping with the theme of this edited volume, this chapter will focus on the cognitive basis of OCD and MDD. The next section will provide some background by very briefly considering the diagnostic link between major depression and OCD. Following this I will

Cognitive Approaches to Obsessions and Compulsions – Theory, Assessment, and Treatment
Copyright © 2002 by Elsevier Science Ltd.
All rights of reproduction in any form reserved.
ISBN: 0-08-043410-X

examine in some detail the points of overlap and distinction in the cognitive processes that characterize obsessions, compulsions and depression. Particular attention will be given to the six OCD belief domains of inflated responsibility, overimportance of thoughts, control of thoughts, threat estimation, intolerance of uncertainty and perfectionism proposed by the Obsessive–Compulsive Cognitions Working Group (OCCWG, 1997), and whether these beliefs are manifest in some form in clinical depression. A consideration of the very limited published empirical research comparing cognition in OCD and depression will be reviewed. I conclude with a summary and possible directions for future research on OCD and depression.

OCD and Major Depression: Diagnostic Considerations

Rachman and Hodgson (1980) provided a detailed review and analysis of the research literature available at that time on the relationship between obsessions, compulsions and depression. Their conclusion was that: (a) in most cases there is a close association between obsessions, compulsions, and depression, although OC symptoms can vary independently of depression; (b) the incidence of obsessions often increases during episodes of depression; (c) persistent obsessional symptoms can facilitate the onset of depression; and (d) depression may help maintain OC symptoms, as evidenced by a positive correlation between severity of depression and increased frequency of obsessions and compulsions.

OCD and major depression have a pattern of high syndromal comorbidity. Estimates of the percentage of patients with a principal diagnosis of OCD who also meet diagnostic criteria for a secondary major depression range from 24 percent to 43 percent (Antony, Downie, & Swinson, 1998; Lensi et al., 1996; Sanderson, Di Nardo, Rapee, & Barlow, 1990). In the Epidemiologic Catchment Area Study, 32 percent of individuals with a positive DSM-III diagnosis of OCD also met criteria for lifetime history of major depression as assessed by the Diagnostic Interview Schedule (Karno & Golding, 1991). Brown, Moras, Zinbarg, and Barlow (1993) reported that 23 percent of their sample with a principal Axis I diagnosis of OCD had co-occurring major depression, 26 percent had dysthymia and 10 percent had depression NOS. Crino and Andrews (1996) found that 50 percent of the 108 individuals with lifetime diagnosis of OCD were comorbid for DSM-III-R major depression and 19 percent were comorbid for dysthymia. In her review Gibbs (1996) noted that individuals with OCD are seven times more likely to have comorbid depression than non-OCD persons. Interestingly, fewer patients (estimates range from four percent to 15 percent) with a principal diagnosis of major depression present with co-existing OCD (Brown & Barlow, 1992; Sanderson & Beck, 1990). In terms of the temporal course, one-half to two-thirds of cases with comorbid OCD and depression report that obsessive and compulsive symptoms precede the onset of depression (for reviews see Antony et al., 1998; Rachman & Hodgson, 1980). In these cases, then, the depression appears as a consequence of the severity of obsessional symptoms.

There is also a high degree of symptom co-occurrence in OCD and major depression. OCD patients frequently report depressive symptoms of sufficient severity to place them within the clinical range. For example, in many studies OCD samples produce Beck Depression Inventory (BDI) group mean scores within the moderate to severe range (i.e., 16–25), and these scores do not differ substantially from the means seen in depressed outpatient samples (e.g., Calamari, Wiegartz, & Janeck, 1999; MacDonald, Antony, MacLeod, & Ritcher, 1997; Shafran, Thordarson, & Rachman, 1996). Di Nardo and Barlow (1990) found that patients with a principal diagnosis of OCD did not differ significantly from patients with a principal diagnosis of major depression on the Hamilton Ratings Scales of Depression or Anxiety.

It has also been shown that individuals with unipolar major depression obtain scores on OCD symptom measures that fall midway between the scores of OCD patients and normal controls (Kendell & Discipio, 1970). Earlier studies found that a significant number of non-OCD patients with depression (14–25 percent) exhibit obsessions or compulsions during the acute phase of depression (Gittleson, 1966; Vaughan, 1976). In a recent unpublished pilot study, a sample of mainly depressed non-obsessional outpatients ($n = 38$) scored significantly higher than non-clinical community adults and students on a new self-report measure of obsessions, although they did not differ significantly from the controls on the compulsion subscale (Clark, 1999a). Jennings, Ross, Popper, and Elmore (1999) found that 41 percent of depressed mothers had thoughts of harming their infant and 24.5 percent were afraid of being alone with the baby. However, Woody, Taylor, McLean, and Koch (1998) found that their samples of outpatients with panic disorder or major depression endorsed very few obsessive compulsive cognitions. It is apparent, then, that depressive symptoms are very common in OCD patients but less is known about the frequency of obsessional symptoms in major depression. It may be, as suggested by Rachman and Hodgson (1980), that obsessions in depression have a different content. For example, depressed patients may more often report aggressive types of obsessions than OCD patients. It is likely that compulsive behavior and possibly other neutralizing activities are quite uncommon, but obsessive ruminations may be more prevalent in major depression. Ricciardi and McNally (1995) reported that OCD patients who were comorbid for depression had significantly more severe obsessional but not compulsive symptoms than OCD patients without major depression. This finding raises the possibility that depression may be correlated with specific aspects of obsessions and compulsions. Whether the presence of obsessional ruminations in depressed patients who do not meet diagnostic criteria for OCD has any diagnostic or treatment implications must await further investigation.

The close symptomatic relationship between mood disturbance and OCD is also apparent in the moderate correlation between OCD and depression symptom measures. OCD symptom measures such as the Padua Inventory, Maudsley Obsessive Compulsive Inventory and Yale–Brown Obsessive Compulsive Scale (YBOCS) correlate equally, or even higher, with self-report depression measures ($r = 0.33–0.55$) than they do with anxiety symptom measures (McKay, Danyko, Neziroglu, & Yaryura-Tobias, 1995; Sternberger & Burns, 1990; Van Oppen, Hoekstra, & Emmelkamp, 1995; Woody, Steketee, & Chambless, 1995; for review see Taylor, 1995, 1998). Foa, Kozak, Salkovskis, Coles, and Amir (1998) found that the distress but not frequency subscale of their new self-report measure of obsessions and compulsions correlated with the Hamilton Rating Scale of Depression. Overall, the findings from this literature suggest that a moderate association exists between mood disturbance and the severity, if not frequency, of obsessions and, possibly, compulsions.

One reason for the connection between OCD and depression is that a significant number of symptoms are common to both disorders. Alloy, Kelly, Mineka, and Clements (1990), for example, argued that "certain helplessness", or the perceived certainty that one can not influence the occurrence of significant future outcomes, is common to both anxiety and depression. Consequently, symptoms associated with "certain helplessness" such as dysphoria, passivity, decreased energy, rumination and obsessions, worry, indecisiveness, self-preoccupation, and negative self-evaluation will be found in mixed or comorbid states of anxiety and depression. However, it is not clear whether "certain helplessness" is a common feature of OCD and depression because in OCD misinterpretations of helplessness over anticipated future threatening events may be less apparent. As Kozak and Foa (1997) point out, the person with OCD concludes that a situation might be dangerous more on the basis of an absence of "certain safety" rather than on indicators of possible threat. For example, a public payphone might be considered contaminated, not because of indicators of possible contamination, but because of the likelihood that cleanliness or sterility can not be assumed. Rituals, then, are performed to reduce possible risk of threat and maximize safety. If obsessional persons believed they were helplessness to prevent anticipated future threat, then they would not engage in compulsive behavior. Unfortunately rigorous empirical research has not been done to determine which symptoms, such as helplessness, most commonly overlap in OCD and major depression. What is needed is a detailed comparison at the symptom level of individuals with a single diagnosis of OCD and persons with a single diagnosis of major depression.

The association between depression and OCD is also evident in the treatment strategies advocated for both disorders. In separate publications, the American Psychiatric Association Practice Guidelines for treatment of major depression and later for OCD recommended the use of SRIs for pharmacotherapy of both disorders (APA, 1993, 1997). Beck's cognitive therapy was originally developed as a treatment for depression (Beck, Rush, Shaw, & Emery, 1979). Although his therapy protocol was refined and elaborated to deal with a number of psychological disorders, Beck felt that cognitive interventions may have little to offer OCD (Hollon & Beck, 1986). However we have recently seen a number of interesting adaptations of cognitive therapy for the treatment of obsessions by Freeston, Rhéaume, and Ladouceur (1996), Salkovskis (1985), van Oppen and Arntz (1994), and Whittal and Mclean (1999). Intervention strategies such as educating the client in the cognitive model of OCD, identification of faulty appraisals or automatic thoughts of the obsession, cognitive restructuring of faulty interpretations, and empirical hypothesis-testing of dysfunctional obsession-related beliefs have all been borrowed from Beck's cognitive therapy. Thus, we see increasing similarities in the both the somatic and psychological treatment protocols for OCD and major depression. Having established that MDD and OCD are linked at the syndromal, symptom and treatment levels, it is reasonable to assume that the two disorders may have a number of common cognitive characteristics.

Cognitive Profile of Depression

According to Beck's cognitive model, depression is characterized by an information processing system that is biased for selecting, encoding, remembering and interpreting negative information about the self, personal world and future (Beck, 1967; Clark, Beck, & Alford, 1999). This pervasive bias for negative self-referent information is the result of negative mental representations or schemas about the self that are activated by external circumstances and, once activated, dominate the information-processing system during the depressed state. The stored contents of depression-relevant schemas consist of core beliefs about the self involving memories, interpretations and evaluations of loss, deprivation and failure. Beliefs about one's acceptance by or relationship with others, referred to as sociotropy, and beliefs about one's achievement, independence and mastery, labelled autonomy, are considered important areas of concern in depression (Beck, 1983; J. S. Beck, 1995). From a cognitive perspective, the various symptoms of depression are intricately linked to the activation of these latent negative self-referent schemas of social loss or goal-directed failure (for reviews see Clark *et al.*, 1999; Haaga, Dyck, & Ernst, 1991; Teasdale & Barnard, 1993).

Beck (1967) proposed that a distinct cognitive profile is associated with each psychopathological state including depression (see also Beck & Clark, 1988; Clark *et al.*, 1999). The *content-specificity hypothesis* states that depression is characterized by pervasive, absolutistic negative automatic thoughts involving themes of personal loss, failure and deprivation. Prepotent maladaptive self-referent schemas or beliefs involving interpersonal rejection, abandonment and criticism (i.e., sociotropic loss) or beliefs about one's failed achievements, loss of mastery or dependency on others (i.e., autonomous loss) are themes that characterize depression at the cognitive structural level. The activation of sociotropic and/or autonomous loss schemas will lead to certain cognitive processing errors (e.g., dichotomous thinking, personalization, overgeneralization, selective abstraction, etc.) whose end result is the selective processing of negative self-referent information. Experimental information processing studies over the last decade indicate that the biased information processing in depression may be most evident at the later conscious strategic, elaborative stage of information processing rather than at the earlier, preconscious attentional processing level (Williams, Watts, MacLeod, & Mathews, 1997).

Cognitive Profile of Obsessions and Compulsions

In recent years cognitive formulations have been advanced for obsessions and compulsions by Salkovskis (1985, 1989, 1998), Rachman (1997, 1998), Freeston *et al.* (1996), and Clark (2002). Although each of these formulations is different, they share basic underlying assumptions about the cognitive basis of OCD (Clark, 1999b). They begin with the assumption that obsessions have their origin in the unwanted, distressing, ego-dystonic intrusive thoughts, images and impulses that are a normal part everyone's stream of consciousness. These intrusive thoughts may be unwanted "noise", a by-product of an active, problem-solving, creative mind (Salkovskis, 1996).

Although the origin and function of unwanted intrusive thoughts are only speculative, the critical cognitive process in the pathogenesis of obsessions occurs at the automatic thought or appraisal level. Unwanted intrusive thoughts of unacceptable sex, aggression, dirt, contamination, errors, or asymmetry may be erroneously appraised or interpreted by obsession-prone individuals as: (a) having great *personal significance* that portends threat or danger (Rachman, 1997, 1998); (b) signifying a heightened sense of *responsibility* to prevent anticipated negative outcomes for one's self or others (Salkovskis, 1985, 1998); (c) equivalent to undesirable actions or beliefs about the self and therefore more likely to result in feared outcomes (*thought–action fusion*, Rachman, 1993); (d) highly important because the thoughts increase the probability of threat (i.e., overinterpretation of threat, Freeston *et al.*, 1996), (e) highly threatening because of the feared consequences of *failed thought control* (Clark, 2002); or (f) *violating* important personal values and features of the self (Purdon & Clark, 1999). At the present time it is not clear how distinctive these appraisal constructs are from each other. There is considerable overlap between them and they certainly are not mutually exclusive. The occurrence of these faulty appraisals will increase the frequency and salience of the unwanted, distressing intrusive thought. It may be that faulty appraisals heighten attentional focus on the intrusion, or attentional focus could be a consequence of faulty interpretations of the intrusion. Whatever the case, it is likely that faulty appraisals will lead to various control efforts to suppress the thought or to neutralize the anticipated harm or inflated responsibility associated with the thought.

Normal thought suppression strategies might be used along with covert and overt neutralization or compulsions, and/or avoidance. Although neutralization results in temporary relief of the anxiety associated with the obsessive intrusive thought because it reduces threat appraisals, in the longer term it acts to increase the salience of the intrusion and so is a self-defeating strategy for dealing with the obsession. The misinterpretation of unwanted intrusions and the futile attempts to control or neutralize these cognitive phenomena are due to the activation of certain underlying dysfunctional schemas or beliefs involving inflated responsibility, over importance of thoughts, control of thoughts, overestimation of threat, intolerance of uncertainty, and perfectionism (OCCWG, 1997). The presence of mood disturbance, such as dysphoria or depression, may be a by-product of the escalation of obsessions, but it also reduces even further the person's control over the obsession (see Beevers, Wenzlaff, Hayes, & Scott, 1999).

Contemporary cognitive models of OCD are still in the development stage and so very little has been written on how cognitive structures, processes and products of OCD differ from other psychopathological states. Salkovskis (1985) did provide an interesting contrast between negative automatic thoughts (NATs) or appraisals and obsessional intrusive thoughts. He noted that NATs tend to be less accessible, less intrusive, rational, ego-syntonic, and processed in parallel to the stream of consciousness. Obsessive intrusive thoughts, on the other hand, are highly accessible, intrusive, irrational, ego-dystonic, and intrude into the stream of consciousness. Although helpful in distinguishing unwanted intrusions from their associated appraisal processes, this comparison does not directly deal with the distinctive cognitive basis of OCD and depression because negative automatic thoughts (later called appraisals) are seen in both disorders.

A number of cognitive features of OCD distinguish it from other disorders. First content-specificity is evident in the source of threat in OCD. The obsession-prone individual appraises internal mental stimuli or products of the mind as threatening or dangerous, although the threat most often is also considered senseless and improbable. Moreover the intrusion has a distinct ego-dystonic nature in light of its inconsistency with important values and perceptions of the self (Purdon & Clark, 1999; Purdon, 2000). As noted above, depression is oriented toward loss of valued resources, which is considered entirely ego-syntonic or characteristic of the self. Thus specificity is evident in the content or theme of the threat, although the actual threatening content of the obsession can be highly idiosyncratic across obsessional patients.

Second, we would expect OCD to be distinguished by the presence of certain appraisal processes associated with unwanted intrusive thoughts, images or impulses. Salkovskis (1998), for example, argued that the appraisal of particular types of intrusive thoughts as indicating responsibility for the occurence or prevention of harm to self or others is what distinguishes obsessions from anxious and depressive cognitions. Thus the tendency to understand one's unwanted intrusions in terms of high or inflated personal responsibility is specific to OCD. Rachman (1993, 1997), on the other hand, proposed that the catastrophic misinterpretation of the significance of one's intrusive thoughts for causing negative, untoward consequences and the psychological fusion of thoughts and actions (i.e., thinking something is as bad as doing it) are unique appraisal processes in the pathogenesis of obsessions.

Clark (2002) proposed that the specific cognitive appraisal process in OCD is the misinterpretation of failed thought control. If an individual perceives that he or she cannot control an unwanted intrusion and then misinterprets the outcome of this failed thought control as signifying an increased possibility of dreaded consequences (e.g., rapid escalation in the obsession, intense anxiety, loss of complete control, etc.), then greater efforts, including neutralization and overt compulsions, will be used to deal with the obsessional intrusion. The end result will be increased salience, frequency and uncontrollability of the intrusive thought. Purdon (2000), on the other hand, noted that obsession-prone individuals might have a tendency to misinterpret unwanted intrusions as representing a threat or extreme inconsistency with one's self-view or normal patterns of behaviour (i.e., ego-dystonicity). In addition, certain maladaptive beliefs about one's cognitive capability (i.e., meta-cognitive beliefs) may be unique to OCD. As discussed in other chapters in this volume, beliefs such as responsibility, overimportance and control of thoughts may be specific to OCD.

Empirical Evidence for Cognitive Specificity in OCD and Depression

Throughout this chapter evidence has been presented of a strong link between depression and the presence of obsessions and compulsions. Moreover, cognitive models have proposed that specific cognitive content, appraisal processes and beliefs will distinguish depression and OCD. On the other hand, it is very likely that many cognitive variables will manifest themselves in both disorders. In this section I examine the scant empirical work that has compared the cognitive features evident in OCD and depression. However, before reviewing this literature, I consider evidence that depressed mood or dysphoria has a direct influence on the frequency, intensity and controllability of unwanted intrusive thoughts in clinical and non-clinical populations.

Correlational studies have examined the relationship between dysphoria and various parameters of obsessive, anxious and depressive cognitions. Presence of a dysphoric mood is associated with more frequent negative cognitions regardless of the actual thought content. That is, dysphoria is associated not only with an increase in negative self-referent thoughts of loss and failure, but also anxious, worrisome thoughts and obsessive-like unwanted intrusive thoughts (Clark, 1992; Freeston, Ladouceur, Thibodeau, & Gagnon, 1992; Niler & Beck, 1989; Rachman & De Silva, 1978; Reynolds & Salkovskis, 1991). Rachman (1981) concluded that presence of anxiety increases the frequency of intrusions whereas dysphoria tends to prolong the duration of unwanted intrusive thoughts.

Depressed mood may be associated with an increase in faulty appraisals of unwanted intrusions (Freeston et al., 1992; Freeston, Ladouceur, Provencher, & Blais, 1995), although the effect of mood on appraisal may be complex and too few studies have directly tested this effect to know whether dysphoria has a direct, unique influence on thought appraisal. Freeston et al. (1992, 1995) found that intensity of dysphoria was related to ratings of responsibility, disapproval, guilt, intensity of the intrusion and probability that the thought would come true in real life (thought–action fusion; TAF). In addition dysphoria but not anxiety was associated with ratings that one's thought control strategies were less efficient (Freeston et al., 1996). In fact, there is much stronger evidence from the thought suppression literature that individuals have less control over unwanted cognitions when in a general dysphoric mood state or when the intrusion causes an increased level of distress or dysphoria (Clark, 1986; Conway, Howell, & Giannopoulos, 1991; Howell & Conway, 1992; Reynolds & Salkovskis, 1991, 1992; Sutherland, Newman, & Rachman, 1982; Wenzlaff, Wegner, & Klein, 1991; Wenzlaff, Wegner, & Roper, 1988). However dysphoria appears unrelated to the type of thought control strategy that may be employed to suppress unwanted intrusions or obsessions (Amir, Cashman, & Foa, 1997; Freeston & Ladouceur, 1997). Of course we can expect that this relationship will be reciprocal with persistent, uncontrollable, distressing cognitions causing a decline in mood state. Also depressed mood will play a secondary role in the persistence of intrusions when anxious mood or distress are also assessed (Clark & de Silva, 1985).

A fairly coherent picture is beginning to emerge about the role of dysphoria in unwanted intrusive thoughts. Depressed mood does reduce one's ability to exercise some degree of control over intrusive thoughts. This reduced controllability may be due to an increased tendency to engage in faulty appraisals of the obsession during depression, particularly moral TAF (i.e., Shafran, Thordarson, & Rachman, 1996), although too few studies have examined the role of dysphoria on specific appraisal variables. The poorer control over intrusive thoughts during depressed mood is not due to the selection of particular thought control strategies. All strategies are utilized with less effectiveness during depressed mood. Rachman (1981) noted that dysphoria may primarily influence the duration of unwanted intrusions. Whatever the precise mechanisms, most cognitive theories of OCD recognize that depressed mood plays a crucial role in the pathogenesis of obsessions.

Given the findings from studies on dysphoria and intrusive thoughts, an important issue for cognitive theories of OCD is whether distinct cognitive processes can be identified for OCD that are independent of depression. Are there specific cognitive structures or schemas that are unique to OCD? In many ways, the integrity of the new cognitive models depends on achieving an adequate level of conceptual specificity. However, empirical research at this level is scarce because the cognitive determinants of OCD have only recently been precisely defined and elaborated. Nonetheless, some preliminary findings are beginning to emerge from various laboratories in North America and Europe.

Responsibility

Most of the studies to date have reported correlations between self-report measures of OCD-related beliefs and measures of depressive, obsessive, and compulsive symptoms. Probably the most extensively investigated of the newer cognitive constructs of OCD is inflated responsibility. In a clinical sample, Rachman, Thordarson, and Radomsky (1995) found that the Responsibility subscale of the Revised Maudsley Obsessive Compulsive Inventory (MOCI-R) correlated 0.42 with the BDI and 0.55 with the original MOCI Total Score. In a study that included OCD patients, non-OCD anxious and non-clinical controls, Steketee, Frost, and Cohen (1998) reported that the Responsibility subscale of the in 129-item Obsessive Compulsive Beliefs Questionnaire (OCBQ) correlated 0.39 with the BDI, and Salkovskis' Responsibility Scale, also a measure of beliefs, correlated 0.44 with the BDI. Correlations with the YBOCS and Padua Inventory were generally greater than with the BDI. In a student sample, Wilson and Chambless (1999) reported that various measures of responsibility appraisals and beliefs had higher correlations with self-reported obsessional symptoms than with negative affect in a sample of 167 undergraduates. However, Rachman, Thordarson, Shafran, and Woody (1995) found that their measure of inflated responsibility for physical or social harm coming to other people was unrelated to self-reported OCD or depressive symptoms in a student sample. Based on their semi-idiographic measure of inflated responsibility, Rhéaume, Ladouceur, Freeston, and Letarte (1994) found that responsibility appraisals correlated more highly with self-reported obsessional symptoms ($r = 0.56$) than with depression symptoms ($r = 0.33$). Finally, in an analysis of stage two OCCWG data (OCCWG, 2001), the responsibility subscales of the Obsessional Beliefs Questionnaire (OBQ) and the Interpretation of Intrusions Inventory (III) correlated 0.50 and 0.32, respectively, with the BDI. Partial correlations controlling for the BDI and Beck Anxiety Inventory revealed that OBQ and III Responsibility both continued to correlate with the Padua Inventory Total Score. In stage three analyses by the OCCWG (in preparation) comparable correlations of the OBQ and III responsibility subscale with the BDI were somewhat lower (0.3 range), and were similar to correlations with OCD symptom measures. Thus, responsibility was not more strongly associated with OCD than with depression. Together these findings suggest that inflated responsibility may be a specific cognitive feature of OCD. However, Rachman and Shafran (1998) noted in their review that exaggerated responsibility may be more characteristic of compulsive checkers than compulsive cleaners. Also it may be that certain aspects of responsibility, such as (TAF), are more characteristic of OCD than other aspects of the construct, such as concern over harm coming to others (see Chapter two in this volume).

In the study by Rachman, Thordarson, and Radomsky (1995), the TAF subscale of their responsibility measure emerged as the only significant cognitive dimension that had a strong relationship to OC symptoms (MOCI Total score 0.45 and BDI 0.38). In a further study of TAF based on an OCD sample, Shafran *et al.* (1996) found that the

TAF Moral, Likelihood-Others and Likelihood-Self subscales were as highly correlated with the BDI as with the MOCI Checking subscale. In fact after partialling out depression, the only TAF subscale to retain a significant correlation with obsessional checking was the Likelihood-for-others subscale. In our own research on appraisals associated with ego-dystonic intrusive thoughts in non-clinical samples, we found that ratings of the belief or worry that the intrusive thought could be acted upon or otherwise come true in real life was one of the primary significant predictors of the frequency and uncontrollability of intrusions (Clark & Claybourn, 1997; Purdon & Clark, 1994a, b). However we did not find that TAF beliefs, as assessed by Clark and Purdon's Meta-Cognitive Beliefs Questionnaire, a precursor to the OBQ, was uniquely associated with the Obsessional Thoughts Checklist (Clark, 1997). Together these results suggest that beliefs and appraisals of TAF may be a specific cognitive appraisal bias of OCD that increases the frequency and uncontrollability of the obsession. However it is not clear how level of mood disturbance in OC patients unduly influences TAF. For example, could depression cause an increase in the strength of belief in moral TAF (i.e., "thinking is as bad as doing")? It also may be that a specific aspect of TAF, in particular beliefs that harm-related thoughts about significant others may increase the likelihood of negative consequences happening to significant others, is more closely aligned to obsessionality than other facets of the construct.

Perfectionism

Perfectionistic beliefs have been implicated in both depression (e.g., Hewitt & Flett, 1991) and OCD (Frost, Marten, Lahart, & Rosenblate, 1990; Rhéaume, Freeston, Dugas, Letarte, & Ladouceur, 1995). However, Frost et al. (1990) found that certain features of perfectionism, in particular concern over mistakes and doubts about actions were significantly associated with self-reported obsessive–compulsive symptoms, whereas there was less evidence of a unique relationship between perfectionism and depressive symptoms. Hewitt and Flett (1993), on the other hand, found that high self-oriented perfectionism, an achievement-based need to attain high self-standards, interacted with negative achievement events to predict depressive symptoms. Rhéaume et al. (1995) found that perfectionism accounted for a small amount of additional variance in the Padua Inventory total score, even after controlling for inflated responsibility. They concluded that although inflated responsibility is a more important construct in OCD, perfectionism is a distinct concept that should be considered more carefully. They suggested redefining pathological perfectionism as "a belief that a perfect state exists" (Rhéaume et al., 1995, p. 792). However they also concluded that perfectionism is evident in many forms of psychopathology and may not be specific to OCD. The OCCWG (2001, in preparation) reported that the perfectionism subscale of the OBQ correlated moderately strongly with OCD symptoms and also correlated similarily with depression. The correlation with depression appeared to be moderated by OCD symptoms. In sum there is evidence that perfectionism is an important cognitive construct in OCD as well as depression. It may be that one aspect of perfectionism, high self-definitional standards of performance, is important in depression and other aspects of perfectionism, concern over mistakes or doubting one's actions, are critical for OCD (see Chapter six in this volume). Also the relationship between perfectionism and other key cognitive constructs of OCD, such as inflated responsibility or control of thoughts, is not well understood.

Other Types of Beliefs

The remaining cognitive constructs of OCD proposed by the OCCWG have received very little research attention to date. Subscales of the OBQ and III assess beliefs and appraisals that unwanted intrusive thoughts are important and should be controlled. Steketee *et al.* (1998) found that the Need to Control Thoughts subscale, a precursor to the OBQ Control of Thoughts subscale, correlated 0.63 with the Padua Inventory total score and 0.43 with the BDI. In the Stage two data analysis by the OCCWG (2001), OBQ Control of Thoughts, Importance of Thoughts, and Tolerance of Uncertainty subscales correlated almost as highly with the BDI total score as they did with the Padua total score. In the stage three analyses, (OCCWG, in preparation), again these subscales were as strongly associated with depressive symptoms as with OCD symptoms. Purdon and Clark (1999) found that the MCBQ Control of Thoughts was the only significant predictor associated with the Obsessional Thoughts Checklist. At this point, then, we do not know the level of specificity for many of the newer cognitive constructs of OCD.

Summary and Future Directions

Psychiatry has long recognized a close relationship between obsessions, compulsions and depression. In this chapter we have seen that OCD and depression are associated at a number of levels. Half to two-thirds of OCD patients present with a comorbid clinical depression that meets diagnostic criteria for major depression, dysthymia or depression NOS. The two disorders share a number of symptoms such as helplessness, excessive guilt, indecisiveness, perfectionism, doubt, and self-blame. Self-report measures of obsessions and compulsions have a moderate correlation with measures of depressive symptoms. Moreover the two disorders may share a common genetic diathesis and family background characteristics (Billett *et al.*, 1998; Coryell, 1981). Similarities can be seen in the medication regimens and, more recently, psychological treatments recommended for major depression and OCD. Hudson and Pope (1990) concluded that OCD is an affective spectrum disorder along with major depression, bulimia, panic disorder and a few other disorders. More recent psychological research has found that depressed mood increases the frequency, distress and uncontrollability of unwanted intrusive or obsessive thoughts, images or impulses.

Despite the close connection between depression and OCD, very little is known about the underlying psychological mechanisms that covary with these conditions or the treatment implications of a secondary depression in OCD. Tallis (1995) noted that no studies have been conducted on the phenomenological differences between non-OCD depression and depression secondary to OCD. It is evident that in most OCD cases depression develops as a result of persistent and severe obsessional problems that are associated with substantial distress, social isolation and functional impairment (Rachman

& Hodgson, 1980; Tallis, 1995). In return, the presence of major depression intensifies OC symptoms and complicates the treatment process. The treatment implications of a comorbid depression are still unclear. Steketee and Shapiro (1995) concluded from their review of the behavioral treatment outcome literature that presence of mild to moderate depressive mood did not interfere with successful treatment of OCD, although presence of symptoms severe enough to meet diagnostic criteria might interfere with treatment gains. Salkovskis (1985) recommended that cognitive therapy be implemented to address depressive symptoms.

It may be that the recent emphasis on the cognitive basis of OCD and depression will provide greater understanding of the psychological mechanisms behind these disorders and how they can be more effectively treated. Table 13.1 presents a summary of the common and distinct cognitive constructs that may be associated with OCD and clinical depression. Unfortunately the cognitive similarities and differences between depression

Table 13.1: Common and distinct cognitive constructs of OCD and Major Depression.

Obsessive Compulsive Disorder	Major Depression
Distinct Cognitive Features	
Cognitive content focuses on internal threatening thoughts, images or impulses (i.e., ego-dystonic material).	Cognitive content focuses on thoughts of past loss, failure or deprivation (i.e., ego-syntonic material).
Cognitive appraisals of responsibility, thought– action fusion, catastrophic misinterpretation of personal significance or failed thought control.	Negative cognitive appraisals of the self, personal world and future.
Maladaptive beliefs of inflated responsibility, thought–action fusion likelihood-others, concern about mistakes (perfectionism), importance of thought control and tolerance of uncertainty.	Maladaptive beliefs of interpersonal loss, rejection, isolation or non-acceptance (sociotropic loss); beliefs of failed mastery, achievement, or independence (autonomous loss).
Common Cognitive Features	
Heightened self-focused attention; increased frequency of negative self-referent cognitions; elevated frequency of unwanted intrusive thoughts and images	
Cognitive processing errors involving dichotomous thinking, overgeneralization, personalization, selective abstraction, arbitrary inference, and minimization/ maximization	
Maladaptive beliefs involving the personal significance of unwanted intrusive thoughts, overimportance of thoughts, self-blame, and need to meet high personal standards (conscientiousness).	

and OCD are largely speculative at this time because there is little empirical research that has directly compared cognitive functioning in depression and OCD. The moderate correlation between OCD cognition measures and depression measures indicates that there is some overlap. However, measures of inflated responsibility, TAF, perfectionism, and need for thought control tend to relate more closely to OCD symptoms than depression symptoms, thus supporting their convergent and discriminant validity.

There are a number of questions about the cognitive links between depression and OCD that require further investigation. Studies are needed that directly compare the cognitive functioning of individuals with a primary OCD and those with Major Depression without comorbid OCD to disentangle the distinct and common cognitive features of each disorder. A fine-grained analysis will be needed for many of the cognitive variables implicated in OCD. For example, certain aspects of perfectionism, such as concern about mistakes or beliefs that a perfect state exists, may be characteristic of OCD, whereas other aspects of the construct, such as striving to meet excessively high standards of personal performance, may be indicative of depression. Also, little is known about how depressed mood affects the appraisal of unwanted intrusive thoughts or obsessions. Are obsession-prone individuals more likely to engage in and believe faulty appraisals of unwanted intrusions when they are dysphoric? Does dysphoria result in the utilization of less effective thought control strategies, or in greater efforts to control unwanted intrusions? Do dysphoric individuals appraise their failed attempts to control unwanted cognitions in a more catastrophic fashion?

At the schema level, a number of dysfunctional beliefs in areas of responsibility, over-importance of thoughts, control of thoughts, perfectionism, tolerance of uncertainty, and threat estimation have been proposed as important belief systems in OCD. However it is not clear which of these beliefs is necessary or sufficient to promote faulty appraisals of intrusions or which are specific to OCD itself. Moreover, it may be that some of these constructs, such as perfectionism or responsibility, will require a more detailed analysis to discern which features of the construct are applicable to obsessions and compulsions, and which may be more relevant to mood disturbance. A good example of this was a recent study by Shafran, Watkins, and Charman (1996) in which they found that guilt correlated as highly with symptom measures of depression as it did with OC measures. They argued for a more elaborate definition of guilt, with OCD-related guilt characterized by specificity to particular intrusions, an association with responsibility and close ties to obsessional symptoms. Depressive guilt, on the other hand, is more pervasive, highly affective, rarely triggered by specific stimuli and accompanied by somatic complaints. Obviously more refined distinctions in our cognitive constructs will result in more precise assessment tools of cognitive functioning and better targeted cognitive interventions for obsessions and compulsions. Although many questions remain about the cognitive mechanisms involved in the link between depression and OCD, it is evident that mood state plays an important role in understanding and treating pathological obsessions and compulsions.

References

Alloy, L. B., Kelly, K. A., Mineka, S., & Clements, C. M. (1990). Comorbidity of anxiety and depressive disorders: A helplessness–hopelessness perspective. In J. Maser & R.C. Cloninger (eds), *Comorbidity of mood and anxiety disorders* (pp. 499–543). Washington, DC: American Psychiatric Press.

American Psychiatric Association (1952). *Diagnostic and statistical manual of mental disorders.* Washington, DC: Author.

American Psychiatric Association (1987). *Diagnostic and statistical manual of mental disorders, (3rd ed. rev).* Washington, DC: Author.

American Psychiatric Association (1993). American Psychiatric Association: Practice guidelines for major depressive disorder in adults. *American Journal of Psychiatry, 150 (suppl.),* 1–26.

American Psychiatric Association (1997). The expert consensus guideline series: Treatment of obsessive–compulsive disorder. *Journal of Clinical Psychiatry, 58 (suppl. 4),* 5–72.

Amir, N., Cashman, L., & Foa, E. B. (1997). Strategies of thought control in obsessive–compulsive disorder. *Behaviour Research and Therapy, 35,* 775–777.

Antony, M. M., Downie, F., & Swinson, R. P. (1998). Diagnostic issues and epidemiology in obsessive–compulsive disorder. In R. P. Swinson, M. M. Antony, S. Rachman, & M. A. Richter (eds), *Obsessive–compulsive disorder: Theory, research and treatment* (pp. 3–32). New York: Guilford.

Beck A. T. (1967). *Depression: Causes and treatment.* Pennsylvania Press: University of Pennsylvania Press

Beck, A. T. (1976). *Cognitive therapy of the emotional disorders.* New York: New American Library.

Beck, A. T. (1983). Cognitive therapy of depression: New perspectives. In P. J. Clayton & J. E. Barrett (eds), *Treatment of depression: Old controversies and new approaches* (pp. 265–290). New York: Raven Press.

Beck, A. T., & Clark, D. A. (1988). Anxiety and depression: An information processing perspective. *Anxiety Research, 1,* 23–36.

Beck, A. T., Rush, A. J., Shaw, B. F., & Emery, G. (1979). *Cognitive therapy of depression.* New York: Guilford.

Beck, J. S. (1995). *Cognitive therapy: Basics and beyond.* New York: Guilford.

Beevers, C. G., Wenzlaff, R. M., Hayes, A. M., & Scott, W. D. (1999). Depression and the ironic effects of thought suppression: Therapeutic strategies for improving mental control. *Clinical Psychology: Science and Practice, 6,* 133–148.

Billett, E. A., Richter, M. A., & Kennedy, J. L. (1998). Genetics of obsessive–compulsive disorder. In R. P. Swinson, M. M. Antony, S. Rachman, & M. A. Richter (eds), *Obsessive–compulsive disorder: Theory, research and treatment* (pp. 181–206). New York: Guilford.

Brown, T. A., & Barlow, D. H. (1992). Comorbidity among anxiety disorders: Implications for treatment and DSM-IV. *Journal of Consulting and Clinical Psychology, 60,* 835–844.

Brown, T. A., Moras, K., Zinbarg, R. E., & Barlow, D. H. (1993). Diagnostic and symptom distinguishability of generalized anxiety disorder and obsessive–compulsive disorder. *Behavior Therapy, 24,* 227–240.

Calamari, J. E., Wiegartz, P. S., & Janeck, A. S. (1999). Obsessive–compulsive disorder subgroups: A symptom-based clustering approach. *Behaviour Research and Therapy, 37,* 113–125.

Clark, D. A. (1986). Factors influencing the retrieval and control of negative cognitions. *Behaviour Research and Therapy, 24,* 151–159.

Clark, D. A. (1992). Depressive, anxious and intrusive thoughts in psychiatric inpatients and outpatients. *Behaviour Research and Therapy, 30,* 93–102.

Clark, D. A. (1997). *Hypervalent cognitions and beliefs in OCD: A case of forgotten identity?* Paper presented at the Anxiety Disorders of America Conference, New Orleans.

Clark, D. A. (1999a). *Preliminary study of a self-report screening instrument for OCD*. Department of Psychology, University of New Brunswick.

Clark, D. A. (1999b). Cognitive–behavioral treatment of obsessive–compulsive disorder: A commentary. *Cognitive and Behavioral Practice,* vol. 6, pp. 408–415.

Clark, D. A. (2002). Controlling obsessions and compulsions: New approaches from a cognitive perspective.

Clark, D. A., & Claybourn, M. (1997). Process characteristics of worry and obsessive intrusive thoughts. *Behaviour Research and Therapy, 12,* 1139–1141.

Clark, D. A., & de Silva, P. (1985). The nature of depressive and anxious thoughts: Distinct or uniform phenomena? *Behaviour Research and Therapy, 23,* 383–393.

Clark, D. A., Beck, A. T. (with Alford, B.) (1999). *Scientific foundations of cognitive theory and therapy of depression*. New York: Wiley.

Conway, M., Howell, A., & Giannopoulos, C. (1991). Dysphoria and thought suppression. *Cognitive Therapy & Research, 15,* 153–166.

Coryell, W. (1981). Obsessive–compulsive disorder and primary unipolar depression: Comparisons of background, family history, course, and mortality. *Journal of Nervous and Mental Disease, 169,* 220–224.

Crino, R. D., & Andrews, G. (1996). Obsessive–compulsive disorder and Axis I comorbidity. *Journal of Anxiety Disorders, 10,* 37–46.

Di Nardo, P. A., & Barlow, D. H. (1990). Syndrome and symptom co-occurrence in the anxiety disorders. In J. Maser & R.C. Cloninger (eds), *Comorbidity of mood and anxiety disorders* (pp. 205–230). Washington, DC: American Psychiatric Press.

Foa, E. B., Kozak, M. J., Salkovskis, P. M., Coles, M. E., & Amir, N. (1998). The validation of a new obsessive–compulsive disorder scale: The Obsessive–Compulsive Inventory. *Psychological Assessment, 10,* 206–214.

Freeston, M. H., & Ladouceur, R. (1997). What do patients do with their obsessive thoughts? *Behaviour Research and Therapy, 35,* 335–348.

Freeston, M. H., Ladouceur, R., Provencher, M., & Blais, F. (1995). Strategies used with intrusive thoughts: Context, appraisal, mood, and efficacy. *Journal of Anxiety Disorders, 9,* 201–215.

Freeston, M. H., Ladouceur, R., Thibodeau, N., & Gagnon, F. (1992). Cognitive intrusions in a non-clinical population. II. Associations with depressive, anxious, and compulsive symptoms. *Behaviour Research and Therapy, 30,* 263–271.

Freeston, M. H., Rhéaume, J., & Ladouceur, R. (1996). Correcting faulty appraisals of obsessional thoughts. *Behaviour Research and Therapy, 34,* 433–446.

Frost, R. O., Marten, P., Lahart, C., & Rosenblate, R. (1990). The dimensions of perfectionism. *Cognitive Therapy and Research, 14,* 449–468.

Gibbs, N. A. (1996). Nonclinical populations in research on obsessive–compulsive disorder: A critical review. *Clinical Psychology Review, 16,* 729–773.

Gittleson, N. L. (1966). The fate of obsessions in depressive psychosis. *British Journal of Psychiatry, 112,* 705–708.

Haaga, D. A. F., Dyck, M. J., & Ernst, D. (1991). Empirical status of cognitive theory of depression. *Psychological Bulletin, 110,* 215–236.

Hewitt, P. L., & Flett, G. L. (1991). Dimensions of perfectionism in unipolar depression. *Journal of Abnormal Psychology, 100,* 98–101.

Hewitt, P. L., & Flett, G. L. (1993). Dimensions of perfectionism, daily stress, and depression: A test of the specific vulnerability hypothesis. *Journal of Abnormal Psychology, 102,* 58–65.

Hollon, S. D., & Beck, A. T. (1986). Cognitive and cognitive–behavioral therapies. In

S. L. Garfield & A.E. Bergin (eds), *Handbook of psychotherapy and behavior change*, 3rd ed. (pp. 443–482). New York: Wiley.

Howell, A., & Conway, M. (1992). Mood and the suppression of positive and negative self-referent thoughts. *Cognitive Therapy and Research, 16*, 535–555.

Hudson, J. I., & Pope, H. G. (1990). Affective spectrum disorder: Does antidepressant response identify a family of disorders with a common pathophysiology? *American Journal of Psychiatry, 147*, 552–564.

Jennings, K. D., Ross, S., Popper, S., & Elmore, M. (1999). Thoughts of harming infants in depressed and nondepressed mothers. *Journal of Affective Disorders, 54*, 21–28.

Karno, M., & Golding, J. M. (1991). Obsessive–compulsive disorder. In L. N. Robins & D. A. Regier (eds), *Psychiatric disorders in America: The Epidemiologic Catchment Area Study* (pp. 204–219). New York: Free Press.

Kendell, R. E., & Discipio, W. J. (1970). Obsessional symptoms and obsessional personality traits in patients with depressive illness. *Psychological Medicine, 1*, 65–72.

Kozak, M. J., & Foa, E. B. (1997). *Mastery of obsessive–compulsive disorder: A cognitive–behavioral approach. Therapist guide*. San Antonio, TX: Graywind Publications.

Lensi, P., Cassano, G. B., Correddu, G., Ravagli, S., Kunovac, J. L., & Akiskal, H. S. (1996). Obsessive–compulsive disorder: Familial–developmental history, symptomatology, comorbidity and course with special reference to gender-related differences. *British Journal of Psychiatry, 169*, 101–107.

MacDonald, P. A., Antony, M. M., MacLoed, C. M., & Richter, M. A. (1997). Memory and confidence in memory judgements among individuals with obsessive–compulsive disorder and non-clinical controls. *Behaviour Research and Therapy, 35*, 497–505.

March, J. S., Frances, A., Carpenter, D., & Kahn, D. A. (1997). Expert Consensus Guideline for Treatment of Obsessive–Compulsive Disorder. *The Journal of Clinical Psychiatry, suppl(4)*, 5–72.

McKay, D., Danyko, S., Neziroglu, F., & Yaryura-Tobias, J. A. (1995). Factor structure of the Yale–Brown Obsessive–Compulsive Scale: A two dimensional measure. *Behaviour Research and Therapy, 33*, 865–869.

Niler, E. R., & Beck, S. J. (1989). The relationship among guilt, anxiety and obsessions in a normal population. *Behaviour Research and Therapy, 27*, 213–220.

Obsessive–Compulsive Cognitions Working Group (1997). Cognitive assessment of obsessive–compulsive disorder. *Behaviour Research and Therapy, 35*, 667–681.

Obsessive–Compulsive Cognitions Working Group (2001). Development and initial validation of the Obsessive–Beliefs Questionnaire and the Interpretation of Intrusions Inventory. *Behaviour Research and Therapy, 39*, 987–1006.

Obsessive–Compulsive Cognitions Working Group (in preparation). Psychometric validation of the Obsessive Beliefs Questionnaire and the Interpretation of Intrusions Inventory : Part I. Manuscript submitted for publication.

Purdon, C. (2000). Cognitive–behavioral models of obsessive–compulsive disorder. In M. H. Freeston & S. Taylor (eds), *Cognitive approaches to treating obsessions and compulsions: A clinical casebook*. New York: Erlbaum.

Purdon, C., & Clark, D. A. (1994a). Obsessive intrusive thoughts in nonclinical subjects. Part II. Cognitive appraisal, emotional response and thought control strategies. *Behaviour Research and Therapy, 32*, 403–410.

Purdon, C., & Clark, D. A. (1994b). Perceived control and appraisal of obsessional intrusive thoughts: A replication and extension. *Behavioural and Cognitive Psychotherapy, 22*, 269–285.

Purdon, C., & Clark, D. A. (1999). Metacognition and obsessions. *Clinical Psychology and Psychotherapy, 6*, 102–110.

Rachman, S. J. (1981). Part I. Unwanted intrusive cognitions. *Advances in Behaviour Research and Therapy, 3*, 89–99.

Rachman, S. J. (1993). Obsessions, responsibility and guilt. *Behaviour Research and Therapy, 31*, 149–154.

Rachman, S. J. (1997). A cognitive theory of obsessions. *Behaviour Research and Therapy, 35*, 793–802.

Rachman, S. J. (1998). A cognitive theory of obsessions: Elaborations. *Behaviour Research and Therapy, 36*, 385–401.

Rachman, S. J., & de Silva, P. (1978). Abnormal and normal obsessions. *Behaviour Research and Therapy, 16*, 233–248.

Rachman, S. J., & Hodgson, R. J. (1980). *Obsessions and compulsions*. Englewood Cliffs, NJ: Prentice-Hall.

Rachman, S. J., & Shafran, R. (1998). Cognitive and behavioural features of obsessive–compulsive disorder. In R. P. Swinson, M. M. Antony, S. Rachman, & M. A. Richter (eds), *Obsessive–compulsive disorder: Theory, research and treatment* (pp. 51–78). New York: Guilford.

Rachman, S. J., Thordarson, D. S., & Radomsky, A. S. (1995, July). *A revision of the Maudsley Obsessional–Compulsive Inventory (MOCI-R)*. Paper presented at the World Congress of Behavioural and Cognitive Therapies, Copenhagen, Denmark.

Rachman, S. J., Thordarson, D. S., Shafran, R., & Woody, S. R. (1995). Perceived responsibility: Structure and significance. *Behaviour Research and Therapy, 33*, 779–784.

Reynolds, M., & Salkovskis, P. M. (1991). The relationship among guilt, dysphoria, anxiety and obsessions in a normal population — An attempted replication. *Behaviour Research and Therapy, 29*, 259–265.

Reynolds, M., & Salkovskis, P. M. (1992). Comparison of positive and negative intrusive thoughts and experimental investigation of the differential effects on mood. *Behaviour Research and Therapy, 30*, 273–281.

Rhéaume, J., Freeston, M. H., Dugas, M., Letarte, H., & Ladouceur, R. (1995). Perfectionism, responsibility and obsessive–compulsive symptoms. *Behaviour Research and Therapy, 33*, 785–794.

Rhéaume, J., Ladouceur, R., Freeston, M. H., & Letarte, H. (1994). Inflated responsibility in obsessive–compulsive disorder: Psychometric studies of a semi-idiographic measure. *Journal of Psychopathology and Behavioral Assessment, 16*, 265–276.

Ricciardi, J. N., & McNally, R. J. (1995). Depressed mood is related to obsessions, but not to compulsions, in obsessive–compulsive disorder. *Journal of Anxiety Disorders, 9*, 249–256.

Salkovskis, P. M. (1985). Obsessional–compulsive problems: A cognitive–behavioral analysis. *Behaviour Research and Therapy, 23*, 571–583.

Salkovskis, P. M. (1989). Cognitive–behavioral factors and the persistence of intrusive thoughts in obsessional problems. *Behaviour Research and Therapy, 27*, 677–682.

Salkovskis, P. M. (1996). Cognitive–behavioral approaches to the understanding of obsessional problems. In R.M. Rapee (ed.), *Current controversies in the anxiety disorders* (pp. 103–133). New York: Guilford.

Salkovskis, P. M. (1998). Psychological approaches to the understanding of obsessional problems. In R. P. Swinson, M. M. Antony, S. Rachman, & M. A. Richter (eds), *Obsessive–compulsive disorder: Theory, research and treatment* (pp. 33–50). New York: Guilford.

Sanderson, W. C., & Beck, A. T. (1990, November). *Comorbidity in patients with major depression and dysthymia*. Paper presented at the annual meeting of the Association for the Advancement of Behavior Therapy, San Francisco.

Sanderson, W. C., Di Nardo, P. A., Rapee, R. M., & Barlow, D. H. (1990). Syndrome comorbidity in patients diagnosed with a DSM-III-R anxiety disorder. *Journal of Abnormal Psychology, 99*, 308–312.

Shafran, R., Thordarson, D. S., & Rachman, S. J. (1996). Thought–action fusion in obsessive–compulsive disorder. *Journal of Anxiety Disorders, 10*, 379–391.

Shafran, R., Watkins, E., & Charman, T. (1996). Guilt in obsessive–compulsive disorder. *Journal of Anxiety Disorders, 10*, 509–516.

Steketee, G., Frost, R. O., & Cohen, I. (1998). Beliefs in obsessive–compulsive disorder. *Journal of Anxiety Disorders, 12*, 525–537.

Steketee, G., & Shapiro, L. J. (1995). Predicting behavioral treatment outcome for agoraphobia and obsessive–compulsive disorder. *Clinical Psychology, 15*, 317–346.

Sternberger, L. G., & Burns, G. L. (1990). Obsessions and compulsions: Psychometric properties of the Padua Inventory with an American college population. *Behaviour Research and Therapy, 28*, 341–345.

Sutherland, G., Newman, B., & Rachman, S. J. (1982). Experimental investigations of the relations between mood and intrusive unwanted cognitions. *British Journal of Medical Psychology, 55*, 127–138.

Tallis, F. (1995). *Obsessive–compulsive disorder: A cognitive and neuropsychological perspective*. Chichester: Wiley.

Taylor, S. (1995). Assessment of obsessions and compulsions: Reliability, validity, and sensitivity to treatment effects. *Clinical Psychology Review, 15*, 261–296.

Taylor, S. (1998). Assessment of obsessive–compulsive disorder. In: R. P. Swinson, M. M. Antony, S. Rachman & M. A. Richter (eds), *Obsessive–compulsive disorder: Theory, research and treatment* (pp. 229–257). New York: Guilford.

Teasdale, J. D., & Barnard, P. J. (1993). *Affect, cognition and change: Remodelling depressive thought*. Hove, UK: Erlbaum.

van Oppen, P., & Arntz, A. (1994). Cognitive therapy for obsessive–compulsive disorder. *Behaviour Research and Therapy, 32*, 79–87.

van Oppen, P., Hoekstra, R. J., & Emmelkamp, P. M. G. (1995). The structure of obsessive–compulsive symptoms. *Behaviour Research and Therapy, 33*, 15–23.

Vaughan, M. (1976). The relationships between obsessional personality, obsessions in depression, and symptoms of depression. *British Journal of Psychiatry, 129*, 36–39.

Wenzlaff, R. M., Wegner, D. M., & Klein, S. B. (1991). The role of thought suppression in the bonding of thought and mood. *Journal of Personality and Social Psychology, 60*, 500–508.

Wenzlaff, R. M., Wegner, D. M., & Roper, D. W. (1988). Depression and mental control: The resurgence of unwanted negative thoughts. *Journal of Personality and Social Psychology, 55*, 882–892.

Whittal, M. L., & Mclean, P. D. (1999). CBT for OCD: The rationale, protocol, and challenges. *Cognitive and Behavioral Practice, 6*, 383–396.

Williams, J. M. G., Watts, F. N., MacLeod, C., & Mathews, A. (1997). *Cognitive psychology and emotional disorders*, 2nd ed. Chichester, England: Wiley.

Wilson, K. A., & Chambless, D. L. (1999). Inflated responsibility and obsessive–compulsive symptoms. *Behaviour Research and Therapy, 37*, 325–335.

Woody, S. R., Steketee, G., & Chambless, D. L. (1995). Reliability and validity of the Yale–Brown Obsessive–Compulsive Scale. *Behaviour Research and Therapy, 33*, 597–605.

Woody, S. R., Taylor, S., McLean, P. D., & Koch, W. J. (1998). Cognitive specificity in panic and depression: Implications for comorbidity. *Cognitive Therapy and Research, 22*, 427–443.

Chapter 14

Obsessive Compulsive Disorder and Schizophrenia: A Cognitive Perspective of Shared Pathology

Jose A. Yaryura-Tobias and Dean McKay

Introduction

We begin with the assumption that cognition is a neuropsychological faculty altered by the presence of obsessive compulsive disorder (OCD) and schizophrenia (SCZ). The site of this faculty is the brain, an organ that is the sum of several subsystems constituting a complex construct. The brain operates by evaluating external and internal sensory information and by executing actions based on this input. This informative language may not always be translated if an operational deficit caused by a mental disorder is present, creating a cognitive crisis manifested when cerebral evaluation and execution begin to fail.

Accepting the brain as an indivisible organ represented by a neural grid allows the assumption that many different functions involved in psychopathology have a common root. Consequently, it is possible to speculate on the presence of a unified mental disease (Griesinger, 1867) encompassing the entire mental pathology. The concept of disease progression in time and space is considered not only within a distinct condition but also across different disorders (e.g., OCD and SCZ). If various functions are involved in pathological conditions, then disease progression evolves not only temporally, with certain modifications in learning, brain structure and functioning, but also spatially across different but interrelated and affected systems. The net result of such temporal and spatial disease progression may manifest itself as an apparent continuity in psychopathology. This might be exemplified by OCD and its associated disorders (Yaryura-Tobias & Neziroglu, 1983).

Clinical observations point to disease progression or coexistence from SCZ into OCD and vice versa (e.g., Hwang & Hollander, 1993; Insel & Akiskal, 1986; Jenike, Baer, & Carey, 1986; Stengel, 1931; Bermanzhon et al., 1997; Yaryura-Tobias, Stevens, Neziroglu, & Grunes, 1997). These studies are based on the general nosological concept of OCD and SZC without attention to possible subcategories. Other studies indicate pathology in thought and perceptual processes in primary OCD and primary SCZ without comorbidity (Yaryura-Tobias, Campisi, McKay, & Neziroglu, 1995), and in some similarities in

Cognitive Approaches to Obsessions and Compulsions – Theory, Assessment, and Treatment
Copyright © 2002 by Elsevier Science Ltd.
All rights of reproduction in any form reserved.
ISBN: 0-08-043410-X

cognitive and behavioral symptoms for both conditions (Yaryura-Tobias, Stevens, & Neziroglu, 1998).

With regard to personality pathology, some writers have suggested that obsessive compulsive characters may evolve into paranoid ones and vice versa (e.g., Shapiro, 1965) and that avoidant personality may decompensate into schizotypal personality disorder (Sperry, 1995; Reid, 1989). The purpose of this chapter is to examine the overlapping features of OCD and schizophrenia, with particular attention to beliefs and interpretations of external and internal events, and to compare the cognitive functioning of these two groups.

Definitions and Pathology of OCD

OCD may be defined as a heterogeneous neuropsychiatric syndrome with a large mosaic of symptoms of which five stand out. These are obsessions, compulsions, doubting, perceptual changes, and motor impairment. In addition, restricted affective experience and social isolation are commonly experienced. An early description by Westphal (1872) indicated that obsessions are intrusive, forceful, parasitic and repetitive thoughts that dwell in the mind and cannot be rejected. Compulsions are mental or motor urges that cannot be postponed and require immediate action. Any attempt to block the urge causes severe anxiety. Doubting is a state of mind that deprives the individual of making decisions and is a reflection of the loss of free will. Chronic doubting in OCD may be masked by the presence of iterative questioning or double-checking. Perception is the awareness of endogenous or exogenous physical sensations. This function may be altered in OCD and may affect any of the five senses (Yaryura-Tobias *et al.*, 1995). Perceptual changes are manifested by the presence of sounds, melodies, taste modifications, or touch pathology that appear as part of the cohort of OCD psychopathology. These perceptual symptoms may be known as "reasoning hallucinations" or eidolic hallucinations (Ey & Brisset, 1978; Yaryura-Tobias *et al.*, 1995).

In this vein, magical thinking, a thought process in which thought becomes action without any personal intervention, is common to both OCD and SCZ. Contemporary theorists have revisited this concept and applied it specifically to OCD under the rubric of "thought–action fusion" (Shafran, Thordarson, & Rachman, 1996). Recent research supports a role for thought–action fusion in the maintenance of OCD. Specifically, as thought–action fusion increases, individuals are at increased risk for experiencing difficulties in eliminating unwanted intrusive thoughts. This has been recently examined in a series of experiments where thought–action fusion predicted the ability to suppress thoughts (Greisberg & McKay, 2000; see also Chapter two in this volume). This concept is discussed further below in comparing OCD and SCZ on cognitive functioning.

The most recent version of the Diagnostic and Statistical Manual (DSM-IV; American Psychiatric Association, 1994) has expanded the taxonomy of OCD to indicate the extent of insight that the patient possesses at the time of evaluation. This is denoted by the specifier "with poor insight" and is similar in function to describing the patient as having overvalued ideas (for review, see Kozak & Foa, 1994). Insight is a central aspect of the overlap of OCD and SCZ and is detailed in the next section.

Definition and Pathology of Schizophrenia

Schizophrenia is currently defined as a heterogenous syndrome typically involving delusions, hallucinations, and disorganized verbal and motor behavior, as well as restricted affect and social isolation (Bentall, 1990; Torrey, 1988; Wong *et al.*, 1993). Schizophrenic phenomenology manifests itself in different characteristic symptoms, identified as paranoid, delusional, schizoaffective, or brief psychotic symptom clusters manifested as a loss of control, choice and will (Torrey, 1988). Leonard (1979) extensively classified this heterogeneous syndrome in his study of endogenous psychoses. Various subtypes have been isolated, including paranoid, catatonic, and hebephrenic types, which are distinguished primarily on the predominance of certain symptom clusters to the relative exclusion of others, following the classic works of Kraepelin (1889) and Kleist and Driest (1937). In his studies, Leonard (1979) seemed to imbricate syndromes that nowadays could be considered comorbid or associated conditions. A similar conceptual framework of SCZ psychopathology, emphasizing the variability of schizophrenic manifestations (Huber & Gross, 1989; Strauss, Carpenter, & Bartko, 1974), Type II SCZ (Crow, 1980), and negative SCZ (Andreasen & Olsen, 1982) has been posited ever since.

While these subtypes have distinct features, obsessive-compulsive and schizophrenic symptomatology can overlap when they are temporally contiguous. In addition, the central phenomenology of OCD and SCZ also suggests spatial continuity between related areas and systems of the brain involved in producing the symptomatology (Yaryura-Tobias & Neziroglu, 1997a). This spatial continuity suggests the presence of a unified psychopathology that eventually may represent a single condition (Yaryura-Tobias & Neziroglu 1997a; Yaryura-Tobias *et al.*, 2000). Cognitive processing impairments associated with OCD and SCZ that bear on brain morphology are discussed later in this chapter.

Co-occurrence of OCD and SCZ

Several studies have documented the frequency with which clinically significant OCD symptoms appear in schizophrenic patients. Estimates in recent studies ranged from 13 percent (Fenton & McGlashan, 1986) to 30 percent (Berman, Kalinowski, Berman, Lengua, & Green, 1995) and to 46 percent based on a more thorough assessment during a diagnostic interview (Porto, Bermanzohn, Pollack, Morrissey, & Siris, 1997). The rate of a full OCD diagnosis among schizophrenic and schizoaffective patients was, of course, somewhat lower, ranging from eight percent (Eisen, Beer, Pato, Venditto, & Rasmussen, 1997) to 24 percent (Porto *et al.*, 1997). Patients whose SCZ was associated with OC symptoms were less functional (more socially isolated, worse employment histories) and required longer hospitalizations. They had a worse prognosis overall.

Researchers agree that an important problem in studying the overlap of OCD and SCZ is deciding whether to classify certain mental features as obsessions or delusions. The distinction between an obsession, especially one with loss of insight, and a delusion is not always clear. Porto *et al.*'s (1997) study of 50 long-term patients with chronic schizophrenia or schizoaffective illustrates the complexity in making these distinctions. They administered the Yale–Brown Obsessive Compulsive checklist to identify obsessions, asking participants to differentiate between their psychotic and OC symptoms and to comment on the interconnection, if any, of these symptoms, as well as their level of insight. The most frequent symptom themes for obsessions were aggressive (34 percent), miscellaneous (32 percent), and religious (20 percent).

Of Porto *et al.*'s 13 schizophrenic patients who also met criteria for OCD, four described their obsessional symptoms as quite unrelated to psychotic symptoms. Five considered their OC symptoms related but not restricted to their psychotic symptoms, as in the case of a man whose obsession about blurting out obscenities was linked to ideas that others could read his mind, but cleaning and arranging compulsions were independent. For the remaining four patients, obsessions lay on a continuum with psychotic symptoms; they were incorporated into delusions in an actively psychotic state, but persisted in a non-delusional form when psychotic symptoms abated. Thus, in these patients the degree of insight waxed and waned. Illustrative is Porto and colleagues' example of a man with multiple obsessions and compulsions whose fears that he was not a good person and might have AIDS became, in their psychotic form, a conviction that he was possessed by the devil and heard voices telling him he was HIV positive.

In some contrast to the findings of studies of SCZ, reports suggest that OCD is less frequently associated with psychosis. Eisen and Rasmussen (1993) found hallucinations, delusions and thought disorder, but not necessarily a diagnosis of schizophrenia or another psychotic disorder, in 14 percent of a large sample of OCD patients. This reduced frequency is likely due to greater attention to psychotic symptoms that overshadow the presence of OCD. Further, OCD has been defined as a condition in which the individual recognizes the senselessness of the symptoms (is aware of reality and not delusional), yet feels compelled to engage in rituals or avoidance as a means of coping with anxiety. Thus, patients with both complaints are more likely to receive a diagnosis of psychosis with OC symptoms than the reverse.

This discussion begs the question of how psychotic forms of OCD appear, and what constitutes a difference between this presentation and the more traditional non-psychotic type. The primary distinction lies in the descriptions of symptoms offered by sufferers and the intact nature of ideas surrounding their condition. As in other psychotic conditions, there is considerable cognitive decline in patients suffering from psychotic forms of OCD. This may be manifest in inability to describe symptoms, loss of rational understanding of the relation between obsessions and associated avoidance or rituals, as well as the extent to which the patient feels that the symptoms are necessary or reasonable (insight).

Likewise, distinguishing OCD and SCZ manifestations may prove difficult, given certain similarities in cognitive manifestations. Anyone who has spent time with individuals diagnosed with schizophrenia presumably would know the difference from OCD. Yet we have heard of many OCD clients being misdiagnosed with schizophrenia, so perhaps this is not as clear as we would like to believe. Table 14.1 lists impairment in various areas of cognitive functioning in OCD and SCZ. Differences are particularly evident in attention, memory, and reasoning and less so in categories of perception, judgement, intellect and mood. Table 14.2 provides an additional view of overlapping and distinctive features of OCD and SCZ in the areas of thought, perception and motor behavior. The similarities and differences in manifestation and cognitive function are detailed further below.

Table 14.1: Typical cognitive functioning in OCD and SCZ.

Cognitive Function	Obsessive Compulsive Disorder	Schizophrenia
Attention	Emotionally biased	General Disturbance
Memory	Emotionally biased	General Disturbance
Reasoning	Intact	Impaired
Perceptual Functioning	Impaired: Hearing, visual, tactile	Impaired: All five senses
Judgment	Minor impairment	Major impairment
Intelligence	Intact	Intact during residual phases, impaired during acute phases
Mood	Impaired	Impaired
Meta-cognition	Intact	Variable

Table 14.2: Overlapping and distinctive features of OCD and SCZ.

OCD	Schizophrenia
Thought	
Obsessions	Delusions
Magical Ideation/Thought–Action Fusion	Magical Ideation/Thought Disorder
Perception	
Images	Hallucination
Melodies	Sensations of anatomical position
Sounds	
Tactile	
Olfaction	
Motion	
Tics	Grimacing
Twitches	Catatonia
Slowness	Parakinesis

Cognitive Features of OCD and SCZ

Thought Pathology

Certain elaborated mental observations or perceptions that are accepted in exaggerated and bizarre ways to the exclusion of other observations (Wernicke, 1900) may be applicable to both OCD and SCZ thought pathology. Thought pathology in OCD entails a process that may shade the rationality of the obsessional thought which then becomes an overvalued idea or a rudimentary delusion, thus starting the direction to a delusional mechanism. Historically, an overvalued idea is a strong irrational belief with an underlying affective component (Wernicke, 1900; Jaspers, 1913). A rudimentary delusion, on the other hand, is a weak delusion much like the concept of "rudimentary psychosis" as it was used to describe the pathogenesis of dysmorphophobia (Morselli, 1891).

Thought pathology in SCZ includes delusions, deliroid ideas, and fixed ideas. Delusions are thoughts that cannot be readily modified by using logic or judgment. Deliroid ideation involves a transient belief including misinterpretations, melancholic and manic beliefs (e.g., delusions of sinful nihilism and impoverishment), as well as overvalued ideas (Jaspers, 1913). Fixed ideas are immalleable and encapsulated thoughts that do not tend to affect one's everyday life, whereas delusions are the result of a primary pathological experience or drastic personality change that challenges the individual's capacity to reason. The transition from normal thought to various gradients of thought pathology in OCD and SCZ seems compatible with the various nosologies that have a point of confluence with both OCD and SCZ. Perhaps overvalued ideas or lack of insight provide the pars intermedia between the two disorders and their spectra (Neziroglu, Yaryura-Tobias, McKay, Stevens, & Todaro, 1999).

Insight.   An important way in which OCD and SCZ may be distinguished is the degree of conviction in the need to complete various tasks that are compulsive, or the degree of belief in the accuracy of the obsessions. Discussed earlier as insight and also known as "overvalued ideas" (Kozak & Foa, 1994), this feature has been identified as a poor prognostic sign in OCD (Kozak & Foa, 1994; Neziroglu, Stevens, Yaryura-Tobias, & McKay, 2001). However, overvalued ideas have been considered part of a continuum from rational ideas that are obsessive on the one side, to delusions on the other. Therefore, when the symptoms of OCD are experienced in a delusional manner, they more closely approximate schizophrenia proper. In SCZ, insight has been more broadly defined as awareness of illness (Amador, Strauss, Yale, & Gorman, 1991), suggesting that insight refers to rational evaluation of a broad range of schizophrenic symptoms, not merely the content of particular thoughts, beliefs or images, as for OCD.

We conceptualize overvalued ideas as linked not only to fixity of thought but to a strong affective experience that contributes to the stability of this belief or conviction. Therefore, it is not sufficient for a person to have a strong belief in an idea or need to complete a behavior, but it must be accompanied by an emotional load. This would then create greater difficulty in challenging primary beliefs associated with obsessive compulsive behavior, such as magical ideas or excessive responsibility. Figure 14.1 depicts emotional state and fixity of ideation with regard to various subtypes of OCD, OCPD, and SCZ.

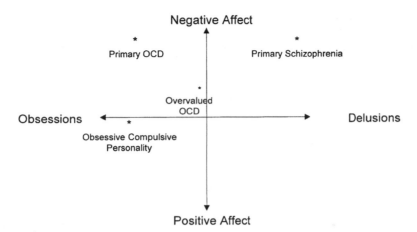

Figure 14.1: Affect and Overvalued Ideas.

Confusing Thought with Action

Thoughts generally, and thought–action fusion specifically, have been considered highly important in understanding the nature of OCD (Obsessive Compulsive Cognitions Working Group, 1997). Although thought–action fusion has been examined in OCD (Rachman & Shafran, 1998), it has not been explicitly studied in schizophrenia. However, there are several points of overlap. First, individuals with SCZ likely also experience a fusion of thinking with actions. This is evidenced by their trouble distinguishing rational from delusional thinking and fear of images that may occur to them (as in the case of paranoid schizophrenia). Second, the link between thoughts and external events is likely elevated in SCZ, based upon direct observations. For example, it would not be unusual for an individual with SCZ to report concerns that other individuals could hear their thoughts, and that this would result in certain feared outcomes. Third, in both groups magical thinking is frequently tied to fears of external events.

Interestingly, although confusion of thought with action is a common feature of SCZ, few writers have discussed the relevance of magical thinking to OCD, although clinical observations support the presence of this aspect of cognitive functioning (Yaryura-Tobias & Neziroglu, 1997a, b). These aspects are further linked not only by a belief system, but by possible deficits in conceptual flexibility in OCD (Savage, 1998; Storzbach & Corrigan, 1996). As we discuss later, deficits in executive functioning are apparent among individuals with OCD, as well as those with schizophrenia, the distinction lying in the presence of thought disorder.

OCD and Schizotypal Personality

Among patients with OCD, schizotypal personality disorder is occasionally a comorbid condition. As such, it represents a significant impediment to treatment (Minichiello, Baer,

& Jenike, 1987; Stanley, Turner, & Borden, 1990). It appears that when this combination is present, standard behavioral interventions are either ineffective (Minichiello *et al.*, 1987) or create a worsening of symptoms (see Walker, Freeman, & Christensen, 1994). The reason for this may rest with a general impairment in cognitive processing necessary for positive treatment effects when exposure-based treatments are used for OCD (Foa & Kozak, 1986). Accordingly, when schizotypal personality is present, the difficulties in information processing override any effect associated with exposure for OCD. At this point, research indicates that patients with schizotypal personality share considerable neurocognitive deficits with patients with schizophrenia (Gruzelier & Doig, 1996).

Shared Phenomenology and Clinical Aspects of OCD and SCZ

At the core of both OCD and SCZ is thought pathology, distorted perception, verbal and motor impairment, restricted affective experience, and social isolation. We have partly addressed some aspects of thought and perceptual problem. Here our focus will be limited to thought process and language emission, as well as motor behaviors.

Language and Thought Impairment

In the mentally ill, language becomes the bridge between thought and the outside world. This connection permits the person to express and communicate attitudes, feelings, and beliefs. How important is language in the cognitive process of OCD and SCZ? Researchers describe two essential modes of thought; one in which thought processes are immediate, pre-logical, and irrational and stimulus bound; and another in which thought is deliberate, symbolic and rule governed. These modes seem to initially operate simultaneously, although the latter mode predominates and eventually separates from the former as normal language development progresses (Lazarus, 1991). With the dissociation and predominance of the deliberate, symbolic and rule-governed mode of thought, language becomes an acquired tool by which reality and the self are constructed and interpreted. In short, internal and external sensations are perceived and then labeled and interpreted in accordance with the consensus of the verbal community (Skinner, 1957). This shaping appears to ultimately be responsible for the construction of schemas or rules that later guide perception, cognition, and consequent action (Matlin, 1989). The self, in turn, remains consistent throughout variable stimulus contexts (Kohlenberg & Tsai, 1995).

The self is an integrated construction of invariants throughout time and space and is experienced as stable. However, when pathology affects thought, perception, verbal and motor behavior, affect and social functioning, language (whether symbolic and capable of generating rules or prelogical and fantastic) not only reflects this pathology (e.g., in word salad, neologisms, chants, repetitive prayers, repetitive questioning, stammering) but is also used as a mechanism to explain it. In addition, with restricted affective experience and social isolation, important consensual and corrective feedback from other members of the verbal community is absent. The abnormality is incorporated into the schema, which in turn guide perception, cognition, affect and behavior. Language, it appears, is the fulcrum for this sequence to take place. The neuropsychiatric pathology involved in producing the symptoms of OCD and SCZ, whether structural or functional and whether genetic or learned, essentially destroys the adaptive functions of language, interpersonal interaction and the ability to use memory, knowledge and judgment to attend to and evaluate internal and external stimulation (Bentall, 1990).

Language in patients with OCD comprises an unusual amount of the first pronoun and active verbs (Balken & Masserman, 1940). In OCD (and possibly OCPD since diagnostic criteria were not as clear before DSM-III), written language is symmetric, very precise, and without misspellings (Montserrat-Esteve, 1995).

In patients with SCZ, symptoms of disorganization, length of hospitalization, and premorbid adjustment are related to language disturbance (Shean, 1999). Hoffman, Stopek, and Andreason (1986) proposed a cognitive model of SCZ language dysfunction based in coherent organization output. Furthermore, thought disorder affects the semantic system (Goldberg, Patterson, Tappu, & Wilder, 1998). Others have found decreased fluency in patients with negative symptoms (Gruzelier, Seymour, Wilson, Jolley, & Hirsch, 1998), although it is customary to consider language disturbances in SCZ to be positive symptoms. Impairment in the speech process may be related to verbal memory deficits and verbal learning dysfunction. Still, the basic functions of language in SCZ typically remain intact (Levin, Hall, Knight, & Alpert, 1985), as also occurs in OCD.

The development of thought may have its roots in perceptual imagery, and this imagery may be a non-verbal form of thought process (Schilder, 1942). Images are common in the pathology of both OCD and SCZ. Therefore, obsessional images and visual hallucinations should be considered closely in the cognitive approach to these two conditions. Behaviorally, it seems that patients with OCD and SCZ return to "egocentric childish thinking," with a tendency to display grandiose thoughts and even divine thinking or magical thinking, in which thoughts are equivalent to actions.

Thought pathology and distorted perception, in turn, are related to the verbal impairments seen in people with both OCD and SCZ. In persons with OCD, verbal impairment may manifest itself in repetitive prayers and chants, which could be functionally shaped as part of the person's learning history to reduce the distress and discomfort associated with the obsessional content. In addition, the expression of doubt may be cognitive and due to retroactive inhibition (Matlin, 1989) or perceptual and due to abnormal proprioceptive feedback mechanisms. In SCZ, the verbal impairments may be observed in phenomena such as word salad and neologisms. In addition, verbal impairment in schizophrenics, similar to that in OCD, is manifested in observations of how such individuals talk to and reassure themselves in attempts to make sense of their delusional and hallucinatory experiences (Bentall, 1990; Chadwick & Lowe, 1990; Lowe & Chadwick, 1990).

Motor Impairment

Motor behavior is a form of non-verbal language. In fact, it is impossible to speak without producing subtle motor activity. Vernadsky (1930) has articulated concepts relating to matter transformation in the biosphere in which we live. This transformation is represented by change and movement (Bergson, 1944). Within this line of thought, Yakovlev (1948) proposed that behavior is movement, a concept that may be extended to include thought as a form of movement (Yaryura-Tobias & Neziroglu, 1983). Accordingly, thought, language, and motor activity may work in association in the pathology of OCD and SCZ, and thus, must be considered when cognitive therapy is applied.

Verbal or motor impairment is usually seen in persons with OCD as they respond motorically with obsessional slowness or freezing (Yaryura-Tobias *et al.*, 1998) or according to rigid verbal rules that dictate conduct during rituals. Motor impairments may also be related to verbal impairments in schizophrenics, for example, as evident in catatonic behavior or seemingly bizarre and excited psychomotor responses to tightly associated, internally cued stimuli (Salzinger, 1996).

The pathology in thought and in verbal impairment seems interrelated within these conditions. However, these shared aspects can easily be seen as dissimilar and unrelated when only extreme manifestations of each symptom's content are compared. Thus, gender identity obsessions may be seen as totally unrelated to a delusion of being a member of the opposite sex when only symptom content is considered. The thought process involved (e.g., an obsession versus a delusion) may exist and evolve within that continuum. Overall, OCD and SCZ both involve an awareness surrounding the illusion of free will, of having a choice and the ability to control internal and external events. Specifically, compulsive rule governed behaviors seen in OCD may represent attempts to re-establish a sense of control and mastery of the individual over the self and the environment. Conversely, in the disease progression of SCZ, individuals are often aware of their own lack of control, of choice and of free will. This deficit is more profound and observable when the patient attempts to re-establish a sense of control and mastery rather than merely attempting to describe the immediate sensory experiences.

Experimental Psychopathology and Cognition Research

Recent years have witnessed an explosion in the number of experiments addressing basic cognitive processes in the anxiety disorders. These have used the Stroop effect (Williams, Mathews, & MacLeod, 1996), memory (Dalgleish & Watts, 1990), and other cognitive processing paradigms (Williams, Watts, MacLeod, & Mathews, 1997). Taken together, this research has examined in large part cognitive processing either in relation to itself, or with normal control participants. This research has strongly suggested that in OCD attention biases are manifest for threatening information (Williams *et al.*, 1997), specific memory biases are not due to neuropsychological impairment (e.g., Radomsky & Rachman, 1999), and these biases may be ultimately inferred to arise from problematic formation of schemas or at least some higher order cognitive function.

Despite the wealth of experimental data that has accumulated determining level and extent of cognitive biases present in OCD, comparisons to psychotic conditions have been few, although cognitive processing research has an extensive history in the psychotic disorders and schizophrenia. For example, the parallel distributed processing (PDP) model that is considered a dominant means of explaining the Stroop color interference effect, arose in part from research in schizophrenia (Cohen, Dunbar, & McClelland, 1990). This model has been instructive in explaining the emotional Stroop effect as applied to the anxiety disorders. Although space prevents a detailed explanation of the PDP, briefly it is a framework that allows determination of differential attention allocation on the basis of word reading and color naming. Along this path, the reading of the word (which is automatic) activates schemas that interfere with the actual color naming of the word. A general model of cognitive processing of anxiety-related information has been offered by Mathews and Mackintosh (1998). It incorporates attention bias and suggests that weak anxiety cues trigger emotional processing in persons suffering from anxiety disorders, but only strong anxiety cues produce an effect in non-anxiety disordered individuals.

Despite the fecundity of literature that has emerged connecting cognitive bias to thematically-related information in persons with anxiety disorders, and OCD specifically, very few direct links to psychotic conditions have been established. This does not suggest the absence of a connection, but only that the current cognitive theory (i.e., Beck, 1976) does not readily lend itself to supporting such a connection. Enright (see Enright, 1996 for comprehensive coverage of this research), however, has shown that for more basic attention tasks, the performance of patients with OCD is similar to that of psychotic individuals, and different from that of individuals with other anxiety disorders. This leads to the conclusion, as Enright (1996) suggests, that perhaps OCD is part of a different set of conditions, or even a condition unto itself.

Through a series of modified Stroop experiments, Enright (1996) shows that OCD patients exhibit deficits in what he refers to as negative priming tasks. Negative priming is an extension of the task used in the original Stroop task, wherein information presented in one trial is necessary in the next trial. In this case, patients with OCD were slower in naming the letter-color of color words when the color and the word did not match (i.e., the word "red" printed in blue). Although similar to that of a group of patients with schizophrenia or schizotypal personality disorder, OCD participants' performance was significantly different from patients with other anxiety disorders, such as panic disorder, social phobia, and post-traumatic stress disorder. Although Enright (1996) suggested that the findings support a different diagnostic label due to links to deficient inhibitory processing, it is also possible that patients with OCD merely present with more neuro-cognitive deficits. Indeed, whereas Enright's research has shown similarities between OCD and SCZ-like disorders, others have not found the type of neuropsychological deficits expected if OCD were included as a member of this class of conditions (i.e., Radomsky & Rachman, 1999). Further, other emotional Stroop tasks have shown a consistent performance bias toward threat words, in a manner similar to other such studies using anxiety disorder patients (Foa, Ilai, McCarthy, Shoyer, & Murdock, 1993; Tata, Leibowitz, Prunty, Cameron, & Pickerling, 1996).

Patients with OCD show attention biases similar to performance on emotional Stroop tasks that other anxiety disorders show, whereas data from studies on memory bias have been varied. Many studies have shown that explicit memory tasks have failed to uncover a memory bias among patients with OCD (for review see Williams *et al.*, 1997; but also see Radomsky & Rachman, 1999). However, other research has suggested that a difference frequently occurs between explicit and implicit memory among anxiety disorder patients (Williams *et al.*, 1997), and this has been observed also in OCD (Dalgleish & Watts, 1990). This suggests that differential encoding may occur, mostly at an automatic processing level.

This difference in encoding is noteworthy since, as in other anxiety disorders, patients with OCD exhibit greater attention to threat related information. However, this bias is only evident under automatic processing memory task. This apparent difference has been explained by motivated avoidance within the cognitive structures responsible for retrieving information (Mogg, Bradley, DeBono, & Painter, 1997).

What most of this research does not account for is the presence of varying levels of overvalued ideas (see Chapter ten in this volume), where one would expect more impaired performance. In fact, it is reasonable to expect performance on cognitive processing tasks to be similar to the performance of patients with psychosis as levels of overvalued ideas increase. This gradient of change has not been examined, but research may begin to investigate these relationships given the appearance of instruments that reliably and validly assess overvalued ideas in OCD (Neziroglu *et al.*, 1999; Eisen *et al.*, 1998) and insight in schizophrenia (Amador *et al.*, 1991).

In the area of cognitive functioning, specific deficits in procedural memory have been recently examined in individuals with OCD (Rauch & Savage, 2000). These appear promising in determining specific brain areas for cognitive deficits associated with OCD, and may indirectly shed light on connections between OCD and SCZ. According to various neuropsychological tests, other areas where individuals with OCD exhibit deficits (as do individuals with schizophrenia, although to generally greater degrees) are nonverbal memory, visuospatial skill, and executive function (Greisberg & McKay, 2002; Savage, 1998). Although the deficits observed in OCD for these functional areas are more specific, they represent areas that are especially problematic for individuals with schizophrenia as well. What remains to be done is identify specific points that distinguish individuals with OCD from those with schizophrenia (such as particular tasks that are collectively part of executive functioning or different memory assessments).

Cognitive–Behavior Therapy

It appears that, given the noted information processing deficits associated with psychotic forms of OCD, treatment for patients with OCD and schizophrenic symptoms should begin with interventions aimed at ameliorating psychosis before attempting exposure with response prevention. Although cognitive therapy may be of value in preparing the patient for exposure-based treatment (Neziroglu, 1994), it may be futile unless cognitive rehabilitation is undertaken first. For example, McKay and Neziroglu (1996) demonstrated that social skill training was an effective alternate treatment in a case of OCD with comorbid schizotypal personality. The value of conducting therapy aimed at improving information processing lies in the ultimate goal of engaging the patient in exposure-based interventions, as well as more effectively undertaking cognitive therapy.

Conclusions

It appears that there are several functional similarities between OCD and SCZ. However, the differences between the conditions are noteworthy, particularly in the area of cognitive functioning. On the one hand, there are several cognitive processing tasks where both groups perform comparably. However, the intactness of cognitive functioning overall is clearly superior among patients with OCD. A possible common link tying the conditions to one another lies in varieties of language disturbance. This area has gone relatively unexplored, but the connection to cognitive function and bias is readily apparent.

Regarding treatment, there are occasions when OCD and SCZ or SCZ-type symptoms co-occur. Under these circumstances, it appears that treatment must be focused more upon social functioning and methods of controlling schizophrenia spectrum symptoms before attention may be paid to OCD symptoms. Clearly, this is an area that warrants additional research.

References

Amador, X. F., Strauss, D. H., Yale, S. A., & Gorman, J. M. (1991). Awareness of illness in schizohrenia. *Schizophrenia Bulletin, 17,* 113–132.

American Psychiatric Association. (1994). *Diagnostic and Statistical Manual, 4th Edition.* Washington DC: Author.

Andreasen, N., & Olsen, S. (1982). Negative vs positive schizophrenia: Definition and validation. *Archives of General Psychiatry, 39,* 789–794.

Balken, E. R., & Masserman, J. H. (1940). The language of phantasy: III. The language of the phantasies of patients with conversion hysteria, anxiety state, and obsessive–compulsive neuroses. *Journal of Psychology, 10,* 75–86.

Beck, A. T. (1976). *Cognitive therapy and the emotional disorders.* New York: International Universities Press.

Bentall, R. P. (1990). The illusion of reality: A review and integration of psychological research on hallucinations. *Psychological Bulletin, 107,* 882–95.

Bergson, H. (1944). *Creative evolution,* Authur Mitchel (trans.). New York: Modern Library.

Berman, I., Kalinowski, A., Berman, S. M., Lengua, J., & Green, A. I. (1995). Obsessive and compulsive symptoms in chronic schizophrenia. *Comprehensive Psychiatry, 36,* 6–10.

Bermanzohn, P. C., Porto, L., Arlow, P. B., Axelrod, S. Stronger, R., Martino-Beyer, J., Pollack, S., & Siris, S. G. (1997). Obsessions and delusions: separate and distinct, or overlapping? *CNS Spectrums, 2,* 58–61.

Chadwick, P. D. J., & Lowe, C. F. (1990) Measurement and modifications of delusional Belief. *Journal of Consulting and Clinical Psychology, 58,* 225–232.

Cohen, J. D., Dunbar, K., & McClelland, J. (1990). On the control of automatic processed: A parallel distributed processing account of the stroop effect. *Psychological Review, 97,* 332–361.

Crow, T. J. (1980). Positive and negative schizophrenic symptoms and the role of dopamine. *British Journal of Psychiatry, 137,* 383–386.

Dalgleish, T., & Watts, F. N. (1990). Biases of attention and memory in disorders of anxiety and depression. *Clinical Psychology Review, 10,* 589–604.

Eisen, J. L., & Rasmussen, S. A. (1993). Obsessive–compulsive disorder with psychotic features. *Journal of Clinical Psychiatry, 54,* 373–379.

Eisen, J. L., Beer, D. A., Pato, M. T., Venditto, T. A., & Rasmussen, S. A. (1997). Obsessive–compulsive disorder inpatients with schizophrenia or schizoaffective disorder. *American Journal of Psychiatry, 154,* 71–273.

Eisen, J. L., Phillips, K. A., Baer, L., Beer, D. A., Atala, K. D., & Rasmussen, S. A. (1998). The

Brown Assessment of Beliefs Scale: Reliability and validity. *American Journal of Psychiatry,* *155,* 102–108.

Enright, S. J. (1996). Obsessive–compulsive disorder: Anxiety disorder or schizotype? In R. Rapee (ed.), *Current controversies in the anxiety disorders* (pp. 161–190). New York: Guilford.

Ey, H., & Brisset, B. Ch. (1978). *Tratado de Psiquiatria (8th ed.).* Paris: Masson Cie.

Fenton, W. S., & McGlashan, T. H. (1986). The prognostic significance of obsessive–compulsive symptoms in schizophrenia. *American Journal of Psychiatry, 143,* 437–441.

Foa, E. B., & Kozak, M. J. (1986). Emotional processing of fear: Exposure to corrective information. *Psychological Bulletin, 99,* 20–35.

Foa, E. B., Ilai, D., McCarthy, P. R., Shoyer, B., & Murdock, T. (1993). Information processing in obsessive–compulsive disorder. *Cognitive Therapy and Research, 17,* 173–189.

Goldberg, J. O., & Cook, P. E. (1996), Cognitive rehab for negative symptoms. In P. W. Corrigan & S. C. Yudofsky (eds), *Cognitive rehab for neuropsychiatric disorders* (pp. 349–369). Washington, DC: American Psychiatric Press.

Goldberg, T. E., Patterson, K. J., Tappu, Y., & Wilder, K. (1998). Capacity limitations in short-term memory in schizophrenia: Tests of competing hypotheses. *Psychological Medicine, 28,* 665–673.

Greisberg, S., & McKay, D. (2000). *Thought–action fusion and the rebound effect: Links to obsessive–compulsive disorder.* Submitted for publication.

Greisberg, S., & McKay, D. (2002). *Neuropsychology of obsessive–compulsive disorder: A review with links to clinical presentation.* In preparation.

Griesinger, W. (1867). *Mental pathology and therapeutics.* New York: Hafner (translated 1965).

Gruzelier, J. H., & Doig, A. (1996). The factorial structure of schizotypy: Part II. Asymmetry, arousal, handedness, and sex. *Schizophrenia Bulletin, 22,* 621–634.

Gruzelier, J., Seymon, K., Wilson, L., Jolley, A., & Hirsch, S. (1998). Impairment on neuro-psychological tests of temperohippocampal and frontohippocampal functions and word fluency in remitting schizophreia and affective disorders. *Archives of General Psychiatry, 45,* 623–629.

Hoffman, R. E., Stopek S., & Andreason, N. (1986). A discourse analysis comparing manic versus schizophrenic speech organization. *Archives of General Psychiatry, 43,* 831–838.

Huber, G., & Gross, G. (1989). The concept of basic symptoms in schizophrenic and schizoaffective psychoses. *Recent Progress in Medicine, 80,* 646–652.

Hwang, M. Y., & Hollander, E. (1993). Schizo-obsessive disorders. *Psychiatric Annuals, 23,* 396–401.

Insel, T. R., & Akiskal, H. S. (1986). Obsessive–Compulsive disorder with psychotic features: A phenomenologic analysis. *American Journal of Psychiatry, 143,* 1527–1533.

Jaspers, K. (1913). *Psicopatologia general (General psychopathology).* Translated by R. O. Saubidet. Buenos Aires: Beta.

Jenike, M. A., Baer, L., & Carey, R. L. (1986) Coexistent obsessive–compulsive disorder and schizotypal personality disorder: A poor prognostic indicator. *Archives of General Psychiatry, 43,* 296.

Kleist, K., & Driest W. (1937) Die Katatonien auf grund katamnestischer untersuchungen. *Zeitschrift neurologie, 157,* 479.

Kohlenberg, R. J., & Tsai, M. (1995). I speak, therefore I am: A behavioral approach to understanding problems of self. *The Behavior Therapist, 18,* 113–116.

Kozak, M. J., & Foa, E. B. (1994). Obsessions, overvalued ideas, and delusions in obsessive–compulsive disorder. *Behaviour Research and Therapy, 32,* 343–353.

Kraepelin, E. (1889). Psychiatrie. Ein Lehrbuch für Studierende und Ärzte, 6th ed. Leipzig: Barth.

Lazarus, R. S. (1991). *Emotion and adaptation.* New York: Oxford.

Leonard, K. (1979). *The classification of endogenous psychoses.* (5th ed). New York: Irvington.

Levin, S., Hall, J. A., Knight, R. A., & Alpert, M. (1985). Verbal and nonverbal expressions of affect in speech of schizophrenia and depressed patients. *Journal of Abnormal Psychology, 94,* 487–497.

Lowe, C. F., & Chadwick, P. D. J. (1990). Verbal control of delusions. *Behavior Therapy, 21,* 461–479.

Mathews, A., & Mackintosh, B. (1998). A cognitive model of selective processing in anxiety. *Cognitive Therapy and Research, 22,* 539–560.

Matlin, M. W. (1989). *Cognition,* 2nd Ed. Fort Worth: Holt, Rinehart and Winston.

McKay, D., & Neziroglu, F. (1996) Social skills training in a case of obsessive–compulsive disorder with schizotypal personality disorder. *Journal of Behaviour Therapy and Experimental Psychiatry, 27,* 189–194.

Minichiello, W. E., Baer, L., & Jenike, M. A. (1987). Schizotypal personality disorder: A poor prognostic indicator for behavior therapy in the treatment of obsessive–compulsive disorder. *Journal of Anxiety Disorders, 1,* 273–276.

Mogg, K., Bradley, B. P., DeBono, J., & Painter, M. (1997). Time course of attentional bias for threat information in non-clinical anxiety. *Behaviour Research and Therapy, 35,* 297–303.

Montserrat-Esteve, S. (1995). *Lenguaje del Enfermo Obsessivo.* Barcelono, Spain: Mason.

Morselli, E. (1891). Sulla dismorfofobia e sulla tafcfobia. *Bolletinno della R accademia di Genova, 6,* 110–119.

Neziroglu, F. (1994). Complexities and lesser known aspects of obsessive–compulsive and related disorders. *Cognitive and Behavioral Practice, 1,* 133–156.

Neziroglu, F., & Stevens, K. (2002). Insight. In R.O. Frost & G. Steketee (eds), *Cognitive Approaches to Obsessions and Compulsions: Theory, Assessment and Treatment,* (pp. 183–193). Oxford: Elsevier.

Neziroglu, F., Stevens, K., Yaryura-Tobias, J. A., & McKay, D. (2001). Predictive validity of the Overvalued Ideas Scale: Outcome in obsessive-compulsive and body dysmorphic disorders. *Behaviour Research and Therapy, 39,* 745–756.

Neziroglu, F., Yaryura-Tobias, J. A., McKay, D., Stevens, K. P., & Todaro, J. (1999). An overvalued ideas scale for obsessive–compulsive disorder: its reliability and validity. *Behaviour Research and Therapy, 37,* 881–902.

Obsessive–Compulsive Cognitions Working Group. (1997). Cognitive assessment of obsessive–compulsive disorder. *Behaviour Research and Therapy, 35,* 667–681.

Porto, L., Bermanzohn, P., Pollack, S., Morrissey, R., & Siris, S. G. (1997). A profile of obsessive–compulsive symptoms in schizophrenia. *CNS Spectrums, 2,* 21–25.

Rachman, S., & Shafran, R. (1998). Cognitive and behavioral features of Obsessive–Compulsive Disorder. In R.P. Swinson, M.M. Antony, S. Rachman, & M.A. Richter (eds), *Obsessive–compulsive disorder: Theory, research, and treatment* (pp. 51–78). New York: Guilford.

Radomsky, A., & Rachman, S. (1999). Memory bias in obsessive–compulsive disorder (OCD). *Behavior Research and Therapy, 37,* 605–618.

Rauch, S. L., & Savage, C. R. (2000). Investigating cortico-striatal pathophysiology in obsessive–compulsive disorders: Procedural learning and imaging probes. In W.K. Goodman, M.V. Rudorfer, & J.D. Maser (eds), *Obsessive–compulsive disorder: Contemporary issues in treatment* (pp. 133–154). Mahwah, NJ: Erlbaum.

Reid, W. (1989). *The treatment of psychiatric disorders, revised for the DSM-III-R.* New York: Brunner & Mazel.

Salzinger, K. (1996). Reinforcement history: A concept underutilized in behavior analysis. *Journal of Behavior Therapy and Experimental Psychiatry, 27,* 199–207.

Savage, C. R. (1998). Neuropsychology of obsessive–compulsive disorder: Research findings and treatment implications. In M.A. Jenike, L. Baer, & W.E. Minichiello (eds), *Obsessive–compulsive disorders: Practical management* (pp. 254–275). St. Louis, MO: Mosby.

Schilder, P. (1942) *Mind: Perpeception and thought in their constructive aspects.* New York: Columbia University Press.

Shapiro, D. (1965). *Neurotic styles.* New York: Basic Books.

Shafran, R., Thordarson, D., & Rachman, S. (1996). Thought–action fusion in obsessive–compulsive disorder. *Journal of Anxiety Disorders, 10,* 379–392.

Shean, G. D. (1999). Syndromes of schizophrenia and language dysfunction. *Journal of Clinical Psychology, 55,* 233–240.

Skinner, B. F. (1957). *Verbal behavior.* New York: Appleton–Century–Crofts.

Sperry, L. (1995). *Handbook of diagnosis and treatment of the DSM-IV personality disorders.* New York: Brunner & Mazel.

Stanley, M. A., Turner, S. M., & Borden, J. W. (1990). Schizotypal features in obsessive–compulsive disorder. *Comprehensive Psychiatry, 31,* 511–518.

Stengel, E. (1931). The relationships between obsessional neurosis and paranoia. *Archiv Fuer Psychologie, 95,* 8–23.

Storzbach, D. M., & Corrigan, P. W. (1996). Cognitive rehabilitation for schizophrenia. In P. W. Corrigan & S.C. Yudofsky (eds), *Cognitive rehabilitation for neuropsychiatric disorders* (pp. 299–328). Washington, DC: American Psychiatric Press.

Strauss J. S., Carpenter, W. T., & Bartko, J. J. (1974). The diagnosis and understanding of schizophrenia. Part III: speculations on the process that underlie schizophrenic symptoms and signs. *Schizophrenia Bulletin, 11,* 61–75.

Tata, P. R., Leibowitz, J. A., Prunty, M. J., Cameron, M., & Pickerling, A. D. (1996). Attentional bias in obsessional compulsive disorder. *Behaviour Research and Therapy, 34,* 53–60.

Torrey, E. F. (1988). *Surviving schizophrenia.* New York: Harper & Row.

Vernadsky, V. I. (1930). *La biosphere.* Paris: Felix Alcan.

Walker, W. R., Freeman, R. F., & Christensen, D. K. (1994). Restricting environmental stimulation (REST) to enhance cognitive–behavioral treatment for obsessive–compulsive disorder with schizotypal personality disorder. *Behavior Therapy, 25,* 709–719.

Wernicke, C. (1900). *Grundrisse der Psychiatrie* (Foundations of Psychiatry). Leipzig: Verlag.

Westphal, C. (1872). *Ueber Zwangsvorstell* (On obsessional ideation). Berliner Klinischen Wochenschrift.

Williams, J. M. G., Mathews, A., & Macleod, C. (1996). The emotional stroop task and psychopathology. *Psychological Bulletin, 120,* 3–24.

Williams, J. M. G., Watts, F. N., Macleod, C., & Mathews, A. (1997). *Cognitive psychology and emotional disorders (2nd ed.).* Chichester, UK: Wiley.

Wong, S. E., Martinez-Diaz, J. A., Massel, H. K., Edelstein, B. A., Wiegand, W., Bowen, L., & Liberman, R. P. (1993). Conversational skills training with schizophrenic inpatients: A study of generalization across settings and conversants. *Behavior Therapy, 24,* 285–304.

Yakovlev, P. I. (1948). Motility, behavior and the brain: Sterodynamic organization and neural coordinates of behavior. *Journal of Nervous and Mental Disease, 107,* 313–335.

Yaryura-Tobias, J. A., & Neziroglu, F. (1983). *Obsessive–compulsive disorders. Pathogenesis, diagnosis, treatment.* New York: Marcel Dekker.

Yaryura-Tobias, J. A., & Neziroglu, F. (1997a). *Obsessive–compulsive disorder spectrum. Pathogenesis, diagnosis, and treatment.* Washington, DC: American Psychiatric Press.

Yaryura-Tobias, J. A., & Neziroglu, F. (1997b). *Biobehavioral treatment of obsessive–compulsive spectrum disorders.* New York: Norton.

Yaryura-Tobias, J. A., Campisi, T. A., McKay, D., & Neziroglu, F. (1995). Schizophrenia and obsessive–compulsive disorder: Shared aspects and pathology. *Neurolology, Psychiatry and Brain Research, 3,* 143–148.

Yaryura-Tobias, J. A., Grunes, M. S., Todaro, J., McKay, D., Neziroglu, F. A., & Stockman, R.

(2000). Nosological insertion of Axis I disorders in the etiology of Obsessive–Compulsive Disorder, *Journal of Anxiety Disorder, 14*, 19–30.

Yaryura-Tobias, J. A., Stevens, K. P.,& Neziroglu, F. A. (1998). Motor disturbances in the obsessive–compulsive disorder and its spectrum. *Neurology, Psychiatry and Brain Research, 5*, 79–84

Yaryura-Tobias, J. A., Stevens, K. P., Neziroglu, F., & Grunes, M. (1997). Obsessive–compulsive disorder and schizophrenia; A phenomenological perspective of shared pathology. *CNS Spectrums, 2*, 21–25.

Chapter 15

Cognitions in Compulsive Hoarding

Michael Kyrios, Gail Steketee, Randy O. Frost and Sophie Oh

Introduction

Phenomenology of Compulsive Hoarding

Hoarding refers to the stocking or amassing of possessions, a phenomenon encountered commonly throughout the community (Frost & Gross, 1993; Frost, Hartl, Christian, & Williams, 1995). Although hoarding behaviors are often widely accepted or dismissed as inconsequential by society, compulsive hoarding is a serious psychiatric problem that disrupts the lifestyle of hoarders and often the lives of friends, family and the community in general. Frost and associates (Frost & Gross, 1993; Frost & Hartl, 1996) have defined compulsive hoarding as the acquisition of and failure to discard possessions that are useless or of limited value, resulting in clutter that renders living spaces unusable for their intended purpose, and causing significant distress and impairment. Definitions of hoarding from a clinical perspective also incorporate dimensions such as impediment and/or hazard (Frost & Gross, 1993; Thomas, 1997). For instance, clutter resulting from hoarding typically reaches a point where rooms cannot be used for their designated purpose, or where safety and hygiene are compromised (Thomas, 1997).

Frost and colleagues (Frost & Hartl, 1996; Frost, Krause, & Steketee, 1996; Frost & Steketee, 2000) have outlined a number of ways in which hoarding is manifested. Most definitions of hoarding focus on the failure or inability to discard and the tendency to keep objects despite their limited usefulness. Furby (1978) described several character-istics of objects or possessions that differentially motivate individuals to save them. Firstly, some objects are seen to have instrumental or practical value, and are considered to have some actual or potential use in the present or future. Alternatively, some objects have sentimental value that prompts an emotional attachment to them. Finally, some objects are seen as having intrinsic value or meaning, although they do not have any particular use or emotional meaning attached to them (e.g., they are "too perfect" or "too pretty" to throw away). For hoarders, the decision to discard objects with limited or no utility is fraught with discomfort, anxiety, sadness or guilt. Hence, avoidance behaviors develop so that objects and possessions are saved.

A less acknowledged but related aspect of hoarding is the tendency to compulsively acquire possessions, either through excessive and impulsive buying or through less direct methods, such as actively collecting objects that others have discarded or picking up free samples. The relationship of compulsive buying to more general aspects of compulsive acquisition is not yet clear (Frost *et al.*, 1998).

An additional component of recent conceptualizations of hoarding (Frost & Hartl, 1996) concerns purported deficits in information processing and organizational capacity among hoarders. While the appropriation and retention of a large volume of possessions results in the loss of livable spaces, information processing and organizational deficits result in chaos and clutter within living spaces and among the individual's possessions. The manifestation of these cognitive deficits is discussed in more detail below. Nonetheless, it should be noted that, along with acquisition and saving, cognitive deficits contribute to overall distress and impairment among hoarders.

The Significance of Compulsive Hoarding

Hoarding behaviors have been observed in a range of non-clinical populations, including students, community controls and the elderly (Frost & Steketee, 1998; Steketee, Frost, & Kim, 2001). Hoarding is closely associated with obsessive–compulsive disorder (OCD; Baer, 1994; Frost *et al.*, 1996; Leckman *et al.*, 1997) occurring in 20 percent to 30 percent of patients with OCD. It also constitutes one of several symptoms of obsessive–compulsive personality disorder (OCPD; American Psychiatric Association, 1994), and has been observed in a range of other clinical conditions, including: anorexia nervosa (Frankenburg, 1984); depression (Shafran & Tallis, 1996); other personality disorders (Frost, Steketee, Williams, & Warren, 2000); and geriatric, psychotic and organic mental disorders (Greenberg, Witztum, & Levy, 1990; Hwang, Tsai, Yang, Liu, & Lirng, 1998; Rosenthal, Stelian, Wagner, & Berkman, 1999; Tracy *et al.*, 1996).

Phenomenological research has identified hoarding to be a robust and independent phenomenon that is related to, but distinct from, other OCD sub-types. For instance, hoarders frequently do not view their behavior as unusual and exhibit less insight into their behavior than those with other OCD symptoms (Black *et al.*, 1998; Frost & Gross, 1993; Frost *et al.*, 1996). Supporting this conceptualization, statistical analyses of obsessive compulsive symptoms repeatedly identify hoarding as a separate factor (Baer, 1994; Calamari, Wiegartz, & Janeck, 1999; Damecour & Charron, 1998; Leckman *et al.*, 1997; Mataix-Cols, Rauch, Manzo, Jenike, & Baer, 1999; Summerfeldt, Richter, Antony, & Swinson, 1999). Some researchers have gone so far as to describe hoarding as a biologically and phenomenologically distinct subset of OCD (Black *et al.*, 1998).

Despite a range of available interventions such as pharmacotherapy and cognitive-behavior therapy designed for OCD, clinically significant hoarding remains resistant to treatment. In fact, in OCD, presence of hoarding is likely to indicate a poor prognosis (Black *et al.*, 1998; Fitzgerald, 1997; Mataix-Cols *et al.*, 1999). Such clinical difficulties are reflected in the growing research focus on hoarding as a distinct syndrome and the interest in developing specific conceptualizations of hoarding (Frost & Gross, 1993; Frost & Hartl, 1996; Stein, Seedat, & Potocnik, 1999). Notwithstanding a body of theoretical literature about the etiology of hoarding and of related conditions such as OCD, recent clinical research supporting the ineffectiveness of current treatments reflects obvious limitations in our understanding of hoarding. While etiological models of OCD have been embraced as the basis for managing hoarding, poor treatment outcomes support the need to develop specific conceptualizations of compulsive hoarding behaviors to help guide these interventions. The recent emergence of specific cognitive-behavioral models of etiology for compulsive hoarding has led to empirical investigation of its behavioral manifestations, associated phenomena, markers of vulnerability for its development and/or maintenance, and the development of more effective psychological treatments (Frost & Hartl, 1996; Frost & Gross, 1993; Frost, Steketee, & Greene, in press; Hartl & Frost, 1999).

In keeping with the aims of the current volume, this chapter describes the cognitive correlates of compulsive hoarding. Results from ongoing studies will be presented, including information on OCD-related cognitive factors relevant to hoarding. While acknowledging a range of etiological influences on hoarding, we argue that current cognitive-behavioral conceptualizations offer a finer delineation of hoarding symptoms and associated features, provide a useful distinction between hoarding-specific and hoarding-relevant cognitions, and contribute to the development and testing of focused psychological treatments.

Models of Compulsive Hoarding

Etiological Theories of Compulsive Hoarding

In the past, theories of clinical hoarding have been formulated primarily in reference to OCD or personality disorders such as OCPD. For instance, Freud (1908) understood hoarding to represent a failure in psychosexual stage progression, particularly related to anal fixation. Hoarding was thought to symbolize fecal retention and to be related to wider anal fixation on parsimony, orderliness and obstinacy. Fromm (1947) suggested that acquisition is a core aspect of character and a means of relating to the wider environment. He suggested that a hoarding orientation constitutes one of four types of non-productive character, distinguished by withdrawal and remoteness from others, compulsiveness, suspiciousness, extremes of order, and concerns about cleanliness and punctuality. Hoarders were thought to derive a sense of security from collecting and saving things, forming attachments to possessions in lieu of attachments to others.

Such psychodynamic theories have been useful in the identification of developmental, affective, behavioral and cognitive influences on hoarding (e.g., focus on attachment, need for control, orderliness and perfectionism). However, because of the absence of empirical evidence supporting such conceptualizations of hoarding and the lack of subsequent effective treatments, such characterological theories have not been widely adopted. Theoretical discourse has turned away from such psychological conceptualizations and towards more biologically-oriented accounts.

A great deal of research evidence is cited in support of biological models of compulsive behavior. However, these biological models seldom refer to compulsive human hoarding behavior specifically. Rather, biological models of hoarding are extensions of OCD research and animal studies. Animal studies usually refer to the maximizing of food stores or to cortical abnormalities involving either the nucleus accumbens (Stern & Passingham, 1994; Whishaw & Kornelsen, 1993) or the prefrontal cortex (de Brabanden, de Bruin, & van Eden, 1993). Human OCD studies have implicated several factors, varying from serotonergic dysregulation to neurophysiological deficits or abnormalities (for a thorough review see Hohagen & Berger, 1998). Although some biological models of hoarding offer the potential for pharmacological remedies, available drug programs have remained essentially ineffective, particularly for the long-term treatment of compulsive hoarders (Black *et al.*, 1998; Mataix-Cols *et al.*, 1999).

From an evolutionary perspective, Rapoport (1989) has likened hoarding to an instinctive nesting behavior. This model proposes that hoarding is evidence of a compulsive manifestation of fixed action patterns. In a variation of the evolutionary theme, Blurton-Jones (1988) proposed that hoarding is an evolved survival instinct and is part of the natural ecology of human and animal behavior. This conceptualization of hoarding is based on an assumed contest for resources. Such an interpretation is readily applicable to animal hoarding because animals have a tendency to hoard only foodstuffs.

Although conceptualizations from animal models may prove useful in some situations, there are limitations in their application to wider compulsive hoarding phenomena in humans because of the heterogeneity of objects collected and the absence of competition. Biological and ethological theories fail because the majority of cases of human compulsive hoarding involves non-foodstuffs, considered by most people to be useless or of limited value. Furthermore, such theories do not account adequately for the emotional attachments to objects and other affective components of hoarding (Frost *et al.*, 1995). Moreover, biologically based theories do not account adequately for sociocultural and historical influences that may be important in the manifestations of hoarding (Greenberg *et al.*, 1990; Kottler, 1999).

Because cognitive-behavioral therapy (CBT) has offered success in the treatment of OCD and related conditions (Abramowitz, 1997; van Balkom *et al.*, 1994, 1998), it has been argued that cognitive and behavioral processes play central etiological or maintenance roles. The lack of specific cognitive-behavioral models for hoarding until recently may account for poor treatment outcomes for hoarders (Shafran & Tallis, 1996). Nonetheless, cognitive-behavioral models of OCD and OCPD offer great heuristic value in improving our understanding of hoarding and its management (Hartl & Frost, 1999), although this contention has remained untested. These psychological models and their possible relevance to hoarding are discussed below.

Cognitive-Behavioral Models of Obsessive-Compulsive Problems

Cognitive-behavioral models of psychopathology ascertain that maladaptive responses to stimuli (e.g. objects, situations, internal and external events) are generated on the basis of beliefs and appraisals about those stimuli, rather than by the stimuli themselves. Most cognitive-behavioral research on obsessions and compulsions has been conducted with OCD subjects and normal controls. However, because hoarding is associated with both OCD and OCPD, it could be argued that aspects of the conceptual models relating to the etiology of both these conditions are applicable to compulsive hoarding.

Cognitive-behavioral model of OCD.   OCD is a heterogeneous condition and, although a number of sub-types have been differentiated, subjects with cleaning or checking compulsions have dominated research. As a result, OCD presentations of hoarding, counting, repeating or obsessions accompanied by only mental rituals have been under-represented in research studies (Ball, Baer, & Otto, 1996). Despite this, cognitive-behavioral models, which explain the development and maintenance of a range of OCD symptoms, are evident in the literature.

The theoretical work of Salkovskis (1985) and Rachman (1993, 1997, 1998) has been particularly influential, and had led to the identification of a range of beliefs associated with obsessional and compulsive phenomena, including: (a) an inflated sense of personal responsibility; (b) a belief in the importance of one's thoughts, including the unwarranted fusion between thought and action; (c) an inflated need for mental control; (d) a tendency towards over-estimating threat; (e) an intolerance of uncertainty; (f) high levels of perfectionism; (g) lack of confidence about capacity to cope and tolerance of discomfort; and (h) core beliefs about self-worth and identity (see Chapters one to six for a thorough review of OCD-related beliefs). Such beliefs are thought to influence the appraisal of specific intrusions, leading to maladaptive emotional, behavioral and cognitive responses (i.e., distress, obsessions, compulsions and other neutralization strategies, avoidance and other safety patterns).

The Obsessive-Compulsive Cognitions Working Group (OCCWG, 1997, 2001) has developed measures of many of these beliefs and the appraisals of specific intrusions thought to stem from such beliefs. These instruments, the Obsessional Beliefs Questionnaire (OBQ) and the Interpretation of Intrusions Inventory (III), are described in detail in Chapter seven of this volume, and are produced in the appendices. Research with OCD and other anxious cohorts has indicated the association between the OBQ, III and measures of OCD severity (OCCWG, 2001). However, to date, few studies have examined the relationship of such OCD-related beliefs and appraisals to hoarding behavior. This chapter includes some preliminary research on this issue.

Cognitive-behavioral conceptions of OCPD.   Relatively little research has investigated specific cognitive patterns in OCPD, although cognitive therapists have identified a number of beliefs, cognitive distortions and behaviors that characterize the obsessive-compulsive personality. Beck and Freeman (1990) determined that people with an obsessive-compulsive personality exhibit rigidity in thinking, typically use dichotomous thinking, over-attend to detail, and apply inflexible rules. They also exhibit a strong belief in correct solutions, demanding that mistakes and failures be avoided at all cost. Mistakes or failures are mis-perceived as intolerable, and dealt with through the use of self-punitive measures. Those with OCPD are inherently concerned about criticism, engage in extremes of personal criticism, set up unrealistic expectations for themselves and others in many domains, and think in terms of "shoulds" and "musts". They over-compensate for low self-esteem and perceived criticism through over-achievement. They are perfectionistic and often exhibit an inflated sense of personal responsibility, resulting in extremes of worry, morality and scruples. If the perfect course of action is not clear, they often regard it best to do nothing, frequently resulting in procrastination. They over-estimate the amount of risk, particularly in relation to the experience of emotion, hence over-emphasizing the need for emotional and behavioral self-control. Their need for control also generalizes to the external world where they insist on certainty, rules and regulations or well-practiced rituals, and are often regarded as dogmatic, opinionated and inflexible.

Post-rationalist cognitive behavioral models of OCPD have emerged incorporating developmental and intra-psychic concepts such as attachment, parenting practices, and morphological organization. For instance, Guidano and Liotti (1983) posited that a ritualistic and perfectionistic yearning for certainty is fostered by an ambivalent sense of self which derives from rejecting parental attitudes camouflaged by an outward mask of absolute devotion. While this theoretical model is relevant to OCPD, it is unclear to what extent it also relates to OCD. The obsessive-compulsive personality is accorded an ambiguous concept of self, with a fear that unacceptable intrusions reflect badly on the type of person he/she is. Therefore, to salvage a positive self and public image, compulsions are generated as attempts to minimize personal responsibility over the possible occurrence of feared outcomes.

Integrating notions from cognitive-behavioral and post-rationalist literature, Kyrios (1998) identified five areas of cognition that could explain the behavioral and affective manifestations of OCPD:

a) *Personal self-worth*: Those exhibiting obsessive compulsive phenomena can be conceptualized as utilizing maladaptive means to preserve their sense of personal self-worth, in the face of a perceived hostile social world which induces a sense of worthlessness (Bhar & Kyrios, 1999).

b) *Trust*: By lacking consistent early childhood experiences of unconditional positive regard, people with obsessive-compulsive personality not only develop low self-worth, but also learn to distrust the external world and themselves for not being able to induce positive engagement.

c) *Control*: Having rarely experienced a sense of security internally or externally, the obsessive-compulsive personality also fears disorganization or even uncertainty, and over-compensates by establishing unrealistic, unattainable and/or unsustainable control strategies for themselves and the external world. The net result is often procrastination, a lack of creative freedom, and a poor range of problem-solving options.

d) *Social roles*: Through their procrastination, those with OCPD may secure role diffusion. Alternatively, through their obsession with control and certainty, they might develop extremes of role cohesion by taking on inflexible and ultimately unsatisfying roles. Such strategies relate to identity, self-perceptions and self-expectations.

e) *Morality*: Individuals who have not been able to achieve satisfying roles often attempt to acquire a sense of self through their adherence to rules and regulations, particularly those relating to morality and personal and social responsibility. Such adherence simplifies life for those with OCPD by averting the need to account for the complexity and confusion of reality. However, the resulting sense of self is vulnerable, unstable and ambivalent. The moral high ground compensates for an ambivalent self-image because it allows identification with external authority that requires no defense. However, inflexible adherence to moral imperatives consistently produces self-doubts and, hence, maintains an ambivalent sense of self in the obsessive-compulsive personality.

Although the study of developmental and intra-psychic factors in hoarding and other obsessive–compulsive disorders is in its infancy, such concepts may further improve our understanding of meta-vulnerability factors underlying compulsive hoarding, and may lead to more effective preventative, corrective, and management strategies.

The challenge for hoarding research.   Hoarding provides a number of challenges for cognitive-behavioral and post-rationalist models of OCD and OCPD. Etiological models of compulsive hoarding need to account for the contribution of beliefs relating to wider obsessive-compulsive concerns and for hoarding-specific cognitive features. With the significant overlap in many features of OCD, OCPD and hoarding (e.g., perfectionism, control, responsibility), elements of cognitive-behavioral models for OCD and OCPD could be applied to our understanding of hoarding. However, it is unlikely that obsessional beliefs possess a consistent focus across obsessive-compulsive conditions or even across subtypes of the same condition. For instance, a large body of psychological literature indicates the important role of perfectionism in a number of psychopathological conditions. It has been related to general symptoms of anxiety in non-clinical samples (Minarik & Ahrens, 1996), social phobia and depression (Antony, Purdon, Huta, & Swinson, 1998), and suicidal behavior (Dean & Range, 1996; Hewitt, Flett, & Turnbull, 1993; Hewitt, Newton, & Flett, 1997), as well as OCPD (Frost *et al.*, 1996), OCD (Rhéaume, Freeston, Dugas, Letarte, & Ladouceur, 1995) and hoarding (Frost & Hartl, 1996). Although perfectionism is acknowledged as a component of psychological vulnerability to these disorders, it does not necessarily determine the exact nature of the consequent condition (Frost & Steketee, 1997).

Disorders may be associated with a particular focus for a specific belief. For instance, while OCD may be associated with concerns about perfect order and symmetry, hoarders may be more concerned about making perfect decisions (Frost & Gross, 1993). On the other hand, subtypes of the same disorder may differ in the salience of a specific belief or the focus of that belief. For instance, while OCD checkers may exhibit excessive responsibility for the safety of others, OCD hoarders might be more concerned about their responsibility for possessions or for ensuring availability of possessions when others may need them. In addition, specific disorders may be associated with idiosyncratic belief systems. For instance, although hoarding has been associated with beliefs about the importance of possessions (Frost *et al.*, 1995), such beliefs have not generally been linked to OCD (OCCWG, 1997). Conversely, beliefs relating to unrealistic mental control may not necessarily relate to hoarding, but concerns about decision-making and memory for possessions may be relevant (Hartl *et al.*, 2000; Frost & Shows, 1993). A number of studies have now examined the cognitive profile of compulsive hoarders, leading to the development of a specific cognitive-behavioral model by Frost and colleagues. This is described below.

Emotional and Cognitive Features of Compulsive Hoarding

Frost and Hartl (1996) have proposed a model asserting that hoarding is a multi-faceted problem stemming from conditioned emotional responses associated with hoarding-specific cognitive patterns. Acquisition of and failure to discard possessions are seen as a means of avoiding the perceived consequences and difficulties associated with throwing away or not possessing objects. Information processing deficits include difficulty with decision-making and categorization of possessions, and memory problems. Because of emotional attachments to possessions, saving behavior and the possessions themselves come to attain a comforting and pacifying quality. Compulsive hoarding problems are further compounded by beliefs about the nature of possessions that drive hoarders to acquire and keep objects in response to their sense of responsibility, wish to remember, and need to control. Facets of the model are described below.

Attentional, Information Processing, Organizational and Memory Deficits

Possessions trigger a narrowing of a hoarder's attention and cognitive functions, and a rich associative network focuses on the nature and potential use of possessions. The potential value of an object is a central component in decision-making deficits experienced by compulsive hoarders. Compulsive hoarders evaluate the potential and inherent worth of an item as greater than the worth others ascribe to it. They also typically perceive objects to be associated with some opportunity that must not be missed. Thus, possessions are accumulated for their potential value.

Pathological hoarders appear to possess a higher threshold for deciding what to discard (Frost & Hartl, 1996; Salzman, 1973). For instance, they may require more reasons for discarding possessions, or they may focus on reasons for keeping objects. Research from animal studies originally suggested that hoarders focus on the cost of discarding items, with little thought to the cost of saving or the benefits of not having objects (Smith, 1990). Salzman (1973) has suggested that hoarders keep possessions because of high levels of anxiety experienced subsequent to the thought of throwing away something that may be needed at some time in the future. However, Frost *et al.* (1998) concluded that, although hoarders spend more time thinking of reasons to save, they do not spend less time on reasons to discard than non-hoarders.

Over-estimation of the importance of remembering information is not unique to hoarding (Guidano & Liotti, 1983), but appears to be linked to some specific beliefs held by hoarders. Compulsive hoarders place excessive importance on remembering unrealistic amounts of seemingly superfluous information. Based on case studies, hoarders often report a belief in their ability or obligation to read, absorb, remember, and retain all the information presented, including useless and temporarily relevant information. Such beliefs frequently refer to information contained in newspapers and junk mail. For instance, one hoarder collected all the newspapers she could acquire for over 20 years to secure as much information as possible about bicentennial celebrations in her home city, information that she felt obliged to pass on to her estranged daughter should they ever be reconciled. Any less than this she considered a personal failure. The sheer amount of information hoarders expect themselves to recall places high demands on their memory. Hoarding becomes a means of postponing failure to remember by keeping the papers. Through their attempts to access and control their possessions, hoarders believe that they can hold on to any relevant information relating to those possessions. Hence, the retention of possessions may compensate for an over-extended memory (Frost & Hartl, 1996).

While there is ample evidence of specific non-verbal memory deficits in OCD using standard neuropsychological tasks (Purcell, Maruff, Kyrios, & Pantelis, 1998; Savage *et al.*, 2000), few such studies have been undertaken with hoarders. Findings from a recent study suggest that hoarders exhibit poorer recall for verbal and visual information than non-hoarders (Hartl *et al.*, 2000). As a number of factors may influence performance on memory tasks (e.g., lowered confidence in memory, unrealistic performance demands and evaluation, low tolerance for uncertainty, depression and anxiety), it has not been clear whether such performance deficits reflect a true memory deficit, or whether they may signify the influence of factors such as compromised metamemory or negative affect (Kyrios, Wainwright, Purcell, Pantelis, & Maruff, 1999). However, Purcell *et al.* (1998) found that OCD-related memory deficits were not found in depressed, panic or normal controls. Furthermore, Hartl *et al.* (2000) indicated that memory deficits in hoarders were not accounted for by lack of confidence in their memory, or for their tendency to keep possessions in sight (Hartl *et al.*, 2000).

Memory difficulties in hoarders could also be further compounded by deficits in the categorization and organization of information. Each hoarded possession is considered to be so unique that a hoarder typically considers it to belong to a class by itself. Hence, even similar objects are not grouped or placed together, leading to disorganization, clutter and chaos. In order to satisfy the perceived inherent usefulness of specific possessions, hoarders place them at the top of their pile, hoping to remember their location. As new possessions are placed on top of older ones, piles are merely churned, changing the placement of objects and adding extra demands on memory.

Churning may also result from indecisiveness. For instance, unable to decide where to place or what to do with a possession they have picked up, hoarders may set it down again and move onto the next possession. Indecisiveness has been found strongly related to compulsive hoarding behaviors (Frost & Shows, 1993). The indecisiveness characteristic of hoarders appears to be a behavioral manifestation of several cognitive processes. Rather than representing a single, discrete psychological mechanism, indecisiveness has been linked to a perfectionistic fear of making mistakes and to uncertainty over the value of possessions (Frost & Hartl, 1996; Frost, Marten, Lahart, & Rosenblate, 1990; Frost & Shows, 1993). The indecisiveness exhibited by pathological hoarders is consistent with the conceptualization of hoarding as an avoidance behavior whereby saving possessions circumvents the need to determine what to discard. Further, saving behavior enables hoarders to alleviate or avoid their exaggerated concern over mistakenly throwing away potentially valuable possessions.

Emotional Attachment Difficulties

Further to the work of Bowlby (1969, 1973), a number of researchers have indicated the potential importance of attachment and early developmental influences such as parenting styles in the emergence of personality traits (i.e., obsessive-compulsive) commonly associated with hoarding (Guidano & Liotti, 1983; Kyrios, 1998). Dysfunctional attachment to objects may be a defense against intra-psychic conflict resulting from anxious or ambivalent attachments. Certainly, emotional attachments to inanimate objects are common (c.f., the transitional objects of childhood) and are not necessarily problematic. However, research indicates that specific emotional attachments are involved in compulsive hoarding. For instance, compared to non-hoarders, hoarders show greater levels of emotional attachment to objects and cite more sentimental reasons for saving (Frost & Gross, 1993; Frost *et al.*, 1995). The tendency for hoarders to anthropomorphize and to view possessions as extensions of themselves may increase their degree of emotional attachment (Greenberg, 1987). It has also been proposed that the disposal of possessions becomes akin to losing a loved one (Frost & Hartl, 1996).

A number of case studies and anecdotal evidence suggest the existence of another form of emotional attachment that is a consequence of the association between possessions and a sense of comfort and preparedness. Objects come to be valued as safety signals because of the sense of security derived from them. For example, Frost and Hartl (1996) reported that one hoarder's response to a difficult day was the desire to go home and gather her treasures around her. Another described her sleeping area surrounded by piles of papers and objects as her "bunker". A third deliberately placed piles near the entrance to her apartment to protect herself from intruders, even though she realized that this was ludicrous. A related sense of comfort may also be gained from the acquisition of items. Although no studies have investigated the explicit nature of the relationship between hoarding and acquisition, a positive association has been found between compulsive buying and compulsive hoarding (Frost *et al.*, 1998). It is possible that hoarders both acquire and are unable to dispose of their possessions because of strong comfort and safety needs.

Beliefs About the Nature of Possessions

Hoarders hold several types of beliefs about the nature of possessions related to those associated with OCD. Beliefs about the necessity for maintaining control over possessions, about responsibility for possessions and about the necessity for perfection seem to distinguish hoarders from non-hoarders (Frost & Hartl, 1996). Hoarders commonly express a need to maintain control over possessions and typically become agitated when possessions are moved or even touched without authorization (Greenberg, 1987). Beliefs about the necessity for maintaining control over possessions may reflect a number of different underlying cognitive processes. Furby (1978) concluded that control over possessions provided hoarders with a sense of control over their environment. Combined with heightened emotional attachment to objects, hoarders may perceive unauthorized touching of possessions as equivalent to undermining their control of self and environment, and a violation of privacy and safety. Unauthorized touching may also aggravate the elaborate responsibilities hoarders hold towards their possessions.

The hoarding of possessions may be a response to an exaggerated sense of responsibility. Inflated levels of responsibility are not unique to hoarding and have been increasingly identified as central to OCD (Rachman, 1993; Salkovskis, 1985). The onus of responsibility experienced by hoarders refers in part to their wish to be prepared for future needs. Hoarders have been found to buy more things to avoid being caught without

(Frost & Gross, 1993). Possessions are kept because they are perceived as having utility in possible future scenarios and, characteristically, hoarders acquire and carry extra possessions in case they will be needed. Likewise, hoarders may express a sense of responsibility for having items available that other people might want or need, and a corresponding feeling of guilt if someone needs an item they do not have.

Consistent with the tendency to anthropomorphize, compulsive hoarders feel a sense of responsibility to protect their possessions from harm. The human-like quality bestowed onto possessions necessitates the need for protection in the mind of the hoarder. Premised on the perception of possessions as extensions of self, protecting the object from harm becomes parallel to defending oneself. In a related vein, Frost and Hartl (1996) suggested that it is often easier for hoarders to sell, recycle or give away possessions than to discard them as trash.

Severity of Anxiety and Depression in Hoarding

Hoarding has been related to significantly increased anxiety and heightened levels of depression (Frost *et al.*, 2000; Shafran & Tallis, 1996; Winsberg, Cassic, & Koran, 1999), as has compulsive buying (Christenson *et al.*, 1994; Lejoyeux, Tassain, Solomon, & Ades, 1997). Nonetheless, few studies have investigated the explicit pathogenic relationship between hoarding and negative mood states. Negative mood states may result from the impairment associated with compulsive hoarding, or are themselves underlying vulnerabilities in the etiology and maintenance of hoarding. Although anxiety is intuitively a symptom integral to avoidance behaviors, it does not distinguish cases of compulsive hoarding. Furthermore, while depression may be a precursor of compulsive buying (Lejoyeux *et al.*, 1997), there is no published data on the temporal relationship between depression and hoarding.

It is also possible that anxiety, depression and hoarding share common underlying cognitive features that act as vulnerability factors for each disorder. For instance, OCD subjects with comorbid generalized anxiety disorder have been found to display elevated indecisiveness and pathological responsibility, both of which are components of cognitive behavioral models of OCD and hoarding (Abramowitz & Foa, 1998). Belief systems that emphasize perfectionism, the need to control events and the prevention of unexpected dangers have been associated with all anxiety disorders except specific phobias (Antony *et al.*, 1998).

The study of cognitions in obsessive-compulsive, hoarding and mood disorders may help to delineate which belief systems are shared by these disorders, and whether there are unique cognitive components to each disorder. In light of suggestions that the efficacy of CBT is dependent on the specificity of the dysfunctional beliefs that are challenged and restructured (van Oppen & Arntz, 1994), this is an important issue. To date, such research has been limited by the lack of relevant cognitive measures. Nonetheless, recent advances have led to the development of various cognitive measures with important theoretical and practical applications.

Recent Studies of Hoarding-Specific Cognitions

Research Issues

Frost's model has been successful in organizing and assimilating anecdotal evidence and a range of findings from earlier studies. However, a number of research issues require attention. Firstly, the relative contribution of each component of the model to hoarding needs to be established. From a treatment perspective, it is important to identify those factors requiring intervention in order to make the greatest impact on hoarding behaviors. Secondly, the specificity of these beliefs to hoarding needs to be established. This is important given that hoarding has been associated with a range of other psychological conditions (e.g., anxiety, depression, OCD and OCPD), and that the beliefs associated with hoarding may also be apparent in these conditions. It is possible that a common cognitive vulnerability (e.g., perfectionism) to all or some conditions exists that makes an important contribution to hoarding-specific cognitions. If hoarding is distinct from OCD, then hoarding-specific cognitions should make a relatively greater contribution than OCD-related beliefs.

Investigation of the relative predictive utility of each of the components of the model has been hampered to date by the lack of measures assessing not only the range of cognitive factors associated with hoarding, but also the severity and range of hoarding-related behaviors. While numerous measures of OCD-related behaviors and cognitions have been developed, including the OBQ and III, none are specific to hoarding. However, this situation is currently being remedied with the development of a number of such measures outlined in the next section.

Measures of Hoarding Behavior and Hoarding-Related Cognitions

Steketee, Frost, and Kyrios (1999, 2001) described the development of various measures assessing hoarding behaviors (e.g. the Savings Inventory [SI], and the Compulsive Acquisition Scale [CAS]), and hoarding-related cognitions (e.g., the Saving Cognition Inventory [SCI] and the Frost Indecisiveness Scale [FIS]). A summary of each measure is presented below.

Savings Inventory (SI).   This version of the SI is a 28-item questionnaire designed to measure various aspects of hoarding, including: saving behaviors, time spent on saving behaviors, emotional responses to saving and throwing things away, utility of possessions, and the extent to which saving behaviors interfere with daily living and social relations. Reliability for the SI has been shown to be satisfactory in USA and Australian samples with alpha coefficients for the Total Score greater than 0.88 (Kyrios & Oh, 2000; Steketee *et al.*, 1999, 2001).

The Compulsive Acquisition Scale (CAS).   The CAS is an 18-item self-report measure of compulsive buying (12 items) and acquisition of free items (six items). Satisfactory internal consistency (α coefficients around 0.90) has been reported in studies using Australian and

American undergraduate samples, and clinical cohorts (Frost *et al.*, 1998; Kyrios & Oh, 2000; Steketee *et al.*, 1999).

Saving Cognition Inventory (SCI). The SCI is a 31-item questionnaire devised to measure beliefs represented in the Frost and Hartl (1996) model of hoarding: memory for possessions, value of possessions, control over possessions, responsibility for possessions, emotional comfort from possessions, and fears about loss of opportunities. Using a seven-point Likert Scale, subjects rate the extent to which a thought influences their decision on whether to discard a possession. The SCI consists of four subscales (Steketee *et al.*, 2001), developed on the basis of factor analysis: (a) Emotional Attachment to Possessions; (b) Memory for Possessions; (c) Control over Possessions; and (d) Responsibility for Possessions. The total scale and all subscales have shown satisfactory internal consistency in clinical and non-clinical cohorts in both the USA and Australia, with alpha coefficients of internal consistency in the 0.70 to 0.97 range (Kyrios & Oh, 2000; Steketee *et al.*, 1999, 2001).

Frost Indecisiveness Scale (FIS). The FIS is a 15-item scale containing two subscales. The Positive Attitudes subscale measures positive attitudes about decision-making, while the Fears subscale was designed to measure fears about making decisions. Internal consistencies of the subscales in both clinical and non-clinical cohorts have been reported as satisfactory with alphas around 0.90 (Kyrios & Oh, 2000; Steketee *et al.*, 1999, 2001). The FIS Fears subscale has been found to be related to hoarding and obsessive compulsive symptoms (Steketee *et al.*, 2001).

Research Findings

Steketee *et al.* (1999, 2001) examined the specificity of hypothesized hoarding-specific cognitions to hoarding behavior, as well as the relationship of more general OCD beliefs to hoarding symptoms. Data were collected from 64 subjects who reported hoarding as their main complaint (Hoarders), 21 with clinician-diagnosed OCD but no hoarding (OCD), and 40 community controls with no psychiatric symptoms. In the results reported below, although we use the terms "hoarders" and "OCD" subjects, it is important to remember that hoarders also exhibited OCD symptoms. Subjects completed a range of symptom measures (including hoarding, compulsive acquisition, OCD, depression and anxiety) and measures of OCD-related and hoarding-specific cognitions. The OBQ and III (OCCWG, 1997, 2001) were used to assess OCD-related beliefs, while the SCI and FIS Fears evaluated hoarding-specific beliefs. OCD symptoms were measured with the self-report version of the Yale–Brown Obsessive Compulsive Scale (YBOCS: Goodman *et al.*, 1989) and the Padua Inventory (Sanavio, 1988), and anxiety and depression were assessed with the Beck inventories (Beck & Steer, 1987, Beck, Epstein, Brown, & Steer, 1988).

  Hoarders exhibited higher levels of depression than OCD subjects who, in turn, were rated as more depressed than community controls. However, hoarders were not more anxious than OCD subjects, though both groups were more anxious than community controls. As expected, hoarders consistently scored higher than community controls and

OCD participants on all of the hoarding measures (SI, CAS, and SCI). OCD and community controls did not differ on these measures, with the exception of SCI Control Over Possessions on which OCD subjects scored higher than community controls. The FIS Fears subscale also discriminated hoarders from OCD and community controls, with hoarders reporting greater decision-making fears. No gender differences were found on any of these measures.

In contrast, the OBQ subscales did not discriminate hoarders from the OCD cohort, supporting the relevance of OCD-related beliefs to this group of hoarders. The hoarding subjects scored consistently higher on these measures than controls.

Convergent validity for the SCI and FIS Fears was investigated through correlations and partial correlations with symptom measures. As expected, SCI subscales correlated strongly with both measures of hoarding symptoms (i.e., SI and CAS) with correlations ranging from 0.69 to 0.74 (mean correlation of 0.71). The FIS Fears exhibited moderate correlations (0.57 and 0.52) with both hoarding measures. SCI correlations with OCD symptom measures (YBOCS and Padua Inventory) were in the moderate range (0.34 to 0.63, with a mean of 0.46). The FIS Fears also correlated moderately with the same measures (0.40 and 0.51). SCI correlations with measures of anxiety and depression were also in the moderate range, although the FIS Fears correlated in the moderate-to-high range.

A further test of convergent validity was to examine the relationships between hoarding and OCD cognition measures. The SCI exhibited moderate-to-high correlations with the OBQ (ranging from 0.32 to 0.62 with a mean of 0.45), although correlations with the III were a little lower (ranging from 0.24 to 0.46 with a mean of 0.31). Correlations were generally highest for SCI Control of Possessions. Overall, most OCD- and hoarding-related beliefs showed moderate-to-high correlations with hoarding, OCD and affective measures. As expected, the strongest relationship was between hoarding cognitions and hoarding behaviors.

Partial correlations were used to test the specificity of hoarding- and OCD-related beliefs to hoarding behaviors. When measures of depression and anxiety were partialled out, the SCI maintained moderate-to-high correlations with hoarding measures (mean partial correlation of 0.58), and moderate but lower magnitude correlations with measures of OCD symptoms and cognitions (mean partial correlation of 0.32). Likewise, when measures of OCD symptoms were partialled out, the SCI still maintained moderate-to-high correlations with hoarding measures (mean partial correlation of 0.54), but low magnitude correlations with measures of depression and anxiety (mean partial correlation of 0.12). This suggests that the relationship of hoarding cognitions to mood was better accounted for by its link to OCD. When measures of depression, anxiety and OCD symptoms were partialled out, OCD-related cognitive measures no longer correlated significantly with hoarding measures. Overall, the specificity of hoarding cognitions to hoarding behaviors and not to OCD or negative mood symptoms was confirmed. Although OCD-related beliefs were associated with hoarding behaviors, the specificity of OCD-related cognitions to hoarding behaviors was not supported; rather, OCD-related beliefs are more closely associated with OCD and affective symptoms.

Hierarchical regression using the total sample indicated that hoarding behavior was predicted by hoarding beliefs even after controlling for the effect of age, gender, mood states, obsessive compulsive symptoms, and OCD-related cognitions. In particular, emotional attachment to possessions, and concerns about memory, excessive responsibility, and control over possessions were all related to hoarding behavior. While there were some minor differences in the cognitive patterns of acquisition versus hoarding, more similarities than differences were evident. However, this study may be limited by the lack of a clinician-diagnosed hoarding cohort.

A similar Australian study with a non-clinical student sample also aimed to find evidence of a relationship between hoarding-specific cognitions and hoarding behaviors, and to examine the specificity of hoarding-related cognitions to hoarding, OCD and mood states (Kyrios & Oh, 2000). Moderate-to-high correlations were again found between hoarding behavior (SI) and hoarding-related beliefs (SCI). As expected, these correlations did not diminish when measures of anxiety, depression and obsessive compulsive symptoms were partialled out. Regression analysis revealed that emotional attachments to objects, concerns about lost opportunities and control of possessions were the best predictors of hoarding behavior.

Hierarchical regression revealed that hoarding behaviors were predicted by hoarding specific cognitions even after controlling for the effect of age, gender, mood states, obsessive compulsive symptoms and perfectionism. Although greater depression predicted more severe hoarding, hoarding cognitions were better predictors in the final regression model. In general, this study replicated findings from the USA (Steketee *et al.*, 2001). Hence, support for Frost's cognitive behavioral model has been found across similar cultural contexts, and with analogue and clinical samples.

Future Directions

Despite preliminary support for recent cognitive-behavioral conceptualizations of hoarding, a number of research issues require further attention. Frost's cognitive-behavioral model of hoarding is still in a process of development and has some limitations. For instance, it is apparent that there are substantial associations between hoarding and factors traditionally unrelated to cognitive behavioral models, such as attachment, self-concept, identity and mood. Future research will need to examine early developmental influences and related issues, including child-rearing patterns, early trauma, loss, quality of attachments, and identity.

Unpublished data using new measures assessing memories of parenting, quality of attachments and self-perceptions has supported Guidano and Liotti's (1983) post-rationalist model of obsessionality (Bhar & Kyrios, 2000; Kyrios & Bhar, 2000; Frost *et al.*, 1999). Specifically, ambivalent parenting, ambivalent and avoidant attachments, and an uncertain sense of self have been found to be associated with measures of OCD, OCPD, and hoarding. Such factors may act as underlying vulnerabilities that influence the development of relevant dysfunctional beliefs (Bhar & Kyrios, 2000). It remains unclear, however, whether such influences constitute a general vulnerability, whether they are relevant across the range of obsessional problems, or whether they pertain to the spectrum of hoarding behaviors or hoarding subtypes. For instance, while compulsive acquisition and hoarding have been found to exhibit many cognitive similarities, important differences may exist in meta-vulnerabilities. It also seems reasonable to expand the model to accommodate compulsive buying which is associated with the qualities of both obsessive-compulsive and impulse-control disorders (Schlosser, Black, Repertinger, & Freet, 1994).

Questions about social, cultural or historical influences on hoarding also need to be further addressed. Do current results reflect the characteristics of Western culture with its individualistic and materialistic orientation? Would the model be supported within more collectivist cultures (e.g., Southern European) or those with less emphasis on materialism (e.g., Eastern/Asian)? Some hoarding studies have also implicated traumatic historical events or periods, such as the Great Depression, World War II or the Holocaust, as important to the development of hoarding (Greenberg *et al.*, 1990; Shafran & Tallis, 1996; Thomas, 1997), although Frost and Gross (1993) failed to find a correlation between hoarding and material deprivation early in life. Future research will need to investigate how the experience of such events and traumas influences hoarding behavior and cognitions, and how such experiences may influence cross-cultural differences in hoarding.

Replications of recent studies need to be conducted across clinical and more representative community samples. In particular, studies with clinical cohorts have been rare. The factor structure of the SCI needs to be replicated across clinical versus non-clinical cohorts, and across different cultures. Furthermore, the structure and influence of OCD-related cognitions should be examined within cohorts exhibiting solely hoarding symptoms, as distinct from OCD cohorts with hoarding symptoms. For instance, do OCD non-hoarders, OCD hoarders, and hoarders without OCD differ in their cognitive patterns and structures? If so, differences between such groups may have important treatment implications.

The treatment implications of the Frost's model need to be examined and resulting treatments evaluated. Although initial results indicate some support (Hartl & Frost, 1999; Steketee, Frost, Wincze, Greene, & Douglas, 2000), further research is required, particularly cross-culturally. The heuristic value of the cognitive-behavioral model of hoarding lies ultimately in its ability to help us understand vulnerability factors in the development, maintenance and treatment of hoarding behaviors. Cross-cultural research can only supplement our knowledge and aid in the validation of such models.

Finally, as with most research on OCD-related cognitions, hoarding research relies on self-report and questionnaire-based methodology. Virtually no research has been undertaken using experimental methods, despite the fact that notions about associative networks, memory difficulties, and information processing deficits are closely associated with etiological models of compulsive hoarding. As outlined in earlier chapters, a rich array of experimental paradigms can be used in future research endeavors.

In summary, until recently, the study of hoarding has been neglected or encapsulated in studies of related disorders and their associated cognitive styles. This chapter has summarized studies providing evidence that hoarding is a discrete phenomenon with independent cognitive features. The empirical findings support the specificity and predictive utility of the cognitions identified in the Frost cognitive-behavioral model. Further, newly devised measures of hoarding cognitions have been developed which can be used in conjunction with the OCCWG cognitive measures in the identification of cognitive patterns relevant to individual patients presenting with hoarding in the presence or absence of OCD.

References

Abramowitz, J. (1997). Effectiveness of psychological and pharmacological treatments for obsessive–compulsive disorder: A quantitative review. *Journal of Consulting and Clinical Psychology, 65*, 44–52.

Abramowitz, J. S., & Foa, E. B. (1998). Worries and obsesions in individuals with OCD, with and without comorbid generalised anxiety disorder. *Behaviour Research and Therapy, 36*, 695–700.

American Psychiatric Association (1994). *Diagnostic and Statistical Manual of Mental Disorders (4th ed.)*. Washington DC: Author.

Antony, M. M., Purdon, C. L., Huta, V., & Swinson, R. (1998). Dimensions of perfectionism across anxiety disorders. *Behaviour Research and Therapy, 36*, 1143–1154.

Baer, L. (1994). Factor analysis of symptom sub-types of obsessive–compulsive disorder and their relation to personality and tic disorders. *Journal of Clinical Psychiatry, 55*, 18–23.

Ball, S. G., Baer, L., & Otto, M. W. (1996). Symptoms sub-types of OCD in behavioral treatment studies: A quantitative review. *Behaviour Research and Therapy, 34*, 47–51.

Beck, A. T., Epstein, N., Brown, G., & Steer, R. (1988). An inventory for measuring clinical anxiety: Psychometric properties. *Journal of Consulting and Clincal Psychology, 56*, 893–897.

Beck, A. T., & Freeman, A. (1990). *Cognitive Therapy of Personality Disorders*. New York: Guilford.

Beck, A. T., & Steer, R. (1987). *Beck Depression Inventory Manual*, NY: The Psychological Corporation, New York: Harcourt Brace Jovanovich.

Bhar, S., & Kyrios, M. (1999). Cognitive personality styles associated with depressive and obsessive compulsive phenomena in a non-clinical sample. *Behavioural and Cognitive Psychotherapy, 27*, 329–343.

Bhar, S., & Kyrios, M. (2000) *Ambivalent self-esteem as meta-vulnerability for Obsessive–Compulsive Disorder*. Paper presented at the International Conference in Self Concept: Theory, Research & Practice: Advances for the New Millennium, Sydney, Australia.

Black, D. W., Monahan, P., Gable, J., Blum, N., Clancy, G., & Baker, P. (1998). Hoarding and treatment response in 38 nondepressed subjects with OCD. *Journal of Clinical Psychiarty, 59*, 420–425.

Blurton-Jones, N. G. (1988). Tolerated theft, suggestions about the ecology and evolution of sharing, hoarding and scrounging. *Social Science Information, 26*, 31–54.

Bowlby, J. (1969). *Attachment and loss: Volume 1 Attachment*. New York: Basic Books.

Bowlby, J. (1973). *Separation and loss*. New York: Basic Books.

Calamari, J. E., Wiegartz, P. S., & Janeck, A. S. (1999). Obsessive–compulsive disorder subgroups: A symptom-base clustering approach. *Behaviour Research and Therapy, 37*, 113–125.

Christenson, G. A., Faber, R. J., de Zwall, M., Raymond, N. C., Specker, S. M. Ekern, M. D., Mackenzie, T. B., Crosby, R. D., Crow, S. J., Eckert, E. D., Mussell, M. P., & Mitchell, J. E. (1994). Compulsive buying: Descriptive characteristics and psychiatric comorbidity. *Journal of Clinical Psychiatry, 55*, 5–11.

de Brabander, J. M., de Bruin, J. P., & van Eden, C. G. (1993). Ineffectiveness of GM1 and ORG2766 on behavioral recovery after prefrontal cortical lesions in adult rats. *Pharmacology, Biochemistry and Behavior, 44*, 565–572.

Damecour, C. L., & Charron, M. (1998). Hoarding: a symptom, not a syndrome. *Journal of Clinical Psychiarty, 59*, 267–272.

Dean, P. J., & Range, L. M. (1996). The escape theory of suicide and perfectionism in college students. *Death Studies, 20*, 415–424.

Fitzgerald, P. B. (1997). "The bowerbird symptom": A case of severe hoarding of possessions. *Australian and New Zealand Journal of Psychiatry, 31*, 597–600.

Frankenburg, F. (1984). Hoarding in anorexia nervosa. *British Journal of Medical Psychology, 57*, 57–60.

Freud, S. (1908). Character and anal erotism. *In Collected Papers. (Vol.II)*. London: Hogarth.

Fromm, E. (1947). *Man for himself: An inquiry into the psychology of ethics*. New York: Rinehart.

Frost, R. O., & Gross, R. C. (1993). The hoarding of possessions. *Behaviour Research and Therapy, 31*, 367–381.

Frost, R. O., & Hartl, T. L. (1996). A cognitive–behavioral model of compulsive hoarding. *Behaviour Research and Therapy, 34*, 341–350.

Frost, R. O., Hartl, T. L., Christian, R., & Williams, N. (1995). The value of possessions in compulsive hoarding: Patterns of use and attachment. *Behaviour Research and Therapy, 33*, 897–902.

Frost, R. O., Kim, H., Morris, C., Bloss, C., Murray-Close, M., & Steketee, G. (1998). Hoarding, compulsive buying and reasons for saving. *Behaviour Research and Therapy, 36*, 657–664.

Frost, R. O., Krause, M. S., & Steketee, G. (1996). Hoarding and obsessive compulsive symptoms. *Behavior Modification, 20*, 116–132.

Frost, R. O., Krause, E., White, L., Ax, E., Chowdhry, F., Williams, L., Franz, A., Roy, K., Cote, J., Steketee, S., & Kyrios, M. (1999, November). *Compulsive hoarding: Patterns of attachment to people and possessions*. Poster presented at the meeting of the Association for Advancement of Behaviour Therapy, Toronto, Canada.

Frost, R. O., Marten, P., Lahart, C., & Rosenblate, R. (1990). The dimensions of perfectionism. *Cognitive Therapy and Research, 14*, 449–468.

Frost, R. O., & Shows, D. (1993). The nature and measurement of compulsive indecisiveness. *Behaviour Research and Therapy, 31*, 683–692.

Frost, R. O., & Steketee, G. (1997). Perfectionism in obsessive–compulsive disorder patients. *Behaviour Research and Therapy, 35*, 291–296.

Frost, R. O., & Steketee, G. (1998). Compulsive hoarding: Clinical aspects and treatment strategies. In M. A. Jenike,. L. Baer, & W. E. Minichiello (eds), *Obsessive–Compulsive Disorders: Practical Management*. St. Louis: Mosby.

Frost, R. O., & Steketee, G. (2000). Issues in the treatment of compulsive hoarding. *Cognitive and Behavioral Practice, 6*, 397–407.

Frost, R. O., Steketee, G., & Greene, K. A. I. (in press). Cognitive and behavioral treatment of compulsive hoarding. In M. H. Freeston & S. Taylor (eds), *Cognitive approaches to treating obsessions and compulsions: A clinical casebook*. Rahway, NJ: Erlbaum.

Frost, R. O., Steketee, G., Williams, L. F., & Warren, R. (2000). Mood, personality disorder symptoms and disability in obsessive compulsive hoarders: A comparison with clinical and non-clinical controls. *Behaviour Research and Therapy, 38*, 1071–1081.

Furby, L. (1978). Possessions: Toward a theory of their meaning and function throughout the life cycle. In P. B. Bates (ed.), *Life-Span Development and Behavior (Vol. 1 pp. 297–336)*. New York: Academic Press.

Goodman, W. K., Price. L. H., Rasmussen, S. A., Maqure, C., Fleischmann, R. L., Hill, C. L., Heninger, G. R., & Charney, D. S. (1989). The Yale–Brown Obsessive Compulsive Scale: Development, use, and reliability. *Archives of General Psychiatry, 46*, 1006–1011.

Greenberg, D. (1987). Compulsive hoarding. *American Journal of Psychotherapy, 41*, 409–416.

Greenberg, D., Witztum, E., & Levy, A. (1990). Hoarding as a psychiatric symptom. *Journal of Clinical Psychiatry, 51*, 417–421.

Guidano, V. F., & Liotti, G. (1983). *Cognitive Processes and Emotional Disorders*. New York: Guildford.

Hartl, T. L., & Frost, R. (1999). Cognitive–behavioral treatment of compulsive hoarding: A multiple baseline experimental case study. *Behaviour Research and Therapy, 37*, 451–461.

Hartl, T. L., Savage, C. R., Frost, R. O., Allen, G. J., Deckersbach, T., Steketee, G., & Duffany, S. R. (2000). Actual and perceived memory deficits among individuals with hoarding symptoms. Unpublished manuscript.

Hewitt, P. L., Flett, G. L., & Turnbull-Donovan, W. (1993). Perfectionism and suicide potential. *British Journal of Clinical Psychology, 31*, 181–190.

Hewitt, P. L., Newton, J., & Flett, G. L. (1997). Perfectionism and suicide ideation in adolescent psychiatric patients. *Journal of Abnormal Child Psychology, 25*, 95–101.

Hohagen, F., & Berger, M. (1998). New perspectives in research and treatment of obsessive–compulsive disorder. *British Journal of Psychiatry, 173* (suppl. 35), 1–6.

Hwang, J. P., Tsai, S. J., Yang, C. H., Liu, K. M., & Lirng, J. F. (1998). Hoarding behaviour in dementia: A preliminary report. *American Journal of Geriatric Psychiatry, 6*, 285–289.

Kottler, J. A. (1999). *Exploring and Treating Acquisitive Desire: Living in the Material World.* Thousand Oaks, CA: Sage Publications.

Kyrios, M. (1998). The cognitive and behavioural treatment of obsessive compulsive personality and other phenomena. In. C. Perris & P. D. McGorry (eds), *Cognitive Psychotherapy of Psychiatric and Personality Disorders* (pp. 351–378). West Sussex: Wiley.

Kyrios, M., & Bhar, S. (2000). *Patterns of attachment, identity and memories of parenting in obsessive-compulsive and related disorders: Exploring theoretical associations using the Early Developmental Influences Inventory (EDII) in a non-clinical sample.* Paper in preparation.

Kyrios, M., & Oh, S. (2000). *Specific cognitive patterns associated with hoarding in a non-clinical sample.* Paper presented at the meeting of the Australian Association for Cognitive and Behavioral Therapies, Melbourne, Australia.

Kyrios, M., Wainwright, K., Purcell, R., Pantelis, C., & Maruff, P. (1999, November). *Neuropsychological predictors of outcome following cognitive-behavior therapy for obsessive–compulsive disorder: A pilot study.* Paper presented at the meeting of the Association for the Advancement of Behavior Therapy, Toronto.

Leckman, J. F., Grice, D. E., Boardman, J., Zhang, H., Vitale, A., Bondi, C., Alsobrook, J., Peterson, B. S., Cohen, D. J., Rasmussen, S. A., Goodman, W. K., McDougle, C. J., & Pauls, D. L. (1997). Symptoms of OCD. *American Journal of Psychiatry, 154*, 911–917.

Lejoyeux, M., Tassain, V., Solomon, J., & Ades, J. (1997). Study of compulsive buying in depressed patients. *Journal of Clinical Psychiatry, 58*, 169–173.

Mataix-Cols, D., Rauch, S., Manzo, P., Jenike, M., & Baer, L. (1999). Use of factor-analyzed symptom dimensions to predict outcome with serotonin reuptake inhibitors and placebo in the treatment of obsessive–compulsive disorder. *American Journal of Psychiatry, 156*, 1409–1416.

Minarik, M. L., & Ahrens, A. H. (1996). Relations of eating behaviour and symptoms of depression and anxiety to dimensions of perfectionism among undergraduate women. *Cognitive Therapy and Research, 20*, 155–169.

Obsessive Compulsive Cognitions Working Group (1997). Cognitive assessment of obsessive–compulsive disorder. *Behaviour Research and Therapy, 35*, 667–681.

Obsessive Compulsive Cognitions Working Group (2001). Development and initial validation of the Obsessive Beliefs Questionnaire and the Interpretation of Intrusions Inventory. *Behaviour Research and Therapy, 39*, 987–1006.

Purcell, R., Maruff, P., Kyrios, M., & Pantelis, C. (1998). Neuropsychological deficits in obsessive–compulsive disorder: A comparison with unipolar depression, panic disorder, and normal controls. *Archives in General Psychiatry, 55*, 415–423.

Rachman, S. (1993). Obsessions, responsibility and guilt. *Behaviour Research and Therapy, 31*, 149–154.

Rachman, S. (1997). A cognitive theory of obsessions. *Behaviour Research and Therapy, 35*, 793–802.

Rachman, S. (1998). A cognitive theory of obsessions: Elaborations. *Behaviour Research and Therapy, 36*, 385–401.

Rapoport, J. L. (1989). *The boy who couldn't stop washing: The experiences and treatment of obsessive–compulsive disorder.* New York: E. P. Dutton.

Rhéaume, J., Freeston, M. H., Dugas, M. J., Letarte, H., & Ladouceur, R. (1995). Perfectionism, responsibility and OC symptoms. *Behaviour Research and Therapy, 33*, 785–795.

Rosenthal, M., Stelian, J., Wagner, J., & Berkman, P. (1999). Diogenes syndrome and hoarding in the elderly: Case reports. *Israel Journal of Psychiatry and Related Sciences, 36*, 29–34.

Salkovskis, P. M. (1985). Obsessive-compulsive problems: A cognitive–behavioral analysis. *Behaviour Research and Therapy, 23*, 571–584.

Salzman, L. (1973). *The obsessive personality: Origins, dynamics and therapy.* NY: Jason Aronson.

Sanavio, E. (1988). Obsessions and compulsions: The Padua Inventory. *Behaviour Research and Therapy, 26*, 169–177.

Savage, C. R., Deckersbach, T., Wilhelm, S., Rauch, S. L., Baer, L., Reid, T., & Jenike, M. A. (2000). Strategic processing and episodic memory impairment in obsessive–compulsive disorder. *Neuro-psychology, 14*, 141–151.

Schlosser, S., Black, D. W., Repertinger, S., & Freet, D. (1994). Compulsive buying: Demography, phenomenology, and comorbidity in 46 subjects. *General Hospital Psychiatry, 16*, 205–212.

Shafran, R., & Tallis, F. (1996). Obsessive compulsive hoarding: A cognitive–behavioral approach. *Behavioural and Cognitive Psychotherapy, 24*, 209–221.

Smith, J. P. (1990). *Mammalian behaviour: The theory and the science.* Tuckahoe, NY: Bench Mark Books.

Stein, D. J., Seedat, S., & Potocnik, F. (1999). Hoarding: A review. *Israel Journal of Psychiatry and Related Sciences, 36*, 35–46.

Steketee, G., Frost, R. O., & Kim, H. J. (2001). Hoarding by elderly people. *Health and Social Care, 26*, 176–184.

Steketee, G., Frost, R. O., & Kyrios, M. (1999, November). *Cognitive Features of Hoarding.* Paper presented at the meeting of the Association for Advancement of Behavior Therapy, Toronto, Canada.

Steketee, G., Frost, R. O., & Kyrios, M. (2001). Beliefs and Decision-making about Possessions among Compulsive Hoarders. Manuscript submitted for publication.

Steketee, G., Frost, R. O., Wincze, J., Greene, K. A. I., & Douglas, H. (2000). Group and individual treatment of compulsive hoarding: A pilot study. *Behavioural and Cognitive Psychotherapy, 28*, 259–268.

Stern, C. E., & Passingham, R. E. (1994). The nucleus accumbens in monkeys (Macaca fascicularis): I. The organization of behaviour. *Behaviour Brain Research, 61*, 9–21.

Summerfeldt, L. J., Richter, M. A., Antony, M. M., & Swinson, R. P. (1999). Symptom structure in obsessive–compulsive disorder: A confirmatory factor analytic study. *Behaviour Research and Therapy, 37*, 297–311.

Thomas, N. D. (1997). Hoarding: Eccentricity or pathology: When to intervene? *Journal of Gerontological Social Work, 29*, 45–55.

Tracy, J. I., de Leon, J., Qureshi, G., McCann, E. M., McGrory, A., & Josiassen, R. C. (1996). Repetitive patterns in schizophrenia: A single disturbance or discrete symptoms? *Schizophrenia Research, 20*, 221–229.

van Balkom, A., de Haan, E., van Oppen, P., Spinhoven, P., Hoogduin, K. A. L., & van-Dyck, R. (1998). Cognitive and behavioral therapies alone versus in combination with fluvoxamine in the treatment of obsessive–compulsive disorder. *Journal of Nervous & Mental Diseases, 186*, 492–499.

van Balkom, A., van Oppen, P., Vermeulen, A., van Dyck, R., Nauta, M., & Vorst, H. (1994).

A meta-analysis on the treatment of obsessive–compulsive disorder: A comparison of anti-depressants, behavior and cognitive therapy. *Clinical Psychology Review, 14*, 359–381.

van Oppen, P., & Arntz, A. (1994). Cognitive therapy for obsessive–compulsive disorder, *Behaviour Research & Therapy, 32*, 79–87.

Whishaw, I. Q., & Kornelsen, R. A. (1993). Two types of motivation revealed by ibotenic acid nucleus accumbens lesions: Dissociation of food carrying and hoarding and the role of primary and incentive motivation. *Behaviour Brain Research, 55 (Special Issue)*, 283–295.

Winsberg M. E., Cassic, K. S., & Koran, M. (1999). Hoarding in obsessive–compulsive disorder: A report of 20 cases. *Journal of Clinical Psychiatry, 60*, 591–597.

Commentary on Cognition in Disorders Related to Obsessive Compulsive Disorder

Martin M. Antony

Distinguishing Obsessive Compulsive Disorder (OCD) from other conditions is often a challenge, in part because of the heterogeneous nature of this condition as well as the symptom overlap between OCD and other psychological disorders. The chapters in this section discuss the relationship between OCD and several other conditions including body dysmorphic disorder (BDD), eating disorders, depression, schizophrenia, and compulsive hoarding. The focus in each of these chapters is on the similarities and differences between OCD and each of these conditions, with a special emphasis on cognitive features. Depression is relevant primarily because of its frequent co-occurrence with OCD. Other problems, such as BDD and eating disorders, have been considered by some researchers to be variants of OCD. Schizophrenia and psychotic disorders are discussed with respect to their continuity with OCD, particularly on the dimension of insight. Finally, compulsive hoarding, although often considered a feature of OCD, also has unique characteristics and can occur in the context of other psychological disorders such as obsessive compulsive personality disorder (OCPD) and eating disorders (Kyrios, Steketee, Frost, & Oh, 2002).

Several relevant topics were not included among the chapters in this section. First, a number of disorders usually considered part of the obsessive compulsive (OC) spectrum are not featured in this volume. The most important of these include tic disorders, hypochondriasis, and certain impulse control disorders (e.g., trichotillomania, compulsive skin picking) (see Black, 1998; Goldsmith, Shapira, Phillips, & McElroy, 1998). In addition, this section of the book does not include a chapter on the relationship between OCD and other anxiety disorders often associated with it, such as social phobia and generalized anxiety disorder (see Brown, 1998).

Determining the Boundaries of the OC Spectrum

For more than a decade, it has been recognized that a wide range of disorders are related to OCD, both with respect to clinical features and in some cases shared etiologies. Eric Hollander (Hollander, 1998; Hollander & Wong, 2000), one of the most influential proponents of the notion of an OCD spectrum, has described three broad categories of OC spectrum disorders: (a) disorders involving preoccupation with bodily appearance and sensations (e.g., BDD, eating disorders, hypochondriasis); (b) impulse control disorders

Cognitive Approaches to Obsessions and Compulsions – Theory, Assessment, and Treatment
Copyright © 2002 by Elsevier Science Ltd.
All rights of reproduction in any form reserved.
ISBN: 0-08-043410-X

(e.g., pathological gambling, trichotillomania, sexual compulsions, self-injurious behaviors, kleptomania, compulsive shopping); and (c) neurological disorders with compulsive features (e.g., autism, Tourette's disorder). In Hollander's previous writings (e.g., Hollander & Wong, 1995), OCD was seen to overlap with as many as eight different broad categories of psychological disorder.

Hollander (2000) argued that inclusion in the OC spectrum should be based on overlap with OCD on five primary dimensions: (a) symptom profile (e.g., intrusive thoughts, repetitive behaviors); (b) associated features (e.g., demographics, family history, course, comorbidity); (c) neurobiology; (d) response to empirically-supported OCD treatments; and (e) etiology (e.g., genetics, environmental factors). What is clear from the relevant chapters in this volume is that overlap in the underlying cognitive features of the disorder with OCD should also play a role in determining whether a particular problem belongs in the OC Spectrum. For example, Yaryura-Tobias and McKay (2002) highlight some of the cognitive features shared by individuals with OCD and schizophrenia, including disordered thinking, confusion of thought with action, and superstitious thinking.

Although Hollander (2000) described five dimensions that can be used to determine whether a particular disorder should be considered part of the OC spectrum, it is unclear whether some dimensions are more important than others. One of the challenges in deciding whether a particular disorder belongs in the OC spectrum is determining whether the relationship between OCD and the other disorder reflects a shared etiology (and perhaps a tendency to respond to similar treatments), versus simply a more superficial overlap in symptoms. For example, although substance use disorders, like OCD, are associated with ruminative thoughts (e.g., about obtaining the substance) that motivate repetitive behaviors (e.g., excessive use of the substance), most investigators agree that substance use disorders do not belong in the OC spectrum. OCD and substance use appear to be related to different psychological and biological processes, and they respond to somewhat different treatments. In addition, substance use disorders are not particularly prevalent among OCD sufferers, relative to individuals with other anxiety disorders.

For other conditions, such as tic disorders (e.g., Tourette's Syndrome), the relationship with OCD is better established. Tic disorders and OCD appear to run in the same families, respond to similar medications, and often occur comorbidly (see Koran, 1999 for a review). In fact, the rates of OCD are higher in relatives of Tourette's sufferers even when the relatives do not themselves have Tourette's. This is not the case for most other psychological disorders, suggesting that the relationship between OCD and Tourette's may have a particularly strong genetic basis (Pauls, Leckman, & Cohen, 1994).

Future Directions for Research on OC Spectrum Disorders

Although there is much speculation about the relationship between OCD and various conditions included in the OC spectrum, much more work needs to be done to establish which of these disorders is truly related to OCD in a meaningful or relevant way. Understanding the relationship between OC spectrum disorders and OCD is likely to lead to an improved understanding of the underlying factors that contribute to OCD and spectrum conditions, development of better treatments for these disorders, and development of unique treatments for individuals suffering from both OCD and one or more spectrum disorders. In particular, we need to develop an improved understanding of the similarities and differences between OCD and spectrum disorders with respect to heritability and familial transmission, developmental factors, course, patterns of comorbidity, cognitive features, and response to psychological and pharmacological treatments.

The study of OC spectrum disorders may also help us to identify important dimensions and subtypes that comprise OCD. For example, the study of the relationship between OCD and psychotic disorders should lead to a better understanding of OCD patients with poor insight and the best ways to treat these individuals. Similarly, studying the relationship between OCD and OCPD should improve our understanding of OCD features that are shared with OCPD, such as perfectionism, a need for symmetry, order, and exactness, and a drive to experience a "just right" feeling.

An important question that has not been adequately addressed is whether OC spectrum disorders are uniquely related to OCD or whether they are also related to other forms of psychopathology. For example, although there is evidence that certain spectrum disorders occur more frequently in people with OCD than in non-clinical samples, very few studies have examined the frequency of OC spectrum disorders in OCD versus other anxiety disorders. An exception is a recent study by Richter, Summerfeldt, Antony, and Swinson (2001), which found that although there were no differences in the frequency of eating disorder symptoms across groups of individuals with OCD, social phobia, and panic disorder, features of tic disorders (e.g., motor tics, vocal tics) and impulse control disorders (e.g., skin picking, hair pulling) were more common among individuals with OCD than among those with social phobia and panic. Nonetheless, some investigators have questioned whether trichotillomania should be considered part of the OC spectrum. Stanley, Swann, Bowers, Davis, and Taylor (1992) argued that trichotillomania is not best considered a variant of OCD, based on a comparison of the clinical features. Himle, Bordnick, and Thyer (1995) drew similar conclusions in a subsequent study.

Investigators have also raised questions about whether there is a unique relationship between BDD and OCD. Although BDD shares features with OCD (e.g., checking, avoidance, preoccupation and rumination, occasional poor insight), its features also overlap considerably with social phobia (Wilhelm & Neziroglu, 2002). In fact, Wilhelm, Otto, Zucker, and Pollack (1997) found that BDD was most commonly diagnosed among individuals with social phobia (12 percent) and less often in other anxiety disorders such as OCD (7.7 percent), GAD (6.7 percent), and panic disorder (1.5 percent). These findings confirmed those from a previous study (Brawman-Mintzer et al., 1995) in which the percentage of individuals with social phobia who also had BDD was 11 percent. The figures for OCD and panic disorders were 8 percent and 2 percent, respectively. No patients with GAD, major depression, or normal controls had BDD (Brawman-Mintzer et al., 1995).

One question raised by Shafran (2002) is whether OCD patients who are high in perfectionism develop other perfectionism-related disorders. If this is true, it is also possible that perfectionism is an underlying causal feature shared by various OC spectrum disorders as well as disorders that often co-occur with OCD. Comorbidity data from our Center and others support a relationship among disorders associated with perfectionism. OCD is frequently associated with social phobia, depression, and eating disorders (Antony, Downie, & Swinson, 1998; Sanderson, Di Nardo, Rapee, & Barlow, 1990; Yaryura-Tobias *et al.*, 1996), and all of these conditions have been shown to be associated with elevated levels of perfectionism (Antony, Purdon, Huta, & Swinson, 1998, Garner, Olmstead, & Polivy,1983; Hewitt & Flett, 1993).

Summary and Conclusion

In summary, there are several challenges to be met in the area of OC spectrum disorders. First, the boundaries of the OC spectrum need to be better defined. More systematic research is needed on the relationship between OCD and various spectrum disorders, especially with respect to etiology, treatment response, and other theoretically important features. In addition, future studies need to address the question of whether OC spectrum disorders are uniquely associated with OCD, or whether they overlap with other conditions as well. We also need to better understand the variables that may contribute to the frequent co-occurrence of OCD and related disorders, such as perfectionism.

Finally, new integrated treatments need to be developed for individuals who suffer from both OCD and one or more related disorders. To date, treatment protocols have tended to focus exclusively on one particular disorder, despite the fact, that most people with OCD have considerable comorbidity. Treatments that target multiple problems may lead to greater improvement, both in the short term and over the long term.

References

Antony, M. M., Downie, F., & Swinson, R. P. (1998). Diagnostic issues and epidemiology in obsessive compulsive disorder. In R. P. Swinson, M. M. Antony, S. Rachman, & M. A. Richter (eds), *Obsessive compulsive disorder: Theory, research and treatment* (pp. 3–32). New York: Guilford.

Antony, M. M., Purdon, C., Huta, V., & Swinson, R. P. (1998). Dimensions of perfectionism across the anxiety disorders. *Behaviour Research and Therapy*, *36*, 1143–1154.

Black, D. (1998). Recognition and treatment of obsessive compulsive spectrum disorders. In R. P. Swinson, M. M. Antony, S. Rachman, & M. A. Richter (eds), *Obsessive compulsive disorder: Theory, research, and treatment* (pp. 426–458). New York: Guilford.

Brawman-Mintzer, O., Lydiard, R. B., Phillips, K. A., Morton, A., Czepowicz, V., Emmanuael, N., Villareal, G., Johnson, M., & Ballenger, J. C. (1995). Body dysmorphic disorder in patients with anxiety disorders and major depression: A comorbidity study. *American Journal of Psychiatry*, *152*, 1665–1667.

Brown, T. A. (1998). The relationship between OCD and other anxiety-based disorders. In R. P. Swinson, M. M. Antony, S. Rachman, & M. A. Richter (eds), *Obsessive compulsive disorder: Theory, research, and treatment* (pp. 207–228). New York: Guilford.

Garner, D. M., Olmstead, M. P., & Polivy, J. (1983). Development and validation of a multidimensional eating disorder inventory for anorexia nervosa and bulimia. *International Journal of Eating Disorders*, *2*, 15-34.

Goldsmith, T., Shapira, A., Phillips, K. A., & McElroy, S. L. (1998). Conceptual foundations of obsessive compulsive spectrum disorders. In R. P. Swinson, M. M. Antony, S. Rachman, & M. A. Richter (eds), *Obsessive compulsive disorder: Theory, research, and treatment* (pp. 397–425). New York: Guilford.

Hewitt, P. L., & Flett, G. L. (1993). Dimensions of perfectionism, daily stress, and depression: a test of a specific vulnerability hypothesis. *Journal of Abnormal Psychology, 102*, 58–65.

Himle, J. A., Bordnick, P. S., & Thyer, B. A. (1995). A comparison of trichotillomania and obsessive compulsive disorder. *Journal of Psychopathology and Behavioral Assessment, 17*, 251–260.

Hollander, E. (1998). Treatment of obsessive compulsive spectrum disorders with SSRIs. *British Journal of Psychiatry, 173* (suppl. 35), 7–12.

Hollander, E., & Wong, C. M. (1995). Introduction: Obsessive compulsive spectrum disorders. *Journal of Clinical Psychiatry, 56* (suppl. 4), 3–6.

Hollander, E., & Wong, C. M. (2000). Spectrum, boundary, and subtyping issues: Implications for treatment-refractory obsessive compulsive disorder. In W. K. Goodman, M. V. Rudorfer, & J. D. Maser (eds), Obsessive compulsive disorder: Contemporary issues in treatment (pp. 3–22). Mahwah, NJ: Erlbaum.

Koran, L. M. (1999). *Obsessive compulsive and related disorders in adults: A comprehensive clinical guide.* New York: Cambridge University Press.

Kyrios, M., Steketee, G., Frost, R. O., & Oh, S. (2002). Cognitions in compulsive hoarding. In R. O. Frost & G. Steketee (eds), *Cognitive approaches to obsessions and compulsions: Theory, assessment and treatment.* (pp. 269–289). Oxford: Elsevier.

Pauls, D. L., Leckman, J. F., & Cohen, D. J. (1994). Evidence against a genetic relationship between Tourette's syndrome and anxiety, depression, panic and phobic disorders. *British Journal of Psychiatry, 164*, 215–221.

Richter, M. A., Summerfeldt, L. J., Antony, M. M., & Swinson, R. P. (2001). *Obsessive compulsive spectrum conditions in obsessive compulsive disorder and other anxiety disorders.* Submitted for publication.

Sanderson, W. C., Di Nardo, P. A., Rapee, R. M., & Barlow, D. H. (1990). Syndrome comorbidity in patients diagnosed with a DSM-III-R anxiety disorder. *Journal of Abnormal Psychology, 99*, 308–312.

Shafran, R. (2002). Eating disorders and obsessive compulsive disorder. In R. O. Frost & G. Steketee (eds), *Cognitive approaches to obsessions and compulsions: Theory, assessment and treatment.* (pp. 215–231). Oxford: Elsevier.

Stanley, M. A., Swann, A. C., Bowers, T. C., Davis, M. L., & Taylor, D. J. (1992). A comparison of clinical features in trichotillomania and obsessive compulsive disorder. *Behaviour Research and Therapy, 30*, 39–44.

Wilhelm, S., & Neziroglu, F. (2002). Cognitive model of body dysmorphic disorder. In R. O. Frost & G. Steketee (eds), *Cognitive approaches to obsessions and compulsions: Theory, assessment and treatment.* (pp. 203–214). Oxford: Elsevier.

Wilhelm, S., Otto, M. W., Zucker, B. G., & Pollack, M. H. (1997). Prevalence of body dysmorphic disorder in patients with anxiety disorders. *Journal of Anxiety Disorders, 11*, 499–502.

Yaryura-Tobias, J., & McKay, D. (2002). OCD and schizophrenia: A cognitive perspective of shard pathology. In R. O. Frost & G. Steketee (eds), *Cognitive approaches to obsessions and compulsions: Theory, assessment and treatment.* (pp. 251–267). Oxford: Elsevier.

Yaryura-Tobias, J. A., Todaro, J., Grunes, M. S., Mckay, D., Stockman, R., & Neziroglu, F. A. (1996, November). *Comorbidity versus continuum of Axis I disorders in OCD.* Paper presented at the annual meeting of the Association for Advancement of Behavior Therapy, New York, NY.

Section D

Cognition in Selected OCD Populations

Chapter 16

Cognitive Aspects of Obsessive Compulsive Disorder in Children

Ingrid Söchting and John S. March

Introduction

Obsessive compulsive disorder (OCD) in children and adolescents looks remarkably similar to the disorder in adults. Indeed, the diagnostic criteria according to the Diagnostic and Statistical Manual of Mental Disorders (DSM-IV; American Psychiatric Association, 1994) are identical, with the exception of the criterion of insight. Unlike adults, children are not required to have insight into their obsessions and compulsions. In other words, children are not expected to recognize that their obsessions and compulsions are unreasonable and due to a psychiatric disorder.

Prevalence of OCD among children and adolescents has been assessed using both community samples and clinical samples. Prevalence estimates using community samples have ranged from 1.9 percent in a United States sample comprised of 9th to 12th grade students (Flament et al., 1988) to 4.1 to 10 percent in a Danish sample of 11–17-year-old school children (Thomsen, 1993). Prevalence estimates using clinical samples have been somewhat lower, ranging from 0.2 to 1.2 percent in a United States sample (Hollingworth, Tanguay, Grossman, & Pabst, 1980) to 1.3 percent in a Danish sample (Thomsen & Mikkelsen, 1991) and 5 percent in a Japanese sample (Honjo et al., 1989). These estimates are likely to be somewhat lower than the population prevalence rate considering that only 25 percent of youth with OCD present for treatment from a mental health professional (Whitaker et al., 1990).

In clinical samples, the average age of onset has ranged from 7.5 to 11.6 years (Hollingworth et al., 1980; Thomsen & Mikkelsen, 1991). In patients seen at the National Institute of Mental Health, the modal age at onset was seven and the mean age at onset was 10.2, implying an early onset group and a group with onset in adolescence (Swedo, Rapoport, Leonard, Lenane, & Cheslow, 1989). Boys were more likely to have pre-pubertal onset and to have a family member with OCD or Tourette's disorder, whereas girls were more likely to experience the onset of OCD during adolescence. In the Flament et al. epidemiological study of 9th to 12th grade students, the ratio of males to females was 1:1 (Flament et al., 1988). This is equivalent to the ratio in adults and likely reflects the tendency for the male to female ratio to equalize during adolescence. For unclear reasons,

OCD is more common in Caucasian than African-American children in clinical samples, although epidemiological data suggest no differences in prevalence as a function of ethnicity or geographic region (Rasmussen & Tsuang, 1986).

As is the case for adults, the course of OCD in children is usually gradual and waxes and wanes depending on perceived stress in the child's life. In the absence of treatment, spontaneous recovery is rare, and, in fact, a diagnosis of OCD in childhood is associated with an increased risk for developing other anxiety, mood or personality disorders (Thomsen & Mikkelsen, 1993).

Although there is strong empirical support for the efficacy of cognitive–behavioral treatment for adults with OCD, the support for this treatment modality in children and adolescents is preliminary at this time due to insufficient controlled studies evaluating treatment outcome. Cognitive–behavioral treatment for children and adolescents has included mainly behavioral interventions in the form of graded exposure to the feared stimulus with prevention of the compulsive behavior, that is, exposure and response prevention (ERP). Single case studies have suggested that behavioral interventions based on the principles of exposure and response prevention may be successful in substantially reducing OCD symptoms during a three month treatment period (Francis, 1988; March & Mulle, 1995). Although the behavioral treatment of children is often referred to as cognitive-behavioral, the behavioral component is the primary driving force. To date, there is limited information regarding children that specifically addresses cognitive interventions as distinct from exposure and response prevention in children. In contrast, the research literature pertaining to cognitions in adult OCD is more extensive.

Based on the formulation of the cognitive model of OCD (Salkovskis, 1985, 1989), several cognitive features, most importantly the faulty appraisals of obsessions, have been identified and are in the process of further examination as a result of the work of the Obsessive Compulsive Cognitions Working Group (OCCWG, 1997). This work may lead to the development of cognitive interventions that specifically target faulty appraisals. The term 'faulty appraisal' refers to the process of appraising or evaluating the presence and/or content of obsessions in a manner that is unrealistic and illogical. For example, an OCD patient may have a faulty appraisal involving a belief that having an image of a loved one being in a car accident makes it more likely to occur in reality; and that the more images he or she has about the accident, the greater the likelihood of the accident actually occurring. An appropriate cognitive intervention would be to design an experiment with the patient to test the belief that thoughts can influence actual outcomes. The patient may be asked to think about a toaster breaking down and then assess whether this thought, in fact, caused the toaster to malfunction. The outcome of the experiment would be reviewed with the patient who would be assisted in drawing more realistic conclusions about the powers of his or her thoughts.

This chapter will review the role of cognitions in children and adolescents who have been diagnosed with OCD. We will then discuss possible avenues for including cognitive strategies in both the assessment and treatment of children with OCD. Of particular note will be the ways in which cognitive interventions may play a role in the motivation of children to adhere to an exposure and response prevention treatment regime. We conclude by offering some recommendations for future work on the role of cognitions in childhood OCD. Throughout the chapter we will use the term childhood OCD or child when referring to both children and adolescents. Although we recognize that the disorder may look quite different in a 6-year-old compared to a 16-year-old, the majority of the existing work on this topic has not made distinctions between younger and older children.

Cognitive Features of OCD in Children

The cognitive phenomenology of OCD, with particular attention to risk assessment and personal responsibility, has received increasing amounts of attention since Salkovskis' (1985) initial formulation. Faulty beliefs seen in adults include an inflated misperception of the chance that one may be responsible for serious harm to others either by engaging in certain risky activities or by failing to take preventive measures. Although faulty beliefs related to inflated responsibility have been, and continue to be, the primary focus of attention from a research perspective, other kinds of OCD-related beliefs have been identified as well. For example, an over-estimation of danger and the over-importance attached to certain thoughts (obsessions) are other kinds of faulty beliefs leading to an urge to neutralize by engaging in compulsive rituals. So far, six kinds of faulty beliefs have been identified and summarized by the Obsessive Compulsive Cognitions Working Group (OCCWG; 1997): (a) over-importance of thoughts; (b) importance of controlling one's thoughts; (c) perfectionism; (d) inflated responsibility; (e) over-estimation of threat; and (f) intolerance of uncertainty .

In addition to these general belief domains which are believed to be consistent across contexts, certain domains also capture appraisals or interpretations of proximal intrusive thoughts, images or impulses. The OCCWG (1997, 2001) has proposed three such domains: responsibility, importance of thoughts, and control of thoughts. That is, when cognitive intrusions (thoughts, images, or impulses) are actively occurring, they are likely to be misinterpreted by those with OCD as signaling that this particular idea is very important, that the person is responsible for the thought or its outcome, and that he/she should control the thought. It is possible that other belief domains, in addition to the three so far identified by the OCCWG, may also be problematic for OCD appraisal processes. In particular, general beliefs involving an over-estimation of threat appear to also give rise to specific (mis)interpretations of intrusive thoughts, images or impulses.

From our work with children, the following examples demonstrate that OCD in children may involve equivalent faulty beliefs or appraisals, although the content will obviously be child-appropriate. A 13-year-old boy was brought to treatment due to obsessions without overt rituals. His obsessions involved recurring images of a dead animal he and his family had encountered once when driving in their car. The images were sufficiently frequent and severe to consume up to five hours per day and interfered with his arriving at school on time and completing assignments in a timely manner. He felt he had no control over the images and attempted to neutralize them by engaging in a mental ritual of rewinding the image. This neutralizing would, at times, lead to new obsessions regarding whether he had rewound the image "perfectly". Treatment proceeded using primarily behavioral interventions of exposure to the image using both visual expressions as well as loop tapes. During the course of therapy, concerns regarding responsibility emerged. He expressed fears about whether he was responsible for the death of the animal because he had failed to warn the driver of the car (inflated responsibility). He rated the strength of his belief in being responsible for the animal's death as 50 percent. To address this problem, cognitive interventions were subsequently incorporated into the behavioral ones. In addition to demonstrating that children may engage in faulty appraisals of their obsessions much like adults, this example also highlights the benefit of inquiring during initial assessment about the meaning (i.e., the appraisal or interpretation) a child attaches to a particular obsession. The example also shows that cognitive appraisals and faulty beliefs may be fairly subtle and not readily apparent in the content of a particular obsession.

Another example involved a 14-year-old boy whose OCD required him to repeat routine activities such as putting on socks and shoes in order to prevent a bad outcome. The bad outcome was becoming a loser and an unpopular person in school. The belief identified in this case was an over-estimation of the probability of a feared outcome occurring (over-estimation of threat). Finally, an example of thought–action fusion, a subtype of beliefs about over-importance of thoughts, was identified in a 16-year-old boy who had images of causing harm to others. This was extremely upsetting as he believed that having these thoughts made them more likely to come true. This had negative implications for his social interactions at an age where such interactions are important for social adjustment and identity development.

Developmental Issues Pertaining to Cognitive Distortions in OCD

Surprisingly, little attention has been devoted to how cognitive development may influence the etiology of the obsessional process. Is there a cognitive developmental pathway to OCD? Drawing on what we know to date about normal cognitive development in children, some researchers have suggested the possibility that children at risk for developing OCD may be stuck at what could be termed a pre-rational stage of cognitive development.

In normal cognitive development, the child progresses through a series of stages involving moving from viewing the world in fairly concrete ways to an ability to understand abstract concepts and reasoning. According to Strauman and Higgins (1993), a child's cognitive development can also be characterized by being increasingly able to differentiate himself/herself from others and the external world. In the pre-school child, egocentricity prevails and the distinction between self and reality is blurred. This inevitably involves the problem of over-estimating the influence of one's own and other's actions on the environment. For example, young children are prone to thinking that by "kissing it better", the pain in a body part will disappear. Or, they may ask their mother to "stop the rain". In pre-adolescence and adolescence, children are progressively better able to separate their own perspectives from the external reality. Also, the world is perceived as complex, but both this complexity and ambiguity are tolerated. This is evident in how healthy adolescents can offer complex inferences about the psychological states of others and about causal attributions (Damon & Hart, 1986). For example, unlike the adolescent described above, a healthy 13-year-old will typically not attribute the accidental death of an animal on the road to himself or herself (over-estimation of responsibility), but will likely list several factors contributing to the accident.

In contrast to the above scenario of healthy development, clinicians have long noted that children afflicted with OCD are different. As early as 1966, Zetzel proposed that the obsessive compulsive child thinks in terms of inexorable either-or categories as a result of a failure to integrate emotions that are initially experienced as mutually exclusive, such as love and hate. As pointed out by Kessler (1988), the obsessive compulsive child tries to establish a simplicity characteristic of a very young child. According to Bolton (1996) who conducted a comprehensive review of developmental issues in OCD, this pre-rational and simplistic way of thinking, characteristic of young children, is quite similar to the thinking of both children and adults with OCD. Just as pre-schoolers tend to over-estimate their influence on their environment and rely on magic for solutions to some problems, so does the OCD patient. The OCD patient holds an illusion of control by engaging in ritualized actions in order to solve problems. One hypothesis, then, according to Bolton (1996), is that young children respond to negative, uncontrollable events by adopting a magical system of cognition in which they believe they can influence events by ritualized action. If the anxiety and the perceived threat of danger are intense and unresolved, and if rationality failed to modify the pre-rational strategy, the result would begin to look something like OCD.

Although this account of OCD as a failure to abandon a pre-rational approach to the world is fairly consistent with our current cognitive model for OCD, we are still not in a position to explain the mechanism by which this would occur. We also cannot account for late onset OCD, unless it is assumed that an earlier pre-rational strategy can become re-activated at a later time. Our current cognitive interventions are, however, logically consistent with this developmental account of OCD in that they include teaching and modeling of more rationally-based coping strategies (Kendall *et al.*, 1991). Indeed, as will be apparent in the section on treatment, all cognitive interventions are designed to promote coping strategies based on rational and logical reasoning.

Cognitive Assessment

Based on a survey of the literature to date, no assessment methods specifically target the cognitive features of OCD in children, with perhaps one exception. Hence, information about the cognitive features in each child-OCD case is gathered using existing methods such as a comprehensive clinical interview and standardized tests assessing symptom presence and severity. However, expanding the standard clinical interview and the standard tests with a cognitive-behavioral case formulation may provide a useful way to gather more information about the particular beliefs and faulty appraisals involved in a child's OCD. Below, we briefly review standard assessment methods which do not specifically inquire about beliefs, followed by a description of the case-formulation approach which specifically addresses cognitive phenomena such as beliefs about the meaning of obsessions.

Initially, the child is assessed using a clinical interview that includes both the child and the parents and covers Axis I through V of the DSM-IV (see March & Mulle, 1998). March and his team also use the Conners-March Developmental Questionnaire (Conners & March, 1996) sent to the family for completion prior to the initial assessment session. This questionnaire covers information pertaining to both the presenting problem and its history, as well as to the child's and the family's psycho-social history and adjustment. It is useful to review as much information as possible prior to the assessment in order to be both more efficient and effective.

As part of the clinical interview, we recommend that the Children's Yale–Brown Obsessive Compulsive Scale (CY-BOCS) be included. This measure is a semi-structured interview administered and rated by the clinician and includes both a Symptom Checklist and Severity Ratings. The Symptom Checklist is similar in format to the adult version, with minor differences, such as specifically mentioning parents under the symptoms "rituals involving other persons." The adult YBOCS has been found to have good reliability and validity (Goodman *et al.*, 1989a, 1989b; Taylor, 1995), and the CY-BOCS appears to be equally sound psychometrically (Scahill *et al.*, 1997).

The Symptom Checklist inquires first about the range of both past and current obsessions, including contamination, aggression, sexual obsessions, hoarding/saving obsessions, magical thoughts/superstitious obsessions, somatic obsessions, religious obsessions, and miscellaneous obsessions. After the presence of obsessions have been established, the Checklist is used to establish the presence of compulsions (e.g., cleaning, checking, repeating, counting, ordering, hoarding/saving, excessive games/superstitious behaviors, rituals involving another person, and miscellaneous compulsions). Following the completion of the Symptom Checklist, severity ratings are used to rate five dimensions of both the obsessions and the compulsions: amount of time consumed on a daily basis, interference with other non-OCD activities, distress, degree of resistance, and degree of control. The final score is composed of the sum of all of the severity-related items and then classified as indicative of mild, moderate, severe or extreme OCD. Degree of insight is also assessed.

It is apparent that the most widely used assessment measure, the CY-BOCS, does not include items or scales pertaining to the six cognitive domains currently being investigated by the Obsessive Compulsive Cognitions Working Group (1997, 2001). At present only one measure taps some information related to cognitions in childhood OCD: the Multidimensional Anxiety Scale for Children (MASC; March, 1998a). The MASC, a 39-item self-report scale that uses 4-point Likert ratings, has undergone extensive psychometric evaluation (March, 1998b) and is particularly useful for evaluating salient OCD-related cognitions in that it contains a robust perfectionism factor in addition to covering other areas of pediatric anxiety. Specifically, the MASC main and sub-factors include: (a) physical symptoms (tense/restless and somatic/autonomic); (b) social anxiety (humiliation/rejection and public performance fears); (c) harm avoidance (anxious coping and perfectionism); and (d) separation anxiety. The MASC contains two other empirically-derived sub-scales: a 10-item unifactorial short form (MASC-10) intended for use in epidemiological and treatment outcome studies, and a 12-item anxiety disorder index useful for diagnostic clarification purposes (March, 1998b).

Case-formulation in Childhood OCD

Although much information is gathered using an extensive symptom-focused interview approach with appropriate coverage of the child's psycho-social history, the clinician generally adopts a cognitive–behavioral case-formulation approach when conceptualizing the case. A cognitive case-formulation approach is valuable when attempting to identify salient cognitions that may be involved in the child's OCD. A treatment plan can subsequently be developed that includes strategies for addressing any faulty appraisals, in addition to the exposure and response prevention treatment program.

A case-formulation approach consists of identifying a model to explain the causal and the maintenance factors related to the client's specific problem(s). Using such an approach (see, for example, Persons & Tompkins, 1997; Taylor, Thordarson, & Söchting, in press), predisposing, precipitating, and perpetuating factors are considered and integrated in the case-formulation. Predisposing factors are vulnerability factors such as dysfunctional beliefs developed early in life. Precipitating factors are stimuli or circumstances immediately preceding the onset of the OCD. Perpetuating factors are those that maintain the problems, such as neutralizing behaviors including compulsions and avoidance. The following case example involving a 14-year-old boy illustrates the case-formulation approach.

The clinical interview and the Children's Yale–Brown Obsessive Compulsive Scale revealed that this patient, Paul, suffered from the "just right" OCD sub-type. His obsessions included a fear of something bad happening, like turning into an unpopular person, if he did not repeat certain routine activities until it felt "just right". Data from the interview indicated that the onset of his OCD followed a drop in his grades from an A student to a B student at age 13. According to the parents, he had only mild symptoms prior to age 13 involving ordering items in his room. It was also apparent that Paul held high, perfectionistic expectations regarding his performance both in sports and in school. He had excelled in many sports and was described as a star athlete by his parents who were noticeably proud of his achievements and very concerned about the degree to which his OCD symptoms interfered with his school performance.

Predisposing factors may include a patient's dysfunctional beliefs, as well as psychosocial factors that shaped these beliefs. For Paul, these beliefs can be viewed as faulty appraisals when applied specifically to his obsessive compulsive behaviors. Questions that are particularly useful in identifying faulty appraisals include the following: (a) What bothers or worries the patient most about their intrusive thoughts or obsessions? (b) What does the patient think the obsessions might lead to? and (c) What does the patient think will happen if he or she does not perform compulsions or avoid obsession-triggering stimuli? In this case, Paul became distressed by the possibility of his obsessions coming true and fearing that they would lead to a personal disaster if he did not engage in preventive measures, i.e., compulsive behaviors. Paul's and his parents' high expectations for both his athletic and academic performance likely increased his vulnerability to becoming distressed when falling below these standards. His perfectionistic tendencies were also reflected in the way he preferred to keep his room from an early age. This need, however, seemed to have been mostly ego-syntonic and perceived by him as pleasurable.

Precipitating factors trigger the onset of the patient's problems. Cognitive–behavioral case-formulations suggest that problem onset or exacerbation arises when dysfunctional beliefs interact with psychosocial stressors. For Paul, the increasing demands in school and the decline in his grades were perceived by him as highly stressful. Interestingly, several cognitive biases or errors in thinking led Paul to become increasingly distressed. Often, general cognitive biases noted primarily in the panic disorder literature (Clark,

1989) can also be identified as either predisposing or precipitating factors in OCD. For example, Paul engaged in catastrophic thinking, immediately imagining the worst case scenario: "what if I fail — I will be a loser forever". He also engaged in the fortune-telling cognitive error by arbitrarily predicting that things would turn out badly for him. Finally, his thinking about his drop in grades was black-and-white in that he only saw two options for himself: a perfect star or a loser. Because he was vulnerable to these cognitive biases, his thoughts about school performance rapidly became profoundly distressing, to the point of becoming a clinical obsession with associated compulsions as described by Salkovskis (1996, 1999). The cognitive biases reflected in Paul's case overlap with several of the OCD belief domains including perfectionism and probability over-estimation.

According to Salkovskis (1996, 1999), neutralizing strategies such as compulsions and avoidance are perpetuating factors for OCD. These strategies prevent the faulty appraisals from being disconfirmed. Paul believed that his obsessions had sufficient power to become true, and that the probability of their becoming true was considerable (90 percent). Hence, he invested much time and energy in neutralizing them. The fact that his neutralizing strategies became increasingly time-consuming and prevented his arriving at school on time and concentrating in the classroom exacerbated his fears. He became stuck in a vicious cycle wherein he began to fall behind as a result of his symptoms which only confirmed, in his mind, the validity and veracity of his beliefs about needing to do things perfectly.

These faulty beliefs were related to both the etiology and maintenance of his obsessions and rituals. For example, Paul's belief that it was important to be the best athlete and to do things perfectly increased his vulnerability to develop an exaggerated fear of falling below a certain standard. At the point where his behavior was diagnosable as OCD, he also held the belief that certain rituals would prevent this fear from coming true. Hence, by believing that his neutralizing behaviors worked to prevent him from becoming a loser, he did not allow opportunities to challenge and to disconfirm his beliefs. Consequently, his over-estimation of the probability of becoming a loser was maintained.

It is apparent in the above case that at least three of the six faulty beliefs identified for adults were operating. First, like adults who over-estimate the importance of their thoughts, Paul thought that the simple occurrence of his intrusive thought about being a loser implied both an important message to him, and the likelihood that this negative thought would lead to a bad outcome. Second, Paul's perfectionism reflected a belief that even minor mistakes may have serious consequences and that doing something perfect is both possible and necessary. Paul believed that it was necessary to be perfect in his academic and athletic performance. Interestingly, he also applied this belief to his compulsions by repeating them (e.g., taking his shoes on and off, pulling up his socks) until they were done correctly. Finally, Paul's belief that there was a 90 percent chance of turning into an unpopular person reflects a tendency to over-estimate this threat.

Although there is reason to assume that children and adolescents with OCD develop much the same faulty beliefs and appraisals as adults, they may be somewhat harder to detect due to their earlier stage of development. However, early identification of faulty beliefs and appraisals may have positive implications for treatment planning and outcome.

Treatment Implications

Treatment of childhood OCD typically follows the cognitive-behavioral approach used for adults. The emphasis, however, is on the behavioral component, that is, classic exposure and response prevention. To date, there is no published comprehensive treatment approach specifically targeting the alteration of OCD-related beliefs or appraisals in children. However, this does not imply that the cognitive component is non-existent in treatment. In this section, we will focus on the research pertaining to treatment of childhood OCD with particular attention to cognitive treatment interventions as they may pertain to the six belief domains. It is apparent that this literature is extremely scant and that not all of the six cognitive domains have been addressed in the child literature. We will first discuss the cognitive domains for which there is some research evidence. These domains include over-estimation of threat, intolerance of uncertainty, and over-importance of thoughts. We will conclude this section by discussing some possible reasons for the absence of research supporting the other cognitive domains.

Over-estimation of threat has been addressed in a single case experimental design by Kearny and Silverman (1990). They used an alternating treatments design in which they compared classic response prevention to cognitive therapy. The patient was a 14-year-old male with a fear of contracting rabies from bats. The response prevention treatment involved instructing the adolescent to reduce the frequency of checking for the presence of bats. The cognitive treatment involved assisting him in challenging the unrealistic nature of his catastrophic fears by providing education about rabies and finding evidence to refute his threat estimate. In this study, only the combined treatment effects were evaluated, and it is therefore not possible to comment on the relative efficacy of each treatment component. Most likely, the overt emphasis on the realistic probability of contracting rabies (cognitive intervention) would have had a positive influence on the patient's felt urge to check for bats (response prevention intervention). Based on post-treatment and follow-up assessments, the patient was considered a treatment success through a six month follow-up assessment.

Various strategies can be helpful in addressing a child's over-estimation of threat. These strategies are all based on the adult OCD literature. In particular, the work by van Oppen and colleagues (1995) has been useful in addressing this faulty belief. March and Mulle (1998) recommend using standard cognitive interventions similar to those used for a variety of anxiety disorders in adults. In children, cognitive restructuring involves moving back and forth between what "OCD says" and what the child actually estimates as a reasonable probability. For example, in the case described previously, Paul initially rated his belief in turning into a loser at 90 percent. As he began to see these fears coming from a monster who was provoking him to a fight, he was able to counter his obsessions, and his belief in becoming a loser declined steadily over time. Since it worked for Paul to view the OCD as an enemy with whom to do battle, a more bellicose terminology was adopted. Paul began to keep track of the number of battles fought in a day; and he would tally how many he won compared to the monster. Paul increased his arsenal of weapons and became a better strategist. He also increased his awareness of where his safety zones were. For example, he found that the monster was less likely to bother him when he played video games or talked to his friends on the phone. His motivation appeared to increase when both these specific cognitive restructuring exercises and the more general concept of detachment (discussed below) were fully integrated into the exposure treatment program.

The cognitive domain involving intolerance of uncertainty has not been explicitly addressed using cognitive interventions. However, one study has addressed this domain using traditional behavior therapy. Francis (1988) used a withdrawal design (A-B-A-B) to assess the efficacy of an extinction procedure designed to eliminate reassurance-seeking behavior in an 11-year-old boy with OCD who could not tolerate uncertainty about health-related concerns. Specifically, the boy had obsessions about illness and death that led him to ask his parents for excessive reassurance about his health. For example, he repeatedly asked if he had a tumor or was going blind. Treatment involved instructing the parents to ignore all reassurance-seeking behaviors exhibited by their son by looking away or re-directing the conversation. The symptoms were eliminated after six days of treatment but returned when treatment was withdrawn. Following the completion of the entire course of treatment the boy was symptom-free. However, as pointed out by Francis, it is unclear whether this treatment approach would result in lasting benefits given that no long-term follow-up data were provided.

In this case, a cognitive intervention would have included evaluating advantages and disadvantages, aimed at helping the boy understand that he was engaging in a fruitless pursuit that had far more costs to him in terms of wasted time and mental energy than benefits. A two-column sheet listing costs and benefits may have proven effective in illustrating the futility of his compulsive reassurance seeking. It would also have been interesting to observe the potential treatment benefits of assisting him in acknowledging the lack of relationship between increased questioning and increased chances of certainty (e.g., guarantee of no tumor). In fact, a behavioral experiment could be designed in which the boy would rate the strength of his feelings of certainty after each compulsive behavior. Most likely, as we have found with adults, he would find that the more he asks, the less certain he actually feels. Again, the aim of a cognitive intervention would be to encourage the boy to develop a more rational approach to his concerns. If successful, such an approach might result in a more fundamental and therefore longer-lasting learning experience than a simple lack of reward approach as in the extinction procedure employed by Francis. However, only future research can address this hypothesis.

The cognitive domain involving over-importance of thoughts is perhaps the most important to date in the childhood literature. The idea of attaching excessive meaning to the presence of an obsession is addressed from the perspective of cultivating detachment. The cognitive component in the standardized treatment manual by March and Mulle (1998) includes cognitive training in the form of cultivating detachment. The idea of cultivating detachment was initially derived from the work of Jeffrey Schwartz and colleagues at the UCLA School of Medicine (Schwartz, Martin, & Baxter, 1992) and later also from the work of Salkovskis (Salkovskis & Campbell, 1994; Salkovskis, Westbrook, Davis, Jeavons, & Gledhill, 1997) and van Oppen (van Oppen & Arntz, 1994; van Oppen *et al.*, 1995).

Integral to the idea of cultivating detachment is the notion that patients learn to create a distance between themselves and their OCD. One general cognitive intervention includes encouraging the child to give his or her OCD a nickname. One child, seen by the first author, made a laminated wallet size card with several statements, e.g., 'OCD is a nasty dragon who is trying to run my life'; 'I can tame this dragon by using my special tricks.' Other cognitive interventions specifically targeting the problem of attaching too much importance to a given obsession includes the approach outlined by March and Mulle (1998). Clinicians working with children are encouraged to assist their patients in viewing their obsessions as brain hiccups. The child is encouraged to view the obsessions as transient (e.g., like a cloud in the sky or a fish swimming by) in order to minimize the child's urge to suppress the unwanted thoughts (obsessions).

There appears to be no published material related to the remaining three cognitive domains of perfectionism, inflated responsibility, and importance of controlling one's thoughts. This may simply be the result of a lack of attention, so far, to cognitive phenomena in childhood OCD. However, perhaps children and adolescents do not possess the same level of cognitive development and awareness as adults. The lack of research on cognitions related to perfectionism in children with OCD may simply be a result of this area of research being in its nascence, whereas the lack of attention to inflated responsibility and importance of controlling one's thoughts may be related to developmental issues.

Although perfectionism in childhood OCD has not been addressed specifically in an empirical manner, most clinicians would likely concur that concerns about perfectionistic standards are often present in presentations of childhood OCD. Examples have been given earlier in the case of the 13-year-old who had to rewind images perfectly and in Paul's perfectionistic repeating rituals. In a study on the relationship between anxiety disorder symptoms and negative self-statements in children, Muris, Mayer, Snieder, and Merckelbach (1998) found that negative self-statements were positively associated with the presence of various anxiety disorders including OCD. It is encouraging that the Multidimensional Anxiety Scale for Children (MASC; March, 1998b) includes a perfectionism factor allowing future research to address empirically the presence of perfectionism in childhood OCD. In the literature on perfectionism in adults, a fear of inadequacy often drives the need for things to be done perfectly. The same may be true for children. It is possible that the negative self-statements noted by clinicians in children engaged in OCD treatment may be associated, in part, with a fear of being inadequate, a fear that becomes generalized to the child's treatment regime. The cognitive domain of perfectionism may thus be important to motivation and adherence to treatment.

No published case studies specifically address a child's inflated sense of responsibility for a bad outcome. An example of this concern was evident in the case of the 13-year-old described earlier who feared he was responsible for the death of an animal. For the most part, however, it seems likely that children and adolescents do not possess the same awareness of others as adults do. In adults with OCD, inflated responsibility typically involves a fear of causing harm to innocent others, often family members. Developmental psychology researchers studying moral development in children and adolescents have consistently found a correlation between age and the ability to consider other people's needs and welfare in addition to one's own (Skoe & Gooden, 1993). Further, if Bolton's (1996) theoretical speculations are correct, children afflicted with OCD may be even more self-focused than children without OCD because of their pre-rational stage of reasoning.

It is possible, then, that the majority of children with OCD are more focused on harm befalling them as a result of their obsessive fears and less focused on harm to others. Guilt about potentially harming others may be correlated with age and social roles that reflect responsibility, such as being an employee or a parent.

Similarly, concerns about the importance of controlling one's thoughts may require a certain level of cognitive development. The belief that "one can and should exercise control over one's thoughts" in order to prevent harm and decrease discomfort has not been linked to childhood OCD in the literature, nor have we found it a salient concern in our clinical experience. Possible reasons may be that this belief can be considered a meta-cognitive belief that involves thinking about thinking. Meta-cognitive beliefs are beliefs about mental events (Clark & Purdon, 1993). In OCD, these beliefs are about the form or content of obsessions. For example, a person with OCD may believe that if he or she can not control the mere presence of an image of being aggressive toward another person, this will increase the chance of the image becoming translated into actual harming behavior. Although the appraisal of the importance of controlling one's thoughts is often related to other appraisals such as, for example, over-importance of thoughts, its absence regarding childhood presentations of OCD may be related to the possibility that meta-beliefs require a certain level of cognitive intellectual sophistication. In normal cognitive development, a child would be expected to engage in abstract and complex reasoning by early adolescence (Strauman & Higgins, 1993). A younger child with OCD may not possess the necessary level of cognitive development to engage in more abstract thinking, such as being able to evaluate one's own thinking as required in the development of meta-cognitions. Moreover, if the development of OCD does involve a failure to abandon a pre-rational cognitive style, as discussed earlier, a child with OCD would be further challenged.

In summary, it is noteworthy that the concept of over-importance of thoughts specifically, and also the other kinds of faulty beliefs and appraisals, are phenomenologically similar to the concept of externalizing the OCD. Both require and involve a conscious evaluation of a mental phenomenon (i.e., the obsession) as irrelevant and without personal meaning despite the fact that the obsession originates in the person's own mind. No attempt has been made to demonstrate empirically if children engage in a variety of faulty appraisals which can be grouped like those in adult OCD sufferers. However, from the work of March and colleagues, it appears that the presentation of childhood OCD may well include various kinds of such beliefs. It also appears that assisting the patient in achieving a cognitive shift may have positive implications for treatment motivation and adherence. A cognitive shift in this context implies the ability to re-evaluate the obsessions as meaningless and as separate from one's personality.

Recommendations

Considering that 50–70 percent of children with OCD continue to suffer from the disorder in adulthood (Bolton, Luckie, & Steinberg, 1995), there is a need to evaluate more rigorously the effectiveness of current behavioral interventions. In addition, further refinement and validation of interventions that incorporate cognitive components addressing obsessive compulsive cognitions are needed. Based on clinical experience and case studies, it appears that children respond positively to cognitive interventions aimed at their faulty appraisals of obsessions. One promising cognitive intervention addresses the faulty appraisal of attaching too much importance to the content of an obsession and encourages the child to distance himself or herself from their obsessions. Exactly what role faulty appraisals play in childhood OCD is not known at present. It would be useful to conduct treatment studies specifically targeting faulty appraisals related to feared outcomes in the absence of compulsive rituals before and after treatment. In order to do so, an appropriate set of cognitive measures would need to be developed. Future plans for the Obsessive Compulsive Cognitions Working Group may include developing and validating a set of measures targeting cognitions in children and adolescents. Once such a set becomes available, several possibilities for addressing further questions arise.

From research on adults with OCD, we know that when a primarily behavioral treatment modality is compared to a primarily cognitive modality, there are no significant differences in the final treatment outcome (e.g., van Oppen *et al.*, 1995). One suggested possibility for this lack of difference is that patients in strict behavioral therapy may interpret their exposure-based experiences in ways that spontaneously produce a cognitive restructuring of their prior faulty appraisals. Because young children typically are not capable of placing their current experiences into a perspective as large as that of adults, children may benefit from cognitive interventions specifically addressing their faulty beliefs and appraisals. Many children do not have sufficient insight into their OCD to allow them to question and challenge their anxiety-provoking beliefs in an unassisted manner. Also, children are more prone to be non-compliant than adults, and, hence, may benefit from the cognitive interventions discussed in this chapter aimed at enhancing their motivation. These questions will need to be addressed in controlled outcome studies.

References

American Psychiatric Association (1994). *Diagnostic and statistical manual of mental disorders* (4th ed.) Washington, DC: Author.

Bolton, D. (1996). Developmental issues in obsessive–compulsive disorder. *Journal of Child Psychology and Psychiatry, 37*, 131–137.

Bolton, D., Luckie, M., & Steinberg, D. (1995). Long-term course of obsessive–compulsive disorder treated in adolescence. *Journal of the American Academy of Child and Adolescent Psychiatry, 34*, 1441–1450.

Clark, D. M. (1989). Anxiety states: Panic and generalized anxiety. In K. Hawton, P. M. Salkovskis, J. Kirk, & D. M. Clark (eds), *Cognitive–Behavior Therapy for Psychiatric Problems* (pp. 52–96). Oxford, UK: Oxford University Press.

Clark, D. A., & Purdon, C. (1993). New perspectives for a cognitive theory of obsessions. *Australian Psychologist, 28*, 161–167.

Conners, C. K., & March, J. S. (1996). *Conners-March Developmental Questionnaire*. Toronto: MultiHealth Systems.

Damon, W., & Hart, D. (1986). Stability and change in children's self-understanding. *Social Cognition, 4*, 102–118.

Flament, M. F., Whitaker, A., Rapoport, J. L., Davies, M., Berg, C. Z., Kalikow, K., Sceery, W., & Shaffer, D. (1988). Obsessive–compulsive disorder in adolescence: an epidemiological study. *Journal of the American Academy of Child and Adolescent Psychiatry, 27*, 764–771.

Francis, G. (1988). Childhood obsessive–compulsive disorder: Extinction of compulsive reassurance seeking. *Journal of Anxiety Disorders, 2*, 361–366.

Goodman, W. K., Price, L. H., Rasmussen, S. A., Mazure, C., Fleischmann, R., Hill, C. L., Heninger, G. R., & Charney, D. S. (1989a). The Yale–Brown Obsessive–Compulsive Scale (Y-BOCS): Part I. Development, use and reliability. *Archives of General Psychiatry, 46*, 1006–1011.

Goodman, W. K., Price, L. H., Rasmussen, S. A., Mazure, C., Fleischmann, R., Hill, C. L., Heninger, G. R., & Charney, D. S. (1989b). The Yale–Brown Obsessive–Compulsive Scale (Y-BOCS): Part II. Validity. *Archives of General Psychiatry, 46*, 1012–1016.

Hollingsworth, C. E., Tanguay, P. E., Grossman, L., & Pabst, P. (1980). Long term outcome of obsessive–compulsive disorder in childhood. *Journal of the American Academy of Child and Adolescent Psychiatry, 19*, 134–144.

Honjo, S., Hirano, C., Murase, S., Kaneko, T., Sugiyama, T., Ohtaka, K., Aoyama, T., Takei, Y., Inoko, K., & Wakabayashi, S. (1989). Obsessive–compulsive symptoms in childhood and adolescence. *Acta Psychiatrica Scandinavia, 80*, 83–91.

Kearney, C. A., & Silverman, W. K. (1990). Treatment of an adolescent with obsessive–compulsive disorder by alternating response prevention and cognitive therapy: an empirical analysis. *Journal of Behavior Therapy and Experimental Psychiatry, 21*, 39–47.

Kendall, P. C., Chansky, T. E., Friedman, M., Kim, R., Kortlander, E., Sessa, F. M., & Siqueland, L. (1991). Treating anxiety disorders in children and adolescents. In P. C. Kendall (ed.), *Child and adolescent therapy: Cognitive–behavioral procedures* (pp. 131–164). New York: Guilford.

Kessler, J. W. (1988). *Psychopathology of childhood*. Upper Saddle River, New Jersey: Prentice — Hall.

March, J. S. (1998a). Cognitive–behavioral psychotherapy for pediatric OCD. In M. A. Jenike, L. Baer & W. E. Minichello (eds), *Obsessive–compulsive disorders: practical management*. (3rd ed., pp. 400–420). Philadelphia: Mosby.

March, J. S. (1998b). *Manual for the Multidimensional Anxiety Scale for Children (MASC)*. Toronto: MultiHealth Systems.

March, J. S., & Mulle, K. (1995). Manualized cognitive–behavioral psychotherapy for obsessive–compulsive disorder in childhood: A preliminary single case study. *Journal of Anxiety Disorders, 9*, 175–184.

March, J. S., & Mulle, K. (1998). *OCD in children and adolescents: A cognitive–behavioral treatment manual*. New York: Guilford.

Muris, P., Mayer, B., Snieder, N., & Merckelbach, H. (1998). The relationship between anxiety disorder symptoms and negative self-statements in normal children. *Social Behavior and Personality, 26*, 307–316.

Obsessive–Compulsive Cognitions Working Group (1997). Cognitive assessment of obsessive–compulsive disorder. *Behaviour Research and Therapy, 35*, 667–681.

Obsessive–Compulsive Cognitions Working Group (2001). Development and initial validation of the Obsessive–Beliefs Questionnaire and the Interpretation of Intrusions Inventory. *Behaviour Research and Therapy, 39*, 987–1006.

Persons, J. B., & Tompkins, M. A. (1997). Cognitive-behavioral case formulation. In T. D. Eells (ed.), *Handbook of psychotherapy case formulation* (pp. 314–339). New York: Guilford.

Rasmussen, S. A., & Tsuang, M. T. (1986). Epidemiology and clinical features of obsessive–compulsive disorder. In M. A. Jenike, L. Baer, & W. E. Minichiello (eds), *Obsessive–compulsive disorders: theory and management* (pp. 23–44). Littleton, MA: PSG.

Salkovskis, P. M. (1985). Obsessional–compulsive problems: A cognitive–behavioral analysis. *Behaviour Research and Therapy, 25,* 571–583.

Salkovskis, P. M. (1989). Cognitive–behavioral factors and the persistence of intrusive thoughts in obsessional problems. *Behaviour Research and Therapy, 27,* 677–682.

Salkovskis, P. M. (1996). Cognitive–behavioral approaches to the understanding of obsessional problems. In R. M. Rapee (ed.), *Current controversies in the anxiety disorders* (pp. 103–133). New York: Guilford.

Salkovskis, P. M. (1999). Understanding and treating obsessive–compulsive disorder. *Behaviour Research and Therapy, 37,* 129–152.

Salkovskis, P. M., & Campbell, P. (1994). Thought suppression induces intrusion in naturally occurring negative intrusive thoughts. *Behavior Research Therapy, 32,* 1–8.

Salkovskis, P. M., Westbrook, D., Davis, J., Jeavons, A., & Gledhill, A. (1997). Effects of neutralizing on intrusive thoughts: an experiment investigating the etiology of obsessive–compulsive disorder. *Behaviour Research Therapy, 35,* 211–219.

Scahill, L., Riddle, M., McSwiggin-Hardin, M., Ort, S., King, R., Goodman, W., Cicchetti, D., & Leckman, J. (1997). Children's Yale–Brown Obsessive–Compulsive Scale: Reliability and validity. *Journal of the American Academy of Child and Adolescent Psychiatry, 36,* 844–852.

Schwartz, J. M., Martin, K. M., & Baxter, L. R. (1992). Neuroimaging and cognitive–behavioral self-treatment for obsessive–compulsive disorder: Practical and philosophical considerations. In I. Hand, W. K. Goodman, & U. Evers (eds), *Obsessive–compulsive disorders: new research* (pp. 82–101). Berling: Springer Verlag.

Skoe, E. E., & Gooden, A. (1993). Ethic of care and real-life moral dilemma content in male and female early adolescents. *Journal of Early Adolescence, 13,* 154–167.

Strauman, T. J., & Higgins, E. T. (1993). The self construct in social cognition: past, present and future. In Z. V. Segal & S. J. Blatt (eds), *The self in emotional distress: cognitive and psychodynamic perspective* (pp. 3–40). New York: Guliford.

Swedo, S. E., Rapoport, J. L., Leonard, H., Lenane, M., & Cheslow, D. (1989). Obsessive–compulsive disorder in children and adolescents. Clinical phenomenology of 70 consecutive cases. *Archives of General Psychiatry, 46,* 335–341.

Taylor, S. (1995). Assessment of obsessions and compulsions: Reliability, validity, and sensitivity to treatment effects. Clinical Psychology Review, 15, 261–296.

Taylor, S., Thordarson, D., & Söchting, I. (in press). Assessment, treatment planning, and outcome evaluation for obsessive–compulsive disorder. In D. H. Barlow, & M. M. Antony (eds), *Handbook of assessment, treatment planning, and outcome evaluation: empirically supported strategies for psychological disorders.* New York: Guilford.

Thomsen, P. H. (1993). Obsessive–compulsive disorder in children and adolescents: Self-reported obsessive–compulsive behavior in pupils in Denmark. *Acta Psychiatrica Scandinavia, 88,* 212–217.

Thomsen, P. H., & Mikkelsen, H. U. (1991). Children and adolescents with obsessive–compulsive disorder: The demographic and diagnostic characteristics of 61 Danish patients. *Acta Psychiatrica Scandinavia, 87,* 456–462.

Thomsen, P. H., & Mikkelsen, H. U. (1993). Development of personality disorders in children and adolescents with obsessive–compulsive disorder: A 6–22-year follow-up study. *Acta Psychiatrica Scandinavia, 87,* 456–462.

van Oppen, P., & Arntz, A. (1994). Cognitive therapy for obsessive–compulsive disorder. *Behaviour Research and Therapy, 32,* 79–87.

van Oppen, P., de Haan, E., van Balkom, A., Spinhoven, P., Hoogduin, K., & van Dyck, R. (1995). Cognitive therapy and exposure in vivo in the treatment of obsessive–compulsive disorder. *Behaviour Research & Therapy, 33,* 370–390.

Whitaker, A., Johnson, J., Shaffer, D., Rapoport, J. L., Kalikow, K., Walsh, B. T., Davies, M., Braiman, S., & Dolinsky, A. (1990). Uncommon troubles in young people: Prevalence estimates of selected psychiatric disorders in a non-referred adolescent population. *Archives of General Psychiatry, 47,* 487–496.

Zetzel, E. R. (1966). Additional notes upon a case of obsessional neurosis: Freud, 1909. *International Journal of Psychoanalyis, 47,* 123–129.

Chapter 17

Cognitive Processes and Obsessive Compulsive Disorder in Older Adults

John E. Calamari, Amy S. Janeck and Teresa M. Deer

Introduction

Chapters in this volume review the burgeoning literature on the importance of cognitive processes to obsessive compulsive disorder (OCD). This body of research has led to new theoretical perspectives on the development and maintenance of OCD symptoms (e.g., Rachman, 1993; Salkovskis, 1985) and has resulted in the formulation of new interventions (e.g., Freeston *et al.*, 1997) and the refinement of established treatments for OCD (e.g., Salkovskis & Westbrook, 1987). Cognitive theory and therapies for OCD hold promise for improving treatment outcome for people with OCD who are unresponsive to established behavioral and pharmacologic therapies.

In this chapter the relationship between cognitive processes and OCD symptoms in older adults is evaluated. Six primary questions are addressed with a focus on how these issues may relate to cognitive dimensions of OCD: (a) What is the prevalence of OCD in older adults?; (b) When OCD symptoms are observed in older adults, do they represent a continuation of a disorder present throughout much of life or can the condition appear for the first time late in life?; (c) Are specific constellations of OCD symptoms (e.g., scrupulosity, hoarding) more characteristic of late-life OCD and what is the relationship between symptoms and appraisals of and beliefs about intrusive thoughts?; (d) Most relevant to cognitive models of OCD, do older adults react differently to negative intrusive thoughts or hold beliefs differing from other age groups regarding the importance of certain types of thought?; (e) Do the cognitive changes and concerns associated with later life (e.g., apprehension regarding memory functioning and other cognitive abilities; Wilson, Bennett, & Swartzendruber, 1997) affect reactivity to intrusive thoughts or alter general beliefs regarding the importance of cognition?; and (f) Do elderly persons respond to cognitive–behavioral interventions for OCD, and what accommodations might need to be made to treatment protocols for this age group?

In the chapter we discuss how developmental issues could interact with appraisals and beliefs relating to intrusive thoughts to precipitate or exacerbate OCD symptoms in older adults. Because the scientific study of OCD in older adults is in its early stages, throughout the review we often only speculate on the answers to many important questions based on clinical observations and case reports. We make suggestions on what studies might be initiated to better understand cognitive dimensions of OCD in the elderly.

The Prevalence of OCD in Older Adults

OCD is a highly prevalent anxiety disorder that may affect three percent of the population at some time during their life (Karno, Golding, Sorenson, & Burnam, 1988). Estimates of the occurrence of OCD in older adults are based on few studies (e.g., Calamari, Faber, Hitsman, & Poppe, 1994; Carmin, Pollard, & Ownby, 1999). Although anxiety disorders are known to occur in older adults at a rate much greater than mood disorders (e.g., Matt, Dean, Wang, & Wood, 1992), anxiety conditions have not received the clinical or empirical attention that the study of depressive disorders has received (e.g., Hersen & van Hasselt, 1992).

Anxiety disorders have generally been found to decrease with age in epidemiological studies (e.g., Flint, 1994; Regier, Narrow, & Rae, 1990). Flint (1994) reviewed prevalence estimates of anxiety problems in the elderly reported in epidemiologic investigations. Flint noted that a point prevalence rate of 5.5 percent was reported for adults 65-years-old or older compared to a rate of 7.3 percent in all adults in the Epidemiologic Catchment Area (ECA) study (Regier *et al.*, 1988). In a Canadian survey, a point prevalence rate of 3.5 percent for elders living in the community and a 5 percent rate for elders living in institutional settings was reported (Bland, Newman, & Orn, 1988). The Canadian survey found a rate of anxiety disorders of 6.5 percent among adults generally. In contrast, in the National Survey of Psychotherapeutic Drug Use (Uhlenhuth, Balter, Mellinger, Cisin, & Clinthorne, 1983), the prevalence of anxiety disorders was slightly higher in older adults: 10.2 percent compared to 9.9 percent in the entire adult sample. The higher rates of anxiety disorders in this survey were accounted for by high rates of generalized anxiety disorder, a condition that was not assessed in the ECA and Canadian surveys (Flint, 1994).

Fuentes and Cox (1997) have identified methodological problems in epidemiologic studies of anxiety symptomatology in older adults and questioned the accuracy of lower prevalence estimates. Fuentes and Cox noted that research instruments used in these studies have not been validated with older adults and that no attempt has been made to adjust diagnostic criteria in response to possible differences in the manifestations of anxiety symptoms in the elderly. Fuentes and Cox concluded that anxiety disorders have been inadequately assessed and underestimated in older adults. Beck and Stanley (1997) pointed out that even if the lower prevalence rate estimates are accurate, in the National Institute of Mental Health ECA studies (Regier *et al.*, 1988; Weissman *et al.*, 1985), anxiety disorders were found to occur four to eight times more frequently than major depression in individuals aged 65 and older. Depressive disorders have been found to occur with sufficient frequency in the elderly to represent a significant public health issue (e.g., Reynolds, Lebowitz, & Schneider, 1993), underscoring the need for additional study of anxiety in older adults.

Prevalence estimates of OCD in older adults have sometimes been low, possibly inhibiting gerontologists' interest in this disorder. For persons over age 65, epidemiologic studies reported a one-month prevalence rate of OCD of 0.8 percent (Regier *et al.*, 1988), and a six-month prevalence rate of 1.5 percent (Bland *et al.*, 1988). The prevalence rate of OCD in older adults living in institutional settings may be considerably higher (Bland *et al.*, 1988), although study of this group has been very limited. Juninger, Phelan, Cherry, and Levy (1993) assessed anxiety disorder prevalence using structured clinical interviews. They found rates of anxiety disorders to be almost three times higher in nursing home residents compared to community residents, and five times greater in their nursing home sample compared to older adults living independently. Unfortunately, their sample size was small.

In summary, OCD appears to occur with regularity in older adults. Prevalence estimates, though, are based on limited study and methodological approaches that may be inadequate for assessing psychological problems in this age group. Additional studies carefully characterizing late-life OCD with methodological approaches sensitive to population issues (e.g., possible difference in the phenomenology of OCD symptoms, structuring the assessment setting to make this age cohort more comfortable discussing psychological symptoms) are needed. Prevalence studies of OCD in elders should target not only older adults living independently, but also residents in supported living situations, including nursing homes where OCD and other anxiety disorders may be more prevalent (e.g., Juninger *et al.*, 1993). Differentiating anxiety and depressive symptoms in this age group will be challenging (Stanley & Averill, 1999) given the extensive overlap of these conditions (Stanley & Beck, 1998). Older adults' reluctance to report psychological problems (e.g., Lasoski, 1986) and their tendencies to attribute anxiety symptoms to physical conditions (Gurian & Miner, 1991) are additional barriers to determining the frequency of OCD in the elderly.

Developmental Issues and the Onset of OCD

To fully understand the cognitive processes underlying OCD in the elderly, the relationship of symptom onset to developmental level needs to be explored. When OCD begins early in life, the psychosocial and biological processes that characterize early life will be most important to understanding the development of OCD. Further, later developmental processes may be most pertinent to the maintenance of the disorder. If onset occurs late in life, developmental processes important in later life may play an essential role in both the onset and maintenance of the disorder.

The typical age of onset of OCD has consistently been reported to be approximately 19 to 25 (Steketee, 1993). Fewer than 15 percent of individuals with OCD are thought to develop symptoms for the first time after age 35 (Goodwin, Guze, & Robbins, 1969; Rasmussen & Tsuang, 1986), although OCD symptoms have rarely been evaluated in older adults. Minichiello, Baer, Jenike, and Holland (1990) assessed age of onset of OCD across major symptom subtypes of the disorder. Significant differences across subtypes were found. Individuals with predominant cleaning compulsions had a significantly later age of onset than persons with checking compulsions or patients described as having mixed rituals. Mean age of onset across all subgroups was young, ranging from 14.4 to 25.6 years. Thyer, Parrish, Curtis, Nesse, and Cameron (1985) evaluated age of onset for anxiety disorders. They reported that among their sample of 27 OCD patients, approximately 14 percent reported initial onset after age 50. Kohn, Westlake, Rasmussen, Marsland, and

Norman (1997) compared reported age of onset of OCD symptoms for older (age 60 or older) and younger OCD patients. Mean age of onset of major OCD symptoms for older patients was significantly later: 33.6 compared to 20.4 for younger patients. Nestadt, Bienvenu, Cai, Samuels, and Eaton (1998) conducted a follow-up evaluation of the Baltimore ECA study participants. Although incidents of OCD were low, two peaks of onset were identified for men and women, both of which were later for females. The second onset peak for women occurred after age 64.

Initial onset of OCD symptoms after age 60 has been documented in several case studies. Bajulaiye and Addonizio (1992) described a 75-year-old woman who, according to family members and self-report, first experienced OCD at age 72. Symptom onset followed an operation for a diverticular abscess and initial obsessions centered on the patient's fear of getting cancer. At the time of treatment the patient had severe contamination obsessions and washing compulsions, as well as doubting obsessions associated with checking behavior. Symptoms were associated with significant life interference.

Colvin and Boddington (1997) described the behavioral treatment of a 78-year-old woman with initial OCD onset in her mid-seventies. The patient had a history of rheumatic fever and Sydenham's Chorea as a child. She had been diagnosed with depression and agoraphobia while in her seventies and had neurologic symptoms that suggested possible epilepsy. A calcified posterior fossa tumor was identified but remained static in size. Initial OCD symptoms developed following the accidental flooding of her apartment by an upstairs neighbor's overflowing bath. At the time of her pre-treatment evaluation, her Yale–Brown Obsessive Compulsive Scale (YBOCS; Goodman *et al.*, 1989a, b) score was 35, suggesting severe OCD. The dominant symptoms involved checking appliances and the locks on her door. A similar case was reported by Gonzalez and Philpot (1998). The authors described a woman whose initial OCD occurred at age 76 in association with startle syndrome (a condition in which an exaggerated startle response is a primary symptom). Brain computerized tomography revealed a calcified mass arising from the inferior tentorium in the right posterior fossa. The patient experienced epileptic symptoms. OCD symptoms involved checking lights, taps and locks, and repetitive hand washing.

Philpot and Banerjee (1998) reported four additional cases of late-life onset OCD associated with neurologic symptoms or disorders. A 74-year-old man experienced intrusive, blasphemous thoughts and doubting obsessions and checking compulsions. Checking behavior consumed three hours per day and precipitated marital discord. An 83-year-old woman had novel rituals involving a need to visualize the faces of television stars and count when passing through doorways. If the ritual was not completed successfully, this severely arthritic patient had to repeat the behavior, a highly time-consuming activity because of her mobility limitations. Philpot and Banerjee (1998) also described an 82 year-old man who experienced intrusive thoughts involving dog faeces and general contamination concerns. A final case reported by these authors involved a 66-year-old man with obsessional slowness.

Age of onset of OCD has been generally under-studied, and very little is known about the likely onset or life course of OCD in older adults. Based on available information, it is probable that for the majority of older adults, OCD symptoms have been present throughout adult life, varying in intensity over time.

A variety of life stressors may cause OCD to become more severe (Steketee, 1993), and the stressors characteristic of later-life may be particularly potent in exacerbating OCD symptoms. Included among the stressful experience associated with later-life are retirement, death of a spouse, and incidents of significant physical illness in the older adult or loved ones, precipitating concern and caretaking responsibilities. Beekman *et al.* (1998) identified the experience of recent life stressors and perceived loneliness as risk factors associated with late-life OCD.

For a minority of older adults seeking treatment for OCD, it appears that the disorder has occurred for the first time late in life. It is not known whether late-life onset is a distinct sub-type with associated differences in etiologic mechanisms, symptom characteristics, or responsiveness to treatment. Late-life onset OCD has been regularly associated with neurologic symptoms or disorders, causing some clinicians to recommend neurological evaluation as a component of the assessment process (Jenike, 1991; Philpot & Banerjee, 1998). The association between neurologic symptoms and late onset OCD may come about for reasons not directly related to nervous system dysfunction. Older adults may respond to the cognitive changes associated with neurologic disorders, or to even the more subtle changes resulting from normal aging processes, with increased concern for cognitive functioning. Increased interest in mental functions may precipitate a hypervigilance for cognitive processing changes. Later in this chapter, we discuss how cognitive changes related to developmental level and hypervigilance for cognitive dysfunction could operate to support beliefs about the over-importance of thoughts and the need for effortful mental control activities. These processes are thought to be important to the development and maintenance of obsessional concerns in cognitive models of OCD (e.g., Freeston, Rhéaume, & Ladouceur, 1996).

Symptoms of Late-life OCD

There is general agreement in the OCD literature that important subtypes of the disorder exist (e.g., Rasmussen & Eisen, 1988), although there is no generally agreed upon framework for defining them (Calamari, Wiegartz, & Janeck, 1999). Differences in the types of obsessions and compulsions experienced by OCD patients have been the most frequently used method for forming subgroups (Calamari *et al.*, 1999). This strategy appears to rest on the assumption that differences in the types of symptoms correspond to important distinctions in the processes underlying the disorder. Differences in symptom sub-types may correspond to differences in the cognitive processes related to OCD, including beliefs promoting appraisals of intrusive thoughts as very important experiences. However, there have been no empirical evaluations of this issue to date.

Do OCD symptoms manifest differently in older adults? Again, the issue has not been systematically studied. Stanley and Averill (1999) suggested that older adults with generalized anxiety disorder, the anxiety disorder that has been most extensively studied in older adults, may present with differences in symptoms. Older adults reported fewer worries overall, but may worry more about health related concerns, and less about work, finances, and social events. Some evidence is reviewed below that certain types of OCD symptoms may be more strongly associated with older age.

Kohn *et al.* (1997) reported the only between-age-group comparison of the clinical features of OCD. The symptom characteristics of 32 elderly (age 60 or older) outpatients with OCD were compared with 601 younger patients. Older patients were better educated, reported a later onset of both minor and major OCD symptoms, and had first contacted a health professional because of their OCD at a later age. Few differences emerged from symptom comparison between age groups. Older patients were more likely to report a fear of having sinned, and ritualized hand washing was more often seen in older adults. Older patients were less likely to report symmetry obsessions, concerns about completing paperwork, preoccupations involving the need to know or remember, fears of AIDS, magical thinking, a need to re-read, and ordering-arranging and touching compulsions.

The relation between age and symptom-based OCD subtypes was evaluated by Calamari *et al.* (1999), although few older adults were included in the sample. Cluster analysis was used to identify symptom-based groupings of 106 OCD patients treated at the Chicago Medical School's anxiety disorders clinic. No significant gender or age differences between subgroups were found, although subgroup sizes were small and standard deviations large. To further explore the relationship between OCD symptoms and age, we conducted additional analyses on an expanded Chicago Medical School data-base ($n = 114$ patients with structured clinical interview diagnosed OCD). Only 12 of the patients in this data-base were of age 50 or older (five were 60 or older). Complete symptom scores and demographic data were available for only 11 participants of age 50 or older and 86 younger adults. Thus, the generalizability of these findings is severely limited. Nonetheless, age group differences between the older and younger patients were explored. These analyses are only exploratory, and future research with larger samples of older adults with OCD is needed.

Symptoms endorsed on the 15 YBOCS checklist categories were quantified as follows: The category was scored zero if the patient did not endorse any symptoms, one if the patient endorsed at least one symptom but the category was not considered primary, or two if symptoms were endorsed and the category was considered a principal problem. Three between-group differences emerged when comparisons were made on reported symptom level across the checklist categories (see Table 17.1). Older adults had significantly greater hoarding obsession scores [$t(95) = 2.99$, $p = 0.004$], hoarding compulsion scores [$t(95) = 2.63$, $p = 0.010$] and significantly lower checking compulsion scores [$t(95) = -2.14$, $p = 0.038$]. Measures of depression, anxiety and anxiety sensitivity did not differ between age groups.

In light of our preliminary finding that there may be an association between older age and hoarding symptoms, we reviewed the literature on this under-studied OCD symptom. An association between older age and this symptom has sometimes been reported. Frost *et al.* (1998) found that a self-identified group of hoarders, five of whom reported being diagnosed with OCD, were significantly older (mean age = 55.7) than a non-hoarding comparison group. However, Frost and Gross (1993) did not find age differences between hoarders and non-hoarders and indicated that hoarding symptoms began in this sample during childhood or adolescence. There are several case reports in the OCD literature where hoarding symptoms have been observed in older adults. Rosenthal, Stelian, Wagner, and Berkman (1999) described two cases of what they described as Diogenes Syndrome, a dementing disorder associated with a tendency to hoard. Both patients were over 80-

years-old. Hwang, Tsai, Yang, Liu, and Lirng (1998) assessed 133 dementia patients (aged 65–91) for hoarding symptoms. Symptoms were identified in 30 patients and the authors concluded that hoarding was a common symptom in dementia patients. Frost and colleagues have recently proposed a comprehensive cognitive–behavioral model of hoarding (Frost & Hartl, 1996). In this model, specific information processing deficits are identified in obsessional hoarders: General decision making problems, categorizing problems involving under-inclusive categorization, an over-focusing of attention on saved items, and deficits in memory confidence, although there is no objective indication of actual memory deficits (Frost & Steketee, 1999).

The association between older age and other types of specific OCD symptoms is based solely on case studies. Obsessional concerns focused on bowel function have sometimes been reported in older adults, although cases in young adults have also been described (e.g., Hatch, 1997). Ramchandani (1990) reported a case involving a 66-year-old man who worried continuously about being able to have a bowel movement. Jenike, Vitagliano, Rabinowitz, Goff, and Baer (1987) reported bowel obsession cases in two women, aged 56 and 57, both of whom feared losing control of bowel function. One of the two cases described by Hatch (1997) was a 69-year-old man who feared loss of control of bowel function in a public setting. Hatch (1997) pointed out that there is disagreement in the literature on whether this symptom should be considered a variant of OCD, a form of social phobia, or an atypical presentation of panic disorder and agoraphobia.

Moral and religious scrupulosity has been reported as a form of elder OCD. Fallon *et al.* (1990) described two such cases. The first case was a 69-year-old man who repeatedly confessed his sins and constantly worried about the morality of his actions. The second case involved a 67-year-old woman, a devout Catholic who attended mass three times per day and had checking and hand washing symptoms. Both cases were responsive to pharmacologic treatments. Other case reports of OCD in elderly patients have involved atypical comorbid presentations. Gordon and Rasmussen (1988) described a 62-year-old man with a 30-year history of OCD with bipolar disorder. Deckert and Malone (1990) reported the occurrence of OCD and non-specific psychotic symptomatology in a 61-year-old woman.

Pollard, Carmin, and Ownby (1997) concluded that there was no convincing evidence that a particular constellation of OCD symptoms was unique to older adults. Symptoms such as hoarding and bowel obsessions have been reported in younger adults, and common OCD presentations (e.g., contamination concerns) have also been seen in elderly patients with OCD. Only one between-age-group comparison of OCD symptoms has been published (Kohn *et al.*, 1997), and in this study, several age group differences in symptoms were identified. Further experimental evaluation of this issue appears warranted.

Although there is limited indication that specific types of OCD symptoms are more strongly associated with OCD in the elderly, evaluation of the relations between the content of obsessions and compulsions and core cognitive dimensions of OCD may be informative. The development of measures of intrusive thought appraisals and obsessional beliefs by the Obsessive Compulsive Cognitions Working Group (OCCWG, 1997; see Chapter seven of this volume) creates an opportunity for investigators to explore possible connections between cognitive dimensions of OCD and OCD symptoms in older adults and other age

Table 17.1: Mean Scores on the Yale–Brown Obsessive Compulsive Scale Symptom Checklist Categories

| | AGE GROUP | | | |
| | Older Adults $n = 11$ | | Adults $n = 86$ | |
	Mean	SD	Mean	SD
Y-BOCS SYMPTOM CATEGORY				
Aggressive Obsessions	0.727	0.905	1.128	0.779
Contamination Obsessions	0.818	0.874	1.012	0.833
Sexual Obsessions	0.272	0.647	0.326	0.541
Hoarding Obsessions*	1.000	0.775	0.419	0.583
Religious Obsessions	0.364	0.809	0.419	0.563
Symmetry or Exactness Obsessions	0.545	0.688	0.686	0.740
Miscellaneous Obsession	0.818	0.751	0.907	0.746
Somatic Obsessions	0.364	0.505	0.535	0.715
Cleaning Compulsions	0.818	0.874	0.953	0.825
Checking Compulsions*	0.727	0.786	1.267	0.803
Repeating Rituals	0.727	0.647	0.756	0.685
Counting Compulsions	0.182	0.405	0.419	0.622
Ordering Compulsions	0.273	0.467	0.465	0.547
Hoarding Compulsions*	0.818	0.874	0.314	0.559
Miscellaneous Compulsions	0.909	0.831	0.826	0.654

Note: * = groups differed at $p < 0.05$.

groups. Such investigations could help in understanding the variability seen in OCD patients' obsessions and compulsions and may help in the refinement of treatment interventions for new sub-types of OCD that may emerge from this type of investigation.

Intrusive Thoughts, Appraisals, and Beliefs in Older Adults

Dysfunctional appraisals of the experience of intrusive thoughts and related beliefs are central to cognitive theories (Carr, 1974; McFall & Wollersheim, 1979; Rachman, 1993; Salkovskis, 1985, 1989). Salkovskis (1985, 1989) offered a detailed cognitive-behavioral theory of obsessions based on two core observations: that cognitive intrusions are universally experienced (e.g., Rachman & de Silva, 1978), and that the difference between clinical and normal intrusions involves the individual's negative appraisal of the experience.

The specific nature of the dysfunctional appraisals and beliefs thought most important to the development or maintenance of OCD has varied across cognitive models. Carr (1974) proposed that all "compulsive neurotics" have abnormally high expectations regarding the occurrence of negative outcomes. Compulsive behavior was thought to develop to reduce the probability of the unfavorable outcome. McFall and Wollersheim (1979) outlined several unreasonable beliefs thought to be central to OCD, including irrational ideas that one should be perfect to avoid criticism or disapproval by others, and that one is powerful enough to prevent disastrous outcomes by rituals. McFall and Wollersheim suggested that rituals reduce uncertainty and anxiety and provide the individual with a sense of control. Salkovskis (1989) proposed that individuals with OCD have dysfunctional beliefs involving blame and excessive responsibility for harm occurring to themselves and others. Compulsive behavior is thought to be a way to reduce potential harm or danger to self or others and avert blame and responsibility.

Experimental methodologies have been developed to identify how individuals appraise the experience of intrusive thoughts and to measure a variety of belief domains thought to be important for OCD. The goal of these experimental investigations has been to identify beliefs and appraisals that distinguish obsessional patients from non-clinicals and from patients with other anxiety disorders. Most often, self-report instruments designed to tap various belief and appraisal domains have been used and between-group differences have been explored. A few researchers have employed experimental methodologies involving the direct manipulation of cognitive domains of interest (e.g., responsibility; Lopatka & Rachman, 1995). None of these methods has been used to investigate obsessional phenomena in older adults.

Responsibility has been a better predictor of OCD symptoms than perfectionism (Rhéaume, Freeston, Dugas, Letarte, & Ladouceur, 1995). However, positive correlations between perfectionism and OCD symptoms have been found in non-clinical (e.g., Frost, Marten, Lahart, & Rosenblate, 1990; Rhéaume *et al.*, 1995) and clinical populations (e.g., Frost & Steketee, 1997). Several studies support the existence of an association between risk aversion and OCD (e.g., Steiner, 1972; Steketee & Frost, 1994) lending support to the notion that OCD patients have elevated expectations regarding danger and threat. Thought–action fusion (the belief that thoughts can influence events or are almost equivalent to actions) has been found to be elevated in samples of OCD patients (Rachman, Thordarson, Shafran, & Woody, 1995; Shafran, Thordarson, & Rachman, 1996). Patients with OCD and with other anxiety disorders differ in their beliefs about the need to control mental activity (Clark & Purdon, 1993) and in their tolerance for uncertainty (beliefs related to doubt about the correctness of their decisions and related conclusions; (e.g., Kozak, Foa, & McCarthy, 1987). Appraisals of responsibility have been successfully manipulated in multiple studies, with corresponding changes in compulsive behavior observed (Ladouceur *et al.*, 1995; Ladouceur, Rhéaume, & Aublet, 1997; Lopatka & Rachman, 1995).

The influence of age on thought appraisal and belief domains has not been directly studied. Age has been included as a variable in two investigations of the relationship between beliefs and OCD symptoms. Steketee, Frost, and Cohen (1998) studied beliefs related to responsibility for harm, control of thoughts, threat estimation, tolerance for uncertainty, discomfort/anxiety, and coping in subjects with OCD, other anxiety disorders (AD), and non-clinical controls. Differences in beliefs among diagnostic groups remained significant after co-varying age. OCD subjects scored higher than the AD group on all belief domains measured. The AD group did not differ from non-clinicals on responsibility for harm, control of thoughts or threat estimation, but did score higher than controls on tolerance for uncertainty, tolerance for anxiety and beliefs about coping. The authors suggested that the last three belief domains may be more prominent in OCD, but perhaps not unique to this disorder. Scarrabelotti, Duck, and Dickerson (1995) examined the relationship between responsibility appraisals, depression, neuroticism, psychoticism and OCD symptoms in a non-clinical sample. Using the Padua Inventory as the dependent measure of OCD symptomatology, regression analysis revealed that responsibility accounted for significant variance even after controlling for other variables including age. Age and gender accounted for a small but significant amount of variance (6 percent) in obsessive compulsive symptoms.

To investigate possible age differences in OCD-related appraisals and beliefs, we conducted a between-age-group analysis of the Stage three data gathered by the OCCWG (in preparation) in their on-going efforts to refine measures of hypothesized core cognitive dimensions of OCD. Only 11 adults aged 55 or older were included in this English speaking sample of 270 patients with OCD. No between-age-group differences were found on the three subscales of the Interpretation of Intrusions Inventory or on the six subscales of the Obsessional Beliefs Questionnaire when the responses of the 11 older adults were compared to 15 randomly selected younger adults.

To date, there has been very limited study of the relationship between cognitive dimensions of OCD and developmental level. Appraisal processes and beliefs about the importance of thoughts have not been studied in an adequate sample of elders with OCD or in non-clinical elderly samples. Beliefs about thought and the appraisal of negative intrusive thoughts may be broadly influenced by developmental processes and evaluation in specific age groups, including elderly samples, is warranted. Age-related changes in cognitive functioning may prove to be important influencers on thought appraisals and beliefs. Evaluation of the OCCWG's large clinical data-base of OCD patients revealed that very few older adults are presenting at major OCD treatment and research centers throughout the world. It appears that concerted efforts will be needed to identify adequate numbers of older adults with OCD for study. Furthermore, it may be that older adults with OCD fail to present for treatment, hindering identification and treatment.

Aging, Cognitive Functioning, and Obsessions

Do the mild cognitive changes associated with normal aging or the more pronounced changes experienced during the initial stages of dementing disease processes interact with other variables to affect reactivity to intrusive thoughts or alter general beliefs regarding the importance of cognition? The cognitive changes observed in normal aging and some affective reactions to these changes are briefly reviewed to explore this issue. Age-related changes in three basic cognitive domains posited to be important in aging are reviewed. These include changes in fluid as opposed to crystallized intelligence, effortful and non-effortful processing of information, and processing or perceptual speed.

Crystallized intelligence represents the ability to perform tasks that are over-learned, practiced, and familiar. Researchers studying this area of aging have found that abilities and knowledge that are crystallized remain highly functional throughout life and that gains in these abilities are seen into the seventh and eight decades (Horn & Donaldson, 1976; Kaufman, Reynolds, & McLean, 1989). Fluid intelligence refers to problem solving and reasoning abilities employed on unfamiliar tasks. Researchers generally agree that a slow decline in fluid intelligence occurs within middle adulthood and that a steeper decrease in ability occurs in the late fifties or early sixties (Kaufman & Horn, 1996; Kaufman *et al.*, 1989).

The related distinction between effortful and non-effortful processing has often been applied to the study of memory. Dobbs and Rule (1989) distinguished between primary memory (the passive capacity to keep things in mind) and working memory (the ability to store and process information at the same time). Dobbs and Rule (1989) reported that older adults did not show primary memory deficits in comparison to younger adults. Reliable age differences were found, however, on working memory tasks when elders were compared to younger individuals. These differences were evident when older adults processed math problems (Babcock & Salthouse, 1990) or spatial information (Salthouse, 1993). Although longitudinal data is limited, older adults appear to experience a decline in working memory abilities as they age (Hultsch, Hertzog, Small, McDonald-Miszczak, & Dixon, 1992). In summary, it appears that automatic, over-learned, abilities are generally age-resistant, whereas abilities more dependent on working memory are vulnerable to the effects of the aging process (Hasher & Zacks, 1979).

Perceptual speed is generally defined as the time required to perform a simple perceptual comparison. Examples of tests that measure this ability include the Digit Symbol Test (Weschler, 1981) and the Symbol Digit Modalities Test (Smith, 1982). In cross-sectional studies, large differences between older adults and other age groups have usually been found on tests of perceptual or processing speed (Wilson *et al.*, 1997). Observed differences appear not to be the result of a general motor behavior slowing, but may be attributable to slowed mental processing or perceptual speed (Salthouse, 1992). Differences in perceptual speed show up early in the aging process and appear to affect most older adults (Salthouse, 1992). Indeed, if age-related differences in perceptual speed are controlled statistically, most memory and higher order cognitive task performance differences between age groups shrink or are eliminated (Salthouse, 1991, 1993).

Older adults have been found to be aware of age-related cognitive change, to be emotionally reactive to such changes, and to be emotionally reactive to their subjective perception of cognitive functioning changes that may or may not closely correlate with objective indicators of cognitive decline. Jorm *et al.* (1994) reported that 71 percent of their community-dwelling sample of adults aged 55 and older complained of memory decline. Subjective memory complaints correlated with objective memory impairment in some studies (Jonker, Launer, Hooijer, & Lindeboom, 1996; Levi-Cushman & Abeles, 1998) and predicted future declines in memory abilities in longitudinal studies (Schmand, Jonker, Geerlings, & Lindeboom, 1997). Other investigations identified no relationships between subjective memory complaints and objective memory problems (West,

Boatwright, & Schleser, 1984). In some studies, subjective memory complaints in older adults were related to general emotional distress (Smith, Petersen, Ivnik, Malec, & Tangalos, 1996), neuroticism (Ponds & Jolles, 1996), depressive symptomatology (Brustrom & Ober, 1998), and general symptoms of anxiety, depression and trait neuroticism (Jorm *et al.*, 1994). Additionally, Jorm *et al.* (1997) observed that subjective memory complaints did not predict future cognitive decline after controlling for the effects of anxiety level and depression.

While the relationships among objective age-related cognitive change, subjective memory complaints and emotional state are complex, some conclusions can be drawn from available information. Older adults are vigilant regarding their cognitive functioning and perceived dysfunction is related to emotional distress. That is, older adults pay close attention to their memory and other cognitive functions and are reactive to change or perceived change. Could these processes set the stage for a type of metacognitive hypervigilance and make the older adult more reactive to common negative intrusive thoughts? As the older adult who is concerned about cognitive functioning, begins to monitor cognitive processes more closely, are negative intrusive thoughts made more salient? Would the increased salience of negative intrusive thoughts lead to effortful thought control strategies? As these effortful strategies to control negative intrusive thoughts fail, does this heighten older adults' fears of cognitive dysfunction or dyscontrol and increase anxiety and other distress that then further increases metacognitive hypervigilance? This hypothesized relation between feared cognitive decline and metacognitive hypervigilance appears analogous to the interrelationships between various feared bodily sensations, common anxiety experiences, apprehension, and panic described by Clark (1986). The relations between objective and subjective measures of cognitive change, beliefs about thought, and obsessional symptoms should be explored in older adults.

Cognitive–Behavioral Treatment of OCD in Older Adults

In their review of the treatment of OCD in older adults, Calamari *et al.* (1994) concluded that there had been very limited evaluation of exposure and response prevention (ERP) with this population. Since then, there have been important additions to the treatment literature, although there has not yet been a large, controlled study of older adults' response to behavioral or cognitive therapies.

Carmin, Pollard, and Ownby (1998) reported the only treatment outcome study involving a comparison between older and younger adults' responses to behavioral therapy for severe OCD. The treatment response of ten older adults (mean age 68) was compared to ten younger adults matched for gender and level of depression. Although the older adults had been symptomatic over twice as long as the younger adult group, they were equally responsive to ERP treatment. Age groups did not differ on their self-rated improvement or in the likelihood of being classified as a treatment responder, rigorously defined as at least a 50 percent reduction in symptoms. Sixty percent of the elderly group and 70 percent of the younger adult group were classified as treatment responders.

Other psychosocial treatment intervention reports of elder OCD have been case study reports. Carmin *et al.* (1999) described two cases successfully treated with ERP. The first case was a 67-year-old woman with no previous psychiatric treatment history. The patient reported checking, arranging and hoarding compulsions motivated by perfectionism, and "just right" obsessions. The patient was responsive to a graduated intensive ERP protocol, an adjustment made because of her chronic obstructive pulmonary disease. The patient was responsive to treatment and gains were maintained at one year follow-up. Carmin *et al.* (1999) described a 71-year-old woman with harming obsessions treated on an inpatient behavior therapy unit with ERP and cognitive therapy. The patient was initially responsive to treatment, but gains were difficult to maintain and the patient discontinued therapy, although a maintenance intervention program was recommended.

Calamari and Cassiday (1999) reported two cases of late-life OCD. They described a 77-year-old woman who was diagnosed with OCD, major depression, and panic disorder with agoraphobia. Her primary OCD symptoms were hoarding, harming obsessions, and checking behavior. The patient presented with her daughter, in treatment for panic disorder herself, who was a significant aid during assessment and treatment. The patient was reluctant to initiate behavioral treatment because of a history of repeated, unsuccessful inpatient hospitalizations. The patient was taught simple anxiety management techniques and coached to use these procedures during ERP. At home, ERP was extensively coached by the patient's daughter with whom she had good rapport. The patient and her daughter judged treatment response to be favorable including a reduction in hoarding behavior.

Calamari and Cassiday's (1999) second case involved severe scrupulosity. The staff at this 87-year-old woman's retirement home complained about her increasingly unusual behavior and was concerned that she was at risk for bladder infection because she avoided urinating until the last possible moment. Additionally, she had begun to listen constantly to religious songs, ate only corn flakes, and was repetitiously checking her dentures and hands. Clinical assessment revealed that the patient's behavior was motivated by a need to try to not think about God while engaged in "dirty" activities (e.g., urinating or eating). Treatment was complicated by a history of involuntary hospitalizations initiated by family members in response to her continuous requests for others to pray with her, repetitive hand washing, and general inability to function at home. The patient refused to allow her son to be a support person in treatment because of embarrassment about her symptoms. Nine therapy sessions involving cognitive therapy and ERP, focused on the excessive nature of scrupulosity behavior, were provided. Significant symptom reduction was reported by the patient and her son, although extensive symptoms remained at treatment termination.

Based on available reports, it appears that older adults are responsive to cognitive–behavioral treatment for OCD, although controlled studies are needed. Older adults with a broad range of symptoms are described in the case report literature, and favorable treatment responses are reported frequently. When a less than complete response to treatment is reported, it appears that less favorable outcome may be associated with forms of OCD considered more difficult to treat in any age group (e.g., scrupulosity) or with more complex patient presentations (e.g., multiple comorbid psychiatric disorders). Controlled study is needed to support or refute these observations.

Some case reports have included discussion of needed adjustments in the assessment or treatment of OCD in older adults. Carmin *et al.* (1999) reviewed the adjustments needed in assessment and treatment protocols for late-life OCD. The authors pointed out that clinicians will be challenged by the need to distinguish OCD from the symptoms of other psychiatric disorders and from symptoms associated with a broad range of physical conditions. Assessment instruments commonly used to evaluate OCD in adults have not been validated with this age group, making the interpretation of findings more difficult. The reticence of older adults to report psychological symptoms may cause them to under-report symptoms or related distress. Sensory impairments may make communication more difficult during the assessment process and during treatment. Treatment protocols may require modification because of co-occurring medical conditions with health problems limiting attendance at treatment sessions and ability to do assignments. Treatment instructions and the general rationale for the treatment approach may need to be repeated with elderly patients. Carmin *et al.* (1999) recommended scheduling regular follow-up sessions with older adults to help maintain treatment gains.

Can the Cognitive Therapies for OCD be Adapted for Older Adults?

Pharmacologic interventions involving selective serotonin reuptake inhibitors, and a specific form of behavior therapy, exposure and response prevention, are well established interventions for OCD in general adults samples (see Stanley & Turner's 1995 review). Although initial evaluations of cognitive therapy treatment of OCD were favorable (Emmelkamp & Beens, 1991; Emmelkamp, Visser, & Hoekstra, 1988), the approach had not attracted extensive attention from clinicians or researchers until recently. The development of the cognitive theories of OCD (Salkovskis, 1985, 1989; Rachman, 1993), and advances in OCD specific cognitive therapy formulations (e.g., Freeston, *et al.*, 1996) have stimulated much greater interest in cognitive therapy for OCD. There is growing evidence for the efficacy of cognitive therapy approaches for the treatment of OCD in adult clients (Emmelkamp & Beens, 1991; Emmelkamp *et al.*, 1988; Freeston *et al.*, 1997; van Oppen, *et al.*, 1995).

There is reason to believe that cognitive therapy procedures can be successfully adapted for use with older adults. Cognitive therapy for late-life depression has been successfully developed and has involved limited modification of standard treatment protocols (e.g., Thompson, Gallagher, & Breckenridge, 1987). Brief cognitive therapy with older adults has been found to produce long-lasting improvements in many participants (Gallagher-Thompson, Hanley-Peterson, & Thompson, 1990). Calamari and Cassiday (1999) reviewed the evolution of OCD-specific cognitive therapy and suggested that these approaches could be adapted for older adults.

A pre-requisite for the development of cognitive interventions for late-life OCD would be the careful characterization of older adults' reactions to and beliefs about negative intrusive thoughts. Out of such experimental work would emerge an understanding of the cognitive dimensions of late-life OCD, — information needed to maximize the effectiveness of intervention. Cognition measures, such as the instruments under development by the OCCWG, will need to be validated with older adult samples as a first step in the completion of this work.

Conclusions

OCD in older adults has been under-studied. Although the disorder appears to occur less often late in life, anxiety disorders generally and OCD specifically occurs frequently in the elderly. Additional efforts involving the careful characterization of OCD in older adults are needed to determine the frequency of clinical and sub-clinical symptoms in this age group. Prevalence estimates of late-life OCD are limited by the use of assessment procedures and instruments that have not been validated with this age group. Refinements in assessment approaches are needed before accurate prevalence estimates of late-life OCD can be obtained. OCD appears to have begun early in life for most older adults presenting for treatment of OCD. For a minority of elderly OCD patients, the disorder will have first appeared after age 60. It is not known how late-onset OCD is related to developmental processes, if the phenomenology of late-onset OCD is different, whether this variant of OCD results from different etiologic processes, if late-onset OCD is associated with different beliefs about the importance of thought, or if the condition responds differently to treatment. It appears that older adults with OCD present with the full range of OCD symptoms. It is not known at this time if some types of symptoms are more prevalent in this age group or generally how different types of obsessions and compulsions might be related to differences in obsessional patients' appraisals of intrusive thoughts.

Cognitive dimensions of OCD have been posited to play a primary role in the development and maintenance of the disorder. These processes have not been evaluated in older adults. The psychometric properties of OCD related cognition measures, including the instruments being developed by the OCCWG, will need to be evaluated with elders as an initial step in the exploration of the cognitive dimensions of OCD in this age group. The possible effects of age-related cognitive change on beliefs about OCD cognitions (e.g., over-importance of thoughts) also remains to be explored. Although available information suggests that older adults are responsive to cognitive–behavioral treatments of OCD, controlled studies are lacking. Older adults with major depression have been successfully treated with cognitive therapy procedures adapted for the needs of this age group. This suggests that cognitive therapy procedures designed to alter OCD-related beliefs may be successfully adapted for use with older adults. Although much work remains to be done, OCD in older adults is a treatable condition that will be made more understandable following completion of much needed empirical work.

References

Babcock, R. L., & Salthouse, T. A. (1990). Effects of increased processing demands on age differences in working memory. *Psychology and Aging, 5*, 421–428.

Bajulaiye, R., & Addonizio, G. (1992). Obsessive–compulsive disorder arising in a 75-year-old woman. *International Journal of Geriatric Psychiatry, 7*, 139–142.

Beck, A. T., Emery, G., & Greenberg, R. (1985). *Anxiety disorders and phobias: A cognitive perspective.* New York: Basic Books.

Beck, J. G., & Stanley, M. (1997). Anxiety disorders in the elderly: The emerging role of behavior therapy. *Behavior Therapy, 28,* 83–100.

Beekman, A. T. F., Bremmer, M. A., Deeg, D. J. H., van Bolkom, A. J. L. M., Smit, J. H., de Beurs, E. D., van Dyck, R., & van Tilberg, W. (1998). Anxiety disorders in later life: A report from the longitudinal aging study Amsterdam. *International Journal of Geriatric Psychiatry, 13,* 717–726.

Bland, R. C., Newman, S. C., & Orn, H. (1988). Prevalence of psychiatric disorders in the elderly in Edmonton. *Acta Psyciatric Scandinavia, 77,* (suppl 338), 57–63.

Brustrom, J. E., & Ober, B. A. (1998). Predictors of perceived memory impairment: Do they differ in Alzheimer's disease versus normal aging? *Journal of Clinical and Experimental Neuropsychology, 20,* 402–412.

Calamari, J. E., & Cassiday, K. L. (1999). Treating Obsessive–Compulsive Disorder in Older Adults: A Review of strategies. In M. Duffy (ed.), *Handbook of counseling and psychotherapy with older adults* (pp. 526–538). New York: Wiley.

Calamari, J. E., Faber, S. D., Hitsman, B. L., & Poppe, B. A. (1994). Treatment of obsessive–compulsive disorder in the elderly: A review and case example. *Journal of Behavior Therapy and Experimental Psychiatry, 25,* 95–104.

Calamari, J. E., Wiegartz, P. S., & Janeck, A. S. (1999). Obsessive–compulsive disorder subgroups: A symptom-based clustering approach. *Behaviour Research and Therapy, 37,* 113–125.

Carmin, C. N., Pollard, C. A., & Ownby, R. L. (1999). Cognitive–behavioral treatment of older adults with obsessive–compulsive disorder. *Cognitive and Behavioral Practice, 6,* 110–119.

Carmin, C. N., Pollard, C. A., & Ownby, R. L. (1998). Obsessive–compulsive disorder: Cognitive–behavioral treatment of older versus younger adults. *Clinical Gerontologist, 19,* 77–81.

Carr, A. T. (1974). Compulsive neurosis: A review of the literature. *Psychological Bulletin, 81,* 311–318.

Clark, D. M. (1986). A cognitive approach to panic. *Behaviour Research and Therapy, 24,* 461–470.

Clark, D. A., & Purdon, C. (1993). New perspectives for a cognitive theory of obsessions. *Australian Psychologist, 28,* 161–167.

Colvin, C., & Boddington, S. (1997). Case report: Behaviour therapy for obsessive–compulsive disorder in a 78-year old woman. *International Journal of Geriatric Psychiatry, 12,* 488–491.

Deckert, D. W., & Malone, D. A. (1990). Treatment of psychotic symptoms in OCD patients. *Journal of Clinical Psychiatry, 51,* 259.

Dobbs, A. R., & Rule, B. G. (1989). Adult age differences in working memory. *Psychology and Aging, 4,* 500–503.

Emmelkamp, P., & Beens, H. (1991). Cognitive therapy with obsessive–compulsive disorder: A comparative evaluation. *Behaviour Research and Therapy, 29,* 293–300.

Emmelkamp, P., Visser, S., & Hoekstra, R. (1988). Cognitive therapy vs. exposure in vivo in the treatment of obsessive-compulsives. *Cognitive Therapy and Research, 12,* 103–114.

Fallon, B. A., Liebowitz, M. R., Hollander, E., Schneier, F. R., Campeas, R. B., Fairbanks, J., Papp, L. A., Hatterer, J. A., & Sandberg, D. (1990). The pharmacotherapy of moral or religious scrupulosity. *Journal of Clinical Psychiatry, 51,* 517–521.

Flint, A. J. (1994). Epidemiology and comorbidity of anxiety disorders in the elderly. *American Journal of Psychiatry, 151,* 640–649.

Freeston, M. H., Ladouceur, R., Gagnon, F., Thibodeau, N., Rhéaume, J., Letarte, H., & Bujold, A. (1997). Cognitive–behavioral treatment of obsessive thoughts: A controlled study. *Journal of Consulting and Clinical Psychology, 65,* 405–413.

Freeston, M. H., Rhéaume, J., & Ladouceur, R. (1996). Correcting faulty appraisals of obsessional thoughts. *Behaviour Research and Therapy, 34*, 433–446.

Frost, R. O., & Gross, R. C. (1993). The hoarding of possessions. *Behaviour Research and Therapy, 31*, 367–381.

Frost, R. O., & Hartl, T. L. (1996). A cognitive–behavioral model of compulsive hoarding. *Behaviour Research and Therapy, 34*, 341–350.

Frost, R. O., Kim, H., Morris, C., Bloss, C., Murry-Close, M., & Steketee, G. (1998). Hoarding, compulsive buying and reasons for saving. *Behaviour Research and Therapy, 36*, 657–664.

Frost, R. O., Marten, P. A., Lahart, C., & Rosenblate, R. (1990). The dimensions of perfectionism. *Cognitive Therapy and Research, 14*, 449–468.

Frost, R. O., & Steketee, G. (1999). Issues in the treatment of compulsive hoarding. *Cognitive and Behavioral Practice, 6*, 397–407.

Frost, R. O., & Steketee, G. (1997). Perfectionism in obsessive–compulsive disorder patients. *Behaviour, Research and Therapy, 35*, 291–296.

Fuentes, K., & Cox, B. J. (1997). Prevalence of anxiety disorders in elderly adults: A critical analysis. *Journal of Behavior Therapy and Experimental Psychiatry, 28*, 269–279.

Gallager-Thompson, D., Hanley-Peterson, P., & Thompson, L. W. (1990). Maintenance of gains versus relapse following brief psychotherapy for depression. *Journal of Consulting and Clinical Psychology, 58*, 371–374.

Gonzales, A., & Philpot, M. P. (1998). Late onset startle syndrome and obsessive–compulsive disorder. *Behavioral Neurology, 11*, 113–116.

Goodwin, D. W., Guze, S. B., & Robins, E. (1969). Follow-up studies on obsessional neurosis. *Archives of General Psychiatry, 20*, 182–187.

Goodman, W. K., Price, L. H., Rasmussen, S. H., Mazure, C., Fleishman, R. L., Hill, C. L., Heninger, G. R., & Charney, D. S. (1989a). The Yale–Brown Obsessive–Compulsive Scale: I. Development, use and reliability. *Archives of General Psychiatry, 46*, 1006–1011.

Goodman, W. K., Price, L. H., Rasmussen, S. H., Mazure, C., Fleishman, R. L., Hill, C. L., Heninger, G. R., & Charney, D. S. (1989b). The Yale–Brown Obsessive–Compulsive Scale: II. Validity. *Archives of General Psychiatry, 46*, 1012–1016.

Gordon, A., & Rasmussen, S. A. (1988). Mood-related obsessive–compulsive symptoms in a patient with bipolar affective disorder. *Journal of Clinical Psychiatry, 49*, 27–28.

Gurian, B. S., & Miner, J. H. (1991). Clinical presentation of anxiety disorders in the elderly. In C. Salzman & B. D. Lebovitz (eds), *Anxiety in the elderly: Treatment and research* (pp. 31–44). New York: Springer.

Hatch, M. L. (1997). Conceptualization and treatment of bowel obsessions: Two case reports. *Behaviour Research and Therapy, 35*, 253–257.

Hasher, L., & Zacks, R. T. (1979). Automatic and effortful processes in memory. *Journal of Experimental Psychology: General, 108*, 356–388.

Hersen, M., & Van Hasselt, V. B. (1992). Behavioral assessment and treatment of anxiety in the elderly. *Clinical Psychology Review, 12*, 619–640.

Horn, J. L., & Donaldson, G. (1976). On the myth of intellectual decline in adulthood. *American Psychologist, 31*, 701–719.

Hultsch, D. F., Hertzog, C., Small, B. J., McDonald-Miszczak, L., & Dixon, R. A. (1992). Short-term longitudinal change in cognitive performance in later life. *Psychology and Aging, 7*, 571–584.

Hwang, J., Tsai, S., Yang, C., Liu, K., & Lirng, J. (1998). Hoarding behavior in dementia: A preliminary report. *American Journal of Geriatric Psychiatry, 6*, 285–289.

Jenike, M. A. (1991). Geriatric obsessive–compulsive disorder. *Journal of Geriatric Psychiatry, 4*, 34–39.

Jenike, M. A., Vitagliano, H. L., Rabinowitz, J., Goff, D. C., & Baer, L. (1987). Bowel obsession responsive to tricyclic antidepressants in four patients. *American Journal of Psychiatry, 144*, 1347–1348.

Jonker, C., Launer, L. J., Hooijer, C., & Lindeboom, J. (1996). Memory complaints and memory impairment in older individuals. *Journal of the American Geriatrics Society, 44*, 44–49.

Jorm, A. F., Christensen, H., Henderson, A. S., Korten, A. E., MacKinnon, A. J., & Scott, R. (1994). Complaint of cognitive decline in the elderly: A comparison of reports by subjects and informants in a community survey. *Psychological Medicine, 24*, 365–374.

Jorm, A. F., Christensen, H., Korten, A. E., Henderson, A. S., Jacomb, P. A., & MacKinnon, A. (1997). Do cognitive complaints either predict future cognitive decline or reflect past cognitive decline? A longitudinal study of an elderly community sample. *Psychological Medicine, 27*, 91–98.

Juninger, J., Phelan, E., Cherry, K., & Levy, J. (1993). Prevalence of psychopathology in elderly persons in nursing homes and in the community. *Hospital and Community Psychiatry, 44*, 381–383.

Karno, M., Golding, J. M., Sorenson, S. B., & Burnam, M. A. (1988). The epidemiology of obsessive–compulsive disorder in five US communities. *Archives of General Psychiatry, 45*, 1094–1099.

Kaufman, A. S., & Horn, J. L. (1996). Age changes on tests of fluid and crystallized ability for women and men on the Kaufman Adolescent and Adult Intelligence Test (KAIT) at ages 17–94 years. *Archives of Clinical Neuropsychology, 11*, 97–121.

Kaufman, A. S., Reynolds, C. E., & McLean, J. E. (1989). Age and WAIS-R intelligence in a national sample of adults in the 20 to 74-year age range: A cross-sectional analysis with educational level controlled. *Intelligence, 13*, 235–253.

Kohn, R., Westlake, R. J., Rasmussen, S. A., Marsland, R. T., & Norman, W. H. (1997). Clinical features of obsessive–compulsive disorder in elderly patients. *American Journal of Geriatric Psychiatry, 5*, 211–215.

Kozak, M. J., Foa, E., & McCarthy, P. (1987). Assessment of obsessive–compulsive disorder. In C. Last & M. Hersen (eds), *Handbook of anxiety disorders* (pp.87–108). New York: Pergamon.

Ladouceur, R., Rhéaume, J., & Aublet, F. (1997). Excessive responsibility in obsessional concerns: A fine-grained experimental analysis. *Behaviour Research and Therapy, 35*, 423–427.

Ladouceur, R., Rhéaume, J., Freeston, M. H., Aublet, F., Jean, K., Lachance, S., Langlois, F., & De Pokomandy-Morin, K. (1995). Experimental manipulations of responsibility: An analogue test for models of obsessive–compulsive disorder. *Behaviour Research and Therapy, 33*, 937–946.

Lasoski, M. C. (1986). Reasons for low utilization of mental health services by the elderly. In T. L. Brink (ed.), *Clinical gerontology: A guide to assessment and intervention* (pp. 1–18). New York: The Haworth Press.

Levi-Cushman, J., & Abeles, N. (1998). Memory complaints in the able elderly. *Clinical Gerontologist, 19*, 3–24.

Lopatka, C., & Rachman, S. (1995). Perceived responsibility and compulsive checking: An experimental analysis. *Behaviour Research and Therapy, 33*, 673–684.

Matt, G. E., Dean, A., Wang, B., & Wood, P. (1992). Identifying clinical syndromes in a clinical sample of elderly persons. *Psychological Assessment, 4*, 174–184.

McFall, M. E., & Wollersheim, J. P. (1979). Obsessive–compulsive neurosis: A cognitive-behavioral formulation and approach to treatment. *Cognitive Therapy and Research, 3*, 333–348.

Minichello, W. E., Baer, L., Jenike, M., A., & Holland, A. (1990). Age of onset of major sub-types of obsessive–compulsive disorder. *Journal of Anxiety Disorders, 4*, 147–150.

Nestadt, G., Bienvenu, O. J., Cai, G., Samuels, J., & Eaton, W. E. (1998). Incidence of obsessive–compulsive disorder in older adults. *The Journal of Nervous and Mental Disease, 186*, 401–406.

Obsessive–Compulsive Cognitions Working Group (1997). Cognitive assessment of obsessive–compulsive disorder. *Behaviour Research and Therapy, 35*, 667–681.

Obsessive–Compulsive Cognitions Working Group (in preparation). *Psychometric Validation of the Obsessive–Beliefs Questionnaire and the Interpretation of Intrusions Inventory: Findings from Stage III Data.*

Philpot, M. P., & Banerjee, S. (1998). Obsessive–compulsive disorder in the elderly. *Behavioural Neurology, 11*, 117–121.

Pollard, C. A., Carmin, C. N., & Ownby, R. (1997). Obsessive–compulsive disorder in later life. *Annals of Psychiatry, 3*, 57–72.

Ponds, R. W. H. M., & Jolles, J. (1996). Memory complaints in elderly people: The role of memory abilities, metamemory, depression, and personality. *Educational Gerontology, 22*, 341–357.

Rachman, S. (1993). Obsessions, responsibility and guilt. *Behaviour Research and Therapy, 31*, 149–154.

Rachman, S., & de Silva, P. (1978). Abnormal and normal obsessions. *Behaviour Research and Therapy, 16*, 233–248.

Rachman, S., Thordarson, D. S., Shafran, R., & Woody, S. R. (1995). Perceived responsibility: Structure and significance. *Behaviour Research and Therapy, 33*, 779–784.

Ramchandani, D. (1990). Trazadone for bowel obsession. *American Journal of Psychiatry, 147*, 124.

Rasmussen, S. A., & Eisen, J. (1988). Clinical and epidemiological findings of significant neuropharmacology rituals in OCD. *Psychopharmacological Bulletin, 24*, 466–470.

Rasmussen, S. A., & Tsuang, M. T. (1986). Epidemiological and clinical findings of significance to the design of neuropharmacologic studies of obsessive–compulsive disorder. *Psychopharmacological Bulletin, 22*, 723–733.

Regier, D. A., Boyd, J. H., Burke, J. D., Rae, D. S., Myers, J. K., Kramer, M., Robins, L. N., George, L. K., Karno, M., & Locke, R. Z. (1988). One-month prevalence of mental disorders in the United States: Based on five epidemiologic catchment area sites. *Archives of General Psychiatry, 45*, 977–986.

Regier, D. A., Narrow, W. E., & Rae, D. S. (1990). The epidemiology of anxiety disorders: The Epidemiologic Catchment Area (ECA) experience. *Journal of Psychiatric Research, 24*, 3–14.

Reynolds, C. F., Lebowitz, B. D., & Schneider, L. S. (1993). The NIH consensus development conference on the diagnosis and treatment of depression in late life: An overview. *Psychopharmacology Bulletin, 29*, 83–85.

Rhéaume, J., Freeston, M. H., Dugas, M. J., Letarte, H., & Ladouceur, R. (1995). Perfectionism, responsibility and obsessive–compulsive symptoms. *Behaviour Research and Therapy, 33*, 785–794.

Rosenthal, M., Stelian, J., Wagner, J., & Berkman, P. (1999). Diogenes syndrome and hoarding in the elderly: A case report. *Israel Journal of Psychiatry and Related Sciences, 36*, 29–34.

Salkovskis, P. M. (1989). Cognitive–behavioral factors and the persistence of intrusive thoughts in obsessional problems. *Behaviour Research and Therapy, 27*, 677–682.

Salkovskis, P. M. (1985). Obsessional-compulsive problems: A cognitive–behavioral analysis. *Behaviour Research and Therapy, 23*, 571–583.

Salkovskis, P. M., & Westbrook, D. (1989). Behaviour therapy and obsessional ruminations:

Can failure be turned into success? *Behaviour Research and Therapy, 27*, 149–160.

Salthouse, T. A. (1991). Mediation of adult age differences in cognition by reductions in working memory and speed of processing. *Psychological Science, 2*, 179–183.

Salthouse, T. A. (1992). What do adult age differences in the Digit Symbol Substitution Test reflect? *Journal of Gerontology: Psychological Sciences, 47*, 121–128.

Salthouse, T. A. (1993). Influence of working memory on adult age differences in matrix reasoning. *British Journal of Psychology, 84*, 171–199.

Sanavio, E. (1988). Obsessions and compulsions: the Padua Inventory. *Behaviour Research and Therapy, 26*, 169–177.

Scarrabelotti, M. B., Duck, J. M., & Dickerson, M. M. (1995). Individual differences in obsessive–compulsive behaviour: the role of the Eysenckian dimensions and appraisals of responsibility. *Journal of Personality and Individual Differences, 3*, 413–421.

Schmand, B., Jonker, C., Geerlings, M. I., & Lindeboom, J. (1997). Subjective memory complaints in the elderly: Depressive symptoms and future dementia. *British Journal of Psychiatry, 171*, 373–376.

Shafran, R., Thordarson, D. S., & Rachman, S. (1996). Thought–action fusion in obsessive–compulsive disorder. *Journal of Anxiety Disorders, 10*, 379–391.

Smith, A. (1982). *Symbol Digit Modalities Test (SDMT) Manual* (Rev.). Los Angeles: Western Psychological Services.

Smith, G. E., Petersen R. C., Ivnik, R. J., Malec, J. F., & Tangalos, E. G. (1996). Subjective memory complaints, psychological distress, and longitudinal change in objective memory performance. *Psychology and Aging, 11*, 272–279.

Stanley, M. A., & Turner, S. M. (1995). Current status of pharmacological and behavioral treatment of obsessive–compulsive disorder. *Behavior Therapy, 26*, 163–186.

Stanley, M. L., & Averill, P. M. (1999). Strategies for treating generalized anxiety in the elderly. In M. Duffy (ed.), *Handbook of counseling and psychotherapy with older adults* (pp. 511–525). New York: Wiley.

Stanley, M. L., & Beck, J. G. (1998). Anxiety disorders. In A. S. Bellack & M. Hersen (Series ed.), & B. Edelstein (Vol. ed.), *Comprehensive clinical psychology: vol. 7. Clinical geropsychology* (pp. 171–191). New York: Elsevier Science.

Steiner, J. (1972). A questionnaire study of risk-taking in psychiatric patients. *British Journal of Medical Psychology, 45*, 365–374.

Steketee, G. S. (1993). *Treatment of Obsessive–Compulsive Disorder*. New York: Guilford.

Steketee, G., Frost, R. O., & Cohen, I. (1998). Beliefs in obsessive–compulsive disorder. *Journal of Anxiety Disorders, 12*, 525–537.

Steketee, G., & Frost, R. O. (1994). Measurement of risk-taking in obsessive–compulsive disorder. *Behavioural and Cognitive Psychotherapy, 22*, 287–298.

Thompson, L. W., Gallagher, D., & Breckenridge, J. S. (1987). Comparative effectiveness of psychotherapies for depressed elders. *Journal of Consulting and Clinical Psychology, 55*, 385–390.

Thyer, B. A., Parrish, R. T., Curtis, G. C., Nesse, R. M., & Cameron, O. G. (1985). Age of onset of DSM-III anxiety disorders. *Comprehensive Psychiatry, 26*, 113–122.

Uhlenhuth, E. H., Balter, M. B., Mellinger, G. D., Cisin, I. H., & Clinthorne, J. (1983). Symptom checklist syndromes in the general population: Correlations with psychotherapeutic drug use. *Archives of General Psychiatry, 40*, 1167–1173.

van Oppen, P., de Haan, E., van Balkom, A., Spinhoven, P., Hoogduin, K., & van Dyck, R. (1995). Cognitive therapy and exposure in vivo the treatment of obsessive–compulsive disorder. *Behaviour Research and Therapy, 33*, 379–390.

Weissman, M. M., Myers, J. K., Tischer, G. L., Holzer, C. E. III, Leaf, D. J., Orvaschel, H., &

Broday, J. A. (1985). Psychiatric disorders (DSM-III) and cognitive impairment among the elderly in a U.S. urban community. *Acta Psychiatric Scandinavica, 71*, 366–379.

Weschler, D. (1981). *Weschler Adult Intelligence Scale-Revised Manual.* New York: Psychological Corporation.

West, R. L., Boatwright, L. K., & Schleser, R. (1984). The link between memory-performance, self-assessment, and affective-status. *Experimental Aging Research, 10*, 197–200.

Wilson, R. S., Bennett, D. A., & Swartzendruber, A. (1997). Age-related change in cognitive functioning. In P. D. Nussbaum (ed.), *Handbook of neuropsychology of aging* (pp. 7–13). New York: Plenum.

Chapter 18

Cognition in Subclinical Obsessive Compulsive Disorder

Ricks Warren, Beth S. Gershuny and Kenneth J. Sher

"Speaking with a score of fellow scientists throughout the week, I elicited anecdote after anecdote of mildly obsessive–compulsive behavior. One researcher said that when she approaches the lab to prepare for a particularly important experiment, she counts to herself and taps the wall as she walks down the corridor. Another 'prefers' prime numbers, and counts to three or to seven before analyzing a sequence of DNA. A third told me that, during the month before grant proposals are due, she repeatedly returns home to check the stove in her apartment, even though she knows that it is turned off".
—*Jerome Groopman (2000, p. 53) writing in the* New Yorker *about the seeming ubiquity of obsessive–compulsive behavior among scientists with whom he is acquainted.*

Introduction

Cognitive and behavioral phenomena that are similar in form and content to obsessions and compulsions are not limited to individuals with obsessive compulsive disorder (OCD) and appear often in persons with no diagnosable disorder. In our research on college students (e.g., Gershuny & Sher, 1995; Goodwin & Sher, 1992; Sher, Mann, & Frost, 1984), we found it is not uncommon for an individual to report checking his/her alarm clock more than once to make sure it is set properly the evening before an important morning meeting, to report checking to make sure keys and wallets were in place in one's pocket or purse, checking to make sure electrical appliances are turned off, etc. It is also not uncommon for an individual to occasionally experience unbidden thoughts or images that can be difficult to dispel and that are not unlike those reported by patients with OCD (see below).

Most research on obsessive compulsive symptoms in community and student samples has sought to characterize the nature and correlates of these symptoms to understand better OCD (Burns, Formea, Keortge, & Sternberger, 1995; Gibbs, 1996). Much reported research has relied on non-clinical (i.e., not treatment-seeking) or sub-clinical (i.e., exhibition of symptoms that do not meet criteria to receive a diagnosis of OCD) samples as analogues for studying the clinical disorder of OCD (see Gibbs, 1996). Although the extent to which such analog research has informed basic research on OCD remains open for discussion, it is clear that such research is useful, and that there are a number of similarities between obsessive and compulsive phenomena reported by OCD patients and those reported by ostensibly well-functioning individuals in community or university populations (Burns *et al.*, 1995). This chapter will focus on data obtained from non-clinical and sub-clinical samples with an emphasis on cognitive domains. To this end, much of the initial sections of this chapter will focus on obsessions rather than compulsions because of the cognitive nature of obsessions and the focus of this book.

Obsessions and Related Phenomena

It is likely that an understanding of the nature of obsessions and their causes (and perhaps cognitive compulsions such as mental rituals) may tell us much about the structure and dynamics of human cognition (e.g., James, 1890/1950; Nowalk, Vallacher, Tesser, & Borkowski, 2000) and attempts to control thought content (e.g., Wegner, 1989). Questions such as, 'How do individuals maintain or dispel thoughts in working memory?' are fundamental to the area of cognition, but little research has attempted to utilize the study of obsessional phenomena to understand cognitive processes involved in the regulation of thought (Baddeley & Della Sala, 1998).

We can think of obsessions as one sub-class of mental phenomena similar to other sub-classes of pathological preoccupation that characterize phenotypically diverse forms of psychopathology.[1] For example, the worry of generalized anxiety disorder, the craving associated with abstinence attempts in substance dependence and pathological gambling, the intrusive and repetitive thoughts of post-traumatic stress disorder, the rumination of major depression, the persistent health concerns of hypochondriasis, the inability to ignore or habituate to pain in chronic pain syndromes, and the preoccupation with delusions in some psychotic conditions all to varying degrees represent an apparent failure of self-regulatory processes to disengage from or inhibit cognitions that have never had or long since ceased to have adaptive value.

Some scientists have attempted to provide a model of the functional relations among conceptually similar cognitive phenomena. For example, Salkovskis (1985) proposed a model whereby intrusive thoughts (characterized by highly noticeable intrusions in the stream of consciousness, perceived irrationality, and ego-dystonicity) trigger automatic cognitions that "run parallel" to the stream of consciousness, are not perceived as intrusive, and are seemingly rational and ego-syntonic. In turn, these automatic cognitions lead to cognitive or behavioral self-regulatory efforts that can have the effect of maintaining that

---

[1]Rachman (1973) distinguished between "obsessional ruminations" and "morbid preoccupations" (similar to worry), noting the similarities with respect to intrusiveness and repetitiveness but also noting differences in that obsessions are more associated with guilt, abhorrence, and active resistance. We use the term "pathological preoccupation" to describe a super-ordinate category that subsumes both obsessions and worry-related cognitions.

obsession. From this perspective, spontaneous cognitive intrusions are a normal, non-pathological phenomenon[2] that can lead to complications in the presence of pathogenic belief systems.

Although this and other taxonomies of intrusive, unwanted and disturbing thoughts appear reasonable, they are not without problematic inconsistencies (e.g., Jakes, 1989a, 1989b), and the extent to which intrusive cognitions are fundamentally distinct from non-intrusive cognitions associated with anxiety and depression remains an open and important research question. For example, Clark (1992) found that his measure of intrusive thoughts correlated 0.75 with his measure of anxious thinking but only correlated 0.39 with the Maudsley Obsessional Compulsive Inventory (MOCI) in the normal group. (Note, however, that MOCI item content tends to be centered primarily on compulsions rather than obsessions). Moreover, the overall pattern of associations between various measures of cognition and symptoms did not yield an unambiguous interpretation.

Although a later study (Purdon & Clark, 1993) ostensibly yielded a more interpretable pattern of findings, it is unclear to what extent predictor/criterion overlap rendered the key observation artifactual. It is probably fair to say that the fundamental similarities and differences among various forms of pathological preoccupation have not been systematically charted, and a well-articulated anatomy of persistent and distressing thoughts that characterize various psychological disorders and pathological states still lies in the future. For example, intrusive thoughts underlying the construct of PTSD may be similar to intrusive thoughts underlying the construct of OCD in that they are thoughts perceived as uncontrollable, frequent, and distressing. Such PTSD- and OCD-related intrusive thoughts may also be different, however, in that PTSD-related intrusive thoughts are characteristic of particular trauma material and memories and thus based in reality (e.g., ruminative thoughts about aspects of an assault) whereas OCD-related thoughts are not characteristic of particular traumatic experiences and generally are not based on reality (e.g., ruminative thoughts about contamination from neutral, safe objects). It is also worth noting that many facets of "normal" but distressing psychological states (e.g., guilt, jealousy, mourning, reality-based concerns for one's safety and the safety of loved ones) can have a clear obsessional flavor.

Although the boundaries between obsessional cognitions and related phenomena are fuzzy, for research and clinical purposes, it is necessary to provide conceptual definitions that are easily operationalized. To this end, Rachman and Hodgson (1980) proposed that "the necessary and sufficient conditions for defining a thought, impulse, or image as obsessional are intrusiveness, internal attribution, unwantedness, and difficulty of control" (p. 251). Similarly, Clark (1992) suggested that research on cognitive intrusions be limited to "thoughts, images, or impulses that not only intrude upon consciousness in an uncontrollable fashion but that are clearly ego-dystonic, highly unacceptable and involve an obvious loss of impulse controls" (p. 101).

In reviewing a number of published studies, the extent to which all reported obsessions

---

[2]It is clear from experimental studies that exposure to films portraying threatening content (e.g., woodshop accidents, male genital mutilation) can evoke intrusive and repetitive thinking for a period of time following stimulus presentation in most individuals (Horowitz, 1975). It is not clear under what conditions such environmentally-provoked intrusions can become persistent, functionally autonomous obsessions.

in non-clinical populations would be consistent with Rachman and Hodgson's (1980) and Clark's (1992) definition is unclear, but most authors attempt to employ criteria that are somewhat restrictive and limited to unwanted and intrusive thoughts. Although adoption of clear conceptual definitions is desirable for many research questions, restricting the domain of distressing thoughts along any dimension means that it is not possible to study the importance or correlates of that dimension except in a limited way. Thus, if we prematurely definitionally restrict the construct we may miss important aspects we hope to characterize by defining out meaningful sources of variation.

Obsessional Thinking is Not Just for Obsessionals

Much of the interest in obsessions in non-clinical populations can be traced to a seminal publication by Rachman and de Silva (1978). In a series of studies, these authors set out to determine whether and how often individuals in a non-clinical sample (composed primarily of students at various levels of higher education and health-related professionals) experienced "intrusive, unacceptable thoughts and impulses, their frequency, and about whether or not these could be easily dismissed" (p. 233). They concluded that obsessions were reported by 84 percent of the sample, and that obsessive thoughts were more common than obsessive impulses. They also found that most obsessive thoughts and impulses were easily dismissed, and the majority of participants reported that they were somewhat infrequent (i.e., occurred 10 times a month or less). The main finding, though, is that obsessions are very common in individuals with no readily apparent diagnosable psychological disorders.

Rachman and de Silva (1978) next attempted to characterize the content of the obsessions to determine whether their content was distinguishable from that of individuals suffering from OCD. The content of the obsessive thoughts and impulses was diverse and included thoughts of anger, harm to self and loved ones, moral indignation, embarrassment, post-traumatic images and impulses to harm self or others (including animals), to be disruptive, to engage in taboo or violent sex acts, or engage in other types of impulsive acts (e.g., making unnecessary purchases). In general terms, the content was similar to those of obsessions reported by clinical obsessionals, and a panel of clinicians had difficulty in classifying obsessions as coming from patients or non-patients. Rachman and de Silva concluded that "the judges were not able to identify the clinical obsessions too well, but on the other hand, they were moderately good at identifying non-clinical obsessions [and] . . . that clinical obsessions are not as readily discernible even to experienced clinicians — as might be expected" (p. 239).[3]

Although exhibiting roughly similar content, the non-patients reported fewer current

---

[3]Rachman and de Silva characterize the accuracy as poor but given the seemingly difficult nature of the task, other psychologists might view the performance as reasonably good. For example, accuracy ranged from 68 percent to 88 percent and validity kappas for the six raters employed ranged from 0.21–0.70 (*Mdn. = 0.39*). *Additionally, for this set of analyses, each obsession reported by each patient was considered to be a clinical obsession even though it is unclear if each was a source of concern to the patient and related to his/her treatment. That is, this does not allow for the possibility that patients reporting multiple obsessions can have both "clinical" and "non-clinical" obsessions. Thus a case could be made that at least some clinicians can do a reasonable job of distinguishing "normal" from "abnormal" obsessions.*

obsessions, and the average chronicity of the obsessions reported by patients was longer than that reported by non-patients. Perhaps most significant, and not surprising, clinical obsessions were more severe with respect to frequency, duration, and intensity, as well as the extent to which they were ego-dystonic, the associated discomfort, the evoked urge to neutralize, and the ability to be dismissed. Rachman and de Silva (1978) concluded that clinical and non-clinical obsessions were "similar in form and content but not in frequency and intensity, or in their consequences" (p. 244).

Salkovskis and Harrison (1984) attempted to replicate Rachman and de Silva's (1978) findings on samples of polytechnic and nursing students and also found that most reported experiencing obsessions. They similarly noted that less frequent obsessions were easier for individuals to dismiss. There was greater discomfort associated with difficult-to-dismiss obsessions, but the type of intrusion (i.e., impulses vs. thoughts) and obsession frequency were unrelated to discomfort levels. In addition to replicating the very high prevalence of obsessional thoughts in non-clinical samples, these authors highlighted the importance of ease of dismissal as a key dimension in assessing the severity of obsessions.

How Common is the Experience of Obsessive Thoughts?

Following Rachman and de Silva's (1978) and Salkovskis and Harrison's (1984) reports, a number of other investigations provided information on the prevalence of normal obsessions or intrusive cognitions. In general, these studies have indicated that the experience of obsessions in non-clinical samples is common, occurring in the overwhelming majority (England & Dickerson, 1988; Freeston, Ladouceur, Thibodeau, & Gagnon, 1991; Niler & Beck, 1989; Purdon & Clark, 1993). One would expect the apparent prevalence to decrease systematically as increasingly more restrictive definitions are employed. Consistent with this notion, Gibbs (1996) estimated that only 14 percent of non-clinical students were considered obsessive in a study (Salkovskis & Campbell, 1994) where frequency of obsessions (three or more in past month) and associated distress (30 or more on a 100-point scale) both had to exceed a minimum cut-off. Although possibly accurate, Gibbs' estimate appears to assume that all eligible participants were successfully recruited and randomized to study conditions. This seems highly unlikely, and her estimate is probably overly conservative. It would be useful to systematically determine the relative prevalence of obsessions under different configurations of thresholds on key characteristics (e.g., frequency, unwantedness, distress, ease of dismissal).

Although existing studies suggest that obsessions and compulsions are very common in non-clinical populations, the overwhelming majority of people studied involved in these estimates were college students. This is potentially problematic because adolescence and the early college years are associated with marked distress that typically decreases dramatically by the third year of college (Sher, Wood, & Gotham, 1996). Because reports of obsessions and compulsions co-vary with generalized distress (Frost, Sher, & Geen, 1986; Sher, Martin, Raskin, & Perrigo, 1991) and with anxiety phenomena such as worry and physiological symptoms (Sternberger & Burns, 1990a), there is a clear need for population-based epidemiology on a wider range of samples. This will increase confidence in the estimates of prevalence suggested in the literature on non-clinical obsessions. For example, Stanley, Beck, and Zebb (1996) found that older adults scored substantially lower on the Padua Inventory (PI) than implied by norms obtained from college students.

It is noteworthy that scales used to assess obsessions, compulsions, and related symptoms (most notably the Maudsley Obsessive Compulsive Inventory and the PI) have been administered to non-clinical samples in many countries including Australia (Kyrios, Bhar, & Wade, 1996), Hong Kong (Chan, 1990), Italy (Mancini, Gragnani, Orazi, & Petrangeli, 1999), the Netherlands (van Oppen, 1992), and the United States (Sternberger & Burns, 1990a, 1990b). Although these studies suggest differences in mean levels of obsessive compulsive symptoms across national samples, the factor structure of various measures appears comparable across various populations.

Also of importance, from the early work of Rachman and de Silva (1978) and Salkovskis and Harrison (1984) and continuing through much of the current literature, researchers vary as to whether unpleasant, unwanted thoughts of normals should be called "intrusive thoughts" or "normal obsessions". This distinction is important because the high prevalence rates reported in the literature are for intrusive thoughts not obsessions. Recently, cognitive models have more explicitly delineated theoretical and empirical differences between intrusive thoughts and obsessions (e.g., Rachman, 1997; Salkovskis *et al.*, 2000). "The starting point for the theory is the premise that unwanted, intrusive thoughts are the raw material of obsessions, and the finding that these thoughts are almost universally experienced" (Rachman, 1997, p. 793). So, what causes the transition from a "normal" obsession to an "abnormal" obsession? "The mis-interpretation of the intrusive thoughts as being very important, personally significant, revealing and threatening or even catastrophic, has the effect of transformimg a commonplace nuisance into a torment" (Rachman, 1997, p. 794).

Obsessions versus Worry

Both similarities and differences have been proposed between obsessions and worry in clinical and non-clinical populations (Turner, Beidel, & Stanley, 1992). For example, obsessions and worry may be similar in that both are associated with negative mood in clinical and non-clinical populations, and both are higher in frequency and perception of uncontrollability in clinical compared to non-clinical populations (Turner *et al.*, 1992). Obsessions and worry may also differ on key factors. For example, worries may be in response to common-life difficulties or everyday problems (e.g., family, work) (Craske, Rapee, Jackel, & Barlow, 1989) whereas obsessions may occur less often in response to identifiable triggers (Rachman & de Silva, 1978). Further, worries tend to consist primarily of thoughts, whereas obsessions may be comprised of images, impulses, and thoughts. Finally, obsessions are more often avoided and resisted than are worries (Turner *et al.*, 1992).

Though these speculations about similarities and differences between worries and obsessions are interesting and make intuitive sense, there is a paucity of research with non-clinical and sub-clinical samples that has sought to empirically examine these theorized similarities and differences (Brown, Dowdall, Cote, & Barlow, 1994). However, findings from extant studies reported in the literature are notable.

Wells and Morrison (1994) reported the first direct comparison of normal worries and obsessions in a non-clinical population of nurses, undergraduate students, and graduate students. Findings indicated that worries and obsessions did not differ in terms of perceived controllability, intrusiveness, or degree of participants' resistance to them. Wells and Morrison further found that worry was predominantly verbal whereas obsessions were more often imagined and suggested that worries about obsessions may be an integral part of the etiological pathway to OCD. Support for this speculation was demonstrated by Purdon and Clark (1994) whose study revealed that, in non-clinical participants, the appraisal that one might act on intrusive thoughts was significantly associated with intrusive thought frequency and perceived controllability. Similarly, Coles, Mennin, and Heimberg (2000) found that thought–action fusion beliefs distinguished distress associated with obsessive compulsive symptoms from trait worry in a non-clinical sample. Clark and Claybourn (1997) found that non-clinical students' worries about everyday problems were more disturbing to them than their obsessive intrusive thoughts. Further, Wells and Papageorgiou (1998) found that positive beliefs about worry and negative beliefs concerning the uncontrollability and danger of worry predicted pathological worry in a sample of undergraduates.

In a non-clinical analogue sample for GAD and OCD, Gershuny and Sher (1995) compared generally anxious individuals who do not engage in checking behaviors with anxious individuals who do engage in compulsive checking behaviors as determined by an MOCI checking score of five or higher. Findings revealed that compulsive checkers reported higher levels of worry than did generally anxious individuals. Findings from a similar study conducted by Gershuny, Sher, Rossy, and Bishop (2000) corroborated these findings by demonstrating that compulsive checkers reported higher levels of neuroticism (as characterized by a number of facets including worry) than did generally anxious individuals who do not engage in checking behaviors. Abramowitz and Foa (1998) who examined obsessions and worries in patients with OCD, with and without comorbid GAD, conducted a clinical counterpart to the Gershuny, Sher and colleagues' studies. Similar to the non-clinical analogue studies, Abramowitz and Foa found that OCD patients with comorbid GAD reported significantly more worries about common-life problems.

Recently, Langlois, Freeston, and Ladouceur (2000a, b) conducted a two-part series of studies that examined differences between worry and intrusive thoughts in a large sample of undergraduate students. In Study one, Langlois and colleagues (2000a) demonstrated: (a) interference caused by worry appeared more severe than interference caused by obsessions; (b) worry content appeared more unpleasant and disturbing than obsessional content; (c) worry was more often experienced as a vague feeling lingering in the back of the mind; (d) worry was more often related to specific events, and people were more often aware of triggers for worry; (e) worry was more often experienced in verbal form, and obsessions were more frequently experienced as images; (f) greater effort was put forth by participants to dismiss worries compared to obsessions (contrary to Turner *et al.*, 1992); (g) worries were perceived as more disturbing than obsessions; (h) worry was associated with more negative emotions; (i) obsessions elicited a greater sense of responsibility; and (j) worries were more ego-syntonic, and obsessions were more ego-dystonic.

In Study two, Langlois and colleagues (2000b) found that higher levels of intrusiveness and emotional disturbance characterized worry, and greater unpleasant content characterized obsessions. They also found that worry was associated with stronger feelings of insecurity, sadness and guilt, as well as higher levels of responsibility and blame compared to obsessions. Although both worries and obsessions were associated with the perception of reality of the thought, intrusions were also associated with thought content and their ego-dystonicity. Surprisingly, obsessions were associated with greater perception of control than worries, perhaps because of the nature of the non-clinical sample for whom obsessional intrusions may occur less frequently, may seem less probable, and thereby be perceived as more controllable than worries. Worries, on the other hand, may be viewed as more reality-based and more potentially solvable, and thereby be associated with responsibility and blame.

Belief Domains and OCD Symptoms

In recent years, belief domains have been identified to help distinguish OCD from other forms of psychopathology (Obsessive Compulsive Cognitions Working Group, [OCCWG] 1997). These belief domains include inflated responsibility, over-importance of thoughts, control of thoughts, over-estimation of threat, intolerance of uncertainty, and perfectionism; they are reviewed in Chapters two through six of this volume in relation to clinical OCD. Few studies have used non-clinical or sub-clinical samples. Findings from this literature are provided below.

Threat Appraisal

In one of the first cognitive models of OCD, Carr (1974) proposed that unrealistic threat appraisal was a core feature of OCD. Carr hypothesized that patients with OCD over-estimate both the probability and the cost of negative events. Related findings from non-clinical samples are presented below.

Ladouceur, Rhéaume, and Aublet (1997) found that when both perceived threat and personal influence were manipulated, increasing only perceived negative consequences was sufficient to provoke checking, while increasing perceived responsibility was required to produce the further behavioral effects of modifying or redoing tasks. In another non-clinical study, Jones and Menzies (1998) manipulated perceived level of danger in 18 undergraduate volunteers whose Padua Inventory scores were in the top ten percent for washing/contamination items. Results indicated that high danger participants engaged in more avoidance and washing. In a more recent study with introductory psychology students, Menzies, Harris, Cumming, and Einstein (2000) presented participants with a questionnaire containing hypothetical scenarios related to worry about possible negative events related to washing and checking. Participants were randomly assigned to respond to scenarios indicating that either they were personally responsible or that another person was responsible. Results indicated that "personally responsible" participants rated the severity, but not likelihood, of potential negative outcomes as greater than did "other responsible" participants. Menzies *et al.* (2000) proposed that perceived responsibility leads to increased severity of danger ratings and that danger expectancies are the direct mediators of OCD phenomena.

Risk aversion has also been studied in non-clinical samples. Steketee and Frost (1994) found that persons who scored high on obsessive compulsive symptoms were disinclined to take normal every-day risks, such as briefly leaving one's car unlocked. Frost, Steketee, Cohn, and Griess (1994) found that sub-clinical obsessive compulsives (i.e., undergraduate students who scored above six on the MOCI) were less risk-taking than non-obsessive compulsives (students who scored below five on the MOCI). As Steketee, Frost, and Cohen (1998) note, however, risk aversion in itself does not confirm over-estimation of threat.

Over-importance of Thoughts

In presenting his cognitive theory of obsessions, Rachman (1997) stated that "the defining quality of the significance attached to intrusive thoughts is the person's belief that the thought (image, impulse) is meaningful and it is *important*; it is not trivial, it is not meaningless but is revealing about me" (p. 800). Relatedly, Freeston and colleagues (1996) discussed a variety of cognitive biases related to beliefs about the over-importance of thoughts. These biases include distorted Cartesian reasoning, thought–action fusion (TAF; Shafron, Thordarson, & Rachman, 1996), and superstitious or magical thinking. In distorted Cartesian reasoning, individuals assume that the presence of a certain thought indicates the thought is important. "It must be important because I think about it, and I think about it because it is important" (Freeston *et al.* 1996, p. 437). TAF describes the psychological phenomenon in which thoughts are considered either morally equivalent to the related action (TAF-moral) or mental events that in themselves increase the likelihood of engaging in the related act and thereby cause harm to self (TAF-likelihood-for-self) or others (TAF-likelihood-for-others). Magical thinking is a particularly strong form of thought–action fusion in which the obsessive thought content and/or process has no logical relationships to the feared outcome. An example would be that a person believes he/she must look at a loved one's picture a certain number of times before going to bed to keep the loved one from dying.

Overall, evidence indicates that TAF is related to obsessionality (as measured by the MOCI) in patients with OCD, students, and community volunteers (Shafron *et al.*, 1996). In a sample of introductory psychology students, Coles, Mennin, and Heimberg (2000) found that TAF (moral and likelihood-self and others) discriminated between obsessive features and worry such that higher TAF was significantly correlated with higher levels of distress as derived from the Obsessive Compulsive Inventory (OCI; Foa, Kozak, Salkovskis, Coles, & Amir, 1998) but not with levels of worry as derived from the Penn State Worry Questionnaire (PSWQ; Meyer, Miller, Metzger, & Borkovec, 1990). In contrast, Dugas, Francis, Robichaud, and Fioriello (2000), also using undergraduate samples, found that magical thinking TAF was significantly correlated with trait worry, especially when structured interviews were used. Purdon and Clark (1994) found that, in a sample of introductory psychology students, the more individuals believed their most upsetting intrusive thought might be acted upon, the higher the frequency and lower the perceived controllability of the intrusion. In another study conducted with university students, TAF-likelihood was a unique predictor of perceived control of both sexual and non-sexual intrusive thoughts, such that the higher the level of TAF-likelihood, the lower the perception of perceived control over these intrusive thoughts. TAF-moral, in contrast, did not predict perceived control of either sexual or nonsexual thoughts (Clark, Purdon, & Byers, 2000).

Rassin, Muris, Schmidt, and Merckelbach (2000) used structural equation modeling to investigate possible relationships between TAF and thought suppression in a sample of undergraduate psychology students. Results indicated that TAF led to thought suppression attempts, which in turn increased obsessive compulsive symptoms. Rassin and colleagues (2000) concluded that, compared to thought suppression, TAF is a more fundamental cause of obsessive compulsive symptoms.

In an experimental study conducted with undergraduates, Shafron, (1996) elicited harm-related thoughts in participants by instructing them to write sentences such as, " 'I hope my husband has a car accident' ". Following this experimental manipulation, it appeared that the higher the TAF-likelihood, the higher the levels of evoked anxiety and feelings of responsibility and the lower the estimates of perceived control. TAF was not associated with evoked guilt, moral wrongness or urge to neutralize. Results further revealed that after writing the sentences, participants engaged in a variety of neutralizing behaviors (e.g., crossing out the sentence) in an attempt to undo the potential effects of engaging in harm-related thoughts and behaviors. Rachman *et al.* (1996) concluded that "the concept of performing an action that is not realistically connected with the event in order to undo a different action is a normal phenomenon and is not restricted to obsessional patients" (p. 897). Zucker, Craske, Barrios, and Holguin (2000), also working with undergraduates, obtained similar findings. In addition, Zucker *et al.* (2000) demonstrated that a brief educational intervention reduced TAF beliefs in participants selected for high TAF.

In another experimental study, Rassin, Merckelbach, Muris, and Spaan (1999) tested 30 non-treatment-seeking women (mostly high school students) who as part of the study underwent a bogus EEG recording and were told that the apparatus could tell the experimenter when participants were thinking of the word "apple". Participants were also told that "apple" thoughts would result in another person receiving electric shocks (TAF-induction). Control participants were told that the EEG equipment could read simple thoughts and that during the procedure they could "think of anything, for example the word 'apple' " (p. 223). Results from this study indicated that TAF-induced participants reported more intrusions, discomfort, anger, resistance, and neutralizing behavior, compared to controls.

Recently, Thordarson, Whittal, and McLean (2000) reported that, in a sample of 92 OCD treatment study patients classified by Padua Inventory sub-types, TAF was specifically related to repugnant obsessions (involving harm, aggression, sex, and harm) but was not significantly correlated with the washing and checking subscales. In addition, TAF change was related to improvement with treatment only for patients with repugnant obsessions. It would be interesting to explore the importance of TAF in non-clinical samples classified by sub-types.

Purdon and colleagues (1999; Cripps & Purdon, 2000; Purdon, in press) have proposed that ego-dystonicity is a distinguishing feature of obsessional thoughts and an important factor in a theoretical account of the escalation of intrusive thoughts into obsessions. In short, Purdon and Clark propose that ego-dystonic thoughts are those that are perceived as a threat to one's self-view (see Cripps & Purdon (2000) for a more detailed definition of ego-dystonicity and the development of a new instrument for its measurement). In support of their proposals, Purdon and Clark (1994) found that ego-dystonicity was a strong predictor of obsessional but not general anxious or depressive symptoms. More recently, Purdon (in press) found that, in a thought suppression study with non-clinical undergraduate students, in vivo appraisals involving ego-dystonicity, responsibility and, TAF predicted anxiety and poor mood state and increasingly more effort to control thoughts.

Control of Thoughts

Clark and Purdon (1993) proposed that dysfunctional meta-cognitive beliefs about thought control are primary determinants in the development and maintenance of OCD, and that "These beliefs constitute a vulnerability factor that will motivate individuals to exert greater control over their mental life" (Purdon & Clark, 2001, p. 7). The basic dysfunctional belief here is that unwanted, intrusive thoughts can and should be controlled. Inevitable failures in thought control occur, leading to increased control efforts and monitoring for the target intrusive thoughts. This results in an increase in thought frequency, a subsequent decrease in sense of control, with an increase in emotional distress and negative mood, and eventually OCD (Purdon & Clark, 2001). The numerous studies of the effects of various types of thought control are relevant to Purdon and Clark's proposed model. For example, Salkovskis, Westbrook, Davis, Jeavons, and Gledhill (1997) conducted a non-clinical study with university students, screened for reporting frequent intrusions and associated discomfort and use of neutralization strategies. Participants instructed to engage in deliberate neutralization of their intrusive thoughts experienced more discomfort, greater urge to neutralize, and more actual neutralization when presented with subsequent presentations of their intrusive thoughts, compared to participants who were instructed to use a specific distraction strategy.

Thought suppression is one of many types of neutralization that individuals may use to cope with unwanted thoughts. The prediction that attempts at thought suppression result in a paradoxical immediate increase in thought frequency (enhancement) and a surge in the target thought following initial suppression (rebound effect) has been tested in numerous studies, and findings have been inconsistent. For example, in studies with non-clinical participants, Salkovskis and Campbell (1994) and Trinder and Salkovskis (1994) obtained results supportive, while Purdon and Clark (2000) and Purdon (in press) obtained results that were not supportive of paradoxical effects of thought suppression. In a recent meta-analysis of 28 thought suppression studies, Abramowitz, Tolin, Przeworski, Street, and Foa (1999) found that thought suppression resulted in small to moderate rebound effects but not to initial enhancement of the thought. Rebound effects did not vary by types of sample, including non-clinical, sub-clinical, or clinical, the latter consisting of OCD, PTSD, and depressed patients. In naturalistic settings a number of factors may modulate the effects of thought suppression (e.g., the amount of effort devoted to thought suppression, negative mood, type and number of suppression strategies employed, sustained emotional reactivity to the target thought).

Although research with clinical samples of OCD patients has indicated that individuals with OCD score higher on measures of beliefs about control of thoughts than about clinical, community, and student controls (Steketee, Frost, & Cohen, 1998; Chapter seven in this volume), very few studies have tested non-clinical or sub-clinical analogue OCD samples. Relatedly, Purdon and Clark (1998; cited in Purdon & Clark, 1999) tested a sample of undergraduate students not screened for diagnosis, and found that beliefs about the importance of thought control, in conjunction with efforts to suppress thoughts, predicted higher frequency of obsessional thoughts. Similarly, in a study of the in vivo appraisal of recurrences of unwanted thoughts, the perceived necessity of thought control was a unique predictor of suppression efforts. However, thought suppression attempts did not lead to significant immediate or delayed increase in thought frequency (Purdon, in press). Interestingly, Purdon (in press) and Purdon and Clark (2000) found that participants who were instructed not to suppress thoughts, nevertheless reported significant thought control efforts. As noted by Purdon and Clark, these findings call into question the ecological validity of experimental manipulations of thought suppression.

Whether thought suppression contributes significantly to the etiology or maintenance of obsessive compulsive psychopathology, has recently been questioned by Rassin, Merckelbach, and Muris (2000). These authors review evidence suggesting that cognitive factors such as TAF and beliefs about the intolerability of uncertainty may be more primary precursors to the development of obsessions and worry, while thought suppression may be a secondary phenomenon.

Responsibility

A cognitive theory of OCD has proposed that the occurrence and/or content of obsessional intrusions (thoughts, images, impulses and/or doubts) may be interpreted (appraised) by individuals as indicating personal responsibility for harm to themselves or others (Salkovskis, Richards, & Forrester, 2000). An inflated sense of responsibility in OCD may be conceptualized as the belief that one has power which is pivotal to bring about or prevent subjectively crucial negative outcomes (Salkovskis et al., 1996). Studies examining this definition of responsibility have typically operationalized pivotal power as ratings of perceived influence and/or pivotal influence, while subjective crucial negative outcome is represented by ratings of perceived probability and severity.

Studies with non-clinical samples largely support the role of responsibility beliefs in the maintenance of obsessive compulsive symptoms and behaviors, particularly checking (e.g., Rhéaume, Ladouceur, Freeston, & Letarte, 1995; Steketee, Frost, Rhéaume, & Wilhelm, 1998). In one such study, Rhéaume and colleagues (1995) found that, in a sample of undergraduate volunteers, participants' beliefs that their influence on a particular outcome was pivotal was the best predictor of perceived responsibility. In another study conducted by Rhéaume and colleagues (Rhéaume, Freeston, Dugas, Letarte, & Ladouceur, 1995), results from a hierarchical regression analysis indicated that responsibility was a better predictor of obsessive compulsive symptoms than was perfectionism. In yet another study with a non-clinical sample, Wilson and Chambless (1999) also found responsibility to be an important correlate of OCD-type symptoms. They reported that responsibility schemas and automatic thoughts were associated with obsessive compulsive symptoms, and analyses suggested that the impact of responsibility schemas on OCD symptoms was mediated through automatic thoughts. Interestingly, responsibility was equally associated with washing.

In a series of experiments, Ladouceur and colleagues sought to understand the behavioral effects of varying levels of responsibility in non-clinical participants. Under-graduates in a high responsibility (HR) condition were led by the experimenters to believe that their performance on a sound recognition task might influence changes made in the audio system of traffic lights (which had led to several recent severe accidents involving old and blind people). Participants in the low responsibility (LR) condition were only told that the experiment involved a sound recognition practice trial, the results of which would not be analyzed. Participants in the HR condition rated the perceived probability and severity of potential negative consequences (i.e., perceived danger) and perceived responsibility for the negative consequences as higher than did LR participants. However, the responsibility manipulation did not lead to differential effects on behavioral variables, such as checking, errors, and time, believed to be needed for an additional check after the experimental task. A subsequent study attempted to obtain a stronger responsibility effect. HR participants were those who were led to believe that their performance on a task involving rapidly sorting capsules into bottles according to colors could have a serious impact on the manufacture, safety, and distribution of an anti-viral medication to be exported to a poor, uneducated population in Southeast Asia. Results of this study showed more hesitations and checking for high versus low responsibility subjects (Ladouceur *et al.*, 1995).

Using a similar experimental task and instructions, Ladouceur, Rhéaume, and Aublet (1997) examined the relative effects of personal influence and potential negative consequences. Non-clinical adults in an influence condition were told that they were one of three participants whose task performance would be crucial (pivotal) in affecting the safety of the medication. Participants in the negative consequence condition were told they were one of 2000 participants providing data that would be considered in decision-making about the drug's safety. Results indicated that perceived influence was a better predictor of responsibility than was over-estimation of negative consequences. In addition, participants perceived themselves as more responsible when both conditions were increased simultaneously. The combination of perceived influence and negative conse-quences led to increased perceived responsibility and more extensive behavioral reactions (e.g., modifications or redoing of task activities).

Recently, Bouchard, Rhéaume, and Ladouceur (1999) also examined the relationship between responsibility and perfectionism in a non-clinical experimental study, using essentially the same capsule sorting task as described above. Students were divided into a highly perfectionistic group (scores over the 90th percentile on the Perfectionism Question-naire; Rhéaume, Freeston, & Ladouceur, 1995) or a moderately perfectionistic group (scores below the 40th percentile). Overall results suggested a link between perception of inflated responsibility and checking behavior, and a relationship between perfectionism and increased perception of responsibility. That is, the higher the perfectionism, the higher the perceived responsibility, and the higher the perceived responsibility, the more frequent the checking behaviors.

Uncertainty

Poor tolerance of uncertainty has been considered a core feature of OCD (Guidano & Liotti, 1983; OCCWG, 1997; Reed, 1985), and its role in clinical samples has been examined in several studies (e.g., Calamari, Weigartz, & Janeck, 1999; Richter, Summerfeldt, Joffe, & Swinson, 1996; Steketee, Frost, & Cohen, 1998; Summerfeldt, Huta, & Swinson, 1998). However, recent studies indicate that poor tolerance of uncertainty is not unique to OCD (Brigidi, Tolin, Donde, & Foa, 2000; Ladouceur *et al.*, 1999).

In a non-clinical study specifically investigating tolerance of uncertainty, Dugas, Gosselin, and Ladouceur (2001) found that intolerance of uncertainty was more highly correlated with pathological worry than with obsessive features in a college student population. In four studies with non-clinical populations, Freeston, Ladouceur, Gagnon, and Thibodeau (1993) demonstrated that dysfunctional beliefs about obsessions measured by the Inventory of Beliefs Related to Obsession (IBRO) were positively correlated with obsessive compulsive symptoms. A factor analysis of the IBRO revealed three factors: inflated responsibility, over-estimation of threat, and intolerance of uncertainty.

In a second study with college students, IBRO scores were positively correlated with obsessive thoughts. In a third study with students, subjects who used escape/avoidance strategies in response to intrusive thoughts scored higher on the IBRO than subjects who used minimal attention (non-avoidant) tactics. In the fourth study, Freeston *et al.* (1993) recruited adults who were in waiting rooms of family medicine and blood sampling units at a university hospital. IBRO scores in this group were significant predictors of total OCD mental control and contamination scores on the Padua Inventory after a large negative mood state effect was partialled out.

These four studies demonstrated that beliefs related to responsibility, threat and uncertainty are related to obsessive compulsive symptoms in non-clinical populations. Further research is needed to clarify the relative importance of these factors in predicting obsessive compulsive symptoms. A recent clinical study found that the intolerance of uncertainty was a better predictor of severity of OCD factors than were other belief domains (Steketee, Frost, & Cohen, 1998).

A number of non-clinical studies have investigated the role of doubt and indecisiveness, often considered aspects of poor tolerance of uncertainty, in obsessive compulsive phenomenon (Frost & Shows, 1993). In a series of studies with female undergraduate students, higher levels of indecisiveness were associated with higher levels of obsessional thoughts and compulsive checking (but not compulsive washing), greater psychopathology, more procrastination, and greater problems with decision-making in a variety of life domains. General indecisiveness, both hoarding and non-hoarding related, has been shown to be positively correlated with measures of compulsive hoarding in college students and community volunteers (Frost & Steketee, 1998).

In two separate non-clinical samples, one consisting of subjects drawn from social work and engineering graduate students, and the other consisting of female introductory psychology students, Frost *et al.* (1994) investigated personality traits in sub-clinical and non-compulsive volunteers. Subjects were classified as either non-compulsive or sub-clinical obsessive compulsive based on clearly defined criteria (e.g., MOCI and other OCD-related measures). Results indicated that sub-clinical obsessive compulsive subjects scored significantly higher than the non-compulsive groups on a number of personality trait measures, including the Doubts About Actions subscale of the Multi-dimensional Perfectionism Scale (MPS; Frost, Marten, Lahart, & Rosenblate, 1990). Gershuny and Sher (1995) found that introductory psychology students classified as checkers (MOCI-Checking equal to or greater than five) scored higher on doubt (MOCI-Doubting) than did non-checking anxious controls (MOCI-Checking equal to one or zero).

Perfectionism

Perfectionism has played an important if not central role in theories of OCD for almost 100 years. Janet (1903) posited a central role for perfectionism in the psychasthenic state that was characterized by uncertainty, indecisiveness and incompleteness (Summerfeldt *et al.*, 1998). Relative to the other belief domains, several studies with non-clinical samples have tested the role of perfectionism in OCD phenomena.

Perfectionism may be conceptualized as a multidimensional construct, and numerous recent studies have used the MPS to test levels of perfectionism in a variety of samples. Along this multi-dimensional continuum, studies with non-clinical samples have found that higher levels of perfectionism, particularly concern over mistakes and doubts about actions, are associated with higher levels of sub-clinical OCD symptom severity, including checking, hoarding, task performance (Frost & Steketee, 1997) and indecisiveness (Frost & Shows, 1993).

In general, studies with non-clinical and subclinical OCD analogue samples have found that higher levels of perfectionism relate to higher levels of OCD symptoms and behaviors. In a study of subclinical individuals, Frost and colleagues (1994) found that subclinical OCD participants (students) were more perfectionistic than non-compulsive participants. Ferrari (1995) demonstrated that higher levels of perfectionism were related to greater obsessive thoughts, compulsive checking, and compulsive hand-washing.

Rhéaume, Ladouceur, and Freeston (2000) found that higher perfectionism was moderately related to greater OCD tendencies in a non-clinical sample. They also found that perfectionism accounted for a significant proportion of the variance in OCD symptoms above and beyond that accounted for by perceived danger and responsibility. Similarly, in an earlier study, Rhéaume, Freeston, Dugas, Letarte, and Ladouceur (1995) found that perfectionism was a significant predictor of OCD symptoms after controlling for responsibility. Indeed, perfectionism is still a significant predictor of OCD symptoms in non-clinical OCD analogue samples after controlling for depression symptoms as well (Bhar & Kyrios, 1999).

Using a somewhat different, but informative approach, Rhéaume and colleagues (Rhéaume *et al.*, 2000) examined compulsive behaviors in individuals who varied in levels of perfectionism. They found that individuals classified as "dysfunctional perfectionists" reported more OCD behaviors than those classified as "functional perfectionists".

Gershuny and Sher and colleagues (Gershuny & Sher, 1995; Gershuny *et al.*, 2000) incorporated the use of an anxious control group when examining perfectionism (as well as a variety of other variables and factors) in non-clinical compulsive checkers. Gershuny and Sher (1995) found that compulsive checkers were more perfectionistic than anxious controls (anxious individuals who do not engage in compulsive checking behaviors) and than non-anxious controls (individuals who do not engage in compulsive checking behaviors or report high levels of anxiety). In a follow-up study, Gershuny and colleagues (2000) also found that compulsive checkers were more neurotic (including symptoms of perfectionism) than anxious and non-anxious controls. Finally, Coles, Rhéaume, Frost, and Heimberg (2000) found that self-reports of "not-just-right" experiences (NJRE's) were positively associated with perfectionism in college student volunteers.

Cognitive Styles of OCD vs. OCPD

As the categorical approach to personality disorders has given way to investigation of more specific personality traits, cognitive styles, and belief domains, so has the categorical uni-dimensional view of OCD given way to more specific exploration of OCD sub-types (e.g., Baer, 1994; Calamari *et al.*, 1999; Feinstein, Fallon, Petkova, & Liebowitz, 2000; Leckman *et al.*, 1997; Summerfeldt, Richter, Antony, & Swinson, 1999; Rasmussen & Eisen, 1992) and OCD-related phenomena including obsessive compulsive personality disorder (OCPD). To this end, Baer (1994) found that OCD patients with incompleteness are more likely to report and exhibit compulsive personality traits. More specifically, a series of factor analyses identified an OCPD factor (including preoccupation with details, inability to throw things away, indecision, and perfectionism) that was related to an OCD factor (including symmetry, hoarding, repeating, and counting symptoms) (Baer & Jenike, 1998).

In studies of non-clinical samples, a relationship between OCD phenomena and OCPD traits appear likely. Gibbs and Oltmanns (1995) found that in a non-clinical sample, compulsive checking was more associated with OCPD traits than was compulsive washing. They suggested that this association might be due to the strong relationship between checking and OCPD characteristics involving perfectionism and devotion to work. In another non-clinical sample, Rosen and Tallis (1995), partialled out anxiety and depression and found a unique positive relationship between OCPD traits measured by the Personality Diagnostic Questionnaire Revised (PDQ-R; Hyler & Rieder, 1987) and OCD symptoms measured by the MOCI, particularly doubting and checking. Frost and Gross (1993) found that in a sample of college students, compulsive hoarding was correlated with OCPD symptoms, especially perfectionism, though not with overall measures of OCPD.

Summary

Burns, Formea, Keortge, and Sternberger (1995) noted that selection criteria for non-clinical groups has varied from the upper 25 percent to the top two percent of scores on OCD measures (usually the MOCI). Burns and colleagues recommended that because about two percent of the population have OCD, the top two percent of relevant scores should be the criteria for inclusion in non-clinical OCD studies. Unless symptom severity of the non-clinical group is close to that of OCD patients, Burns and colleagues argued, results from non-clinical studies may not increase understanding of OCD. Gibbs (1996) supported this position and, in addition, emphasized the importance of clear definitions of sub-clinical OCD so that research procedures and findings can be replicated. Gibbs delineated samples that are either non-treatment seekers in the general population who meet diagnostic criteria for OCD or samples selected on the basis of elevated OCD symptom scores. Both groups have also been referred to as analogue-clinical. Other researchers have defined additional populations, such as unselected groups who are non-treatment seeking and are not screened for normality or pathology; and non-anxious groups who have been screened and determined to be within the normal range on relevant measures or interview procedures (Molina & Borkovec, 1994).

The majority of studies reviewed in this chapter utilized unselected non-treatment seeking, college students. Though it is unclear whether these research participants had elevated scores on OCD measures similar to OCD patients, they provided important information necessary for exploring the dimensional or continuum model of OCD.

OCD relevant cognitions, when compared with those of OCD patients, may offer hypotheses as to the progression of non-pathological to pathological cognitive and behavioral processes. For example, it seems counter-intuitive at first to find that students were more disturbed by worries than obsessive intrusive thoughts, and that worries were more strongly resisted (Langlois et al., 2000b). Also surprising was Rachman and colleagues' (1996) finding that performing an action not realistically connected with an event in order to undo it occurs in the normal population and not only in OCD patients. It would be useful to see how such phenomena may vary as non-clinical populations screened for varying degrees of obsessive compulsive symptom severity are assessed. As noted above, this type of research, requires that non-clinical groups be clearly defined and screened for normality, symptom severity, and clinical diagnosis.

The growing interest in investigating OCD subtypes appears to be a useful approach for research with non-clinical samples. For example, Gibbs and Oltmanns (1995) found that in non-clinicals, the checking, but not washing, subtype was significantly associated with OCPD traits such as perfectionism. It would be interesting to explore whether or not non-clinical checkers would score higher than non-clinical washers on OBQ items assessing perfectionism and intolerance of uncertainty. Additionally, one might predict that these items might discriminate between non-clinical checkers and non-clinical subjects with non-OCD-related anxiety.

As the evidence appears to suggest, the fear structure of contamination and washing symptoms is more similar to the phobias than are other OCD subtypes (Rasmussen & Eisen, 1992). This may be relevant to Jones and Menzies' (1997) finding that danger expectancies were better predictors of washing-related behavior in OCD patients, than were responsibility and perfectionism; and that in a non-clinical sample, manipulated high perceived danger increased washing and avoidance. Perhaps the OBQ over-estimation of threat subscale would be more associated with persons whose fear of germs and related washing is driven by threat to their own safety, whereas the responsibility subscale would better identify persons who primarily fear causing harm to others.

Summerfeldt (1998) has revised the OCD sub-type model of Rasmussen and Eisen (1992), and has proposed that the two core dimensions of OCD are harm avoidance and incompleteness, the latter involving perfectionism and intolerance of uncertainty. Future research might investigate whether OBQ items would discriminate between persons with harm vs. incompleteness-related symptoms.

Future non-clinical research might profitably continue to explore the interaction of different cognitive domains and OCD symptom severity and behaviors. Studies reviewed in this chapter that have manipulated perceived responsibility and threat estimation (Ladouceur et al., 1997; Menzies et al. 2000), TAF and thought suppression (Rassin et al., 2000), and responsibility and perfectionism (Bouchard, Rhéaume, & Ladouceur, 1999) provide excellent models for conducting this type of research with non-clinical populations.

Studies assessing different kinds of uncertainty might also enhance our understanding of how OCD might differ from other anxiety disorders. For example, how closely associated are the concepts and measures of intolerance of uncertainty that have been shown to be specifically associated with GAD and worry (Ladouceur, Gosselin, & Dugas, 2000) to the OBQ intolerance of uncertainty subscale, and the fear of uncertainty found by Richter et al., 1996 to discriminate between OCD patients and normal controls?

In addition, the importance of including adequate control groups should be noted. For example, when examining differences between non-clinical or sub-clinical obsessive compulsive samples and "controls", including only one control group of participants who do not exhibit OCD symptoms and behaviors is the method most often used but it is a method that is not wholly sufficient. To understand more fundamental differences between groups that cannot be explained by different levels of anxiety rather than the hypothesized differences in levels of obsessive compulsive symptoms, it is necessary to also include an anxious control group that does not exhibit OCD symptoms but does report similar levels of anxiety, as was done in the studies completed by Gershuny and Sher and their colleagues (1995, 2000).

In conclusion, the studies discussed in this chapter are supportive of Burns and colleagues' (1995) and Gibbs' (1996) views on the appropriateness and benefits of the utilization of non-clinical populations in research on OCD. The majority of evidence reviewed is also consistent with the dimensional or continuum model of OCD. Hopefully, increased understanding of vulnerability factors, including cognitive variables, that may explain differences between normals, those with sub-clinical OCD, and OCD patients will contribute to the prevention and amelioration of this prevalent form of human suffering.

References

Abramowitz, J. S., & Foa, E. B. (1998). Worries and obsessions in individuals with obsessive compulsive disorder with and without comorbid generalized anxiety disorder. *Behaviour Research and Therapy, 36*, 695–697.

Abramowitz, J., Tolin, D., Przeworski, A., Street, G., & Foa, E. B. (1999, November). *The paradoxical effects of thought suppression: A meta-analysis.* Poster session presented at the annual meeting of the Association for Advancement of Behavior Therapy, Toronto.

Baddeley, A. D., & Della Sala, S. (1998). Working memory and executive control. In A. C. Roberts *et al.* (eds), *The prefrontal cortex: Executive and cognitive functions* (pp. 9–21). New York: Oxford University Press.

Baer, L. (1994). Factor analysis of symptom sub-types of obsessive–compulsive disorder and their relation to personality and tic disorders. *Journal of Clinical Psychiatry, 55*, 18–23.

Baer, L., & Jenike, M. A. (1998). Personality disorders in obsessive–compulsive disorder. In M. A. Jenike, L. Baer, & W. E. Minichiello (eds), *Obsessive–compulsive disorder: Practical management* (pp. 65–83). St. Louis: Mosby.

Bhar, S. S., & Kyrios, M. (1999). Cognitive personality styles associated with depressive and obsessive–compulsive phenomena in a non-clinical sample. *Behavioural and Cognitive Psychotherapy, 27*, 329–343.

Bouchard, C., Rhéaume, J., & Ladouceur, R. (1999). Responsibility and perfectionism in OCD: An experimental study. *Behaviour Research and Therapy, 37*, 239–248.

Brigidi, B. D., Tolin, D. F., Donde, S., & Foa, E. B. (1999, November). *Intolerance of uncertainty in compulsive checkers.* Poster session presented at the annual meeting of the Association for Advancement of Behavior Therapy, Toronto.

Brown, T. A., Dowdall, D. J., Cote, G., & Barlow, D. H. (1994). Worry and obsessions: The distinction between generalized anxiety disorder and obsessive–compulsive disorder. In G. C. L. Davey, & F. Tallis (eds), *Worrying: Perspective on theory, assessment and treatment* (pp. 229–246). New York: John Wiley and Sons.

Burns, G. L., Formea, S. K., & Sternberger, L. G. (1995). The utilization of non-patient samples in the study of obsessive–compulsive disorder. *Behaviour Research and Therapy, 33*, 133–144.

Calamari, J. E., Wiegartz, P. S., & Janeck, A. (1999). Obsessive–compulsive disorder sub-groups: A symptom-based clustering approach. *Behaviour Research and Therapy, 37*, 113–126.

Carr, A. T. (1974). Compulsive neurosis: A review of the literature. *Psychological Bulletin, 81*, 311–318.

Chan, D. W. (1990). The Maudsley Obsessional–Compulsive Inventory: A psychometric investigation on Chinese normal subjects. *Behaviour Research and Therapy, 28*, 413–420.

Clark, D. A. (1992). Depressive, anxious and intrusive thoughts in psychiatric inpatients and outpatients. *Behaviour Research and Therapy, 30*, 93–102.

Clark, D. A., & Claybourn, M. (1997). Process characteristics of worry and obsessive intrusive thoughts. *Behaviour Research and Therapy, 35*, 1139–1141.

Clark, D. A., & Purdon, C. (1993). New perspectives for a cognitive theory of obsessions. *Australian Psychologist, 28*, 161–167.

Clark, D. A., Purdon, C., & Byers, E. S. (2000). Appraisal and control of sexual and non-sexual intrusive thoughts in university students. *Behaviour Research and Therapy, 38*, 439–456.

Coles, M. E., Mennin, D. S., & Heimberg, R. G. (2000, March). *Distinguishing obsessive features and worries: The role of thought–action fusion.* Poster session presented at the annual meeting of the Anxiety Disorders Association of America, Washington, DC.

Coles, M. E., Rhéaume, J., Frost, R. O., & Heimberg, R. G. (2000, March). *Not-just-right-experiences: Sensory perfectionism.* In P. J. Bieling & R. O. Frost (Chairs), Perfectionism and psychopathology: Linking personality and dysfunctional behavior. Symposium conducted at the annual meeting of the Association for Advancement of Behavior Therapy, New Orleans.

Craske, M. G., Rapee, R. M., Jackel, L., & Barlow, D. H. (1989). Qualitative dimensions of worry in DSM III- R generalized anxiety disorder subjects and nonanxious controls. *Behaviour Research and Therapy, 27*, 189–198.

Cripps, E., & Purdon, C. (2000, November). *Ego-dystonicity as a distinguishing feature of obsessions.* Poster session presented at the annual meeting of the Association for Advancement of Behavior Therapy, New Orleans.

Dugas, M. J., Francis, K., Robichaud, M., & Fioriello, A. (2000, November). *Thought–action fusion in high and low worriers.* Paper presented at the meeting of the Association for Advancement of Behavior Therapy, New Orleans.

Dugas, M. J., Gosselin, P., & Ladouceur, R. (2001). Intolerance of uncertainty and worry: Investigating specificity in a non-clinical sample. *Cognitive Therapy and Research, 25,* 551–558.

England, S. L., & Dickerson, M. (1988). Intrusive thoughts; Unpleasantness not the major cause of uncontrollability. *Behaviour Research and Therapy, 26,* 279–288.

Feinstein, S. B., Fallon, B. A., Petkova, E., & Liebowitz, M. (2000, March). *Factor-derived groups of obsessive–compulsive disorder symptoms: Predictors of treatment outcome.* Poster session presented at the annual meeting of the Anxiety Disorders Association of America: Washington, DC.

Ferrari, J. R. (1995). Perfectionism cognitions with non-clinical and clinical samples. *Journal of Social Behaviour and Personality, 10,* 143–156.

Foa, E. B., Kozak, M. J., Salkovskis, P. M., Coles, M. E., & Amir, N. (1998). The validation of a new obsessive–compulsive disorder scale: The Obsessive–Compulsive Inventory (OCI), *Psychological Assessment, 10,* 206–214.

Freeston, M. H., Ladouceur, R., Gagnon, F., & Thibodeau, N. (1993) Beliefs about obsessional thoughts. *Journal of Psychopathology and Behavioural Assessment, 15,* 1–21.

Freeston, M. H., Ladouceur, R., Thibodeau, N., & Gagnon, F. (1991). Cognitive intrusions in a non-clinical population. I. Response style, subjective experience, and appraisal. *Behaviour Research and Therapy, 29,* 585–597.

Freeston, M. H., Rhéaume, J., & Ladouceur, R. (1996). Correcting faulty appraisals of obsessional thoughts. *Behaviour Research and Therapy, 34,* 433–446.

Frost, R. O., & Gross, R. C. (1993). The hoarding of possessions. *Behaviour Research and Therapy, 31,* 367–381.

Frost, R. O., Sher, K. J., & Geen, T. (1986). Psychological characteristics of compulsive checkers. *Behaviour Research and Therapy, 24,* 133–143.

Frost, R. O., & Shows, D. L. (1993). The nature and measurement of compulsive indecisiveness. *Behaviour Research and Therapy, 31,* 683–692.

Frost, R. O., & Steketee, G. (1998). Hoarding: Clinical aspects and treatment strategies. In M. A. Jenike, L. Baer, & W. E. Minichiello (eds), *Obsessive–compulsive disorders: Practical management* (pp. 533–554). St. Louis: Mosby.

Frost, R. O., & Steketee, G. (1997). Perfectionism in obsessive–compulsive disorder patients. *Behaviour Research and Therapy, 35,* 291–296.

Frost, R. O., Steketee, G., Cohn, L., & Griess, K. (1994). Personality traits in sub-clinical and non-obsessive-compulsive volunteers and their parents. *Behaviour Research and Therapy, 32,* 47–56.

Frost, R. O., Marten, P., Lahart, C., & Rosenblate, R. (1990). The dimensions of perfectionism. *Cognitive Therapy and Research, 14,* 449–468.

Gershuny, B. S., & Sher, K. J. (1995). Compulsive checking and anxiety in a non-clinical sample: Differences in cognition, behavior, personality, and affect. *Journal of Psychopathology and Behavioural Assessment, 17,* 19–38.

Gershuny, B. S., Sher, K. J., Rossy, L., & Bishop, A. K. (2000). Distinguishing manifestations of anxiety: How do personality traits of compulsive checkers differ from other anxious individuals? *Behaviour Research and Therapy, 38,* 229–242.

Gibbs, N. A. (1996). Non-clinical populations in research on obsessive–compulsive disorder: A critical review. *Clinical Psychology Review, 16*, 729–773.

Gibbs, N. A., & Oltmanns, T. F. (1995). The relationship between obsessive–compulsive personality traits and sub-types of compulsive behaviour. *Journal of Anxiety Disorders, 9*, 397–410.

Goodwin, A., & Sher, K. J. (1992). Deficits in set-shifting ability in non-clinical compulsive checkers. *Journal of Psychopathology and Behavioural Assessment, 14*, 81–92.

Groopman, J. (2000, April 10). The doubting disease: When is obsession a sickness? *The New Yorker*, 52–57.

Guidano, V., & Liotti, G. (1983). *Cognitive processes and emotional disorders*. New York: Guilford.

Hyler, S. E., & Rieder, R. O. (1987). *PDQ-R: Personality Diagnostic Questionnaire Revised*. New York: New York State Psychiatric Institute.

Jakes, I. (1989a). Salkovskis on obsessional–compulsive neurosis: A critique. *Behaviour Research and Therapy, 27*, 673–675.

Jakes, I. (1989b). Salkovskis on obsessional–compulsive neurosis: A rejoinder. *Behaviour Research and Therapy, 27*, 683–384.

James, W. (1950). *The principles of psychology*. New York: Dover. (Original work published in 1890).

Janet, P. (1903). *Les obsessions et la psychasthenie* (Vols. 1–2, 2nd ed.), Paris: Alcan.

Jones, M. K., & Menzies, R. G. (1997). The cognitive mediation of obsessive–compulsive hand-washing. *Behaviour Research and Therapy, 35*, 843–850.

Jones, M. K., & Menzies, R. G. (1998). Role of perceived danger in the mediation of obsessive–compulsive washing. *Depression and Anxiety, 8*, 121–125.

Kyrios, M., Bhar, S., & Wade, D. (1996). The assessment of obsessive–compulsive phenomena: Psychometric and normative data on the Padua Inventory from an Australian non-clinical student sample. *Behaviour Research and Therapy, 34*, 85–95.

Ladouceur, R., Dugas, M. J., Freeston, M. H., Rhéaume, J., Blais, F., Boisvert, J. M., Gagnon, F., & Thibodeau, N. (1999). Specificity of generalized anxiety disorder symptoms and processes. *Behaviour Therapy, 30*, 1191–1207.

Ladouceur, R., Gosselin, P., & Dugas, M. J. (2000). Experimental manipulation of intolerance of uncertainty: A study of a theoretical model of worry. *Behaviour Research and Therapy, 38*, 933–942.

Ladouceur, R., Rhéaume, J., & Aublet, F. (1997). Excessive responsibility in obsessional concerns: A fine-grained experimental analysis. *Behaviour Research and Therapy, 35*, 423–427.

Ladouceur, R., Rhéaume, J., Freeston, M. H., Aublet, F., Jean, K., Lachance, S., & Langlois, F. (1995). Experimental manipulations of responsibility: An analogue test of models of obsessive–compulsive disorder. *Behaviour Research and Therapy, 33*, 937–946.

Langlois, F., Freeston, M. H., & Ladouceur, R. (2000a). Differences and similarities between obsessive intrusive thoughts and worry in a non-clinical populations: Study 1. *Behaviour Research and Therapy, 38*, 157–174.

Langlois, F., Freeston, M. H., & Ladouceur, R. (2000b). Differences and similarities between obsessive intrusive thoughts and worry in non-clinical population: Study 2. *Behaviour Research and Therapy. 38*, 175–190.

Leckman, J. F., Grice, D. E., Boardman, J., Zhang, H. Vitale, A., Bondi, C., Alsobrook, J., Peterson, B. S., Cohen, D. J., Rasmussen, S. A., Goodman, W. K., McDougle, C. J., & Pauls, D. L. (1997). Symptoms of obsessive–compulsive disorder. *American Journal of Psychiatry, 154*, 911–917.

Mancini, F., Gragnani, A., Orazi, F., & Pietrangeli, M. G. (1999). Obsessions and compulsions: Normative data on the Padua Inventory from an Italian non-clinical adolescent sample. *Behaviour Research and Therapy, 37*, 919–925.

Menzies, R. G., Harris, L. M., Cumming, S. R., & Einstein, D. A. (2000). The relationship between inflated personal responsibility and exaggerated danger expectancies in obsessive–compulsive concerns. *Behaviour Research and Therapy, 38*, 1029–1038.

Meyer, T. J., Miller, M. L., Metzger, R. L., & Borkovec, T. D. (1990). Development and validation of the Penn State Worry Questionnaire. *Behaviour Research and Therapy, 28*, 487–495.

Molina, S., & Borkovec, T. D. (1994). The Penn State Worry Questionnaire: Psychometric properties and associated characteristics. In G. Davey & F. Tallis (eds), *Worrying: Perspectives on theory, assessment and treatment* (pp. 265–283). New York: Wiley.

Niler, E. R., & Beck, S. J. (1989). The relationship among guilt, dysphoria, anxiety and obsessions in a normal population. *Behaviour Research and Therapy, 27*, 213–220.

Nowalk, A., Vallacher, R. R., Tesser, A., & Borkowski, W. (2000). Society of self: The emergence of collective properties in self-structure. *Psychological Review, 107*, 39–61.

Obsessive–Compulsive Cognitions Working Group (1997) Cognitive assessment of obsessive–compulsive disorder. *Behaviour Research and Therapy, 35*, 667–681.

Purdon, C., & Clark, D. A. (1993). Obsessive intrusive thoughts in non-clinical subjects. Part I. Content and relation with depressive, anxious and obsessional symptoms. *Behaviour Research and Therapy, 31*, 713–720.

Purdon, C., & Clark, D. A. (1994). Perceived control and appraisal of obsessional intrusive thoughts: A replication and extension. *Behavioral and Cognitive Psychotherapy, 22*, 269–285.

Purdon, C., & Clark, D. A. (1998). Thought suppression and appraisal: Implications for cognitive theories of obsessive–compulsive disorder. Manuscript under review.

Purdon, C., & Clark, D. A. (1999). Metacognition and obsessions. *Clinical Psychology and Psychotherapy, 6*, 102–110.

Purdon, C., & Clark, D. A. (2001). Suppression of obsession-like thoughts in non-clinical individuals. Part I. Impact on thought frequency, appraisal and mood state. *Behaviour Research and Therapy, 39*, 1163–1182.

Purdon, C., & Clark, D. A. (2000b). White bears and other elusive intrusions: Assessing the relevance of thought suppression for obsessional phenomena. *Behaviour Modification, 24*, 425–453.

Purdon, C. (in press). Appraisal of obsessional thought recurrences: Impact on anxiety and mood state. *Behaviour Research and Therapy*.

Rachman, S. J. (1997). A cognitive theory of obsessions. *Behaviour Research and Therapy, 35*, 793–802.

Rachman, S. J., & de Silva, P. (1978). Abnormal and normal obsessions. *Behavior Research and Therapy, 16*, 233–248.

Rachman, S. J., & Hodgson, R. J. (1980). *Obsessions and compulsions*. Englewood Cliffs, NJ: Prentice-Hall.

Rasmussen, S. A., & Eisen, J. L. (1992). The epidemiology and clinical features of obsessive–compulsive disorder. *Psychiatric Clinics of North America, 15*, 743–758.

Rassin, E., Merckelbach, H., & Muris, P. (2000). Paradoxical and less paradoxical effects of thought suppression: A critical review. *Clinical Psychology Review, 20*, 973–995.

Rassin, E., Merckelbach, H., Muris, P., & Spaan, V. (1999). Thought–action fusion as a causal factor in the development of intrusions. *Behaviour Research and Therapy, 37*, 231–238.

Rassin, E., Muris, P., Schmidt, H., & Merckelbach, H. C. (2000). Relationships between thought–action fusion, thought suppression and obsessive–compulsive symptoms: A structural equation modeling approach. *Behaviour Research and Therapy, 38*, 889–908.

Reed, G. F. (1985). *Obsessional experience and compulsive behavior: A cognitive-structural approach*. Toronto: Academic Press.

Rhéaume, J., Freeston, M. H., Dugas, M. J., Letarte, H., & Ladouceur, R. (1995). Perfectionism, responsibility, and obsessive–compulsive symptoms. *Behaviour Research and Therapy, 33*, 785–794.

Rhéaume, J., Freeston, M. H., & Ladouceur, R. (1995, June). *Functional and dysfunctional perfectionism: construct validity and a new instrument.* Paper presented at the World Congress of Behavioural Cognitive Therapy, Copenhagen.

Rhéaume, J., Ladouceur, R., Freeston, M. H., & Letarte, H. (1995). Inflated responsibility and its role in OCD II. Psychometric studies of a semi-idiographic measure. *Journal of Psychopathology and Behavioural Assessment, 16,* 265–276.

Rhéaume, J., Freeston, M. H., Ladouceur, R., Bouchard, C., Gallant, L., Talbot, F., & Vallieres, A. (2000). Functional and dysfunctional perfectionists: Are they different on compulsive-like behaviors? *Behaviour Research and Therapy, 38,* 119–128.

Rhéaume, J., Ladouceur, R., & Freeston, M. H. (2000). The prediction of obsessive–compulsive tendencies: Does perfectionism play a significant role? *Personality and Individual Differences, 28,* 583–592.

Richter, M. A., Summerfeldt, L. J., Joffe, R. T., & Swinson, R. P. (1996). The Tridimensional Personality Questionnaire in obsessive–compulsive disorder. *Psychiatry Research, 65,* 185–188.

Rosen, K. V., & Tallis, F. (1995). Investigation into the relationship between personality traits and OCD. *Behaviour Research and Therapy, 33,* 445–450.

Salkovskis, P. M. (1985). Obsessional–compulsive problems: A cognitive–behavioral analysis. *Behaviour Research and Therapy, 25,* 571–583.

Salkovskis, P. M., & Campbell, P. (1994). Thought suppression induces intrusion in naturally occurring negative intrusive thoughts. *Behaviour Research and Therapy, 32,* 1–8.

Salkovskis, P. M., & Harrison, J. (1984). Abnormal and normal obsessions-A replication. *Behaviour Research and Therapy, 22,* 549–552.

Salkovskis, P. M., Rachman, S. J., Ladouceur, R. , Freeston, M. H., Taylor, S., Kyrios, M., & Sica, C. (1996). *Proceedings of the Smith College women's room: An addendum to Toronto Cafeteria.* Unpublished manuscript.

Salkovskis, P. M., Richards, C., & Forrestor, E. (2000). Psychological treatment of refractory obsessive–compulsive disorder and related problems. In W.K. Goodman, M.W. Rudorfer, & J.D. Maser, (eds). *Obsessive–compulsive disorder: Contemporary issues in treatment* (pp. 201–222). Mahwah, NJ: Lawrence Erlbaum Associates.

Salkovskis, P. M., Westbrook, D., Davis, J., Jeavons, A., & Gledhill, A. (1997). Effects of neutralization on intrusive thoughts: An experiment investigating the etiology of obsessive–compulsive disorder. *Behaviour Research and Therapy, 35,* 211–219.

Salkovskis, P. M., Wroe, A. L., Gledhill, A., Morrison, N., Forrester, E., Richards, C., Reynolds, M., & Thorpe, S. (2000). Responsibility attitudes and interpretations are characteristic of obsessive–compulsive disorder. *Behaviour Research and Therapy, 38,* 347–372.

Shafran, R., Thordarson, D. S., & Rachman, S. (1996). Thought–action fusion in obsessive–compulsive disorder. *Journal of Anxiety Disorders, 10,* 379–391.

Shafron, R. (1996). How to remain neutral: An experimental analysis of neutralization. *Behaviour Research and Therapy, 34,* 889–898.

Sher, K. J., Martin, E., Raskin, G., & Perrigo, R. (1991). Prevalence of DSM-III-R disorders among non-clinical compulsive checkers and non-checkers in a college student sample. *Behaviour Research and Therapy, 29,* 479–483.

Sher, K. J., Mann, B., & Frost, R. O. (1984). Cognitive dysfunction in compulsive checkers: Further explorations. *Behaviour Research and Therapy, 22,* 493–502.

Sher, K. J., Wood, P. K., & Gotham, H. J. (1996). The course of psychological distress in college: A prospective high-risk study. *Journal of College Student Development, 37,* 42–51.

Stanley, M. A., Beck, J. G., & Zebb, B. J. (1996). Psychometric properties of four anxiety measures in older adults. *Behaviour Research and Therapy, 34,* 827–838.

Steketee, G., & Frost, R. O. (1994). Measurement of risk-taking in obsessive–compulsive disorder. *Behavioural and Cognitive Psychotherapy, 22,* 269–298.

Steketee, G., Frost, R. O., & Cohen, I. (1998). Beliefs in obsessive–compulsive disorder. *Journal of Anxiety Disorders, 12*, 525–537.

Steketee, G. S., Frost, R. O., Rheaume, J., & Wilhelm, S. (1998) Cognitive theory and treatment of obsessive–compulsive disorder. In M.A. Jenike, L. Baer, & W.E. Minichiello (eds), *Obsessive–compulsive disorder: Practical Management* (pp. 368–399). St. Louis: Mosby.

Sternberger, L. G., & Burns, G. L. (1990a). Maudsley Obsessional–Compulsive Inventory: Obsessions and compulsions in a non-clinical sample. *Behaviour Research and Therapy, 28*, 337–340.

Sternberger, L. G., & Burns, G. L. (1990b). Compulsive Activity Checklist and the Maudsley Obsessional–Compulsive Inventory: Psychometric properties of two measures of obsessive–compulsive disorder. *Behaviour Therapy, 21*, 117–127.

Sternberger, L. G., & Burns, G. L. (1990c). Obsessions and compulsions: Psychometric properties of the Padua Inventory with an American college population. *Behaviour Research and Therapy, 28*, 341–345.

Summerfeldt, L. J. (1998). Cognitive processing in obsessive–compulsive disorder: Alternative models and the role of sub-types. *Unpublished doctoral dissertation*, York University, Canada.

Summerfeldt, L. J., Huta, V., & Swinson, R. P. (1998). Personality and obsessive–compulsive disorder. In R. P. Swinson, M. M. Antony, S. Rachman, & M. A. Richter. (eds), *Obsessive–compulsive disorder: Theory, research, and treatment* (pp. 79–119). New York: Guilford.

Summerfeldt, L. J., Richter, M. A., Antony, M. M., & Swinson, R. P. (1999). Symptom structure in obsessive–compulsive disorder: A confirmatory factor analytic study. *Behaviour Research and Therapy, 37*, 297–311.

Thordarson, D. S., Whittal, M., L., & McLean, P. D. (2000). Thought–Action Fusion in OCD: Differences among OCD sub-types. In M. G. Craske & M. J. Dugas (Chairs), *The fusion of thoughts, actions, and perceptions in psychopathology*. Symposium conducted at the meeting of the Association for Advancement of Behavior Therapy, New Orleans.

Trinder, H., & Salkovskis, P. M. (1994). Personally relevant intrusions outside the laboratory: Long-term suppression increases intrusion. *Behaviour Research and Therapy, 32*, 833–842.

Turner, S. M., Beidel, D. C., & Stanley, M. A. (1992). Are obsessional thoughts and worry different cognitive phenomena? *Clinical Psychology Review, 12*, 257–270.

van Oppen, P. (1992). Obsessions and compulsions: Dimensional structure, reliability, convergent and divergent validity of the Padua Inventory. *Behaviour Research and Therapy, 39*, 631–637.

Wegner, D. M. (1989). *White bears and other unwanted thoughts: Suppression, obsession, and the psychology of mental control.* New York: Viking.

Wells, A., & Morrison, A. P. (1994). Qualitative dimensions of normal worry and normal obsessions: A comparative study. *Behaviour Research and Therapy, 37*, 325–335.

Wells, A., & Papageorgiou, C. (1998). Relationships between worry, obsessive–compulsive symptoms and meta-cognitive beliefs. *Behaviour Research and Therapy, 36*, 899–913.

Wilson, K. A., & Chambless, D. L. (1999). Inflated perceptions of responsibility and obsessive–compulsive symptoms. *Behaviour Research and Therapy, 37*, 325–336.

Zucker, B. G., Craske, M. G., Barrios, V., & Holguin, M. (2000, November). Thought–action fusion: Can it be corrected? In M. G. Craske & M. J. Dugas (Chairs), *The fusion of thoughts, actions, and perceptions in psychopathology*. Symposium conducted at the meeting of the Association for Advancement of Behavior Therapy, New Orleans.

Chapter 19

Cognitions in Individuals with Severe or Treatment Resistant Obsessive Compulsive Disorder

Pamela S. Wiegartz, Cheryl N. Carmin and C. Alec Pollard

Introduction

With advances in pharmacological and behavioral treatments, the prognosis for patients with obsessive compulsive disorder (OCD) has improved significantly over the past decade. However, for a rather large subset of patients who seek treatment, OCD remains a chronic and disabling disorder with potentially devastating effects on work, social functioning, and independent self-care (Calvorcoressi, Libman, Vegso, McDougle, & Price, 1998). To effectively address the needs of individuals with severe and refractory OCD, current treatment strategies may need to be modified or supplemented. Hopefully, a better understanding of factors that influence OCD severity and resilience will lead to innovations in treatment. A promising area of research is the role of cognitive factors in OCD.

One challenge in studying refractory disorders is the difficulty of defining terms. For example, as the understanding of processes underlying OCD has evolved, so have treatment success rates and the definition of what constitutes "treatment-refractory" OCD. Early naturalistic studies suggest that treatment efforts for OCD resulted in minimal success, with around 16 percent of patients indicating significant improvement following treatment (see Rasmussen & Eisen, 1997). It is highly doubtful, however, that the remaining 84 percent of patients in these early studies constituted a "treatment-refractory" group. Rather, it is now evident that adequate treatments did not exist at that time. Subsequent development of behavioral treatments, including exposure and response prevention (ERP), resulted in a remarkable increase in the number of patients noting substantial symptom reduction (up to 75 percent) and, thus, a comparable decrease in the proportion of patients currently considered to have treatment-refractory OCD.

Furthermore, defining the term "treatment-refractory" is problematic because treatment can fail to benefit patients for a number of reasons. Among those patients who have access to and are suitable for behavioral treatment, a substantial portion refuse or discontinue treatment prematurely due to therapeutic constraints. Among those who do complete therapy, 25 percent fail to respond or are unable to maintain treatment gains over time

Cognitive Approaches to Obsessions and Compulsions – Theory, Assessment, and Treatment
Copyright © 2002 by Elsevier Science Ltd.
ISBN: 0-08-043410-X

(Foa & Kozak, 1996). Labeling a case as "treatment-refractory" does not elucidate the nature of or the reasons for an individual's inadequate response to therapy. It is possible that different factors are involved in different types of treatment failure. However, because the literature on refractory OCD is scant, the present review was not limited to a particular type of treatment failure. Any data considered relevant to understanding the relationship between cognition and treatment responsiveness was included.

The role of cognition in OCD has received increasing attention from investigators in recent years. Cognitive research has focused on etiology, psychopathology, and treatment. The purpose of this chapter is to review the existing literature relevant to the relationship between cognition and OCD treatment outcome and severity. Areas for future research are also identified.

Cognitive Domains

One area of cognitive research has examined the relationship between certain types of beliefs, or cognitive domains, and OCD. It is possible that individuals with severe or refractory OCD are more likely to hold certain kinds of beliefs than individuals with more treatment-responsive OCD. There is preliminary evidence that beliefs related to responsibility, danger estimates, and thought–action fusion might be related to OCD symptom severity.

Responsibility and Danger Estimates

Responsibility, or the belief that one possesses the power to provoke or prevent negative consequences, has long been anecdotally associated with obsessive compulsive behaviors (see Chapter four of this volume). Although direct investigations of responsibility and refractory OCD are lacking, some extrapolations may be made based on the extant literature. An interesting study done by Ladouceur, Rhéaume, and Aublet (1997) found that manipulating beliefs resulted in compulsive checking behaviors, and that specific beliefs about perceived control and negative consequences may combine to result in increased severity of observable, checking behaviors in a non-clinical sample. Similarly, Shafran (1997) found that perceptions of responsibility increased the urge to ritualize and resulted in higher levels of discomfort. These findings together suggest that a linear relationship may exist between a person's perceptions of responsibility and both the objective frequency and subjective severity of obsessive-compulsive checking behaviors in normals. Recent clinical studies (Steketee, Frost, & Cohen, 1998) have reported findings directly supporting the notion that a variety of beliefs, including responsibility, are predictive of OCD severity even after controlling for mood state and worry.

Some studies, however, have *not* found an association between responsibility and degree of obsessive compulsive symptoms. Wells and Papageorgiou (1998) found positive correlations between beliefs and a variety of compulsive behaviors in a non-clinical sample. However, no compulsive subtype was particularly associated with beliefs about responsibility. Beliefs about danger and potentially negative consequences predicted washing rituals, a finding also supported by a study of clinically diagnosed OCD subjects (Jones & Menzies, 1997). In a group of 27 DSM-IV diagnosed OCD subjects with washing concerns, estimates of danger were positively associated with high levels of anxiety during a behavioral avoidance task, as well as with strong urges to wash and increased time spent washing. Apart from danger expectancy, no cognitive mediators (i.e., responsibility, perfectionism, anticipated anxiety, self-efficacy) were correlated with the behavioral measures.

These mixed findings suggest the possibility of differentially important beliefs for various subtypes of OCD (i.e., washing, checking). However, this conclusion is at odds with results from clinical studies that find no differences between OCD subgroups (i.e., washers, checkers, ruminators) on measures of responsibility (Ladouceur, Bouvard, Rhéaume, & Cottraux, 1999). While some evidence for the role of cognition in obsessive compulsive symptom severity may be garnered from the positive correlation between beliefs and compulsive behaviors, discrepancies illustrate the need for further research.

Thought–Action Fusion

Thought–Action Fusion (TAF) refers to a failure to recognize critical differences between thought and action as, for example, when the thought of a loathsome act and the act itself are considered morally equivalent. TAF can also refer to instances in which an obsessive thought is believed to increase the probability of a feared event occurring (Rachman & Shafran, 1998). TAF is generally higher in obsessive samples than in non-obsessives and has been noted to correlate strongly with the checking subscale of the Maudsley Obsessive compulsive Inventory (Shafran, Thordarson, & Rachman, 1996).

The relationship between TAF and "magical thinking" is unclear, although the two concepts clearly overlap to a large degree. This overlap is worth noting due to the relationship between OCD and other diagnoses that include this characteristic. For instance, Jenike *et al.* (1986) found that OCD patients with comorbid schizotypal personality disorder exhibited high rates of treatment failure. Interestingly, it was the more schizophrenic-like symptoms such as ideas of reference and suspiciousness, that accounted for the treatment failures. Magical thinking, a concept more closely aligned with TAF, was found in *both* treatment successes and failures. Obviously, more research is needed to determine the impact of TAF on OCD symptom severity, although current data suggest that TAF correlates positively with compulsive behavior. A clearer definition of the relationship between TAF and dysfunctional thought patterns present in other disorders would facilitate interpretation of the literature.

Strength and Fixity of Beliefs

Another aspect of cognition that could be related to severe or treatment-refractory OCD is the strength or fixity of a belief (see Chapter ten in this volume). Much of the research in this area has examined over-valued ideation (OVI) which refers to irrational beliefs held with a high degree of conviction. Depending on the study and the definition of OVI used, it may (e.g., Solyom, DiNicola, Phil, Sookman, & Luchins, 1985) or may not (e.g., Lelliot, Noshirvani, Basoglu, Marks, & Montiero, 1988) indicate poor prognosis. While the idea that closely held beliefs would be more resistant to treatment has high face validity, the data have been largely inconclusive.

One issue complicating the interpretation of these studies is the representation of OVI as a dichotomy (i.e., beliefs either make sense or they do not). As Kozak and Foa (1994) suggest, OVI may be more accurately viewed as a continuum that would include the broad range of insight evident among OCD patients. From this perspective, obsessions would be considered senseless, delusions would be considered sensible, and OVI would cover the beliefs that fall somewhere between.

Attempts to operationalize this continuum are currently underway. Foa, Abramowitz, Franklin, and Kozak (1999) measured the effects of feared consequences and poor insight on behavior therapy outcome. OCD patients reporting high certainty that feared consequences would occur as measured by the Fixity of Beliefs Questionnaire (Foa *et al.*, 1995) evidenced smaller decreases in YBOCS scores following a three-week ERP program than did the low-fixity group. ERP was shown to decrease strength of belief in seven of the nine patients with feared consequences, presumably based on the behavioral provision of corrective information to disconfirm their fears. A case series reported by one of these authors (Abramowitz, 1999) noted similar findings, as well as evidence of differential patterns of habituation depending on level of OVI. Both high and low OVI individuals were found to exhibit within-session habituation during ERP treatment, but this reduction in anxiety did not generalize to between-session exposures and failed to produce long-term habituation in the high OVI patients. As these authors note, their findings are limited due to unknown psychometric properties of their central measure, the Fixity of Beliefs Questionnaire. However, these preliminary results suggest that OVI may influence the effectiveness of standard behavioral treatment and provide clues about the mechanism by which OVI affects treatment success.

A newly developed instrument, the Brown Assessment of Beliefs Scale (BABS; Eisen *et al.*, 1998), provides the opportunity for more valid and reliable assessment of beliefs in OCD. The BABS was designed to measure delusions across a wide range of psychiatric disorders, and some data have been reported on an OCD sample. Eisen *et al.* (1998) found that in 20 DSM-III-R diagnosed OCD subjects who were administered sertraline, the mean change in BABS scores mirrored the change in YBOCS scores from pre- to post-treatment. The correlation between mean change in total YBOCS and BABS scores indicated that improvement in degree of conviction was associated with improvement in severity of OCD symptoms. These results are consistent with those of Foa *et al.* (1999) and suggest that, with the availability of a reliable measure, the role of strength and fixity of beliefs in OCD severity and treatment outcome could be clarified in the near future.

Information Processing

Cognition may also play a role in the expression of OCD through idiosyncrasies in information processing (see Chapter nine in this volume). Recent research has examined how information is perceived, attended to, and recalled by patients with OCD. Data indicate

OCD can be characterized by selective processing of obsessive, content-relevant information (e.g., Foa & McNally, 1986; Lavy, van Oppen, & van den Hout, 1994). Some studies have found that these attentional biases are specific to negative OCD concerns (Foa, Ilai, McCarthy, Shoyer, & Murdock, 1993; Lavy *et al.*, 1994) and disappear following intensive behavior therapy (Foa & McNally, 1986). To our knowledge, no studies have directly examined symptom severity relative to attentional biases. However, the Foa and McNally (1986) study suggests that these deficits in attentional processes are state dependent and may resolve with treatment.

Anecdotal reports and some experimental investigations suggest possible memory deficits in patients with OCD, particularly deficits in non-verbal memory (e.g., Savage *et al.*, 2000). Studies of severe and refractory OCD are lacking, but a handful of studies have reported significant correlations between memory deficits and OCD symptom severity. For instance, Tallis, Pratt, and Jamani (1999) found that attention/concentration was equivalent in OCD checkers and controls, but as general OCD symptom severity increased, so did the number of false positives endorsed on a non-verbal memory task. No significant correlation was found between checking and memory, however, bringing into question the etiologic significance of these observed deficits.

Several authors have made a strong case for normal memory functioning in OCD patients and have suggested that it is *confidence* in memory, rather than memory *per se*, that is impaired in this group (e.g., Foa, Amir, Gershuny, Molnar, & Kozak, 1997; MacDonald, Antony, MacLeod, & Richter, 1997). One study (MacDonald *et al.*, 1997) examining DSM-IV diagnosed OCD checkers, OCD non-checkers and controls found no difference in recall or recognition memory for words across the three groups. However, confidence ratings for recognition memory judgments were significantly lower in the checking group, as was their latency to respond (suggesting uncertainty). It is worth noting that the checking group had significantly higher YBOCS and MOCI scores, raising the possibility that OCD severity, rather than sub-type, may have influenced confidence ratings. This finding expands upon earlier results that also found equivalence in memory between OCD checkers, OCD non-checkers and normal controls, but decreased confidence in memory judgments for the clinical group (McNally & Kohlbeck, 1993).

Implications from Treatment Outcome Studies

Another source of information about the relationship between cognition and severe or refractory OCD is research that examines the effect of cognitive interventions on OCD symptoms. If cognition plays a key role in the severity or treatment-responsiveness of OCD, then interventions specifically designed to modify cognition should be more effective than interventions that do not have a cognitive component. Failure to adequately address cognition might explain some cases that do not respond sufficiently to behavior therapy.

Unfortunately, existing outcome data do not adequately address the questions raised in this chapter. Controlled studies supporting the efficacy of cognitive therapy (e.g., Freeston *et al.*, 1997; van Oppen *et al.*, 1995) do not specifically target severe or refractory OCD. The design of investigations that do focus on this subgroup of OCD sufferers, such as in-patient treatment-outcome studies (Pollard, 2000), do not isolate the cognitive components of treatment. This makes it difficult to draw sound conclusions about the specific contributions of cognitive intervention. Depending on the study, cognitive interventions were either not used at all or were integrated with behavioral interventions (Pollard, 2000).

Data recently reported by Sookman and Pinard (in press) provide preliminary support for the proposition that certain cognitive treatments may be particularly effective with severe or refractory OCD. They administered cognitive therapy to seven OCD patients, five of whom had previously failed to respond to exposure and response prevention and two of whom had refused treatment altogether. Therapy consisted of interventions that targeted domains such as inflated responsibility, perfectionism, over-importance of thoughts, and other cognitive factors believed by the authors to be relevant to OCD. From pre- to post-treatment, mean scores on OCD symptom measures such as the YBOCS had dropped from moderately severe to the sub-clinical level. In six of the seven cases, changes in targeted dysfunctional beliefs seemed to be associated with symptom change. The same investigators have reported similar findings with additional samples of three (Sookman, Pinard, & Beauchemin, 1994) and 15 (Sookman & Pinard, 2000) patients with refractory OCD.

As it currently stands, the treatment outcome literature offers very little information that improves our understanding of the relationship between cognition and the severity or treatment responsiveness of OCD. Only the reports by Sookman and Pinard have specifically examined the use of cognitive interventions with a difficult-to-treat sample of OCD patients. The apparent success of their cognitive treatment suggests that cognitive mechanisms could be involved in determining the severity or resilience of OCD. However, firm conclusions regarding the specific effects of cognitive intervention on severe or refractory OCD must await controlled studies and treatment component analyses involving larger samples of patients.

Conclusions and Future Directions

Few definitive conclusions can be drawn concerning the impact of cognition on OCD severity and treatment-responsiveness. Thus far, no single cognitive domain has been uniquely associated with failure to respond to treatment. Even if a particular type of belief emerges as a major contributing factor, strength and fixity of beliefs may be at least as important as the type of belief. The role of information processing deficits in refractory OCD is unclear and has only begun to be examined. Preliminary research suggests that cognitive intervention may be able to help some individuals who do not respond to ERP alone, but the evidence to date involves uncontrolled studies and only a small number of subjects.

Several important directions for future research are indicated. One area of study is extending investigations that have found a positive relationship between severity of obsessive compulsive symptoms and beliefs involving responsibility, danger, and TAF. The bulk of this research has studied non-clinical samples. While some recent clinical studies have found similar results (e.g., Steketee *et al.*, 1998), further research involving patient samples is clearly needed.

The call for additional clinical research is also applicable to the information processing literature. Studies of this nature will help determine whether attentional biases found in non-clinical individuals who score high on obsessive-compulsive measures are also characteristic of patients who have been formally diagnosed with OCD. Low confidence in memory, rather poor memory itself, appears to be associated with OCD, but additional research is indicated in this area as well. Whether studying attentional biases or memory, future research will have to include individuals who have failed treatment if more is to be learned about the role of information processing in refractory OCD.

Another direction for future research is outcome studies that specifically address questions concerning refractory OCD. Controlled trials that directly compare ERP versus cognitive therapy in individuals designated as treatment resistant or treatment refractory would improve upon prior outcome research that was either uncontrolled or did not specifically focus on refractory OCD. In addition to examining how pre-treatment beliefs and strength of beliefs influence post-treatment outcome, this type of investigation can also shed light on the process of change by measuring beliefs, strength of beliefs, and symptom severity at different points during the course of therapy. Within this domain is the opportunity to explore the contribution of comorbid disorders (e.g., depression, personality disorders) to irrational or strongly held beliefs and subsequent treatment response in this group.

A final area of investigation should include attempts to refine and standardize the definition and assessment of beliefs. Variance among measures used by investigators probably accounts for some of the inconsistencies in prior research findings. Efforts to address the issue are currently underway (e.g., Obsessive Compulsive Cognitions Working Group, 1997; 2001) and could improve the ability of researchers to answer complex questions regarding the relationship between cognition and treatment response. Are certain beliefs differentially important depending on the type of obsessive compulsive symptom? Is it a combination of mal-adaptive beliefs, rather than any single belief, that results in severe or refractory OCD? Will strength or fixity of beliefs, rather than the content of beliefs, turn out to be the best predictor of treatment failure? Recent advances in assessment now emerging will hopefully aid researchers to answer these and the many other remaining questions about the role of cognition in OCD.

References

Abramowitz, J. S. (1999). Over-valued ideation, habituation, and treatment outcome in obsessive–compulsive disorder: A case series. *Psicoterapia Cognitiva e Comportamentale, 5*, 223–232.

Calvorcoressi, L., Libman, D., Vegso, S. J., McDougle, C. J., & Price, L. H. (1998). Global functioning of inpatients with obsessive–compulsive disorder, schizophrenia, and major depression. *Psychiatric Services, 49*, 379–381.

Eisen, J. L., Phillips, K. A., Baer, L., Beer, D. A., Atala, K. D., & Rasmussen, S. A. (1998). The Brown assessment of beliefs scale: reliability and validity. *American Journal of Psychiatry, 155*, 102–108.

Foa, E. B., Abramowitz, J. S., Franklin, M. E., & Kozak, M. J. (1999). Feared consequences, fixity of belief, and treatment outcome in patients with obsessive–compulsive disorder. *Behavior Therapy, 30*, 717–724.

Foa, E. B., Amir, N., Gershuny, B., Molnar, C., & Kozak, M. J. (1997). Implicit and explicit memory in obsessive–compulsive disorder. *Journal of Anxiety Disorders, 11*, 119–129.

Foa, E. B., Ilai, D., McCarthy, P. R., Shoyer, B., & Murdock, T. (1993). Information processing in obsessive–compulsive disorder. *Cognitive Therapy and Research, 10,* 477–485.

Foa, E. B., & Kozak, M. J. (1996). Psychological treatment for obsessive–compulsive disorder. In R. F. Prien (ed.), *Long-term treatments of anxiety disorders* (pp. 285–309). *Washington, DC: American Psychiatric Press.*

Foa, E. B., Kozak, M. J., Goodman, W. K., Hollander, E., Jenike, M. A., & Rasmussen, S. (1995). DSM-IV field trial: Obsessive–compulsive disorder. *American Journal of Psychiatry, 152,* 90–96.

Foa, E. B., & McNally, R. J. (1986). Sensitivity to feared stimuli in obsessive-compulsives: A dichotic listening analysis. *Cognitive Therapy and Research, 10,* 477–485.

Freeston, M. H., Ladouceur, R., Gagnon, R., Thibodeau, N., Rhéaume, J., Letarte, H., & Bujold, A. (1997). Cognitive–behavioral treatment of obsessive thoughts: A controlled study. *Journal of Consulting and Clinical Psychology, 65,* 405–413.

Jenike, M. A., Baer, L., & Carey, R. J. (1986). Co-existent obsessive–compulsive disorder and schizotypal personality disorder: A poor prognostic indicator. *Archives of General Psychiatry, 43,* 296.

Jones, M. K., & Menzies, R. G. (1997). The cognitive mediation of obsessive–compulsive hand-washing. *Behaviour Research and Therapy, 35,* 843–850.

Kozak, M. J., & Foa, E. B. (1994). Obsessions, over-valued ideas, and delusions in obsessive–compulsive disorder. *Behaviour Research and Therapy, 32,* 343–353.

Ladouceur, R., Bouvard, M., Rhéaume, J., & Cottraux, J. (1999). Evaluation of perceived responsibility among obsessive-compulsive patients. *Encephale, 25,* 408–415.

Ladouceur, R., Rhéaume, J., & Aublet, F. (1997). Excessive responsibility in obsessional concerns: A fine-grained experimental analysis. *Behaviour Research and Therapy, 35,* 423–427.

Lavy, E. H., van Oppen, P., & van den Hout, M. A. (1994). Selective processing of emotional information in obsessive–compulsive disorder. *Behaviour Research and Therapy, 32,* 243–246.

Lelliot, P. T., Noshirvani, H. F., Basoglu, M., Marks, I. M., & Montiero, W. O. (1988). Obsessive-compulsive beliefs and treatment outcome. *Psychological Medicine, 18,* 697–702.

MacDonald, P. A., Antony, M. M., MacLeod, C. M., & Richter, M. A. (1997). Memory and confidence in memory judgements among individuals with obsessive–compulsive disorder and non-clinical controls. *Behaviour Research and Therapy, 35,* 497–505.

McNally, R. J., & Kohlbeck, P. A. (1993). Reality monitoring in obsessive–compulsive disorder. *Behaviour Research and Therapy, 31,* 249–253.

Obsessive Compulsive Cognitions Working Group. (1997). Cognitive assessment of obsessive–compulsive disorder. *Behaviour Research and Therapy, 35,* 667–681.

Obsessive Compulsive Cognitions Working Group. (2001). Development and intial validation of the Obsessive–Beliefs Questionnaire and the Interpretation of Intrusions Inventory. *Behaviour Research and Therapy, 39,* 987–1006.

Pollard, C. A. (2000). Inpatient treatment of refractory obsessive–compulsive disorder. In W. K. Goodman & M. V. Rudorfer (eds), *Obsessive–compulsive disorder: Contemporary issues in treatment* (pp. 223–231). Mahwah, N.J. Lawrence Erlbaum.

Rachman, S., & Shafran, R. (1998). Cognitive and behavioral features of obsessive–compulsive disorder. In R. P. Swinson, M. M. Antony, S. Rachman, & M. A. Richter (eds), *Obsessive-compulsive disorder: Theory, research, and treatment* (pp.51–78). New York: Guilford Press.

Rasmussen, S. A., & Eisen, J. L. (1997). Treatment strategies for chronic and refractory obsessive-compulsive disorder. *Journal of Clinical Psychiatry, 58* (Suppl. 13), 9–13.

Savage, C. R., Deckersback, T., Wilhelm, S., Rauch, S. L., Baer, L., Reid, T., & Jenike, M. A. (2000). Strategic processing and episodic memory impairment in obsessive–compulsive disorder. *Neuropsychology, 14,* 141–151.

Shafran, R., Thordarson, D. S., & Rachman, S. (1996). Thought–action fusion in obsessive–compulsive disorder. *Journal of Anxiety Disorders, 10*, 379–391.

Shafran, R. (1997). The manipulation of responsibility in obsessive–compulsive disorder. *British Journal of Clinical Psychology, 36*, 397–407.

Solyom, L., DiNicola, V. F., Phil, M., Sookman, D., & Luchins, D. (1985). Is there an obsessive psychosis? Aetiological and prognostic factors of an atypical form of obsessive–compulsive neurosis. *Canadian Journal of Psychiatry, 30*, 372–380.

Sookman, D., & Pinard, G. (in press). Integrative cognitive therapy for obsessive–compulsive disorders which focuses on multiple schemas. *Cognitive and Behavioral Practice.*

Sookman, D., & Pinard, G. (2000, March). *Assessing change in core beliefs in the treatment of resistant OCD patients.* Paper presented at the annual meeting of the Anxiety Disorders Association of America, Washington D.C.

Sookman, D., Pinard, G., & Beauchemin, N. (1994). Multi-dimensional schematic restructuring treatment for obsessions: Theory and practice. *Journal of Cognitive Psychotherapy: An International Quarterly, 8*, 175–194.

Steketee, G., Frost, R. O., & Cohen, I. (1998). Beliefs in obsessive–compulsive disorder. *Journal of Anxiety Disorders, 12*, 525–537.

Tallis, F., Pratt, P., & Jamani, N. (1999). Obsessive–compulsive disorder, checking, and non-verbal memory: A neuropsychological investigation. *Behaviour Research and Therapy, 37*, 161–166.

van Oppen, P., DeHaan, E., van Balkom, A., Spinhoven, P., Hoogduin, K., & van Dyck, R. (1995). Cognitive therapy and exposure in-vivo in the treatment of obsessive–compulsive disorder. *Behaviour Research and Therapy, 33*, 379–390.

Wells, A., & Papageorgiou, C. (1998). Relationships between worry, obsessive–compulsive symptoms and meta-cognitive beliefs. *Behaviour Research and Therapy, 36*, 899–913.

Chapter 20

Obsessive Compulsive Disorder Cognitions Across Cultures

Claudio Sica, Caterina Novara, Ezio Sanavio, Stella Dorz and Davide Coradeschi

Introduction

It is well known that psychological phenomena are influenced by many factors, such as age, gender, socio-economic and educational background, as well as ethnic and cultural factors. Culture can be defined as "Patterns, explicit and implicit, of and for behavior acquired and transmitted by symbols, constituting the distinctive achievement of human groups, including their embodiments in artifacts; the essential core of culture consists of traditional ideas and especially their attached values" (Kroeber & Kluckhohn, 1952, p. 181). From a behavioral stand-point, culture refers to "aspects of past learning common to members of a society, resulting in shared patterns of behavior (including cognitive, affective, somatic, and motor responses to intra-personal, inter-personal, and physical environmental stimuli) that overlap more with behavior of other members of that society than with members of other societies" (Seiden, 1999, p. 200). With the term "culture" we refer to behavior patterns and value systems shared by a group of people.

According to Tseng (1997), culture may influence psychopathology in a variety of ways. First, culture shapes the phenomenology of psycho-pathology (i.e., the manner by which individuals describe their symptoms). For instance, when a person becomes depressed, he/she may feel guilty for sins committed or ashamed for socially non-compliant performance. Second, cultural factors may affect not only the level of symptom content, but also the syndrome as a whole. In this case, the concept of sub-type or variation of a syndrome needs to be entertained. Third, culture may contribute to the development of a unique psycho-pathology that is observed only in a certain cultural environment. Some examples of such culture-bound syndromes are South Asia *koro* (impotence panic), Egyptian *kabsa* (fear of reproductive infertility attributed to symbolic pollution), or homophobia (fear of homosexuals) typical of Western and Latin countries (Ficarrotto, 1990; Inhorn, 1994; Tseng *et al.*, 1988). Fourth, culture may favor or hinder the development of psycho-pathology. That is, performance demands, beliefs about and, acceptance of the disorders by members of the culture, the availability of social support,

Cognitive Approaches to Obsessions and Compulsions – Theory, Assessment, and Treatment
Copyright © 2002 by Elsevier Science Ltd.
All rights of reproduction in any form reserved.
ISBN: 0-08-043410-X

and the existing care system contribute to the frequency of the disorders in the community. Suicidal behaviors and substance abuse are examples of disorders whose frequency varies among different societies according to the socio-cultural context (Castillo, 1997). Lastly, culture plays a role in how the problem is presented or communicated by the patient, in other words, his or her "problem-presenting style" may dictate if or how symptoms are endorsed.

While research endeavors in this domain may be extremely appealing, cross-cultural research on psycho-pathology encounters a formidable obstacle in the lack of consensus among researchers about models and measures thought to be relevant to and reliable for the phenomenon being studied. In this context, the cognitive measures developed by the Obsessive Compulsive Cognitions Working Group (OCCWG, 1997) represent an international attempt to standardize definitions and instruments to facilitate research concerning obsessive compulsive disorder (OCD). As a result of this collaboration, the OCCWG measures constitute an extraordinary effort to carry out cross-cultural research with instruments that have incorporated cultural sensitivity into their development. The aim of this chapter is to review cross-cultural research on OCD symptoms and cognitions and present cross-cultural data about cognitive phenomena in OCD.

OCD Prevalence Across Cultures

OCD lifetime prevalence rates reported in the literature vary depending on diagnostic criteria adopted and type of interview utilized. Furthermore, the use of lay interviewers and the temporal stability of diagnoses have been criticized by several authors (e.g., Elliot & Rice, 1997; Lewis *et al.*, 1992; Murray, Forde, Geri, & Walker, 1997). The complex nature of this disorder and the methodological problems in epidemiological research have caused some scholars to state that "the OCD of clinicians is not the same as the OCD of epidemiologists" (Bourgeois, 1996, p. 23). However, epidemiological research may disclose differences in OCD prevalence across cultures, and such differences might be considered possible clues regarding cultural influences on this form of psycho-pathology.

The Cross National Collaborative Study (Weissman *et al.*, 1994) examined the lifetime prevalence of OCD across several countries. OCD lifetime prevalence was approximately 2.3 percent in United States, Canada, Puerto Rico, Germany (Munich) and New Zealand; in Korea, OCD prevalence was 1.9 percent and in Taiwan 0.7 percent. Figures similar to those obtained in North America were found in Iceland (Stefannson, 1993). On the other hand, investigations of ethnicity revealed very low OCD rates in African, Afro-Caribbean, Asian, and Australian aborigines groups (Jones & Horne, 1973; Meltzer *et al.*, 1995). The low frequency of OCD reported in sub-Saharan Africa and South East Asia could be explained by particular attitudes (e.g., "optimistic fatalism") and available social support (e.g., extended family) typical of those cultures (German, 1962; Sechrest, 1969).

In the Cross National Collaborative Study (Weissman *et al.*, 1994), OCD prevalence was investigated by the National Institute of Mental Health Diagnostic Interview Schedule (DIS; Robins *et al.*, 1981) based on DSM-III criteria. Nestadt, Bienvenu, Cai, Samuels, and Eaton (1998), traced a cohort originally sampled during the 1981 Epidemiologic

Catchment Area Study (the US part of the Cross National Collaborative Study) and re-interviewed people using a modified version of the DIS that reflected changes in DSM criteria. They found that the threshold for new case identification was higher than in the original study, probably because the DSM-III-R criteria for OCD were more stringent than DSM-III criteria. In addition, a more recent study carried out in Great Britain using ICD-10 diagnostic criteria revealed an OCD lifetime prevalence of approximately 1 to 1.5 percent (Meltzer *et al.*, 1995). Another recent study reported an OCD lifetime prevalence of 0.9 percent in Netherlands (Bijl, Zessen, & Ravelli, 1997).

Epidemiological research also inquired into the demographic variables associated with OCD. OCD in adults appears to have an equal gender distribution, although differences have been reported in some symptom categories, such as contamination/washing which may be more prevalent in women. Obsessive compulsive patients are less likely to be married than age matched controls. Lastly, there is conflicting evidence about the role of intelligence, social class and birth order (Parkin, 1997; Pigott, 1998; Samuels & Nestadt, 1997). It still remains to be determined the extent to which these findings are valid outside Western countries.

Thus, it seems that in Western countries, especially Anglo-Saxon and Anglo-Celtic ones, lifetime prevalence rates of OCD are remarkably consistent at about 1–2 percent, whereas rates vary across Asian and other ethnic groups. However, the lack of data from many countries (e.g., South America, Africa, Europe) and the differences in screening methods utilized make it difficult to draw unequivocal conclusions about the presence of any relationships between culture and OCD and about the socio-demographic factors related with OCD.

Religious Influence on Beliefs and OCD

It is generally acknowledged that OCD and other anxiety disorders may vary across cultures in prevalence and form of expression but not in essential structure (e.g., Good & Kleinman, 1985; Salkovskis, personal communication, 1997). To date, many of the empirical studies have emphasized the relationship between religious beliefs and OCD. Rachman (1997) hypothesized that "people who are taught, or learn, that all their value-laden thoughts are of significance will be more prone to obsessions — as in particular types of religious beliefs and instructions" (p. 798). In fact, several great religious leaders were subject to intrusive obsessions (Rachman & Hodgson, 1980). Rasmussen and Tsuang (1986) observed that if their OCD patients had an inordinately strict or orthodox religious upbringing, these themes were subsequently involved in their obsessive thoughts or compulsive rituals. More recently, Steketee, Quay, and White (1991) contended that religion may play a role in OCD as a medium that partly determines how, although not necessarily whether, symptoms are expressed. These authors found no difference between OCD patients and patients with other anxiety disorders when religiosity was considered. Nonetheless, severity of OCD pathology was positively correlated with religiosity. Furthermore, the OCD patients with religious obsessions were significantly more religious than those who did not report such obsessions. Fitz (1990) suggested that the role of religion in the etiology of obsessive compulsive disorder is not clear. Some evidence indicates that a high degree of religiosity can predispose a person to OCD, but many studies do not recognize the multi-dimensional aspects of religious phenomena and are poorly designed to address this issue.

Sica, Novara, and Sanavio (in press (a)) investigated OCD cognitions and symptoms in a sample of 54 Italian Catholic nuns and friars (Religious group), 47 persons who regularly attended church activities (practicing Catholics) and 64 students not particularly involved with religion (Students). After controlling for anxiety and depression, religious groups scored higher than individuals with a low degree of religiosity on measures of obsessionality, over-importance of thoughts, control of thoughts, perfectionism and responsibility. Moreover, measures of control of thoughts and over-importance of thoughts were associated with OCD symptoms only in religious subjects. This last finding might be explained with regard to the matters of purity inherent in Catholic precepts. For instance, Greenberg (1984) and Rapoport (1989) suggested that religions emphasizing ritual penance and purification may predispose followers to religious obsessions or compulsions. Moreover, the equivalence between thoughts and behaviors, as embodied in the thought–action fusion construct, is a feature of Catholic teachings. The general findings of this study confirmed that specific cognitions linked to OCD phenomena are relevant in Religious and Catholics groups. Future studies are necessary to extend the research on cognitions in religious samples to clinical samples of clergy or various religious groups.

A number of cross-cultural studies seem to support the hypothesis of a strict link between religion and OCD. Early studies found that in Moslem culture in Saudi Arabia the themes of obsessions were more often related to religious practices than were evident in British OCD patients from a mainly Christian culture (Mahgoub & Abdel-Hafeiz, 1991). Akthar (1978) and Khanna and Channabasavanna (1988) observed a preponderance of obsessions concerning dirt and contamination among Hindus with OCD and noted that Indian culture is preoccupied with matters of purity and cleanliness. In another study assessing OCD symptoms in 34 Israeli patients, symptoms linked to religious practices were found in 13 of 19 ultra-orthodox Jewish subjects and in only one of the 15 non-ultra-orthodox Jewish subjects (Greenberg & Witzum, 1994).

Okasha, Saad, Khalil, El-Dawla, and Yehia (1994) noted that in Egypt, both obsessions and compulsions were influenced by the Moslem culture. Compared to British samples, the obsessions of the Egyptian sample were concerned mostly with religious matters, and matters related to cleanliness and contamination. In fact, Moslems are required to pray five times per day, with each prayer preceded by a ritualistic ablution. Strict fundamentalist Moslems may be required to perform a complex ritualistic cleansing process if they should touch a woman. Interestingly, Okasha *et al.* (1994) also noted that there were similarities between the contents of obsessions in Moslems and those reported by Jews.

Studies carried out within a single country can also highlight how religion affects OCD phenomenology. For instance, two investigations conducted in Turkey reported opposite results. One study in Western Turkey did not find a prevalence of religious themes in obsessions despite the influence of Moslem culture (Egrilmez, Gulseren, Gulseren, & Kultur, 1997). The other study, carried out in Eastern Turkey, found that religion was the second most common obsessive theme after dirt and contamination (Tezcan & Millet, 1997). In fact, it is possible that dirt and contamination obsessions also reflected religious concerns within this culture.

The literature reviewed thus far raises the interesting question of whether the differences in symptom presentation are due to "cultural factors" or whether they are largely due to differences in the nature and strength of the person's religious views. In other words, it could be that OCD is likely to be characterized by prominent religion-related symptoms (e.g., blasphemous obsessions and contrition compulsions) when a person is raised in a highly religious community, regardless of the person's country, language and other cultural factors.[1] This last hypothesis is very appealing and deserves further study.

OCD and Superstition

Superstitious beliefs are defined as "central personality dynamism that energizes and organizes individual and collective behavior; (such a dynamism) provides persons and societies with meaning in life, with perceived control, and with resources for adjustment" (Tobacyk, 1995, p. 145). This definition suggests that superstition, which may be considered a form of magical thinking, may influence individual beliefs and behaviors. In fact, in some cultures, superstition is a widespread and accepted attitude.

Two studies have examined the possible links between superstition and OCD. In the first, Leonard, Goldberger, Rapoport, Cheslow, and Swedo (1990), administered a semi-structured interview about superstitions to a group of 38 OCD patients (children) and to a group of 22 matched control individuals. In addition, the parents completed a semi-structured interview about their child's developmental rituals (e.g., doing things exactly the same way, games with specific or elaborate rules, time-consuming hobbies). Although no differences between OCD and normal control groups were found in the frequency of childhood superstitions, the OCD patients were identified by their parents as having significantly more ritualized behaviors in childhood. In the second study, Frost *et al.* (1993) administered a series of questionnaires about superstitious and obsessive compulsive phenomena to 108 female US college students. Their results indicated that super-stitiousness was correlated with compulsive checking (but not compulsive cleaning), perfectionism and responsibility. Not surprisingly, the correlations between OCD cognitions and superstitousness were larger than those observed between superstitiousness and OCD symptoms. The authors hypothesized that both checking and superstitiousness might have a common function with respect to the warding off of events over which one has little perceived control.

A recent investigation to further examine the nature of relationship between superstition and obsessive compulsive cognitions — as measured by the OBQ and the Interpretations of Intrusions Inventory (III, OCCWG, in press), symptoms and other psycho-pathological features was carried out by Sica *et al.* (in press (b)). Italian college students ($n = 258$) completed the OBQ, III, Padua Inventory (PI; Sanavio, 1988), Beck Anxiety Inventory (BAI; Beck, Epstein, Brown, & Steer, 1988), Beck Depression Inventory (BDI; Beck, Steer, & Garbin, 1988) and a questionnaire about superstition. After controlling for anxiety and depression, high superstitious subjects scored higher than low-superstitious subjects on measures of over-estimation of threat, impaired mental control, contamination and

[1]*Note: The authors are indebted with Steven Taylor for this suggestion.*

worry. A logistic regression analysis showed that over-estimation of threat and perfectionism discriminated high from low superstitious subjects over and above anxiety and depression measures. Consequently, the particular content of these domains implies that superstitious people may be more prone to pure obsessions or worry compared to non-superstitious ones. In support of this last hypothesis, Borkovec and Roemer (1995) found that a group of patients with generalized anxiety disorder (GAD) consistently reported that worrying caused them to believe that the feared event was less likely to occur. In other words, GAD patients attributed an excess of importance to their thoughts, an attribution the authors labeled as "superstition". On the other hand it would be difficult to assume that all superstitious individuals in Italy (a substantial part of the population) are more prone to develop OCD compared to non-superstitious individuals. We think that owing to the cultural acceptance of superstitious behaviors and beliefs in Italy, the obsessive and compulsive-like features of superstitious people would not be considered pathological, mitigating the etiological role of appraisals and beliefs in the development of OCD.

In sum, superstitiousness may be a predisposing factor for general instead of specific psycho-pathology, but cultural factors may moderate the relation between superstitiousness and psycho-pathology. Of course, our results need to be confirmed and further elaborated by other studies using both normal and clinical subjects. Nonetheless, these data offer some preliminary hypotheses and open intriguing scenarios within cross-cultural and clinical research.

OCD Cognitions and Cultural Issues

Culture not only provides the categories, explanatory frames, and idioms for responding to physiological symptoms, it may also play a significant role in structuring pathologies of cognitions themselves (Good & Kleinman, 1985). Thus, culture may differently shape beliefs or core cognitive schemas thought to be etiologically relevant to OCD. For instance, beliefs regarding responsibility are probably different in Japan (where, in the past, people could kill themselves if they thought they failed in complying with their moral duties), compared to beliefs regarding responsibility held in other cultures. In countries like Italy, which are deeply influenced by religion, thought–action fusion is a normal feature of the cognitive style. Even for people who are not particularly religious, negative self-referenced thoughts might be regarded as indicative of one's real nature. In countries where superstition is acknowledged and well-accepted, specific mental and behavioral rituals might be considered as a normal occurrence. Unfortunately, the hypothesized link between cultural habits and beliefs and cognitive schema has not been adequately investigated.

To our knowledge, only one study has examined the relationship between OCD cognitions and symptoms across cultures. Kyrios, Liguori, Sanavio, and Bhar (1997) compared Australian (30 percent females) and Italian (50 percent females) college students on several measures of OCD symptoms and cognitions. In this study, the authors considered three dimensions of inflated responsibility (Safety of Others; Blame and Personal Responsibility for Faults and Negative Outcomes; Need to Control, Hinder or Compensate for Negative Outcomes) as measured by the Inflated Responsibility

Questionnaire (IRQ; Kyrios, 1993), three dimensions of perfectionism (Socially-Prescribed; Self-Oriented; and Other-Oriented) drawn from the Multi-dimensional Perfectionism Scale (MPS; Hewitt, Flett, Turnbull, & Mikail, 1991) and five OCD symptoms domains (Impaired Mental Control, Contamination, Checking, Urges/Worries and Overall Obsessionality) included in the Padua Inventory. The results suggested a higher association in the Australian cohort between some specific cognitive domains (Blame and Personal Responsibility and Self-Oriented Perfectionism) and the Padua Inventory scales. Moreover, the major differences in the correlations across the groups were found for the Urges/Worries scale of the Padua Inventory. The authors concluded that, consistent with common stereotypes, Anglo-Celtic culture might be more concerned than Italian culture about personal control issues.

Clearly, more studies are necessary to attain a better understanding about the influences of culture on OCD cognitions. Moreover, the cross-cultural research may help to verify the reliability of the models and measures so far developed. If we find consistency across cultures, we may be entitled to greater confidence in our measures. If there are inconsistencies, the cultural, ethnic, or religious diversity of subjects may allow for greater understanding of the contribution of these variables to obsessive compulsive cognitions.

Cultures and Obsessive Compulsive Cognitions: OCCWG Findings

In the effort to validate the Obsessive Beliefs Questionnaire (OBQ) and the Interpretations of Intrusions Inventory (III), the OCCWG collected data from several countries, including students from Greece, Italy and the USA. The findings are reported in Sica, Frost, and Sanavio (2001). Subjects from these three countries were expressly chosen because they represent distinct ethnic groups. We expected some differences in beliefs among participants from the three countries based on observed differences in cultural style. For example, we anticipated that, given the strong influence of Catholicism, Italians would show more over-importance of thoughts and its component thought–action fusion, as well as more control of thoughts. On the other hand, we expected US subjects to exhibit greater perfectionism.

In order to carry out these cross-cultural comparisons, three basic methodological issues deserve our attention. These issues included translation of instruments (i. e., questionnaires, etc.), homogeneity of a given culture, and selection of statistical method(s) for analyzing data in a reliable way. Translations were done in accordance with guidelines proposed in the methodological literature pertaining to cross-cultural psychology (e.g., Brislin, 1986). With respect to the second issue, people living in the same country were considered culturally homogenous even though we were aware that a particular culture is not necessarily shared by all the members of a single country. For practical purposes, broad cultural attributes such as nationality, ethnicity, and language are usually selected in order to investigate cross-cultural differences, while recognizing the wide range of within-culture variability. Thus, students who were born in the same country and share the same language were considered more similar than different and somewhat representative of a given national culture. Lastly, due to the problems determining the meaning of a group's specific norms (e.g., style of presenting symptoms, response biases, etc.), direct statistical comparisons between test scores of subjects belonging to different cultures are not generally recommended. A better strategy lies in taking in consideration the patterns of co-variations between different measures. As a consequence, we first performed a series of multiple regression analyses on the overall sample. If analyses had revealed a significant effect for country, then we examined the correlations between OBQ, and III scales and measures of OCD symptoms, anxiety, and depression. In this way, possible differences might be better interpreted in terms of cultural peculiarities instead of generic biases (Arrindell *et al.*, 1999; Good & Kleinman, 1985; Warwick & Osherson, 1973).

For this study, 43 Greek students, 348 Italian students and 73 US students completed OBQ, III, BAI, BDI, and Padua Inventory. Italian students were significantly younger than the other two groups and less educated than US students. No significant differences were found with respect to gender.

Across all groups, the OBQ, III, BAI, BDI and Padua evidenced good internal consistencies (0.70–0.90), with the exceptions of the OBQ Control of Thoughts (0.67), and Importance of Thoughts (0.52) Scales and the BAI in the Greek group (0.60), and Padua Urges and Worries Scale (0.44) in the US group. In addition, the major part of item-remainder correlations achieved acceptable values, the lowest acceptable bound being 0.20 (Nunnally, 1978). Again, the Greek group showed lower values compared to the other two groups. Not unexpectedly the US group reported the highest values.

Regression analyses were performed on the overall sample using the Padua Inventory Total scale as the dependent variable and OBQ and III total scores (separately) as independent variables. Three country variables included Greek students (1), not Greek students (0); US students (1), not US students and Italian students (1), not Italian students (0). To discover significant cultural effects, three interaction terms were created by multiplying the country variables (dummy coded) by OBQ total score and three interaction terms by multiplying the variable "country" (dummy coded) by III total score.[1] The interactions terms were then forced in equation after having controlled for OBQ or III total scores alone. The two separate analyses revealed a significant effect of the interaction terms, suggesting the presence of differences among the three countries (the Italian interaction term did not appear in the analyses because it was formed by a linear combination of the other interactions). Instead of interpreting the standardized regression coefficients (i.e., beta) of regression analyses, attention was focused on the product-moment correlations between symptoms and cognitive measures for each group. This pattern of correlations could reveal more information about the differences among the three countries than beta weights because the latter measured the relations between *global* measures of OCD symptoms (Padua Total) and *global* measures of OCD domains (OBQ and III total). In fact, the inspection of correlation patterns between symptoms and cognitive measures disclosed interesting results. In Greek students, each of the cognitive domains was strongly related to the Impaired Mental Control subscale of the PI. However, few other significant relationships were observed. In Italian students, the cognitive domains were consistently associated with depression and with all OCD symptom scales, especially Impaired Mental Control from the PI. However, the OBQ Importance of Thoughts and Responsibility subscales, as well as all three subscales of the III showed a weaker pattern of correlations with OCD symptoms compared to the US group. With few exceptions, the US students showed the highest correlations between belief domains and appraisals and

OCD symptoms. Greek students had the weakest pattern of correlations with Italians somewhat in the middle.

Discussion

Our findings suggest that, with some exceptions, psychometric characteristics of the self-report measures obtained from students from three countries were similar. The absolute magnitude of the correlations appeared, more often than not, clearly different across the three groups. One explanation for these results might be a lack of internal validity (i.e., non-homogenous groups, poor psychometric features of the instruments, different procedures, etc.). In contrast, our results might be tentatively interpreted as indicating cultural specificity, evident in both by correlation patterns and regression analyses outcomes. In Greek students, OCD cognitive domains were unrelated to symptoms of checking and cleaning and the highest correlations were related to depression and impaired mental control. These results are surprising because the OCD domains identified by OCCWG are thought to be relevant to OCD symptoms, as emerged in the correlation pattern of US and Italian groups. When the Italian students were compared with their US counterparts, consistent with some cultural stereotypes, Importance of Thoughts and Responsibility were less correlated with OCD symptoms, depression, and anxiety. The US students appeared more concerned about their own thoughts (as showed by the high correlations between cognitive appraisal measures and OCD symptoms) compared to the other two groups.

In all groups, OCD cognitive domains were strongly related to the Padua Scale of Impaired Control over Mental Activities and to depression. As a matter of fact, the measure of impaired control focuses on cognitive aspects and in US students shares as much as 50 percent of variance with the single OBQ and III scales. On the other hand, the relationship between depression and OCD cognitive domains deserves further study. For example, do the cognitive features measured by OBQ and III reflect mainly depression, OCD symptoms or both? As pointed out by Rachman (1997), the interaction of depression and obsessions is complex.

Only the Over-estimation of Threat scale consistently related to OCD symptoms in Italian and US students. Several authors have indeed proposed that people with OCD symptoms tend to over-estimate the probability and cost of aversive events (OCCWG, 1997). The correlation pattern differed markedly in Greek students compared to US and Italian students; the closeness of Greece to Eastern culture might be advocated as one of the factor explaining these differences. Of course, our interpretations are highly speculative and more studies are needed. However, it remains that large differences were found in these three cultural groups, and these differences appear to be in accordance with ethnic stereotypes.

Conclusion

Although not conclusive, empirical research suggests that certain cultural features affect OCD phenomenology and, in less measure, OCD prevalence. Low prevalence rates of OCD are detected in cultures where there is a low overall rate of psycho-pathology (e.g., Weissman *et al.*, 1994). As a consequence, it is difficult to identify specific cultural factors associated with OCD until additional epidemiological studies are carried out.

The present study highlights four points worthy of further investigation. First, OCD cognitive domains, particularly responsibility, importance of thoughts and the three dimensions of appraisals (control of thoughts, importance of thoughts and responsibility) seem not to have the same relevance (as measured by correlation with OCD symptoms and anxiety) in non-clinical students from different countries. More research is necessary to evaluate if these findings are reliable, applicable to clinical populations and influence the manner in which OCD prevalence is estimated. Available evidence casts doubt upon the universal value of theories asserting the etiologic role of specific beliefs and appraisals in the development of OCD. Future research should therefore establish if OCCWG cognitive domains are culture-bound or in what manner they generalize across various cultural or ethnic groups.

Second, superstition and a high involvement in religion seem to play a particular role in OCD phenomenology. The influence of these factors on OCD etiology is an open issue and needs further examination. We hypothesize that in ethnic groups in which superstitiousness and religion play an important role in ordinary life, some OCD behaviors (e.g., behavioral or mental rituals) may cause less distress because they would be considered culturally congruent/acceptable. As previously pointed out, the mixed findings about the relationship between religion and OCD may be attributed to the lack of attention to the multi-dimensionality of religious experience. It is probable that only a few aspects of religious teachings (e.g., very high moral standards, inflexibility, prohibition, purity) are linked with OCD phenomena.

Lastly, it is necessary to ascertain in which measure the differences in OCD across countries could be attributed to differences in religious practices rather than to other cultural factors. The OBQ and the III seem consistently related to measures of impaired control over mental activities. This finding suggests that the OCCWG measures may have a particular value in predicting pure obsessions and worries because the Padua Inventory Scale of Impaired Control covers features belonging to both pure obsessives and worriers (e.g., Freeston *et al.*, 1994). In fact, Taylor and colleagues (see Chapter seven of this volume) showed that most of the OBQ and III scales measure beliefs and appraisals common to anxiety disorders in general. Lastly, the lack of research into early development influences and family interaction patterns from a cross-cultural perspective makes incomplete any attempt at discovering specific factors relating to OCD. Future studies should address these important topics.

Tseng and Streltzer (1997) note that there are a number of factors limiting our understanding of the link between culture and psycho-pathology. First of all, culture is an abstract concept which may be considered from alternative viewpoints including stereo-typical, actual, ideal, and deviant. Consequently, defining the cultural group can be quite difficult. In the same country, for example, we can find sub-cultures that differ markedly from each other. In addition, psycho-pathology is shaped by many factors other than culture, including individual life experiences and biological pre-disposition. Further, psycho-pathology may be conceptualized as having different degrees of universality or cultural specificity (Castillo, 1997). Some conditions, like dementias, are essentially free of cultural influence whereas other syndromes are shared only by the members of a particular human group. Most syndromes, OCD included, probably lie in between the extremes, having both universal and cultural aspects. Disentangling this skein is not simple as evidenced by contradictory findings.

In conclusion, cross-cultural studies can encourage us to systematically and rigorously assess the cultural bias implicit in our disease categories, as well as in our social and psychological theories. Within this frame of reference, consensus groups like OCCWG may shed some light over complex matters like those addressed in this chapter, making possible an increase of our knowledge of psychological phenomena across the diversity of ethnic and cultural groups.

Acknowledgments

The authors wish to thank the following scholars for their help and advice: Martine Bouvard (France), Paul Emmelkamp (The Netherlands), Randy Frost (USA), Michael Kyrios (Australia), Fugen Neziroglu (USA), Patricia van Oppen (The Netherlands), Gail Steketee (USA) and Steven Taylor (Canada).

References

Akhtar, S. (1978). Obsessional neurosis, marriage, sex and fertility: Some transcultural comparisons. *International Journal of Social Psychiatry, 24,* 164–166.

Arrindell, W. A., Sanavio, E., Aguilar, G., Sica, C., Hatzichristou, C., Eisemann, M., Recinos, L. A., Gaszner, P., Peter, M., Battagliese, G. Kàllai, J., & van der Ende, J. (1999). The development of a short form of the EMBU: Its appraisal with students in Greece, Guatemala, Hungary and Italy. *Personality and Individual Differences, 27,* 613–628.

Beck, A. T., Epstein, N., Brown, G., & Steer R. A. (1988). An inventory for measuring clinical anxiety: Psychometric properties. *Journal of Consulting and Clinical Psychology, 56,* 893–897.

Beck, A. T., Steer R. A., & Garbin, M. G. (1988). Psychometric properties of Beck Depression Inventory: Twenty-five Years of Evaluation. *Clinical Psychology Review, 8,* 77–100.

Bijl, R. V., van Zesen, G., & Ravelli, A. (1997). Psychiatrische morbiditeit onder volwassenen in Nederland: het NEMESIS — onderzoek. II. Prevalentie van psychiatrische stoornissen. Nederlands *Tijdschrift voor Geneeskunde, 141,* 2453–2460.

Borkovec, T. D., & Roemer, L. (1995). Perceived functions of worry among generalized anxiety disorder subjects: Distractions from more emotionally distressing topics? *Journal of Behavior Therapy and Experimental Psychiatry, 26,* 25–30.

Bourgeois, M. (1996). Troubles et syndromes obsessionnels et pathologie de l'humeur. A propos de l'enquete épidémiologique française DRT TOC et SOC. *L'Encéphale, 22,* (Suppl. 1), 23–31.

Brislin, R. W. (1986). The wording and translation of research instruments. In W. J. Lonner, & J.W. Berry (eds.), *Field methods in cross-cultural research* (pp. 137–164). Beverly Hills, CA: Sage.

Castillo, R. (1997). *Culture and mental illness: A client-centered approach.* Pacific Grove, CA: Brooks/Cole.

Dag, I. (1999). The relationships among paranormal beliefs, locus of control and psychopathology in a Turkish college sample. *Personality and Individual Differences, 26,* 723–737.

Egrilmez, A., Gulseren, L., Gulseren, S., & Kultur, S. (1997). Phenomenology of obsessions in a Turkish series of OCD patients. *Psychopathology, 30*, 106–110.

Elliot, N., & Rice, J. (1997). Stability of diagnosis of obsessive–compulsive disorder in the Epidemiologic Catchment Area Study. *American Journal of Psychiatry, 154*, 826–831.

Ficarrotto, T. J. (1990). Racism, sexism and erothophobia: Attitudes of heterosexuals towards homosexuals. *Journal of Homosexuality, 19*, 111–116.

Fitz, A. (1990). Religious and familial factors in the etiology of obsessive–compulsive disorder: A review. *Journal of Psychology and Theology, 18*, 141–147.

Freeston, M. H., Ladoucer, R., Rhéaume, J., Letarte, H., Gagnon, F., & Thibodeau, N. (1994). Self report of obsessions and worry. *Behaviour Research and Therapy, 32*, 29–36.

Frost, R. O., Krause, M. S., McMahon, M. J., Peppe, J., Evans, M., McPhee, A. E., & Holden, M. (1993). Compulsivity and superstitiousness. *Behaviour Research and Therapy, 31*, 423–425.

German, G. A. (1972). Aspects of clinical psychiatry in sub-Saharan Africa. *British Journal of Psychiatry, 121*, 461–466.

Good, B. J., & Kleinman, A. M. (1985). Culture and anxiety: Cross-cultural evidence for the patterning of anxiety disorders. In A. H. Tuma & J. D. Maser (eds), *Anxiety and the anxiety disorders*, (pp. 297–323). New York: Lawrence Erlbaum Associates.

Greenberg, D. (1984). Are religious compulsions religious or compulsive? *American Journal of Psychoterapy, 38*, 524–532.

Greenberg, D., & Witzum, E. (1994). The influence of cultural factors on obsessive–compulsive disorder: Religious symptoms in a religious society. *Israel Journal of Psychiatry and Related Sciences, 31*, 211–220.

Hewitt, P., Flett, G., Turnbull, D. W., & Mikail, S. (1991). The Multidimensional Perfectionism Scale: Reliability, validity and psychometric properties in psychiatric samples. *Psychological Assessment, 3*, 464–468.

Inhorn, M. C. (1994). Kabsa (a.k.a. mushahara) and threatened fertility in Egypt. *Social Science and Medicine, 39*, 487–505.

Jahoda, G. (1969). *The psychology of superstition*. London, WI: Allen Lane The Penguin Press.

Jones, I. H., & Horne, D. J. (1973). Psychiatric disorders among aborigines of the Australian Western Desert. *Social Science and Medicine, 7*, 219–228.

Khanna, S., & Channabasavanna, S. M. (1988). Phenomenology of obsessions in obsessive–compulsive neurosis. *Psychopathology, 20*, 23–28.

Kroeber, A. L., & Kluckhohn, C. (1952). Culture: A critical review of concepts and definition. *Papers of the Peabody Museum of American Archaeology and Ethnology, 47*, 181.

Kyrios, M. (1993). *Inflated Responsibility Questionnaire*. Unpublished manuscript.

Kyrios, M., Lia, L., Sanavio, E., & Bhar, S. S. (1997, September). *Associations between obsessive–compulsive phenomena, affects and beliefs: Cross-cultural comparisons of Australian and Italian data*. XXVII Congress of European Association for Behavioural and Cognitive Therapies, Venice.

Leonard, H. L., Goldberger, E. L., Rapoport, J. L., Cheslow, D. L., & Swedo, S. E. (1990). Childhood rituals: Normal development or obsessive–compulsive symptoms? *Journal of the American Academy of Child and Adolescent Psychiatry, 29*, 17–23.

Lewis, G., Pelosi, A. J., Araya, R. C., & Dunn. G. (1992). Measuring psychiatric disorder in the community: A standardized assessment for use by lay-interviewers. *Psychological Medicine, 22*, 465–486.

Mahgoub, O. M., & Abdel-Hafeiz, H. B. (1991). Patterns of obsessive–compulsive disorders in Eastern Saudi Arabia. *British Journal of Psychiatry, 158*, 840–842.

Matsunaga, H., Kiriike, N., Miyata, A., Iwasaki, Y., Matsui, T., Nagata, T., Takei, Y., & Yamagami,

S. (1998). Personality disorders in patients with obsessive–compulsive disorder in Japan. *Acta Psychiatrica Scandinavica, 98*, 128–134.

Meltzer, H., Gill, B., & Petticrew, M. (1995). *OPCS surveys of psychiatric morbidity in Great Britain. Report n. 1. The prevalence of psychiatric morbidity among adults living in private households.* London: Office of Population Censuses and Surveys.

Murray, S., Forde, D., Geri, A., & Walker, J. (1997). Obsessive–compulsive disorder in the community: An epidemiologic survey with clinical reappraisal. *American Journal of Psychiatry, 154*, 1120–1126.

Nestadt, G., Bienvenu, J., Cai, G., Samuels, J., & Eaton W. E. (1998). Incidence of obsessive–compulsive disorder in adults. *The Journal of Nervous and Mental Disease, 186*, 401–406.

Nunally, J. C. (1978). *Psychometric theory, second edition.* New York: McGraw-Hill

OCCWG (1997). Cognitive assessment of obsessive–compulsive disorder. *Behaviour Research and Therapy, 35*, 667–681.

Okasha, A., Saad, A., Khalil, A., El-Dawla, A., & Yehia, N. (1994). Phenomenology of obsessive–compulsive disorder: A transcultural study. *Comprehensive Psychiatry, 35*, 191–197.

Parkin, R. (1997). Obsessive–compulsive disorder in adults. *International Review of Psychiatry, 9*, 73–81.

Pigott, T. A. (1998). Obsessive–compulsive disorder: Symptom overview and epidemiology. *Bulletin of the Menninger Clinic, 62*, Suppl. A, A5–A32.

Rachman, S. (1997). A cognitive theory of obsessions. *Behaviour Research and Therapy, 35*, 793–802.

Rachman, S., & Hodgson, R. (1980). *Obsessions and compulsions.* Hillsdale, NJ: Prentice-Hall.

Rapoport, J. L. (1989). The boy who couldn't stop washing. *The experience and treatment of obsessive–compulsive disorder.* New York: E.P. Dutton.

Rasmussen, S. A., & Tsuang, M. T. (1986). Clinical characteristics and family history in DSM-III obsessive–compulsive disorder. *American Journal of Psychiatry, 143*, 317–322.

Robins, L. N., Helzer, H. E., Croughan, J. L., Williams, J. B. W., & Spitzer, R. L. (1981). *N. I. M. H. Diagnostic Interview Schedule, version III.* Rockville: MD: National Institute of Mental Health.

Samuels, J., & Nestadt, G. (1997). Epidemiology and genetics of obsessive–compulsive disorder. *International Review of Psychiatry, 9*, 61–71.

Sanavio, E. (1988). Obsession and compulsion: The Padua Inventory. *Behaviour Research and Therapy, 26*, 169–177.

Sechrest, L. (1969). Philippine culture, stress and psychopathology. In W. Candill & T. Y. Lin (eds), *Health research in Asia and the Pacific* (pp. 306–334). Honolulu: East West Center Press.

Seiden, D. (1999). The effect of research on practice in cross-cultural behavior therapy: A single case study (you're the case). *The Behavior Therapist, 22*, 200–201.

Sica, C., Novara, C., & Sanavio, E. (in press (a)). Religiousness and Obsessive-Compulsive Cognitions and Symptoms in an Italian Population. *Behaviour Research and Therapy.*

Sica, C., Novara, C., & Sanavio, E. (in press (b)). Culture and psychopathology: Superstition and obsessive–compulsive cognitions and symptoms in a non-clinical Italian sample. Personality and Individual Differences.

Sica, C., Frost, R. O., & Sanavio, E. (2001). *Different countries, different obsessions? Results from cross-cultural research.* Unpublished manuscript.

Stefannson, J. G. (1993). The lifetime prevalence of anxiety disorders in Iceland as estimated by the United States National Institute of Mental Health Diagnostic Interview Schedule. *Acta Psychiatrica Scandinavica, 88*, 29–34.

Steketee, G., Quay, S., & White, K. (1991). Religion and guilt in OCD patients. *Journal of Anxiety Disorders, 5*, 359–367.

Tezcan, E., & Millet, B. (1997). Phénoménologie des troubles obsessionnels compulsifs. Formes et contenus des obsessions et des compulsions dans l'est de la Turquie. *L'Encéphale, 23,* 342–350.

Tobacyk, J. (1995). Final thoughts on issues in the measurement of paranormal beliefs. *The Journal of Parapsychology, 59,* 141–145.

Tobacyk, J., & Pirttilae-Backman, A. M. (1992). Paranormal beliefs and their implications in university students from Finland and the United States. *Journal of Cross-Cultural Psychology, 23,* 59–71.

Tseng, W. (1997). Overview: Culture and psychopathology. In W. Tseng & J. Streltzer (eds), *Culture and Psychopathology* (pp. 1–27). New York: Brunner/Mazel.

Tseng, W., & Streltzer, J. (1997). Integration and conclusions. In W. Tseng & J. Streltzer (eds), *Culture and Psychopathology* (pp. 1–27). New York: Brunner/Mazel.

Tseng, W. S., Mo, K. M., Hsu, J., Li, L. S., Ou, L. W., Chen, G. Q., & Jiang, D. W. (1988). A sociocultural study of Koro epidemics in Guangdong, China. *American Journal of Psychiatry, 145,* 1538–1543.

Weissman, M. M., Bland, R. C., Canino, G. J., Greenwald, S., Hwu, H., Lee, C. K., Newman, S. C., Oakley-Browne, M. A., Rubio-Stipec, M., Wickramaratne, P. J., Wittchen, H., & Yeh, E. (1994). The cross national epidemiology of obsessive–compulsive disorder. *Journal of Clinical Psychiatry, 55,* supp. 3, 5–10.

Wolfradt, U. (1997). Dissociative experiences, trait anxiety and paranormal beliefs. *Personality and Individual Differences, 23,* 15–19.

Warwick, D. P., & Osherson, S. (1973). *Comparative research methods.* Englewood Cliffs, NJ: Prentice-Hall.

Commentary on Special Populations

C. Alec Pollard

The authors of this section have provided thorough reviews of the research literature and useful suggestions for future research examining the relationship between cognition and obsessive compulsive disorder (OCD) symptoms in various populations. By necessity, much of their discussion is directed at areas in need of additional investigation, as the amount of existing research directly addressing this topic is modest. The authors' thorough treatment of the subject leaves little left for me to add. However, I will comment on a few issues.

Two of the chapters in this section focus on age-related populations, covering each end of the life span (Calamari, Janeck, & Deer, 2002; Söchting & March, 2002). Like many other aspects of OCD, cognition has not been studied in children or the elderly as extensively as it has been examined in the general adult population. The focus of most prior research on the young and middle-aged adult population has obvious ramifications for those who do not fall within this age range. We still do not know the extent to which cognitive behavioral assessment and treatment methods can be successfully applied to children and older adults. Söchting and March (2002) and Calamari *et al.* (2002) agree that treatment adaptations must be made to address relevant developmental issues so that cognitive behavior therapy (CBT) is effective across the lifespan. However, we do not yet fully appreciate what adaptations, cognitive or otherwise, are necessary. Discovering how to adapt CBT to patients of different ages should be a top priority for future treatment outcome research.

Much of the research discussed in the two chapters on age-related populations focuses on the age of participants at the time of the study. However, age at onset in some ways may be a more critical variable than age at time of assessment. I have observed many adult patients with early childhood onset OCD who have difficulty articulating their fears and catastrophic beliefs. Despite extensive probing, they describe engaging in compulsions simply to get rid of an unpleasant feeling. Even though these patients are now adults, attributions concerning the motivation behind their compulsions appear to be more primitive and consistent with the level of cognitive development characteristic of early childhood. Cognition may play a less crucial role in the development of OCD when cognitive capacity is not fully developed, as in the case of a young child. I will be interested to see if future research supports my clinical impression that adults with OCD who present without clearly articulated fears are more likely to have a history of early childhood OCD.

Studying age at onset in individuals at the other end of the lifespan could also be informative. Of particular interest are people with late-life onset OCD. As Calamari and his co-authors point out, OCD does not typically emerge for the first time in later life, but late-life onset OCD does occur. Comparisons of cognitive variables in late versus earlier-onset OCD could help explain how cognition interacts with developmental factors associated with older adulthood and how those interactions might precipitate onset.

Two of the chapters in this section addressed issues relevant to populations defined according to symptom severity (Warren, Gershuny, & Sher, 2002; Wiegartz, Carmin, & Pollard, 2002). Warren and his colleagues examined analogue research on subclinical and non-treatment seeking individuals with at least some OCD features or symptoms. The OCD nonclinical groups are distinguished from the OCD clinical population in that neither have they sought treatment (i.e., the non-treatment seekers) nor do they meet full criteria for OCD (i.e., the sub-clinicals). Although it is understandable why these two groups were considered together in this chapter, I suspect that non-treatment seekers are a very different population than the sub-clinicals. The non-treatment-seeking group is almost certainly a heterogeneous population, owing to the wide variety of reasons different people might not seek treatment. Individuals who do not pursue help because their condition produces only limited interference with functioning may have little in common with severely affected individuals who have not sought treatment because of shame about their symptoms or lack of information about treatment.

This latter group of non-clinicals may have more in common with the other end of the symptom-severity spectrum discussed in the chapter by Wiegartz *et al.* (2002), which focused on OCD clinic patients who were either severely symptomatic or treatment-refractory. These clinically challenging patients offer OCD researchers the opportunity to address some intriguing questions about the relevance of cognition to important clinical variables other than presenting symptoms. Future cognitive research with this population could help shed light on why some individuals with clinically severe OCD do not seek, prematurely withdraw from, or fail to respond to CBT. It is possible that general beliefs or specific beliefs about things other than obsessional stimuli are more relevant to how someone approaches and participates in treatment than are beliefs directly related to OCD.

Wiegartz and colleagues note that no single cognitive domain has emerged as being uniquely associated with highly severe OCD. In other words, there is no specific obsessional belief that is uniquely toxic. It may be necessary to look at other variables, such as strength of conviction or number of obsessional beliefs, to understand the cognitive contribution to symptom severity, but this remains a topic in need of further investigation.

For many years, there was no successful treatment for OCD. Now that a generally effective treatment is available, a high priority for future research should be to search for ways to reach those who have not benefited from therapy. Cognitive models offer some promising clues. My colleagues and I are currently studying whether a cognitive intervention can help treatment-refractory OCD patients return to behavior therapy and successfully participate in exposure and response prevention. Hopefully, in the near future, more outcome research will examine cognitive factors that may be associated with unsatisfactory treatment response, followed closely by research on interventions designed to remediate those factors.

Authors of the final chapter tackle the complex topic of culture (Sica, Novara, Sanavio,

Dorz, & Coradeschi, 2002). Sica and his associates remind us there are many potential sources of cross-cultural variance, including religious, familial, local, and regional influences, to name just a few. In each culture, there are subcultures, and subcultures within subcultures, each of which might contribute alone or in combination to help shape an individual's obsessional beliefs and symptoms and the impact of those symptoms on the person's life. Given the multiple factors involved, the interpretation of cross-cultural research findings presents a sizable challenge. When differences are found between groups, it is difficult to sort out which factors within a group's culture might have influenced the findings.

Not surprisingly, very little cross-cultural research has specifically addressed cognition and OCD. I was very interested to read Sica and his co-authors' initial report of a study comparing responses to the OBQ, III, and several other measures in Greek, Italian, and US samples. They found group differences in the strength of relationships between cognitive domains and OCD symptoms. The authors caution that there are many possible explanations for their findings and that more research is clearly needed. Nonetheless, their results provide preliminary evidence that the relationship between cognition and OCD symptoms is culturally influenced. There is good reason to believe we will learn much more about this topic in the near future. The international membership of the OCCWG suggests we can anticipate many additional cross-cultural studies of cognition and OCD in the years ahead.

The five chapters in this section all address the same fundamental question. Does the relationship between cognition and OCD vary between populations? We have no clear answer. On the one hand, the consistency of the phenomenology and presentation of OCD across populations is notable. Approximately one percent of people from various gender, age, and cultural groups can be found washing their hands to avoid contamination, checking their homes to prevent catastrophe, misinterpreting their intrusive thoughts as dangerous, or engaging in some other OC behavior. Yet, the chapters in this book contain preliminary evidence that some differences between populations do exist and should be explored further. Discovering these differences is vital to gaining an adequate understanding of the nature and treatment of OCD. Any cognitive model that cannot ultimately account for population differences will, at best, be applicable to a limited portion of OCD sufferers.

References

Calamari, J. E., Janeck, A. S., & Deer, T. M. (2002). Cognitive processes and OCD in older adults. In R. O. Frost & G. Steketee (eds), *Cognitive approaches to obsessions and compulsions: Theory, assessment and treatment* (pp. 315–335). Oxford: Elsevier.

Sica, C., Novara, C., Sanavio, E., Dorz, S., & Coradeschi, D. (2002). OCD cognitions across cultures. In R.O. Frost & G. Steketee (eds), *Cognitive approaches to obsessions and compulsions: Theory, assessment and treatment* (pp. 371–384). Oxford: Elsevier.

Söchting, I., & March, J. S. (2002). Cognitive aspects of OCD in children. In R. O. Frost & G. Steketee (eds), *Cognitive approaches to obsessions and compulsions: Theory, assessment and treatment* (pp. 299–314). Oxford: Elsevier.

Warren, R., Gershuny, B. S., & Sher, K. J. (2002). Cognition in subclinial OCD. In R. O. Frost & G. Steketee (eds), *Cognitive approaches to obsessions and compulsions: Theory, assessment and treatment*, (pp. 337–360). Oxford: Elsevier.

Wiegartz, P. S., Carmin, C. N., & Pollard, C. A. (2002). Cognitions in individuals with severe or treatment resistant obsessive–compulsive disorder. In R. O. Frost & G. Steketee (eds), *Cognitive approaches to obsessions and compulsions: Theory, assessment and treatment*, (pp. 361–369). Oxford: Elsevier.

Section E

Therapy Effects on Cognition

Chapter 21

Cognitive Changes in Patients with Obsessive Compulsive Rituals Treated with Exposure in vivo and Response Prevention

Paul M. G. Emmelkamp, Patricia van Oppen and
Anton J. L. M. van Balkom

Introduction

Until the early 1970s, obsessive compulsive disorder (OCD) was considered a treatment-refractory, chronic condition. Neither psycho-dynamic therapy, nor a variety of pharmacological treatments that were available at that time led to significant clinical improvement. Today, substantial evidence suggests that behavior therapy by exposure in vivo and response prevention, is effective in treating this chronic disorder (Foa, Franklin, & Kozak, 1998; van Oppen & Emmelkamp, 1997). Although in the early days exposure in vivo and response prevention were applied in a hospital setting (e.g., Rachman & Hodgson, 1980), studies have shown that such treatment can also be applied in the natural environment of the patient (Emmelkamp, Bouman, & Scholing, 1993). Self-exposure treatment in the natural environment of the patient was found to be as effective as exposure treatment with inpatients in the hospital (van den Hout, Emmelkamp, Kraaükamp, & Griez, 1988).

There is no evidence yet that actual assistance of a therapist during the exposure exercises is necessary in most instances (e.g., Emmelkamp & Kraanen, 1977; Emmelkamp, van Linden, van den Heuvell, Rüphan, & Sanderman, 1989). However, a definite conclusion is not possible, since the number of patients in these studies was rather small. Larger studies are needed before more conclusive recommendations can be made. Further, there is considerable evidence that both exposure to distressing stimuli and prevention of rituals are necessary ingredients in successful treatment of OCD (Foa, Steketee, Grayson, Turner, & Latimer, 1984). Although there is some evidence that the marital relationships of OCD patients are more distressed than the relationship of control couples (Emmelkamp & Gerlsma, 1994), spouse-aided therapy has not yet been found to be more effective than treatment by the patient alone (Emmelkamp & Vedel, 2002).

Foa, Franklin, and Kozak (1998) reviewed 16 outcome studies with OCD patients ($n = 376$) with exposure in vivo in combination with response prevention. They reported

76 percent treatment responders at a long-term outcome follow-up interval of 29 months. Although a combination of pharmacotherapy and exposure and response prevention is often recommended, to date there are no studies to support this notion. Generally, adding pharmacotherapy to exposure in vivo and response prevention does not enhance the effects of exposure in vivo and response prevention (e.g. van Balkom, *et al.*, 1995; van Balkom, *et al.*, 1998; Foa *et al.*, 1998, Kozak, Liebowitz, & Foa, 2000).

Cognitions and OCD

Given the fact that most obsessive compulsive behavior is evoked by thoughts, in recent years some authors have suggested that the role of cognitive factors must be considered (Beck *et al.*, 1985; McFall & Wollersheim, 1979; Salkovskis, 1989). There is considerable evidence that cognitions are related to obsessive compulsive disorder (Emmelkamp & Aardema, 1999). Several authors attribute an important role to inflated responsibility in OCD, particularly for those with checking rituals (e.g., Rachman, 1993; Salkovskis, 1989; van Oppen & Arntz, 1994), and this has indeed been supported in several studies (Ladouceur *et al.*, 1994; Lopatka & Rachman, 1995; Rhéaume, Freeston *et al.*, 1995; Rhéaume, Ladouceur, Freeston, & Letarte, 1995) (see also Chapter four in this volume). Another cognitive distortion described as thought–action fusion (TAF) is defined as the belief that specific intrusive thoughts can directly influence the relevant external event and/or the belief that having these intrusive thoughts is morally equivalent to carrying out a prohibited action (Rachman & Shafran, 1999) (refer to Chapter two in this volume). TAF correlates significantly with measures of obsessionality, guilt and depression (Rachman, Thordarson, Shafran, & Woody, 1995).

Others have argued that OCD is related to perfectionism, but it does seem more likely that perfectionism is a dispositional trait for the development of psycho-pathology in general, rather than for OCD in particular. Further, indecisiveness, magical thinking, aversion to risk-taking and guilt have also been found to be related to OCD (Emmelkamp & Aardema, 1999).

Initially, most of the identified cognitive distortions were thought to be related to OCD in general rather than that domains of beliefs or cognitive processes being related to specific forms of obsessive compulsive behavior; for example, washing, checking, impulsive behavior, rumination and precision. However, Emmelkamp and Aardema (1999) found that beliefs related to contamination play an important role in washing, but not in other obsessive compulsive behaviors. Thought–action fusion appears to be important in washing as well in checking, but not in impulses, precision and rumination. Guilt was found to be related to rumination and checking, but not to other compulsive behaviors. These results suggest that instead of global obsessive beliefs, specific domains of obsessive beliefs account for specific obsessive compulsive behavior in a meaningful way. This finding may also have important implications for the assessment of cognitions in treatment-outcome studies. Global measures of obsessive beliefs may be less appropriate to assess relevant changes in cognitive processes. We will elaborate on this issue below.

Cognitive Therapy Versus Exposure and Response Prevention

Although some have proposed that cognitive therapy may be inappropriate for treating obsessive compulsives, since these patients already over-emphasize their thoughts (e.g., Kendall, 1983; Reed, 1985), there is evidence that cognitive therapy may be effective in treating OCD. In studies of RET with obsessive compulsive patients Ellis' (1962) ABC framework was used (Emmelkamp, Visser, & Hoekstra, 1988; Emmelkamp & Beens, 1991). The therapist challenged the irrational beliefs in a Socratic-like fashion and the patients were instructed to do this on their own as homework. In the first study (Emmelkamp *et al.*, 1988) RET (*n* = 9) was compared with treatment consisting of exposure in vivo and response prevention (*n* = 9). Exposure was self-controlled and applied by means of homework assignments. Treatment in both conditions consisted of ten sessions. On the obsessive compulsive targets (Maudsley Obsessional Compulsive Inventory and Anxiety/Discomfort Scale), the results of cognitive therapy were about equally effective as self-controlled exposure in vivo. Both treatments led to a reduction of social anxiety. On depressed mood, cognitive therapy led to significant improvement, whereas self-controlled exposure did not.

In a second study, Emmelkamp and Beens (1990) investigated whether a combined package (cognitive therapy followed by exposure in vivo) would enhance the effects of exposure in vivo and response prevention. Patients were randomly assigned to two conditions: (1) self-controlled exposure (*n* = 11) and (2) cognitive therapy (*n* = 10). In the first block, half of the patients received cognitive therapy; the other half exposure. In the second block, the patients in the exposure condition received another six sessions of exposure; patients in the cognitive therapy condition received added exposure. A significant time effect during first and second treatment block was found on all obsessive compulsive measures (e.g., MOCI and anxiety/ discomfort). On none of the obsessive compulsive measures was there a significant difference between cognitive therapy and exposure in vivo, thus replicating the findings of the Emmelkamp *et al.* (1988) study in which cognitive therapy was as effective as exposure in vivo. There was, however, no evidence that the effects of a treatment package in which cognitive therapy and exposure in vivo were combined was more effective than exposure in vivo alone.

The primary aim of the third study of van Oppen *et al.* (1995) was to compare the effects of cognitive therapy based on models of Beck and Salkovskis with those of self-controlled exposure in vivo plus response prevention. Seventy-one patients were randomly assigned to cognitive therapy and/or to exposure in vivo plus response prevention. After six sessions an intermediate assessment took place and then behavioral experiments were added to the cognitive therapy. The behavioral experiments were only used to test the empirical basis of the dysfunctional assumptions. After 16 sessions a post-test assessment was held. Fifty-seven patients completed this study. Both treatments led to statistically significant improvement. Multivariate significant differences suggested a superior efficacy of cognitive therapy in comparison to exposure in vivo on the obsessive compulsive measures and on the measures for associated psycho-pathology. However, these differences did not stand up in separate ANCOVA's in which initial differences between conditions were taken into account. These results showed that this form of cognitive therapy is an effective treatment for OCD.

Some have argued that the difference between exposure and cognitive therapy is meaningless (e.g., Foa *et al.*, 1998), since cognitive restructuring is always part of exposure treatment: ". . . in our clinic, therapists routinely discuss patients' mistaken beliefs . . ." (p.267). Thus, in the studies by Foa and colleagues cognitive restructuring has been combined with exposure and response prevention. Perhaps the reason why results of exposure in vivo and response prevention in the studies in which this treatment was compared with cognitive therapy are slightly less effective than in other studies, is because researchers attempted by all possible means to exclude cognitive restructuring procedures from the exposure protocol.

Do Global Irrational Beliefs Change as a Result of Treatment?

It is now well recognized that cognitions should also change to produce enduring effects on emotion and behavior. Unfortunately, very few studies that investigated exposure in vivo and response prevention have attempted to assess obsessive or irrational beliefs of the patients, and the few studies that did so used rather global measures to assess irrational beliefs in general rather than specific obsessional beliefs. Further, most studies rely on pre- and post-test scores, which preclude the study of changes in the course of treatment. Table 21.1, shows the studies that assessed irrational beliefs in OCD patients as outcome measures.

As appears in Table 21.1, improvement in irrational beliefs is modest, even in cognitive therapy. Generally, cognitive therapy leads to slightly greater changes in irrational beliefs than exposure in vivo plus response prevention. In the Emmelkamp *et al.* (1988) study, irrational beliefs as measured by the Irrational Belief Test (IBT-50; Jones, 1968) changed after cognitive therapy but not after exposure. The difference between the two treatments did not reach acceptable levels of significance. Further, a small but significant correlation ($r = 0.44$, $p < 0.05$) was found between improvement on the IBT-50 and improvement on OCD as assessed by the anxiety/discomfort scale. Of course, whether improvement in OCD leads to changes in irrational beliefs or whether changes in beliefs affects obsessive compulsive behavior cannot be determined. In the Emmelkamp and Beens (1991) study a

Table 21.1: Means and standard deviations for cognitive measures in trials of cognitive therapy and exposure in vivo.

Study	Measure	Treatment	Pre-test		Post-test	
			Mean	SD	Mean	SD
Emmelkamp *et al.*, 1988	IBT-50	Cognitive	172.2	11.3	164.0	12.5
		Exposure	165.1	13.9	164.3	16.9
Emmelkamp & Beens, 1991	IBT-30	Cognitive	107.5	12.5	88.8	18.3
		Exposure	106.8	13.9	100.8	21.1
Van Oppen *et al.*, 1995	IBI	Cognitive	158.3	18.0	149.6	21.1
		Exposure	163.2	19.1	159.2	17.4

significant difference between groups was found on the Irrational Belief Test (IBT-30): cognitive therapy led to a greater reduction in irrational beliefs than exposure plus response prevention. Finally, in the van Oppen *et al.* study, cognitive treatment led to improvement in irrational beliefs as assessed by the Irrational Belief Inventory (IBI; Koopmans, Sanderman, Timmerman, & Emmelkamp, 1994), whereas exposure in vivo did not result in significant improvement on this measure. However, the difference between groups was not significant.

In sum, there is some evidence that cognitive therapy leads to changes, albeit limited, in global irrational beliefs; exposure in vivo plus response prevention hardly affects the irrational beliefs of the OCD patients.

Studies of Cognitive Change after Exposure plus Response Prevention

Until recently, only very crude measures were available to assess cognitive aspects of OCD; for example, the IBT and IBI. It is questionable whether such questionnaires are the most appropriate measures to assess the cognitive processes of obsessive compulsive patients. Themes that are characteristic of the thought content of obsessional patients are absent or under-represented in this questionnaire. We will describe two studies by our research teams of the effects of exposure in vivo and response prevention, in which more specific measures to assess obsessive compulsive beliefs were used.

Study one

In a study by Emmelkamp, Hulsteijn, and van Hout (unpublished), a successive series of OCD patients was treated by exposure in vivo and response prevention. All patients fulfilled DSM-III-R criteria for OCD and had for at least one year.

After two introductory and assessment sessions patients received up to 15 sessions of exposure in vivo and response prevention. In the introductory sessions the treatment rationale was explained and the therapist solicited detailed information on the obsessive compulsive behavior in order to construct a hierarchy of exposure exercises. Treatment sessions were conducted in the homes of the patients and lasted 75 minutes.

In each treatment session, patients were confronted with exposure exercises from the hierarchy for about 15 minutes and were not allowed to perform their rituals (active exposure). After the active exposure part of the session, patients had to rest in an easy chair for a full hour (passive exposure) and heart rate was monitored with an ambulatory device in order to investigate the habituation process. Further, every ten minutes, patients were asked to rate their anxiety/tension on zero–ten scales (Subjective Units of Discomfort). In order to reduce elevated heart rates due to physical activity, patients were instructed to keep seated for one hour and not to make sudden movements. The results on heart rate and SUDs will not be discussed here. For the present purposes, we will focus on the obsessive irrational beliefs of the patients.

Assessments were conducted before and after treatment. The Yale–Brown Obsessive

Compulsive Scale (YBOCS, Goodman *et al.*, 1989) was completed by an independent assessor. Patients completed the following questionnaires: Obsessive Compulsive Cognitions List (OCCL, Hoekstra, 1995), Anxiety-Discomfort Scale (Emmelkamp, 1982), and the Padua Inventory — Revised (PI-R; van Oppen, Hoekstra, & Emmelkamp, 1995, van Oppen *et al.*, 1995). In addition, at the end of each session patients had to rate ten idiosyncratic obsessive compulsive beliefs. These beliefs were selected according to the patients' highest scores on the OCCL at the pre-test.

Treatment resulted in significant improvement on the Y-BOCS Obsessions and Compulsions Subscales, Anxiety-Discomfort Scale, PI-R and OCCL. Thus, treatment resulted not only in significant changes in obsessive compulsive behavior, but also in a significant change in obsessive beliefs.

Most improved versus least improved patients.   Further, the five most improved patients were compared with the five least improved patients on cognitive measures. Percentage improvement was based on a composite measure consisting of percentage improvement on the Y-BOCS and percentage improvement on the Anxiety-Discomfort Scale. The percentage improvement for the five most improved patients ranged from 73– 89 percent; for the five least improved patients from 32–51 percent. Obsessive beliefs hardly changed over the course of treatment in the least improved patients. In the most improved patients, however, obsessive beliefs improved during the treatment or were already rather high at the pre-test. If we compare the most improved patients with the least improved patients on the OCCL and two cognitive subscales of the PI-R, a statistically significant difference was found (OCCL $t(8) = -1.87$, $p < 0.05$; Impulses, $t(8) = 2.10$, $p < 0.04$), or a marginally significant difference was evident (Rumination $t(8) = 1.45$, $p < 0.09$). Thus, results of this study suggest that improvement after exposure in vivo and response prevention was related to improvement in obsessive beliefs.

Study two

Preliminary data are presented of an ongoing study of the authors in which the effects of exposure in vivo were studied. Of the 32 patients who started treatment, four dropped out. The data of the remaining 28 patients were used in the data analyses. The mean age was 37 years, (SD 11; range 17–62). Thirty-six percent were males and 64 percent were females. Three patients fulfilled criteria for DSM-IV major depression. Excluded were patients with only obsessions. As a rule, patients with personality disorders were included in the study, but anti-social PD and borderline PD were reason for exclusion; however, none of the referrals had to be excluded for this reason.

Treatment consisted of exposure in vivo and response prevention. In about half of the patients, treatment was conducted in the natural environment (e.g., home) of the patient. Treatment at home consisted of once weekly sessions of 90 minutes. When treatment was provided by means of instructions for homework assignments, sessions took place at the hospital once a week and lasted approximately 30 minutes. Patients were requested to practice exposure exercises between treatment sessions. Patients ($n = 15$) were treated by experienced behavior therapists or ($n = 13$) by clinical psychology students who had taken a course in behavior therapy and who had received advanced training in exposure in vivo and response prevention for the treatment of OCD. All therapists were supervised by the senior author (PE), student therapists weekly and experienced therapists once every two weeks.

Assessments were conducted before and after therapy. The YBOCS was completed by an independent assessor. Patients completed the following questionnaires: PI-R, Obsessional Beliefs Questionnaire (OBQ) and Interpretation of Intrusions Inventory (III) (Obsessive Compulsive Cognitions Working Group [OCCWG], 2001).

Results. Treatment resulted in a significant reduction on the Y-BOCS and the PI-R. Interestingly, treatment resulted also in highly significant changes on the OBQ and III (see Table 21.2). Improvement in obsessive compulsive symptomatology was related to improvement on the cognitive measures. The correlation coefficient between the pre- and

Table 21.2: Comparison of results at pre-test and post-test for measures of OCD symptoms, beliefs, and interpretation of intrusions.

	Pre-test Mean (SD)	Post-test Mean (SD)	*t*
Y-BOCS	25.3 (4.9)	15.4 (8.9)	7.235***
PI-R	64.9 (20.3)	45.8 (25.5)	5.166***
OBQ-Total	277.2 (20.0)	233.4 (35.7)	4.311**
Tolerance of Uncertainty	46.5 (14.5)	39.6 (16.0)	3.434**
Threat estimation	40.8 (15.7)	35.7 (16.7)	2.459*
Control of Thoughts	52.2 (14.0)	43.5 (16.6)	4.776***
Importance of Thoughts	33.0 (13.3)	28.6 (16.0)	2.739**
Responsibility	54.5 (17.4)	43.8 (19.4)	4.077***
Perfectionism	50.2 (21.3)	42.1 (17.5)	2.965**
III-Total	116.6 (50.3)	74.1 (45.5)	5.848***
Control	49.6 (17.2)	33.4 (17.5)	4.798***
Importance of Thoughts	26.7 (16.2)	16.3 (14.4)	3.973***
Responsibility	40.2 (23.2)	24.4 (19.4)	5.100***

$* = p < 0.05;\ ** p < 0.01;\ *** p < 0.001$

PI-R = Padua Inventory Revised
III = Interpretation of Intrusions Inventory
OBQ = Obsessive Beliefs Questionnaire
Y-BOCS = Yale–Brown Obsessive Compulsive Scale

post-test changes on the OBQ and changes on Y-BOCS and PI-R were 0.30 and 0.58 respectively; the correlation between pre- and post-changes on the III and Y-BOCS and PI-R were 0.63 and 0.66 respectively. Further, changes on the OBQ were related to changes on the III ($r = 0.60$). Thus, improvement on the III was more related to improvement in obsessive compulsive behavior than to improvement in obsessional beliefs as measured by the OBQ.

Not all patients are equally dysfunctional in terms of specific belief domain. To study whether obsessive beliefs characteristic for a particular patient changed as a result of treatment, for each patient the most distressing obsessive belief domain at the pre-test was determined. On the OBQ, Tolerance for Uncertainty was the main obsessive belief domain ($n = 12$), followed by Responsibility ($n = 4$), Perfectionism ($n = 4$), Control of Thoughts ($n = 4$), Threat Estimation ($n = 3$), and Importance of Thoughts ($n = 1$). On the III, Control was the main target domain ($n = 12$), followed by Responsibility ($n = 8$), and Importance of Thoughts ($n = 8$). After standardizing the scores on the target domains to permit a comparative statistical analysis, results revealed significant improvement on the target domain of the OBQ ($t(27) = 3.196$, $p < 0.002$). On the target domain of the III, results failed to reach an acceptable level of statistical significance ($t(27) = 1.305$, $p < 0.10$).

Table 21.3: Mean pre-post change scores of treatment responders and non-responders on measures of OCD obsessive beliefs and intrusions.

	Mean (SD) Non-responders	Mean (SD) Responders	*t*
OBQ-Total	23.6 (54.5)	50.6 (53.1)	1.159
Tolerance of Uncertainty	6.8 (9.1)	6.9 (11.2)	0.030
Threat estimation	−0.22 (9.0)	6.8 (11.0)	1.517
Control of Thoughts	7.3 (14.6)	9.2 (7.9)	0.454
Importance of Thoughts	1.1 (12.1)	5.5 (6.9)	1.200
Responsibility	3.6 (13.5)	13.1 (13.5)	1.617
Perfectionism	5.1 (9.8)	9.0 (15.7)	0.617
III-Total	14.5 (19.8)	51.8 (38.8)	2.419*
Control	14.6 (15.6)	16.7 (18.8)	0.264
Importance of Thoughts	−1.1 (7.5)	14.3 (13.5)	3.755***
Responsibility	0.7 (11.7)	20.8 (14.6)	3.290**

* = $p < 0.05$; ** $p < 0.01$; *** $p < 0.001$

OBQ = Obsessive Beliefs Questionnaire
III = Interpretation of Intrusions Inventory

Responders versus non-responders. Responders were defined as patients who improved at least 33.33 percent on the Y-BOCS. According to this criterion, 21 patients (75 percent) were defined as responders and seven patients were defined as non-responders. Thus, treatment was rather successful in terms of number of responders.

Responders and non-responders could be differentiated from each other on the improvement scores on the III as assessed by pre- and post-test change scores. As shown in Table 21.3, improvement status at the post-test was significantly related to improvement on the III total score and improvement on the III subscales Responsibility and Importance of Thoughts. Although on the OBQ-scales non-responders also improved less than responders, this failed to reach statistical significance.

Finally, we wondered whether improvement in severity of OCD symptoms could be predicted by cognitive dysfunction at the pre-test. Only one correlation was significant; stronger beliefs in the need to control thoughts at pre-test predicted less change on the Y-BOCS ($r = -0.40$, $p < 0.02$).

Concluding Remarks

In the earlier studies in which cognitions were assessed with global irrational beliefs measures, such as the IBT and the IBI, no evidence was provided that exposure in vivo and response prevention affected the irrational beliefs of the OCD patients. In the more recent studies presented here, there is some evidence that successful treatment with exposure in vivo and response prevention is related to significant changes in obsessional beliefs and intrusions as assessed with the OCCL, OBQ and III, but results are far from conclusive. For example, we do not know whether the change in specific obsessive beliefs and impulses precede, follow, or co-vary with changes in obsessive compulsive behavior. Alternatively, irrational beliefs may merely be epi-phenomena of changes in mood states rather than changes in deeper cognitive structures. Further, since we have no data from a no-treatment control group, we cannot conclude that improvements on the cognitive measures are the result of improvement in the obsessive compulsive behavior.

Although the development of specific cognitive measures such as the OBQ and III are an improvement over more general cognitive measures, for some purposes, other instruments may be required. For example, for clinical purposes, other assessment procedures, such as thought listing, may be more useful than questionnaires. One could ask patients at various points each day to list the thoughts that have just run through their minds. More adequate assessment of the cognitions of obsessive compulsive patients may lead to a better understanding of these disorders and permit more detailed evaluation of the specific effects of treatment on the thought disorders of these patients.

References

Beck, A. T., Emery, G., & Greenberg, R. L. (1985). *Anxiety disorders and phobias: A cognitive perspective*. New York: Basic Books.

Ellis, A. (1962). *Reason and emotion in psychotherapy*. New York: Lyle-Stuart.

Emmelkamp, P. M. G. (1982). *Phobic and obsessive–compulsive disorders: Theory, research and practice.* New York: Plenum.

Emmelkamp, P. M. G., & Aardema, A. (1999). Metacognition, specific obsessive–compulsive beliefs and obsessive–compulsive behaviour, *Clinical Psychology and Psychotherapy, 6,* 139–145.

Emmelkamp, P. M. G., & Beens, H. (1991). Cognitive therapy with obsessive–compulsive disorder: A comparative evaluation. *Behaviour Research and Therapy, 29,* 293–300.

Emmelkamp, P. M. G., Bouman, T. K., & Scholing, A. (1993). *Anxiety disorders.* Wiley, Chichester.

Emmelkamp, P. M. G., & Gerlsma, C. (1994). Marital functioning and the anxiety disorders. *Behavior Therapy, 25,* 407–429.

Emmelkamp, P. M. G., van Linden, van den Heuvell, C., Rüphan, M., & Sanderman, R. (1989). Home-based treatment of obsessive–compulsive patients: Intersession interval and therapist involvement. *Behaviour Research and Therapy, 27,* 89–93.

Emmelkamp, P. M. G., & Kraanen, J. (1977). Therapist-controlled exposure in vivo versus self-controlled exposure in vivo: A comparison with obsessive–compulsive patients. *Behaviour Research and Therapy, 15,* 491–495.

Emmelkamp, P. M. G., & Vedel, E. (2002). Spouse-aided therapy. In M. Hersen & W. Sledge (eds), *The encyclopedia of psychotherapy.* Academic Press, New York.

Emmelkamp, P. M. G., Visser, S., & Hoekstra, R. J. (1988). Cognitive therapy vs exposure in vivo in the treatment of obsessive-compulsives. *Cognitive Therapy and Research, 12,* 103–144.

Foa, E. B., Steketee, G. S., Grayson, J. B., Turner, R., & Latimer, P. (1984). Deliberate exposure and blocking of obsessive–compulsive rituals: Imediate and long-term effects. *Behavior Therapy, 15,* 450–472.

Foa, E. B., Franklin, M. E., & Kozak, M. J. (1998). Psychosocial treatments for obsessive–compulsive disorder: A literature review. In R. P. Swinson, M. M. Antony, S. Rachman, & M. A. Richter (eds), *Obsessive–compulsive disorder: Theory, research, and treatment.* New York: Guilford.

Goodman, W. K., Price L. H., Rasmussen S. A., Mazure C., Fleischmann, R., Hill, C. L., Henninger, G. R., & Charney, D. S. (1989). The Yale–Brown Obsessive–Compulsive Scale I: development, use, and reliability. *Archives of General Psychiatry, 46,* 1006–1011.

Hoekstra, R. J. (1995). Obsessive–Compulsive Cognitions List. Unpublished scale, Research Office, Faculty of Medicine, Limberg University, Maastricht, The Netherlands.

Jones, R. (1968). *A factored measure of Ellis' irrational beliefs system with personality and maladjustment correlated.* Unpublished doctoral dissertation. Texas Technological University.

Kendall, P. C. (1983). Methodology and cognitive–behavioral assessment. *Behavioural Psychotherapy, 11,* 285–301.

Ladouceur, R., Rheaume, J., Freeston, M. H., Aublet, F., Jean, K., Lachance, S., Langlois, F., & De Pokomandy-Morin, K. (1995). Experimental manipulation of responsibility: an analogue test for models of obsessive–compulsive disorder. *Behaviour Research and Therapy, 33,* 937–946.

Lopatka, C., & Rachman, S. (1995). Perceived responsibility and compulsive checking: an experimental analysis. *Behaviour Therapy and Research, 33,* 673–684.

Koopmans, P. C., Sanderman, R., Timmerman, I., & Emmelkamp, P. M. G. (1994). The Irrational Beliefs Inventory: Development and psychometric evaluation. *European Journal of Psychological Assessment, 10,* 15–27.

Kozak, M. J., Liebowitz, M. R., & Foa, E. B. (2000). Cognitive behavior therapy and pharmacotherapy for obsessive–compulsive disorder: The NIMH-sponsored collaborative study. In I. B. Weiner (Series ed.), W. K. Goodman, M. V. Rudorfer, & J. D. Maser (eds), *Obsessive–compulsive disorder: Contemporary issues in treatment: The LEA series in personality and clinical psychology.* Mahwah, NJ: Lawerence Erlbaum Associates.

McFall, M. E., & Wollersheim, J. P. (1979). Obsessive–compulsive neurosis: A cognitive-behavioral formulation and approach to treatment. *Cognitive Therapy and Research, 3*, 333–348.

Obsessive Compulsive Cognitions Working Group (2001). Development and initial validation of the Obsessive Beliefs Questionnaire and the interpretation of Intrusions Inventory, *Behaviour Research and Therapy, 39*, 987–1006.

Rachman, S. J. (1993). Obsessions, responsibility, and guilt. *Behaviour Research and Therapy, 31*, 149–154.

Rachman, S., & Hodgson, R. J. (1980) *Obsessions and compulsions.* Englewood Cliffs, New York: Prentice.

Rachman, S., & Shafran, R. (1999). Cognitive distortions: Thought–action fusion. *Clinical Psychology and Psychotherapy, 6*, 80–85.

Rachman, S., Thordarson, D., Shafran, R., & Woody, S. (1995). Perceived responsibility: Structure and significance. *Behaviour Research and Therapy, 33*, 779–784.

Reed, G. F. (1985). *Obsessional experience and compulsive behavior: A cognitive structural approach.* Orlando, Fl: Academic Press.

Rhéaume, J., Freeston, M. H., Dugas, M. J., Letarte, H., & Ladouceur, R. (1995). Perfectionism, responsibility, and obsessive–compulsive symptoms. *Behaviour Research and Therapy, 33*, 785–794.

Rhéaume, J., Ladouceur, R., Freeston, M. H., & Letarte, H. (1995). Inflated responsibility and its role in OCD. *Behaviour Research and Therapy, 33*, 159–169.

Salkovskis, P. M. (1989). Cognitive–behavioral factors and the persistence of intrusive thoughts in obsessional problems. *Behaviour Research and Therapy, 27*, 677–682.

van Balkom, A. J. L. M., van Oppen, P., de Haan, E., Spinhoven, P., & van Dyck, R. (1998). Cognitive–behavioral therapies alone versus in-combination with fluvoxamine in the treatment of obsessive–compulsive disorder. *Journal of Nervous and Mental Disease, 86*, 492–499.

van Balkom, A. J. L. M., van Oppen, P., Vermeulen, A. W. A., Nauta, M. M. C., Vorst, H. C. M., & van Dyck, R. (1994). A meta-analysis on the treatment of obsessive–compulsive disorder: A comparison of antidepressants, behavior and cognitive therapy. *Clinical Psychology Review, 14*, 359–381.

van den Hout, M., Emmelkamp, P. M. G., Kraaükamp, J., & Griez, E. (1988). Behavioural treatment of obsessive-compulsives: Inpatient versus outpatient. *Behaviour Research and Therapy, 26*, 331–332.

van Oppen, P., & Arntz, A. (1994). Cognitive therapy for obsessive–compulsive disorder. *Behaviour Research and Therapy, 32*, 79–87.

van Oppen, P., de Haan, E., van Balkom, A. J. L. M., Spinhoven, P., Hoogduin, K., & van Dyck, R. (1995). Cognitive therapy and exposure in vivo in the treatment of obsessive–compulsive disorder. *Behaviour Research & Therapy, 33*, 379–390.

van Oppen, P., Emmelkamp, P. M. G., Balkom, A. J. L. M., & van Dyck, R. (1995) The sensitivity to change of measures for obsessive-compulsive disorder. *Journal of Anxiety Disorders, 9*, 241–248.

van Oppen, P., & Emmelkamp, P. M. G. (1997) Behaviour and cognitive therapy for obsessive-compulsive disorder. In J. A. den Boer & H. G. M. Westenberg (eds), *Focus on obsessive-compulsive spectrum disorders* (pp. 185–204). Synthesis, Amsterdam.

van Oppen, P., Hoekstra, R. J., & Emmelkamp, P. M. G. (1995). The structure of obsessive-compulsive symptoms. *Behaviour Research and Therapy, 33*, 15–23.

Chapter 22

Cognitive Effects of Cognitive–Behavior Therapy for Obsessive Compulsive Disorder

Martine Bouvard

Cognitive Approaches to OCD

Cognitive–behavior therapy (CBT) involves the combination of behavior therapy (exposure plus response prevention) and cognitive therapy. Behavior therapy for OCD most specifically employs exposure (E) and response or ritual prevention (RP). Exposure capitalizes on the fact that anxiety usually attenuates after sufficient duration of contact with the feared stimulus. In order to achieve adequate exposure, it is usually necessary to help the patient block the rituals or avoidance behaviors; a process termed response prevention. In fact, the OCD patient is exposed to stimuli that provoke the obsessive response and helped to desist from avoidance and escape (compulsive) responses. In the particular case of ruminators (OCD without overt compulsions), exposure occurs on a cognitive level because it is focused on the intrusive thoughts while the response prevention deals with the internal mental rituals (neutralization strategies). The use of this adaptation of ERP derives from Salkovskis and colleagues' work (Salkovskis & Warwick, 1988; Salkovskis & Westbrook, 1989).

There are several models of cognitive therapy and thus several different cognitive approaches to intervention. Meichenbaum's (1975) model of cognitive therapy, Self-Instructional Training (SIT), was applied to OCD in a study by Emmelkamp, van der Helm, van Zanten, and Plochg (1980). In SIT, patients were trained to become conscious of their negative self-statements and to substitute positive coping self-statements for the anxiety engendering self-statements. Eight subjects received exposure treatment alone, and seven subjects received exposure plus SIT. There was no evidence that self-instructional training enhanced the effectiveness of ERP. The results revealed that both treatments were roughly comparable on the post-treatment questionnaires measuring anxiety, depression and obsessive compulsive symptoms.

The benefits of Rational Emotive Therapy (RET) were examined for OCD subjects in two studies (Emmelkamp & Beens, 1991; Emmelkamp, Visser, & Hoekstra, 1988). Ellis (1962) developed this alternative form of cognitive therapy. In this technique, patients were trained to record their irrational thoughts and to challenge these irrational beliefs. Attention is paid to ten basic beliefs described by Ellis. In the first study, the authors compared a group of subjects who had received training in exposure and response

Cognitive Approaches to Obsessions and Compulsions – Theory, Assessment, and Treatment
Copyright © 2002 by Elsevier Science Ltd.
All rights of reproduction in any form reserved.
ISBN: 0-08-043410-X

prevention to a group who received RET (Emmelkamp *et al.*, 1988). The cognitive technique produced comparable results to the behavioral methods. Emmelkamp and Beens (1991) replicated this result in their second study in which they compared Ellis' cognitive methods to behavior therapy and to the combination. Furthermore, they showed that when RET was applied in conjunction with ERP, this combination produced results no better than ERP by itself. However, although RET was as effective as self-controlled live exposure on most outcome measures, the combined cognitive-exposure therapy improved irrational beliefs more than did exposure alone. The cognitive technique described by the authors in this last study was closer to the therapy inspired by Beck's model. Therapists encouraged patients to discuss their irrational beliefs, particularly those that related to the OCD theoretical model described by McFall and Wollersheim (1979). This model hypothesized that OCD results from faulty primary appraisals that are produced by four types of beliefs. The beliefs concern the necessity of being perfect (in order to avoid criticism), that making mistakes deserves punishment, that magical rituals can prevent disasters, and that certain thoughts and feelings are unacceptable.

These early studies suggest that cognitive approaches are at least as effective as traditional ERP. At the same time, it is possible that the sample sizes were too small to allow detection of group differences. Still, the efficacy of cognitive techniques was essentially demonstrated for OCD symptoms. The only cognitive measure used in the Emmelkamp and Beens study (1991) was one that focused on Ellis' irrational beliefs and was thus not tailored to OCD. Thus, it is difficult to know whether the RET cognitive therapy produced substantial changes on cognitive beliefs tied to patients' OCD symptoms.

We will not discuss these studies further as the cognitive techniques employed had a different rationale than the cognitive therapy originating from Beck's work. The earlier work focused more on common irrational beliefs in psychiatric patients and did not emphasize the distinction between intrusive thoughts considered to be normal occurrences and automatic thoughts that are reactive to these intrusions. By cognitive therapy, we mean a model based on Beck's work (Beck, Emery, & Greenberg, 1985) which was developed further by Salkovskis for OCD (1985, 1989). This model emphasizes the presence of automatic thoughts that represent an interpretation of intrusive thoughts. The theoretical models underlying recent CT treatments for OCD postulate that appraisal of the thoughts plays a key role in the onset and maintenance of OCD symptoms and should therefore be addressed directly. The general strategies are first, to consider the intrusions as stimuli; second, to identify the distressing thoughts (negative automatic thoughts) that immediately follow the intrusions; third, to challenge these automatic thoughts; fourth, to change these thoughts to non-distressing ones; and finally, to look for the underlying dysfunctional schemas and modify these.

Relationship of Treatment Method to Cognitive Domains

The first step in cognitive therapy for OCD consists of informing the patient that his/her intrusive thoughts (IT) are a normal phenomenon and providing him or her with a list of intrusive thoughts that commonly occur in the general population (Rachman & de Silva, 1978). The therapist emphasizes that these thoughts do not reveal an aspect of the personality but rather a relationship with the individual's value system. A negative interpretation occurs most frequently when the intrusive thought contradicts the person's values (Rachman, 1997; Salkovskis, 1999). The patient then learns that the difference between normal and dysfunctional intrusive thoughts lies in the significance attached to these thoughts. The interpretation of the intrusive thought made by people with obsessions affects the occurrence and/or the content of this thought (Salkovskis, 1989).

An important general cognitive technique used by the therapist to challenge the automatic thoughts is Socratic dialogue (Beck, 1976). The patient is encouraged to question the catastrophic significance of the intrusive thought and to construct alternative less catastrophic interpretations. For example, the patient may identify the pros and the cons of his/her interpretation. Behavioral experiments are commonly used to test the empirical basis of the patient's new interpretation in order to challenge or evaluate the beliefs. Some overviews of cognitive restructuring that describe these techniques for the appraisal of the thoughts have been published (van Oppen & Arntz, 1994; Freeston, Rhéaume, & Ladouceur, 1996).

The number of domains of beliefs examined during cognitive therapy for OCD patients varies according to the investigator. Salkovskis (1985) has described one area of belief, pathological responsibility, whereas a consortium of researchers identified six main types of beliefs (Obsessive Compulsive Cognitions Working Group [OCCWG], 1997). Three types of beliefs might be considered specific to OCD, inflated responsibility, over-importance of thoughts (thought–action fusion and other beliefs about the importance of the thoughts), and importance of controlling one's thoughts. Three other belief domains thought to be related but not specific to OCD are over-estimation of danger, intolerance of uncertainty, and perfectionism.

CBT helps OCD patients construct and test a coherent alternative, less threatening explanation of their problem. Cognitive therapy (CT), which may be added to behavior therapy, addresses such dysfunctional beliefs as faulty estimation of the importance of thoughts, exaggerated sense of personal responsibility and perfectionism often seen in OCD patients. CT may also provide additional benefits by improving compliance with ERP. Cognitive treatment of OCD patients has been detailed in several articles, especially Freeston, Ladouceur, Rhéaume, and Léger (1998); Rachman (1998); Salkovskis (1999); and Freeston, Léger, and Ladouceur (2001). In this chapter, our objective is to review studies that used this form of cognitive therapy.

Therapy Effects on Cognitions and OCD Symptoms: Case Studies

The effectiveness of CBT was first demonstrated in single case studies and in descriptions of case series. Salkovskis and Warwick (1985) presented the first protocol of an individual case using CBT as we have just described it. It concerned a patient for whom the over-importance of thoughts did not allow the immediate use of behavioral techniques. The application of cognitive restructuring followed by ERP significantly modified the patient's evaluation of discomfort, the Maudsley Obsessive Compulsive Inventory (MOCI) and the Beck Depression Inventory (BDI). This combined treatment resulted in almost complete recovery, which was maintained at follow-up at six months.

Simos and Dimitriou (1994) reproduced these results with a patient who ruminated. Cognitive exposure with prevention of mental rituals followed a cognitive technique centered on the re-attribution of responsibility. Improvement was evident on the Yale–Brown Obsessive Compulsive Scale (YBOCS), the revised version of the Symptom Check-List 90 (SCL 90-R) and the BDI. Shafran and Somers (1998) reported on two clinical cases of adolescents. It appeared that demonstrating the paradigm of thought suppression (e.g., trying not to think of white bears as per Wegner [1989]), and demonstrating that normal subjects have the same intrusive thoughts was sufficient to reduce the OCD symptoms. Unfortunately, the authors did not report an outcome evaluation.

Hoarding symptoms can also be successfully treated with a multi-faceted cognitive–behavioral intervention (Hartl & Frost, 1999). The cognitive–behavioral treatment included training in decision making and categorization, exposure and habituation to discarding, and cognitive restructuring. This was applied with success to a 53-year-old patient who had always suffered from this problem. A significant clinical improvement in the amount of clutter was noted, as well as improvement on the YBOCS and on scales measuring hoarding and indecisiveness. This change was maintained at follow-up.

In three of these individual case protocols, the effectiveness of CBT (ERP plus cognitive therapy) was evident for obsessive compulsive symptoms evaluated either by global scales (YBOCS or MOCI) or by questionnaires for specific symptoms (e.g., hoarding, indecisiveness). The effectiveness of CBT was also sometimes evaluated for symptoms associated with OCD, such as depression measured by the BDI, and general pathology assessed via the SCL-90-R. Multiple baseline single case designs allowed testing not only of CBT in general, but also of the specific cognitive components of treatment, such as cognitive correction of inflated responsibility and cognitive restructuring of other faulty beliefs.

The first experimental study of CBT for evaluating the effectiveness of treatment for obsessive thoughts was conducted by Ladouceur, Freeston, Gagnon, Thibodeau, and Dumont (1995). They used a multiple baseline design across subjects. Treatment sessions were based on imagined exposure and covert response prevention (EPR) and on cognitive restructuring techniques (CT). All three subjects reported a clinically significant decrease in discomfort associated with obsessive thoughts. This result was maintained at follow-up.

A second experimental study (Ladouceur, Léger, Rhéaume, & Dubé, 1996) concerned cognitive treatment focused on correction of inflated responsibility. Four patients suffering from checking rituals were treated in a multiple baseline across subjects design. Cognitive correction targeted inflated responsibility without any exposure or response prevention. All four patients showed a clinically significant decrease in interference caused by rituals, on the YBOCS and on Rhéaume's Responsibility Questionnaire (RQ) at post-test. Therapeutic gains were maintained at follow-up for three of the four patients. Thus, cognitive correction of inflated responsibility alone produced a decrease in perceived responsibility and clinically significant changes in checking symptoms.

The goal of a third experimental study was to test, within an experimental single case design, cognitive therapy for six patients with obsessive thoughts (Freeston *et al.*, 2001). The cognitive treatment consisted of an explanation of the cognitive–behavioral model of OCD, the correction of faulty beliefs, and encouragement of patients to act in accordance with their new way of understanding their obsessive thoughts. As in the preceding study, the therapist did not prescribe formal behavioral experiments. The authors worked on several schemas, five of which were identical to the belief domains retained by OCCWG: over-importance of thoughts, inflated responsibility, perfectionism, control, and over-interpretation of threat. The last domain identified by the Laval group referred to feared consequences of anxiety. At the end of treatment, five participants scored lower than the clinical cut-off point on the YBOCS and four of them changed reliably according to the reliable change index (RCI) for this measure. All YBOCS scores were in the non-clinical range at 6 and 12-month follow-ups, and five met the RCI criterion. Further, depressive symptoms decreased in all participants.

In summary, the first experimental study showed that cognitive restructuring with cognitive exposure leads to improvement of the discomfort associated with obsessive thoughts in subjects without overt rituals. The two other studies demonstrated that cognitive therapy based solely on cognitive restructuring improved OCD symptoms, whether they are applied to subjects with checking rituals or patients with obsessive thoughts. In the study of cognitive correction of responsibility, responsibility scores concerning participants' problem situations reduced substantially. The small number of participants in each of these studies limits the generalizability of the findings. However, as evident from the review below, controlled studies have supported these results.

Therapy Effects on Cognitions and OCD Symptoms: Controlled Studies

van Oppen and colleagues (1995) carried out the first controlled study comparing cognitive techniques based on Beck's model (CT) to behavioral techniques (ERP). During the first six sessions, CT was carried out without behavior experiments and ERP without discussion of expected consequences. The second part of the study consisted of 10 additional sessions that included behavioral experiments for CT and discussions of the patient's expected consequences for ERP. CT was as effective as ERP at the end of six weeks. At the end of the study (16 sessions), both groups improved on obsessive compulsive symptoms evaluated by the YBOCS, the Revised Padua Inventory (Padua-R) and the Anxiety Discomfort Scale (ADS) evaluating participants' five main obsessive compulsive targets. No significant change was evident in the ERP group for the SCL 90-R or the Irrational Belief Inventory which measured general irrational beliefs. On the YBOCS scale, CT was not better than ERP on obsessions in much the same way that ERP was not better than CT on compulsions. In conclusion, patients in CT improved on all the variables and those in ERP improved on nearly all the variables. This would imply a slight superiority for CT, in particular on general pathology and general irrational beliefs.

These results have been frequently discussed. According to Foa, Franklin, and Kozak (1998), the reduction of YBOCS in the ERP group (32 percent) in follow-up is less than that usually obtained with exposure therapies. In other words, the ERP treatment may not have been adequate as per usual expectation. They suggested that van Oppen *et al.* compared a less effective version of exposure (self-help exposure) to cognitive therapy which was confounded by additional advice for exposure in vivo (behavioral experiments).

Thus, it is possible that a comparison of therapist-guided exposure in vivo with cognitive therapy might have produced results in favor of exposure (Hand, 1998). Further, the number of subjects who participated in the final analysis were insufficient to allow demonstration of the differences between groups (Freeston, Bouchard, & Ladouceur, 1996).

The same team led by van Balkom and colleagues (1998) carried out another interesting comparison between cognitive therapy and behavior therapy (ERP), a waiting list, and an anti-depressant medication (fluvoxamine) treatment. During the first part of the study (six sessions), CT alone, BT alone, and fluvoxamine alone were compared to a waiting list control. At the end of six sessions, the overall results indicated that, compared to the waiting list control condition, the active treatment conditions showed improvement in OCD symptoms according to the ADS patient-and-assessor rating and the YBOCS. No significant decrease was found on the Padua Inventory Revised. Compared with the waiting list condition, CT alone showed superior efficacy on the patient and assessor rating of the ADS. The BT alone was superior to the waiting list condition on the assessor-rating of the ADS and fluvoxamine showed superior effectiveness over the control condition on the YBOCS. No significant pair-wise differences between the active treatments were found. In the second part of the study (ten sessions), CT alone and BT alone were compared to CT plus fluvoxamine and BT plus fluvoxamine. At the end of 16 treatment sessions, the results suggested that the combination treatments were not superior to the cognitive or behavioral treatments alone. All four treatments produced a significant decrease on all the OCD measures. For the Beck Depression Inventory and the SCL-90-R, significant pre- to post-test differences were found only for CT and the conditions containing fluvoxamine.

Thus, in the first part of this study, the treatments were comparable on the evaluation of the OCD symptoms and showed an improvement in relationship to the waiting list control. However, few sessions (only six) were dedicated to determining the effectiveness of CT and BT. In the second longer part of the study, the results for BT and CT remained the same. The addition of an anti-depressant did not enhance either cognitive therapy or behavior therapy effects on OCD symptoms. The critiques of the first van Oppen *et al.* study can be applied equally to the van Balkom *et al.* study, since some of the subjects were identical. These two studies confirm the effectiveness of cognitive therapy for OCD and associated symptoms. In both studies, cognitive therapy dealt with over-estimation of the probability and consequences of danger on the one hand and with personal responsibility on the other. They did not have a follow-up assessment without additional treatment and did not use measures of cognition specific to OCD.

In another multi-center controlled trial (Cottraux *et al.*, 2001), CBT was compared to behavior therapy (ERP). Fifty-nine patients without major depression participated in the treatments, each of which lasted 20 hours. The CBT consisted of cognitive techniques and cognitive exposure (habituation to intrusive thoughts). The therapists did not receive any particular instructions concerning the operative beliefs during the course of the therapy. The study showed no significant difference in response to CBT and ERP; both were beneficial in decreasing obsessive and compulsive symptoms. Depression improved significantly more in CBT compared with EPR. This multi-center trial thus confirmed the results obtained by van Oppen and collaborators for obsessive compulsive symptoms. These are preliminary results and only concern the principal measures of OCD symptoms (YBOCS) and depression (BDI). Findings for the one-year follow-up study are presently in preparation. The principal finding is that benefits are maintained and both treatments produced equivalent results.

Interventions Focused on Threat Estimation

The cognitive method put forward by Jones and Menzies (1997a; 1998) applies a variety of procedures to reduce the patient's estimation of the consequences of danger. Thus, it focuses on a single cognitive bias, the estimation of danger and deals only with individuals with contamination fears and washing or cleaning compulsions. Danger Ideation Reduction Therapy (DIRT) is a mixture in eight sessions of Ellis' cognitive therapy, of Beck's classic cognitive therapy, and behavior techniques like the viewing of films of anxiogenic stimuli and conducting experiments on contamination.

In the case of three subjects treated in a single case design, the DIRT technique produced satisfying results (Jones & Menzies, 1997b). The authors noted a reduction in the severity of the OCD symptoms according to the patient's and clinician's evaluation and a reduction in standardized measures of OCD from the MOCI and the Padua Inventory. These results were maintained at a three-month follow-up. When the DIRT method was administered in a group format to 11 participants during a controlled study, results were less satisfying. Changes from pre-treatment to after-treatment (post-treatment and follow-up scores were averaged) were significantly greater for the DIRT condition compared to a wait list control condition for all measures. The change in self-rated severity of symptoms after treatment was significant, as was change on the MOCI, the Leyton (measure of overall OCD severity) and the BDI. However, the authors note that post-treatment MOCI scores remained higher than those typically observed at post-treatment using ERP. No significant differences were observed between conditions from post-treatment to follow-up on any measure. That is, participants in the DIRT condition showed little further improvement at follow-up. Three hypotheses may explain the relatively weak effect for DIRT in this study: the size of the group (five–six patients each); the application of the technique in a group which may diminish its impact on individual patients; and the limited number of sessions (eight). Even if only slightly different from Beck's model, this cognitive technique seems interesting and worthy of attention. Findings suggest that patients with washing rituals are sensitive to expectations of danger. The long term effectiveness of this technique remains to be demonstrated.

These first controlled studies have demonstrated the effectiveness of cognitive therapy (CT) and of CBT for the OCD. CBT seems to be as effective as ERP or an anti-depressant treatment for OCD symptoms and symptoms of depression. A limit of these studies is that the evaluation tools were centered on obsessive and compulsive symptoms and none used cognitive measures specific to OCD.

Interventions Focused on Beliefs Associated with OCD

A study by Freeston *et al.* (1997) compared ERP combined with cognitive restructuring to a waiting list control group in obsessive ruminations. The treatment consisted of a detailed explanation of the occurrence and maintenance of intrusive thoughts, exposure to intrusive thoughts, response prevention applied to all neutralizing strategies, cognitive restructuring and relapse prevention. The schemas worked on were those we have described earlier in this chapter, including responsibility, over-importance of thoughts, over-estimation of danger, and perfectionistic beliefs about thoughts and their control. Fifteen subjects received CBT and 14 were assigned to the waiting list control condition. These 14 subjects then received the CBT treatment. When the two groups were compared, significant improvements were evident in obsessive–compulsive symptoms (measured with the YBOCS and the Padua Inventory), current functioning and self-reported anxiety (Beck Anxiety Inventory). When waiting list patients were subsequently treated with CBT, they improved on all measures including depression (BDI). At post-test, 67 percent of the total sample showed clinically significant change on the YBOCS; this figure dropped somewhat to 53 percent at six-month follow-up. Among treatment completers ($n = 22$), the corresponding figures were 77 percent and 59 percent, respectively. For other variables, end-state scores were within the functional distribution for 63 percent to 81 percent (depending on the measure) of completers at post-test.

This study clearly demonstrated the efficacy of cognitive–behavioral treatment of obsessions without overt compulsions. Treatment gains were maintained at six-month follow-up. Among the completer sample, reduction in obsessive symptoms was accompanied by significant improvement in cognitive variables, including appraisal of danger and responsibility, and other irrational beliefs about obsessions (Freeston & Ladouceur, 1995). The Inventory of Beliefs Related to Obsessions (IBRO; Freeston, Ladouceur, Gagnon, & Thibodeau, 1993) and a general irrational belief scale (Malouff & Schutte, 1986) showed that only beliefs about obsessions (IBRO) reduced with changes in obsessive symptoms. The correlation between changes in OCD symptoms and changes in irrational beliefs remained significant, even when changes in depressive symptoms were partialled out. Thus, CBT not only produced relief from OCD symptoms but the degree of improvement was specifically related to changes in beliefs about obsessions, as postulated by cognitive models. This study was the first to establish the improvement in beliefs about obsessions after CBT for patients without overt compulsions using a specific measure of cognitions associated with OCD.

In another study, O'Connor, Todorov, Robillard, Borgeat, and Brault (1999) compared four treatments for patients with overt compulsions. The treatment conditions were CBT without medication, CBT with medication, medication alone and a waiting list control. In a second phase of the study, the medication group and the waiting list group received CBT so that eventually, all groups received this therapy. In addition to classical clinical tools, two belief scales measured the strength of subjects' obsessive beliefs. The primary belief scale measured the strength of the individual's belief that the original obsessive conviction was correct when others did not share it. An example might be: "Now that I've shaken hands, my fingers are contaminated." The second belief scale measured how strongly the person felt that something other than anxiety would occur if she or he did not perform the ritual. For example, the person might believe: "Now I must wash my hands or I will contaminate someone else." The primary and secondary beliefs were recorded for each of the subject's rituals.

The principal clinical finding of O'Connor *et al.*'s study was that CBT alone, CBT with medication, and CBT following medication provided statistically equivalent benefits. Medication alone improved the patients' obsessive symptoms (YBOCS) and depression (BDI). However, only subjects receiving CBT showed reduced strength in their obsessive beliefs, whereas during the waiting period, neither those on medication only nor those on the waiting list showed any change in strength of beliefs. The subsequent administration of CBT to patients on the waiting list also decreased the strength of their primary obsessive beliefs and beliefs about the consequences of not performing the rituals. The value of this study is that it shows that the specific effect of CBT is to dislodge obsessive beliefs. It is limited by the small number of subjects per condition (five–nine maximum), the duration of the treatment (five months), and the absence of follow-up.

The studies of Freeston and colleagues (1997) and of O'Connor and colleagues (1999) both incorporated cognitive measures specifically relevant to OCD. It appears that CBT specifically improves the beliefs related to obsessions or reduces the strength of the belief in the intrusive thoughts (primary belief) and the automatically associated reaction to this thought (secondary belief). These results are important, but it would be interesting to make the comparison on the same variables for a group of individuals receiving ERP.

Recent efforts by the Obsessive Compulsive Cognitions Working Group (OCCWG, 1997; 2001; in preparation) have resulted in new measures of OCD related cognitions. Several recent studies have supported the hypotheses that OCD-related cognitions as measured by the Obsessive Beliefs Questionnaire (OBQ) and the Interpretation of Intrusions Inventory (III) change with successful treatment and that these cognitive changes are correlated with changes in symptoms.

A study by McLean, Whittal, and colleagues (2001) compared CBT with strict exposure and response prevention (EPR) in group and individual treatment. The YBOCS, the OBQ and the III were used to assess the effectiveness of treatment. The group treatment consisted of twelve 90-minute sessions (six–eight patients per two therapists). The individual treatment contained twelve 60-minute sessions. Both CBT and ERP delivered in groups and individually were effective in decreasing OCD symptom severity and produced a decrease in the two cognitive measures (Whittal, Thordarson, & McLean, 2001). There was no differential effect, according to type or form of treatment, on post treatment YBOCS or cognitive measures. However, YBOCS change for CBT subjects appeared to be correlated with more cognitive change compared to subjects treated with ERP. The correlations of change scores in the YBOCS with the six belief dimensions of the OBQ and the three belief dimensions of III showed that the type of treatment played a role in changing beliefs. Only a single correlation of change scores between the YBOCS and the cognitive questionnaire dimensions (OBQ responsibility) was significant for ERP. For CBT, five correlations were statistically significant, including OBQ tolerance for uncertainty, threat estimation, control of thoughts, and responsibility, and III responsibility.

A more recent study compared the group-treated OCD patients from the above trial to 30 OCD patients who were individually treated with CBT or ERP (Whittal *et al.*, 2001). Individual CBT was highly effective in reducing YBOCS scores at post-test and at three-month follow-up, especially for patients with checking rituals. Individual CBT was considerably more effective than group CBT for both OCD symptoms and cognitive changes according to several self-report measures of thought–action fusion, responsibility and OCD beliefs assessed by the III (but not the OBQ). Cognitive changes, especially responsibility beliefs, were correlated with OCD symptom change, although the authors pointed out that the catalyst for change could not be determined since both ERP and CBT delivered individually produced comparable reductions in beliefs.

Another study by Sookman, Pinard, and Grise (1999) reported data on change in beliefs for the III and the OBQ for 15 patients treated with CBT. Treatment consisted of cognitive therapy strategies for symptom-related appraisals and assumptions across several cognitive domains, as well as ERP in the form of behavioral experiments and homework. Patients who did not respond adequately to the above also received schema-focused CT for more general beliefs pertaining to their view of themselves and the world (Sookman, Pinard, & Beauchemin, 1994). Change in compulsions on the YBOCS was correlated with change on all three sub-scales of the III, whereas change on the Padua correlated more consistently with improvement on the OBQ sub-scales. Five subscales of the OBQ correlated significantly with change on Padua (tolerance of uncertainty, threat estimation, control of thoughts, importance of thoughts, responsibility). The group was then divided into responsive ($n = 10$) and non-responsive subjects ($n = 5$). Response to treatment was defined as a greater than 30 percent drop in YBOCS scores. At pre-treatment, responders were comparable to non-responders on all of the study variables. Only the responders reported a significant reduction on the III total score and its sub-scales after therapy. Likewise, on the OBQ, only the responders reported a significant reduction in strength of beliefs on all subscales. The group differences at post-treatment were significant with the exception of subscales measuring tolerance for uncertainty and perfectionism.

Rector, Richter, Gemar, Denisoff, and Cassin (2001) provided a preliminary report on 12 of 30 OCD patients treated with ERP or ERP plus cognitive therapy for 14 weeks in a group format. The analyses of these patients revealed significant reductions in OBQ responsibility, importance of thoughts, and control over thoughts' subscales. In addition, all three subscales of the III were also significantly reduced at post-test. Using an individual format to deliver CBT, Kyrios, Hordern, and Bhar (2001) treated 19 OCD patients for 16 weeks. Treatment resulted in significant changes in OCD symptoms and level of functioning. Change in level of functioning and in global assessment of functioning were significantly correlated with changes in the total OBQ score. Furthermore, change in GAF was significantly correlated with change in the total III score.

Summary and Comment

These findings indicate that a number of different teams of researchers have demonstrated that cognitive change has been brought about by CBT on measures of beliefs considered specific to OCD. Rector *et al.* demonstrated significant pre- and post-changes in selected OBQ and all III sub-scales. The study by Whittal *et al.* (2001) comparing CBT and ERP showed that cognitive changes were greater with CBT. The studies by Sookman and colleagues and Kyrios *et al.* confirmed that changes in beliefs correlated with improvement of OCD symptoms. More research is needed in this area. The concern of the first controlled studies was to show the effectiveness of cognitive therapy or of CBT in relationship to a waiting list or to other active treatments (ERP or anti-depression medicines). The effectiveness of CBT was verified by a reduction of OCD symptoms in all of the relevant studies. Several studies also showed reduction of depression and associated psychopathology. The results were maintained after treatment had stopped. However, long term maintenance of CBT-produced results is still unknown; the longest follow-up of these studies has been one year.

Studies showing that CBT results in a reduction of beliefs about obsessions are more rare. The therapeutic gains obtained appear to be associated with the modification of erroneous beliefs by the OCD patient. The creation of questionnaires evaluating beliefs specific to OCD are very recent compared to the tools evaluating the symptoms. Thus, more studies are needed in this area. It appears that the principal types of obsessions and compulsions can benefit from CBT, particularly for subjects with checking rituals and without overt compulsions.

Few studies have examined cognitive techniques without ERP (see Chapter 21 in this volume). The majority of reported studies ($n = 11$) used CT in association with ERP. Thus, it seems difficult for the moment to differentiate which results come from behavior therapy and which come from cognitive therapy. It has already been suggested that ERP may influence cognition indirectly by providing ideal conditions for the disconfirmation of beliefs associated with obsessive illness. Indeed, the studies described by Emmelkamp, van Oppen, and van Balkom (2001; Chapter 21 in this volume) suggest that ERP changes OCD specific cognitions as measured by the OBQ and III, and these changes are correlated with changes in OCD symptoms. Nevertheless, changes in cognition in the case of behavioral treatment may be more limited than those noted with CBT when specific measures of OCD cognitions are used. Much work remains to be done in order to clarify the results obtained by cognitive techniques alone.

References

Beck, A. T. (1976). *Cognitive therapy and the emotional disorders*. New York: International University Press.

Beck, A. T., Emery, G., & Greenberg, R. L. (1985). *Anxiety disorders and phobias: A cognitive perspective*. New York: Basic Books.

Cottraux, J., Note, I., Yao, S. N., Lafont, S., Note, B., Mollard, E., Bouvard, M., Sauteraud, A., Bourgeois, M., & Dartigues, J. F. (2001). A randomized controlled trial of cognitive therapy versus intensive behavior therapy in obsessive compulsive disorder. *Psychotherapy and Psychosomatics, 70*, 288–297.

Ellis, A. (1962). *Reason and emotion in psychotherapy*. New York: Lyle Stuart.

Emmelkamp, P. M. G., & Beens, H. (1991). Cognitive therapy with obsessive–compulsive disorder: A comparative evaluation. *Behaviour Research and Therapy, 29*, 293–300.

Emmelkamp, P. M. G., van der Helm, M., van Zanten, B. L., & Plochg, I. (1980). Treatment of obsessive–compulsive patients: The contribution of self-instructional training to the effectiveness of exposure. *Behavior Research and Therapy, 18*, 61–66.

Emmelkamp, P. M. G., Visser, S., & Hoekstra, R. J. (1988). Cognitive therapy vs exposure in vivo in the treatment of obsessive compulsives. *Cognitive Therapy and Research, 12*, 103–114.

Foa, E. B., Franklin, M. E., & Kozak, M. J. (1998). Psychosocial treatments for obsessive–compulsive disorder. In R. P. Swinson, M. M Antony, S. J. Rachman, & M. A. Richter (eds) *Obsessive–Compulsive Disorder: Theory, research and treatment* (pp. 258–276). New York: Guilford.

Freeston, M. H., Bouchard, C., & Ladouceur, R. (1996). Traitement cognitif et comportemental du trouble obsessionnel compulsif. Partie 2: Interventions thérapeutiques. *Revue Québècoise de Psychologie, 17,* 1–24.

Freeston, M. H., & Ladouceur, R. (1995, July). *Cognitive change in the treatment of obsessional thoughts.* In S. Rachman, G. Steketee, R. Frost, & P. Salkovkis (chairs), Towards a better understanding of obsessive–compulsive disorder, World Congress of Behavioural and Cognitive Therapies, Copenhagen, Denmark.

Freeston, M. H., Ladouceur, R., Gagnon, F., & Thibodeau, N. (1993). Beliefs about obsessional thoughts. *Journal of Psychology and Behavioral Assessment, 15,* 1–21.

Freeston, M. H., Ladouceur, R., Gagnon, F., Thibodeau, N., Rhéaume, J., Letarte, H., & Bujold, A. (1997). Cognitive behavioral treatment of obsessive thoughts: A controlled study. *Journal of Consulting and Clinical psychology, 65,* 405–413.

Freeston, M. H., Ladouceur, R., Rhéaume, J., & Léger E. (1998). Applications of cognitive models of OCD in clinical practice. In E. Sanavio (ed.), *Behavior and cognitive therapy today: Essays in honor of Hans J. Eysenck* (pp. 117–127). Oxford: Elsevier Science.

Freeston, M. H., Léger, E., & Ladouceur, R. (2001). Cognitive therapy of obsessive thoughts. *Cognitive and Behavioral Practice, 8,* 61–78.

Freeston, M. H., Rhéaume, J., & Ladouceur, R. (1996). Correcting faulty appraisals of obsessional thoughts. *Behaviour Research and Therapy, 34,* 433–446.

Hand, I. (1998). Out-patient, multi-modal behavior therapy for obsessive–compulsive disorder. *British Journal of Psychiatry, 173,* (S. 35), 45–52.

Hartl, T. L., & Frost, R. O. (1999). Cognitive–behavioral treatment of compulsive hoarding: a multiple baseline experimental case study. *Behaviour Research and Therapy, 37,* 451–461.

Jones, M. K., & Menzies, R. G. (1997a). The cognitive mediation of obsessive–compulsive handwashing. *Behaviour Research and Therapy, 35,* 843–850.

Jones, M. K., & Menzies, R. G. (1997b). Danger ideation reduction therapy (DIRT): preliminary findings with three obsessive–compulsive washers. *Behaviour Research and Therapy, 35,* 955–960.

Jones, M. K., & Menzies, R. G. (1998). Danger ideation reduction therapy (DIRT) for obsessive–compulsive washers: A controlled trial. *Behaviour Research and Therapy, 36,* 959–970.

Kyrios, M., Hordern, C., & Bhar, C. (2001, July). *Specific and non-specific changes in cognition associated with cognitive–behavioral treatment of obsessive–compulsive disorder.* Paper presented at the World Congress of Behavioural and Cognitive Therapies, Vancouver, BC.

Ladouceur, R., Freeston, M. H., Gagnon, F., Thibodeau, N., & Dumont, J. (1995). Cognitive–behavioral treatment of obsessions. *Behavior Modification, 19,* 247–257.

Ladouceur, R., Léger, E., Rhéaume, J., & Dubé, D., (1996). Correction of inflated responsibility in the treatment of obsessive–compulsive disorder. *Behaviour Research and Therapy, 34,* 767–774.

Malouff, J. M., & Schutte, N. S. (1986). Development and validation of a measure of irrational beliefs. *Journal of Consulting and Clinical Psychology, 54,* 860–862.

McLean, P. D., Whittal, M. L., Thordarson, D. S., Taylor, S., Sochting, I., Koch, W. J., Paterson, R., & Anderson, K. W. (2001). Cognitive versus behavior therapy in the group treatment of obsessive–compulsive disorder. *Journal of Consulting and Clinical Psychology, 69,* 205–214.

Meichenbaum, D. H. (1975). Self-instructional methods. In F. H. Kanfer, & A. P. Goldstein (eds), *Helping people change: A textbook of methods.* New York: Pergamon Press.

Obsessive–Compulsive Cognitions Working Group. (1997). Cognitive assessment of obsessive–compulsive disorder. *Behaviour Research and Therapy, 35,* 667–681.

Obsessive–Compulsive Cognitions Working Group. (2001). Development and validation of the Obsessive–Beliefs Questionnaire and the Interpretation of Intrusions Inventory. *Behaviour Research and Therapy, 39,* 987–1006.

Obsessive–Compulsive Cognitions Working Group (in preparation). *Psychometric validation of the Obsessive–Beliefs Questionnaire and the Interpretation of Intrusions Inventory: Findings from stage 3 data.* Unpublished manuscript.

O'Connor, K., Todorov, C., Robillard, S., Borgeat, F., & Brault, M. (1999). Cognitive–behavior therapy and medication in the treatment of obsessive–compulsive disorder: A controlled study. *Canadian Journal of Psychiatry, 44,* 64–71.

Rachman, S. J. (1993). Obsessions, responsibility and guilt. *Behaviour Research and Therapy, 31,* 149–154.

Rachman, S. J. (1997). A cognitive theory of obsessions. *Behaviour Research and Therapy, 35,* 793–802.

Rachman, S. J. (1998). Cognitive theory of obsessions: Elaborations. *Behaviour Research and Therapy, 36,* 385–401.

Rachman, S. J., & de Silva, P. (1978). Abnormal and normal obsessions. *Behaviour Research and Therapy, 16,* 233–248.

Rector, N. A., Richter, M. A., Gemar, M., Denisoff, E., & Cassin, S. (2001, July). *Cognitive and behavioral treatment of obsessive–compulsive disorder: The role of cognitive factors in treatment response.* Paper presented at the World Congress of Behavioral and Cognitive Therapies, Vancouver, CA.

Salkovskis, P. M. (1985). Obsessional–compulsive problems: A cognitive–behavioral analysis. *Behaviour Research and Therapy, 23,* 571–583.

Salkovskis, P. M. (1989). Cognitive–behavioral factors and the persistence of intrusive thoughts in obsessional problems. *Behaviour Research and Therapy, 27,* 677–682.

Salkovskis, P. M. (1999). Understanding and treating obsessive–compulsive disorder. *Behaviour Research and Therapy, 37,* S29-S52.

Salkovskis, P. M., & Warwick, H. C. (1985). Cognitive therapy of obsessive–compulsive disorder: Treating treatment failures. *Behavioural Psychotherapy, 13,* 243–255.

Salkovskis, P. M., & Warwick, H. C. (1988). Cognitive therapy of obsessive–compulsive disorder. In C. Perris, I. M. Blackburn, & H. Perris, *Cognitive psychotherapy: Theory and practice* (pp. 376–395). Berlin: Springer Verlag.

Salkovskis, P. M., & Westbrook, D. (1989). Behavior therapy and obsessional ruminations: Can failure be turned into success? *Behaviour Research and Therapy, 27,* 149–160.

Shafran, R., & Somers, J. (1998). Treating adolescent obsessive–compulsive disorder: Applications of the cognitive theory. *Behaviour Research and Therapy, 36,* 93–97.

Simos, G., & Dimitriou, E. (1994). Cognitive–behavioral treatment of culturally bound obsessional ruminations: A case report. *Behavioural and Cognitive Psychotherapy, 22,* 325–330.

Sookman, D., Pinard G., & Beauchemin, N. (1994). Multi-dimensional schematic restructuring treatment for obsessions: Theory and practice. *The Journal of Cognitive Psychotherapy, 8,* 175–194.

Sookman, D., Pinard G., & Grise, P. (1999, November). *Change in dysfunctional appraisals, beliefs and symptoms in OCD patients treated with cognitive behavior therapy.* Paper presented at the third meeting of the Obsessive–Compulsive Cognition Working Group, Toronto.

van Balkom, A. J., De Haan, E., van Oppen, P., Spinhoven, P., Hoogduin, K. A., & van Dyck, R. (1998). Cognitive and behavioral therapies alone versus in combination with fluvoxamine in the treatment of obsessive–compulsive disorder. *The Journal of Nervous and Mental Disease, 186,* 492–499.

van Oppen, P., & Arntz, A. (1994). Cognitive therapy for obsessive–compulsive disorder. *Behaviour Research and Therapy, 32,* 79–87.

van Oppen, P., de Haan, E., van Balkom, A. J. L., Spinhoven, P., Hoogduin, K., & van Dyck, R. (1995). Cognitive therapy and exposure in vivo in the the treatment of obsessive–compulsive disorder. *Behaviour Research and Therapy, 33,* 379–390.

Wegner, D. (1989). *White bears and other unwanted thoughts: Suppression, obsession, and the psychology of mental control.* New York: Penguin Books.

Whittal, M. L., Thordarson, D. S., (1999, November). *OBQ and III: Sensitivity to change according to the format and type of treatment.* Paper presented at the third meeting of the Obsessive Compulsive Cognition Working Group, Toronto.

Whittal, M. L., Thordarson, D. S., & McLean, P. M. (2001, July). *Cognitive change in cognitive and behavioral treatments for OCD.* Paper presented at the World Congress of Behavioural and Cognitive Therapies, Vancouver, BC.

Chapter 23

Group Cognitive Behavioral Therapy for Obsessive Compulsive Disorder

Maureen L. Whittal and Peter D. McLean

Introduction

Obsessive compulsive disorder (OCD) was originally thought to be rare and recalcitrant to treatment. However, OCD is now known to have a lifetime prevalence of one to three percent and of those who are able to complete pharmacological treatment, approximately two-thirds receive some immediate benefit. Of those who are able to complete psychosocial treatment, which to date has primarily been behavioral via exposure plus response prevention (ERP), approximately 75 percent report positive acute effects. However, despite these encouraging results, medication and behaviorally-based treatments are not a panacea. Following medication discontinuation, approximately 90 percent of patients relapse after six weeks. For those who continue on medication, side effects such as weight gain and sexual dysfunction are a life-long problem. Behaviorally-based treatments, as well as medication, are associated with substantial refusal/drop-out rates and the majority of patients are left with significant residual symptoms following treatment.

In sum, although there have been positive steps in the treatment of OCD, patients would clearly benefit from additional treatment options. Cognitive–behavioral therapy (CBT) offers a promising alternative. The purpose of this chapter is to describe how CBT can be delivered in a group setting, the advantages and disadvantages of this treatment modality, and lastly, to present some data regarding the change in symptoms and cognition following group treatment for OCD.

Group Treatment for OCD

There have been eight uncontrolled clinical trials of group treatment for OCD (Enright, 1991; Epsie, 1986; Hand & Tichatzky, 1979; Himle, 2000; Krone, Himle, & Nesse, 1991; Taylor & Sholomskas, 1993; van Noppen, Pato, Marsland, & Rasmussen, 1998; van Noppen, Steketee, McCorkle, & Pato, 1997). Each of these studies used a behavioral treatment protocol that relied on exposure plus response prevention. Table 23.1 illustrates duration

Table 23.1: OCD group treatment outcome studies*

Study	No. of Patients	No. of Sessions	Outcome
Hand & Tichatzky, (1979)	17	25	Variable decrease in OCD symptoms
Epsie, (1986)	5	10	Successful outcome after individual behavior therapy failed
Taylor & Sholomskas, (1993)	6	14	Benefits comparable to individual BT
Enright, (1991)	24	9	Significant benefits for OCD symptoms; 17 percent clinically improved**
Krone, Himle, & Nesse, (1991)	36	7	YBOCS: 21 pre-test, 16 post-test, 12 three-month follow-up
van Noppen et al., (1993)	73	8–10	YBOCS: 22 pre-test, 17 post-test, 16 6-month follow-up
van Noppen et al., (1997)	17	10–12	YBOCS: 24 pre-test, 17 post-test, 14.5 1-year follow-up; 43 percent clinically improved**
Fals-Stewart, Marks, & Schafer, (1993)	30	24 group BT	Group BT = individual BT > relaxation
	31	24 indiv BT	YBOCS: 22 pre-test, 12 post-test, 14 six-month follow-up
	32	24 relaxat	
Himle et al., (2001)	89	7	YBOCS: 22 pre-test, 16 post-test, 13 3-month follow-up (50 percent attrition at three mths)
	24	12	YBOCS: 22 pre-test, 15 post-test, 15 3-month follow-up (37 percent attrition at three mths)
McLean et al., (2001)	31	12 group CBT	YBOCS: 22 pre-test, 16 post-test, 17 three-month follow-up, 16 percent "recovered"
	32	12 group ERP	YBOCS: 22 pre-test, 13 post-test, 13 three-month follow-up, 38 percent "recovered"

* Table reproduced with permission
** Clinically significantly improved according to Jacobson & Truax's, (1991) method
YBOCS = Yale–Brown Obsessive Compulsive Scale, mths = months, BT = behavior therapy

of treatment, sample size, and treatment outcome for these studies in addition to a recent study comparing group CBT to group ERP.

Steketee and van Noppen (1998) reviewed the uncontrolled clinical trials of group treatment for OCD. Since then, one additional study has been published. Himle (2000) conducted an uncontrolled study with 113 patients who were assigned either to a seven-week or a 12-week behavioral group treatment. The first seven sessions of both groups were two hours in duration. The first hour was dedicated to a psychoeducational topic that varied each week (e.g., the principles of behavior therapy, causes of OCD, family life and OCD). The second hour was dedicated to exposure and response prevention, goal setting, and homework assignment. The final five sessions of the 12-week group were one hour in duration and focused on the behavior therapy component of treatment (i.e., exposure). Both groups reported a significant decline as assessed by the Yale–Brown Obsessive Compulsive Scale (YBOCS; Goodman *et al.*, 1989) from pre- to post-treatment. These gains were generally maintained over a three-month and long-term follow-up. Moreover, there was no significant difference between the seven-week and the 12-week groups. Although it is encouraging that such a short group treatment can have a beneficial effect on OCD symptom severity, these results must be interpreted with caution secondary to the high attrition rate. All subjects were available at post-treatment, but at three-month follow-up, the retention rate was approximately 55 percent. At long-term follow-up, 26/113 subjects were available for assessment. Thus, it seems clear that short-term group treatment has positive acute effects, but the maintenance of these effects remains to be seen.

In summary, these uncontrolled trials have demonstrated that behavioral group treatment is effective in decreasing OCD symptom severity. Although the results are not significantly different from those obtained in individual treatment, group treatments tend to produce post-treatment YBOCS scores between 12–15 in contrast to individual post-treatment YBOCS scores of 9–12. The results achieved during acute treatment tend to be maintained by the majority of patients up to one year following treatment, although caution must be used with the Himle (2000) study because of their high attrition rate.

To date, only one controlled trial of behavioral group treatment for OCD has been published (Fals-Stewart, Marks, & Schafer, 1993). Participants in this study were randomly assigned to individual or group behavior therapy or a psychological control. Patients were seen twice weekly for 12 weeks. The individual sessions were 60 minutes, whereas the group sessions were 120 minutes. Both treatment groups reported a significant decline in YBOCS symptom severity, and there was no significant difference between individual and group treatment at post-treatment or at six-month follow-up. However, generalizability of these results is hindered due to the exclusion of subjects who reported Beck Depression Inventory (Beck, Ward, Mendelson, Mock, & Erbaugh, 1961) scores above 22 or those who were diagnosed with comorbid axis II pathology.

McLean *et al.* (2001) have recently completed the only controlled trial comparing contemporary group CBT with standard group ERP. Sixty-one patients were randomly assigned to immediate treatment or wait-list control. Groups were 150 minutes in duration and were conducted once a week for 12 consecutive weeks. Each group contained six to eight patients and was led by two therapists. At post-treatment, both groups reported a significant decline in YBOCS total score. Use of medication was significantly more prevalent in the ERP group (62.5 percent) compared to the CBT group (35.5 percent) and therefore was used as a blocking variable. These analyses resulted in a significant difference in favor of group ERP over group CBT at post-treatment, and this advantage remained at the three-month follow-up. With regard to clinically significant outcomes (i.e., a reliable change of six points on the YBOCS scale and a post-treatment YBOCS score under 12), there was a clear advantage for group ERP over group CBT. At three-month follow-up, 13 percent of the CBT participants met the above criteria compared to 45 percent of the ERP participants. Contamination/washers did particularly poorly in CBT compared to ERP. There were 13 washers in the CBT condition and ten in the ERP condition. At post-treatment none in the CBT group met criteria for a clinically significant change versus 20 percent of those treated in the ERP group.

Principles in Working with OCD Patients

As with CBT of other disorders, therapists need to work collaboratively with OCD patients to establish a working alliance. Socratic questioning and guided discovery are tools that assist therapists in establishing this working alliance which begins during the assessment when the goal is to achieve a shared understanding of the problem. Having a conceptual understanding of their intrusive thoughts and compulsive behavior and agreeing with the rationale for treatment likely promotes homework completion, which has been demonstrated to positively impact treatment outcome (de Araujo, Ito, & Marks, 1996). During the assessment and the ensuing treatment, we provide normalizing information and make it clear to patients that they will never be told that their interpretations are incorrect, but rather we will work together to determine if there is an alternate way to interpret the meaning of their thoughts.

Because the feared consequences are often future-oriented (e.g., going to hell for having blasphemous thoughts or developing cancer from using cellular phones) and not imminent as they often are in panic (e.g., "what if I suffocate and die during this panic attack"), cognitive challenging does not focus on disconfirmation. Rather, Socratic questioning is used whenever possible to assist patients in drawing their own conclusions about their intrusive thoughts. Salkovskis (1999) has expanded on the guidelines and the unique features of working with OCD patients.

Rachman and de Silva (1978) originally demonstrated that more than 90 percent of analogue subjects reported the presence of unwanted intrusive thoughts, although not with the frequency or intensity reported by OCD patients. This result was replicated by Salkovskis and Harrison (1984). Given the ubiquity of intrusive thoughts, removing them is not a target for treatment in CBT. It is not possible to eradicate something that is part of the human condition. The over-arching goal in CBT, for OCD is to give the person alternatives for how they appraise, or attach meaning to, their intrusive thoughts. Although it is tempting for therapists who are new to CBT with OCD, attempting to talk patients out of their intrusions will not work. It becomes similar to giving them reassurance and may increase the strength with which they hold their beliefs. We find it essential to stay focused on the appraisal and not attempt to alter the intrusion. For example, for a patient who is having sexual intrusive thoughts, reviewing the evidence for and against her intrusive thought that she inappropriately touched a child would not be helpful and may be hurtful.

Rather, the cognitive challenging should focus on the appraisal of the intrusive thought (e.g., "I'm a sicko").

Cognitive Behavioral Group Treatment of OCD

Prior to discussing the specifics of cognitive behavioral group treatment for OCD, the role of exposure in treatment must be clarified. In traditional behavioral treatment, ERP is the main technique used by therapists. The goal of ERP is within and between session habituation to the feared stimulus. In cognitive behavioral approaches, as the name suggests, exposure does play a role. However, the function of the exposure is *not* habituation to the feared stimulus (e.g., touching the ground), but rather a behavioral experiment to test the validity of alternate appraisals developed during treatment (e.g., the power of thoughts to foreshadow negative events). Behavioral experiments are one of several tools at the disposal of the cognitive–behavioral therapist.

Although the treatment conducted at our center is manualized, a substantial amount of flexibility is also built in. This flexibility is necessary given the heterogenous symptom-presentation of OCD patients. Moreover, independent of diagnostic status, manualized treatment is not meant to be identical for each patient, but tailored to fit the individual needs of the patient (Kendall, Chu, Gifford, Hayes, & Nauta 1998). Kendall *et al.* (1998) have referred to the art of doing protocol therapy as "breathing life into the manual". At our center we refer to it as "invoking the spirit of the manual".

The Obsessional Belief Questionnaire (OBQ) and the Interpretations of Intrusions Inventory (III) (Obsessive Compulsive Cognitions Working Group, 2001; see appendix) are administered during the assessment phase to identify the cognitive domains that are relevant for each patient. Cognitive challenging begins with the appraisal domain that appears to be the most common among the group members. Although we will present the techniques that we use to challenge the domains in a particular order, note that this order is flexible and should be tailored to meet the needs of the patient or group. In the event that patients endorse multiple cognitive domains as problematic, therapists should begin with the domain that is causing the most concern or is the most central. Also, the challenges that we will present are easily transported to individual treatment as indicated in Chapter 21 of this volume.

In the first session, we provide education regarding obsessions and compulsions, establish goals, and present our model for maintenance of OCD prior to challenging appraisals. Although our model is a template (see Whittal & McLean, 1999 and Whittal, Rachman, & McLean [in press] for a pictorial representation of our model), it is a generic model driven by what patients report. We focus on the importance of the appraisal process and the fact that intrusive thoughts are essentially universal. To reinforce the latter point, we give patients a list of intrusive thoughts, images, and/or urges reportedly experienced by people who did not have OCD (see Rachman & de Silva, 1978 for this list). In some cases, patients are asked to survey their own friends and family (occasionally by anonymous report) to determine if they have ever experienced any of the listed intrusive thoughts and if so, identify the appraisal that accompanied it. The appraisals identified by non-OCD people are typically neutral as opposed to the threatening personally-relevant appraisals made by OCD patients. For example, the thought of a loved one's family dying in a car accident is a common intrusive thought reported by people, with and without OCD. The associated appraisals made by those without are typically not threatening but explanatory (e.g., "that's an unusual thought — I must be upset about something"). However, the appraisals made by people with OCD tend to be more threatening (e.g., "I have to warn them; if I don't and something happens, it will be my fault").

Group treatment provides an immediate opportunity to conduct a survey regarding the importance of the appraisal process. Although all group members have OCD and thus share many similar features, the heterogeneity of their symptoms often provides the opportunity to compare and contrast appraisals. For example, we recently ran a group where one patient had intrusive thoughts and urges to strangle her newborn infant. She believed that having the thought made the action more probable (likelihood thought–action fusion [TAF]) and that she was an evil person and a poor mother for having that thought (moral TAF). Other members in the group had also experienced that intrusive thought/ urge at some point in their lives, but were neutral in their appraisal (e.g., "having a thought can't make me do something I don't want to do"; "I'm having this thought because I'm tired"; "lots of new parents have also experienced these thoughts").

Lastly, the list of intrusive thoughts (Rachman & de Silva, 1978) can be used with each patient in group (or with a patient who is being treated on an individual basis) to identify intrusions they have experienced very occasionally, the ones that they find easy to dismiss. The appraisals associated with these intrusions are compared to those associated with OCD intrusions. Patients discover that the former appraisals are generally neutral, whereas the latter appraisals are threatening and are relevant to them in a negative way. The therapist's goal at this initial stage is to demonstrate the association between appraisals, emotion, and behavior. In contrast to neutral appraisals, threatening, personally-relevant appraisals are associated with compulsive behavior, anxiety, the urge to suppress or control the thought, and/or avoidance.

Many patients find the concept of appraisals difficult to understand and even more difficult to identify. To help them, patients are given definitions and asked to record relevant examples of intrusions and appraisals. To further assist them in developing skills, they are asked to self-monitor intrusions and appraisals in the first and subsequent weeks of treatment.

Often, the appraisals that patients initially identify have additional meaning. A downward arrow procedure, a series of successive questioning, can often be useful in determining underlying appraisals and/or feared consequences. Figure 23.1 illustrates the downward arrow of an obsessive ruminator whose primary concern was being responsible for harm coming to herself or others if she didn't warn people of potential dangers. As is evident in Figure 23.1, the subsequent appraisals are a mix of feared consequences and their emotional sequelae. When completing a downward arrow, we ask patients to attempt to focus not on what they think would happen (i.e., the feared consequences), but on the meaning associated with the feared consequences. We have found that focusing on the feared consequences in the downward arrow method can sensitize patients and reinforce their vigilance and compulsive behavior. For example, in working with a person with contamination/washing symptoms, if the downward arrow reveals the ultimate consequences of death after suffering months of a painful existence, the urge to wash may be greater than ever. However, focusing on the associated meaning of contracting an illness and perhaps passing it on may reveal appraisals of responsibility and poor self-worth.

For some people, it may be too difficult or impossible at this early stage of treatment to focus exclusively on the emotional meaning in their downward arrow, resulting in a mix of feared consequences and the associated appraisals as illustrated in Figure 23.1. It also may be helpful for patients to not take too much time with each response, but rather to attempt to give an immediate response when faced with the question that is repeatedly asked during the downward arrow (i.e., "if that were true, what would that mean about you?"). For many patients the subsequent appraisals they identify are overwhelming things they may not have necessarily thought about before but nevertheless appear valid. This process of uncovering the ultimate fear is often emotionally taxing for patients as they are asked to think about consequences that are horrific for them and that the compulsive behavior is designed to prevent. The goal of the downward arrows is to identify subsequent appraisals that will ultimately be challenged during treatment.

Figure 23.1:

It's my responsibility to prevent something bad from happening
↓
If that were true, what would it mean about me?
If something bad happens to someone, it's my fault
↓
If that were true, what would it mean about me?
Not a good person
↓
If that were true, what would it mean about me?
I'd disappoint my family
↓
If that were true, what would it mean about me?
They couldn't count on me
↓
If that were true, what would it mean about me?
They wouldn't need me and wouldn't interact with me
↓
If that were true, what would it mean about me?
Lonely
↓
If that were true, what would it mean about me?
Not a nice person because I don't have much to offer
↓
If that were true, what would it mean about me?
I'm nothing

Challenging Over-importance of Thoughts

Many of the strategies presented in the subsequent paragraphs are easily transferred to individual treatment and also may be useful for challenging multiple types of appraisals. In challenging overimportance of thoughts, we present the different manifestations (e.g., moral and likelihood TAF) and allow patients to decide which, if any, are important for them. If they believe their thought has merit because it occurred, we suggest that this leads to dwelling on the thought, which further indicates that the thought is important, which leads to further dwelling, etc. The goal with this Socratic questioning is that patients identify the circularity of their thinking. By contrast, thoughts that are not important are not dwelt on and subsequently not attended to. To demonstrate this phenomenon, patients are asked to complete a behavioral experiment in which, on alternate days, they record the frequency of their intrusive thoughts and the associated anxiety as they dwell on their thoughts as they typically do, compared to letting the thoughts come and go as if they were unimportant. This behavioral experiment is similar to testing the need to control thoughts, which will be described later. Prior to engaging in the experiment, patients are asked to make a prediction regarding the frequency of intrusive thoughts and overall anxiety. Patients often predict both will be higher on days when they are attempting to let thoughts come and go.

Challenging likelihood TAF also involves behavioral experiments to test the power of thoughts. Recall that people with likelihood TAF believe that the probability of the outcome increases secondary to the occurrence of the intrusive thought. Initially, we begin by testing the power of the person's thoughts to make neutral things occur (e.g., to make the bus arrive at the stop, to make a light bulb burn out) and increase the difficulty by attempting to make bad things happen to their therapist (e.g., a broken bone, a motor vehicle accident) and ultimately to themselves or their loved ones. When doing these behavioral experiments, patients are testing alternate appraisals that were developed with their therapists. The appraisals are idiosyncratic to the individual patient but generally suggest that thoughts are not powerful and cannot make an event occur.

For a proportion of patients, these thought experiments seem artificial and do not have the same power as naturally-occurring intrusions. If a group contains such a person, each group member is asked to keep a list of "premonitions" or predictions (e.g., thinking about an old friend and recording if they hear from that person in the week or two subsequent to the thought). Periodically, throughout treatment, therapists should inquire about the "hit" and "miss" rate of these predictions, as well as the base rate of this phenomenon (i.e., how common is it to think about an old friend and hear from that person). These experiences (thinking about something and have it subsequently happen) are very common and the goal is to have patients re-evaluate their experience as a normal part of human experience.

Challenging moral TAF can involve presenting continuums that are anchored by the "best person ever" and the "worst person ever". Patients are asked to choose someone they know or know of for these anchors. The patients are then asked to place themselves on this continuum. Typically, if moral TAF is present, the patient will place him/herself near the "worst person ever". The therapist suggests other people who would ultimately cover the range on the continuum (e.g., someone who cheats on their spouse, someone who has thoughts of cheating on their spouse but otherwise remains faithful [note the separation of thought and action in the latter example]). The purpose of constructing the continuum is two-fold: to allow patients to view themselves more objectively and to differentiate between thoughts and actions. One goal is for patients to consider that moral value is based on actions and not thoughts. The latter objective can be a difficult one to discuss with people who have blasphemous obsessions, as it may conflict with the teachings of their religion.

Challenging Control over Thoughts

Helping patients construct an alternate explanation for their behavior may be particularly useful in challenging the need to control thoughts. For example, one of us recently worked with a patient who had intrusive thoughts, images, and urges primarily at night as she was drifting off to sleep (e.g., urges to stab her husband, images of cartoon characters and faceless people, repetition of names that were in the media). She perceived going to sleep as a time when her guard was down and that she was more vulnerable to doing something that she didn't want to do, such as stab her husband. She also had a long-standing belief, prior to her OCD, that she was flawed in some way and that she was vulnerable to losing touch with reality. When these intrusions occurred, she appraised them as indicating that she was going crazy. In an effort to control the intrusions, she hid knives and other potential weapons, sought reassurance from others, attempted to reassure herself by reading about schizophrenia and seeking the opinion of health professionals, attempted to distract herself and suppress the thoughts, and prayed to God that she would not go crazy. Each of these strategies served to make her hyper-vigilant to subsequent intrusions she then expected them to occur as she was drifting off to sleep. Not surprisingly, this patient had developed bouts of insomnia during the ten years she had been having these intrusive thoughts. One of the most helpful strategies for this patient was to understand the process by which she may have increased the frequency of the intrusions. Figure 23.2 illustrates the alternative conceptualization developed with the therapist. She further believed that the OCD would continue to plague her if she maintained her fear of having intrusive thoughts.

Similar to the alternating-days behavioral experiment in over-importance of thoughts, this patient compared the frequency of intrusions when she alternated between trying to control the thoughts, as she had done in the past, and when she let the thoughts come and go. Much to her surprise, she found that letting go of control by not trying to push the thoughts away actually increased her control as the frequency of her intrusions decreased.

Given that attention was such a crucial part of the alternate conceptualization, we agreed that she should do attention experiments. Specifically, she was asked to attend to "for sale" signs for a week. Prior to engaging in this experiment, she was asked to estimate the number of "for sale" signs she had seen. In the subsequent week she was asked to no longer seek out these signs but record the number of times that she happened to see them. As is typical for these patients, she noticed a higher frequency of the target object after training herself to attend to it, even when asked to discontinue attending to the target. In the midst of this experiment, this patient had the image of a "for sale" sign intrude during a period when she was relatively relaxed at home. This event demonstrated to her that she was quite suggestible. This experiment was important in generating evidence for the alternate conceptualization that we developed during treatment, that perhaps it was her

Figure 23.2:

Belief that I'm flawed
↓
Occurrence of normal intrusive thoughts/images/impulses
↓
Evidence that I'm going crazy
↓
Attempt to prevent self from going crazy (reduce temptation by hiding knives, praying, distracting self, suppressing thoughts)
↓
Attempting to reassure self that I'm not going crazy (reading medical books, going to doctors, asking friends and family)
↓
Increased fear of going crazy
↓
Anticipatory anxiety when going to bed
↓
Increased frequency of intrusive thoughts
↓
Strengthened belief that I am flawed and on the edge of losing my mind

efforts at trying to suppress the thoughts and the subsequent hyper-vigilance and attention that resulted in the persistence and increased frequency of the intrusion.

Challenging Responsibility

When a broad view of responsibility is taken, it includes over-importance of thoughts and control of thoughts (Salkovskis, 1999). However, a narrow view of responsibility that directly implies blame (e.g., "it will be my fault if the house burns down or I pass on the AIDS virus") is open to another set of challenges. We have found pie charting to be particularly helpful. In doing a pie chart, patients are asked to identify a situation in which they felt responsible and determine the extent of their perceived responsibility. As a group, participants identify other factors that may have played a role, even if it was small. These factors and their associated percentages are placed into a pie chart of the responsibility, with the actions of the patient coming last. The goal of pie charting is to help patients objectify responsibility and consider that other people/situations may play a role. As a short-hand to pie charting, patients can ask themselves the following: "it's possible that I'm solely to blame for this incident, but what are the other possibilities?"

Figure 23.3 illustrates the pie chart developed with a contamination/washing patient in the week following the break-in of her car. Prior to the pie chart procedure, she believed that she was 85 percent responsible for contracting a disease that may have been left from the person who broke into the car. Following the pie chart in which she and the other group members identified other possible sources to share the blame (e.g., the landlord for

Figure 23.3:

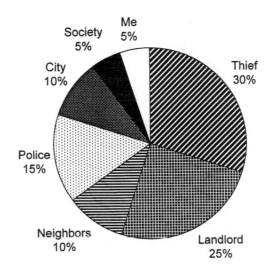

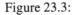

not having secure parking, the person who broke into the car, the city for not having adequate lighting, the police for not having an adequate presence in the neighborhood), she reassessed the extent of her responsibility at five percent.

For a subset of patients, their responsibility provides them with a sense of self worth and makes them better people. To illustrate this concept, a continuum, like the one discussed earlier, is drawn and numerous people the patient knows personally are placed it. A second continuum is drawn directly underneath the first one with the anchors of "least responsible person" and "most responsible person". The patient is asked to rate each of the people on this continuum regarding extent of responsibility. One of two things typically occurs when the second continuum is completed. For themselves, the relationship between self-worth and responsibility is quite high (i.e., reasonably good person and very responsible), whereas the correlation for others tends to be quite low (e.g., good person but irresponsible). The patient's double standard quickly becomes obvious and can lead to a discussion of the qualities of a good and bad person and to the patient surveying others to determine the various definitions of a good and bad person. A second possible outcome from the responsibility continuum is that the patient is using responsibility as a trait to judge the worthiness of others (e.g., "the more responsible you are, the better person you are"). The latter type of moral responsibility may be particularly difficult to challenge, as it is unlikely that they want to change this. However, it may be helpful to have the patient list the behaviors that a responsible person does and compare this list to the list of behaviors by other responsible people in their lives. The latter may help normalize responsiblity.

Over-estimation of Danger

Like many other people with anxiety disorders, people with OCD tend to see danger as more probable compared to people who do not have an anxiety disorder. For example, after leaving the house without checking the stove to ensure it was 'off', they often predict that the stove is very likely 'on' and that the house will burn to the ground. Table 23.2 illustrates logical versus subjective probabilities. This involves listing all possible intermediate steps and their associated probabilities prior to the final feared outcome (e.g., the house burning down). The logical probability is the product of the probabilities associated with the intermediate steps (0.000005 percent) in the example illustrated in Table 23.2). This percentage is compared to the subjective probability, which is ascertained prior to beginning the challenge. We have found it helpful in doing logical probabilities to list the first step (e.g., in Table 23.2, the probability that the stove is 'on'), leave several spaces for other intermediate steps yet to be determined, and list the final step (e.g., that the house will burn down) as this is typically how patients view the situation (i.e., that leaving the stove 'on' is a direct line to having the house burn down). Listing the intermediate steps between the start and end point helps the patient visually re-evaluate the danger in the situation.

Behavioral experiments also may be helpful in assessing threat estimation. Although they can be considered to include exposure, they are conducted for the purpose of gathering evidence for an alternate appraisal. For example, to follow-up the logical probabilities calculated in the previous paragraph, a typical behavioral experiment might be to set the oven timer so the oven will come on during the day when the house is empty or to go to bed with the oven 'on' at a low temperature.

Challenging Tolerance of Uncertainty

OCD patients often report that it is "not knowing for sure" that prompts checking. Slight uncertainty presumably leaves room for error and the potential consequences of that error (e.g., getting a fatal disease) are estimated so high that the risk is also viewed as high. One strategy that we have found helpful is normalizing uncertainty. Specifically, we ask that patients survey 10 friends or co-workers, to determine if they actually remembered locking

Table 23.2: Logical versus subjective probability challenge for a compulsive checker.

Intermediate steps toward the feared outcome	Associated probability
Stove 'on'	1/1000
Something on/near the stove	1/10
Item catches fire and spreads	5/10
Smoke alarm fails to go off or takes several minutes	1/100
Fire department is delayed in responding	1/10

Logical probability of the house burning down = 0.000005 percent their door the last time they left their home and if not, how certain they were the door was locked. Patients are asked to predict the results prior to the survey and are often surprised to learn that the majority of people do not remember locking their door, but their confidence that it is locked is quite high. The goal for patients is to realize that uncertainty is common and does not indicate danger. Similar to the use of exposure as an information-gathering tool, surveys should be done once to fulfill an information deficit and not repeatedly, as this may be construed as reassurance.

Challenging Perfectionism

A downward arrow with perfectionistic people with OCD typically reveals that the perfectionism is related to perception of self-worth (e.g., "the cleaner I am, the better person I am"). Given the egosyntonic nature of these perfectionistic appraisals, they can be difficult to challenge. Fortunately, they are not often the central theme for OCD patients. Similar strategies that were used for people who identified responsibility as a trait that improved their self-worth can be used with perfectionistic people (e.g., continuums, surveys of the characteristics associated with good and bad people, and behavioral experiments).

Advantages and Disadvantages of Group CBT for OCD

Group treatment in other anxiety disorders has been demonstrated effective (e.g., Telch *et al.*, 1993) and in some cases, it is the suggested as the favored method of treatment delivery (e.g., Hope & Heimberg, 1993). In OCD, perhaps more so than for other anxiety disorders, there is a great deal of shame for having unacceptable thoughts and/or engaging in repetitive, senseless behaviors. Perhaps, due to the associated shame, people with OCD are often secretive and have never met another person with OCD. Group treatment can be a powerful experience in normalizing their symptoms. Although we run groups with combined subtypes of OCD, there are considerable similarities amongst participants, which typically fosters a sense of belonging. If the group is cohesive, participants can encourage, motivate, and problem-solve with each other. Clinically, we have observed that patients appear to place a different value on peer encouragement compared to similar suggestions given by the therapist. Using other group members to identify therapy-interfering behaviors, such as avoidance, can help therapists avoid a power differential and potential argument with the patient. The ability of the therapist to use other group members as co-therapists is part of the art of maximizing the non-specific effects of group therapy.

Another benefit of working in groups is that the larger numbers often increase the power of behavioral experiments (e.g., having group members all doing thought experiments) or surveys (e.g., each group member asking their non-OCD friends if they remembered locking their doors). Given the ratio of patients to therapists, there is clearly a therapeutic time advantage in delivering treatment in a group format. Based on a 12-session treatment and seven patients/group, the average therapist time/patient would equal approximately five hours, compared to 12 hours (12 weeks, one hour/week) in individual treatment. In these times of long waiting lists and a paucity of appropriately trained CBT therapists, group treatment has the advantage of providing patients wider access to effective services. If treatment were provided privately, group therapy also has an economic advantage for patients. Again, based on a 12-session treatment, treatment delivered in group would cost patients approximately $600 ($50/session), which would be clearly less expensive than a similar number of individual sessions.

The biggest disadvantage of group treatment is the amount of individual time allotted to each patient. Although most OCD patients share common features, they typically have an idiosyncratic presentation. It is difficult to address the unique features of each group member's OCD and continue to make therapy applicable to the entire group. Presuming that not all members share the same type of appraisals, it is inevitable that some aspects of group treatment may not be helpful for a proportion of group members.

Although most treatment groups are cohesive, there are occasional groups in which members appear not to engage with each other. Similarly, an occasional patient appears substantially different, perhaps due to the severity of their OCD or to inter-personal characteristics. Likewise, group treatment can be demoralizing for the patient who perceives that he or she is not improving at the same rate as other group members. In these cases, we focus on the variable rates of improvement and encourage these patients to make within-person comparisons and focus on the changes that he or she has made since beginning treatment.

Impact of Treatment on OCD Symptoms and Cognitive Processing

Given the minimal data available on treatment outcome using this contemporary form of cognitive behavioral treatment for OCD, the conclusions in this section should be taken with caution. McLean *et al.* (2001) have described the only controlled group trial of OCD. At post-treatment, the mean YBOCS total score for people who were treated with CBT was 16.1 and represented only a 5.8 point drop in YBOCS, compared to pre-treatment levels. Three months later, subjects had slipped somewhat, as reflected by a slight increase in YBOCS total score (17.3). Thus, it appears that subjects treated with group CBT had made little lasting change in their OCD symptomatology and most would meet inclusion criteria for another treatment trial. It was suggested that the group setting provided insufficient time to adequately address the idiosyncratic cognitive processes. A recently completed individual treatment trial at our center supports the previous explanation. Using the same strategies described in this chapter, 30 OCD patients were treated with 12 consecutive 60-minute sessions of CBT. After treatment, their YBOCS score was 10.33. At three-month follow-up, CBT subjects maintained their gains and improved slightly (YBOCS total score = 9.34).

With regard to cognitive processing, it also appears that group CBT is associated with significant declines pre- to post-treatment, but the effect sizes are generally quite small: 0.48 for OBQ Importance of Thoughts sub-scale to 0.89 for III Control of Thoughts subscale; (Whittal & Thordarson, unpublished data). Following group treatment, people reported significantly less need to control their thoughts, and less concern about uncertainty. They no longer viewed their intrusive thoughts as important as they did before treatment, viewed situations as less threatening, and were less concerned with perfectionism. These results continued to hold three months following treatment. Moreover, people who did particularly well in treatment made significantly more change on the above measures compared to people who did not benefit from treatment.

However, similar decreases and maintenance of change are also noted with ERP treatment and in some cases, the effect sizes in behavioral treatment exceeded those in CBT. Compared to the effect sizes noted in the individual treatment study (from 0.76 for OBQ Uncertainty subscale to 1.69 for III Responsibility subscale), group CBT produced relatively small changes in cognitive processing. It is unclear if cognitive change more often precedes behavioral change or if the reverse is true. Some preliminary case data suggests that cognitive change occurs prior to behavioral change (Ladouceur, Rhéume, & Léger, 1996).

Conclusions

CBT for OCD is in its infancy. Although one controlled individual treatment study suggests individual CBT is superior to traditional exposure and response prevention (van Oppen *et al.*, 1995), the McLean *et al.* (2001) study is the only controlled trial of group cognitive behavior therapy for OCD. In that study, patients' symptom severity declined significantly with treatment but patients treated with ERP did significantly better than those treated with CBT. These results await replication. However, if group CBT is relatively ineffective, this does not mean that CBT for OCD should be discarded. It may be that group treatment does not allow for the idiosyncratic focus on the cognitive processes that may be necessary for successful treatment. In an ongoing individual treatment study that we are currently conducting with OCD patients, it appears that individual CBT is significantly better than group CBT.

From a therapist's viewpoint, we believe that CBT is more a complex treatment and requires a higher level of therapeutic skill. Whether it corresponds to an advantage in treatment outcome remains to be established. For purposes of scientific exploration, the CBT studies have been relatively pure (i.e., exposure only in the context of behavioral experiments used to collect evidence for and against an alternate appraisal). However, in clinical practice, the cognitive challenges described in this chapter will likely be combined with existing ERP treatment. Hopefully, these will provide patients additional avenues to obtain lasting change.

References

Beck, A. T., Ward, C. H., Mendelson, M., Mock, J., & Erbaugh, J. (1961). An inventory for measuring depression. *Archives of General Psychiatry, 4*, 561–571.

de Araujo, L. A., Ito, L. M., & Marks, I. M. (1996). Early compliance and other factors predicting out come of exposure for obsessive–compulsive disorder. *British Journal of Psychiatry, 169*, 747–52.

Enright, S. J. (1991). Group treatment for obsessive–compulsive disorder: An evaluation. *Behavioral Psychotherapy, 19*, 183–192.

Epsie, C. A. (1986). The group treatment of obsessive–compulsive ritualizers: Behavioral management of identified patterns of relapse. *Behavioral Psychotherapy, 14*, 21–33.

Fals-Stewart, W., Marks, A. P., & Schafer, J. (1993). A comparison of behavioral group therapy and individual behavior therapy in treating obsessive–compulsive disorder. *Journal of Nervous and Mental Disease, 181*, 189–193.

Goodman, W. K., Price, L. H., Rasmussen, S. A., Mazure, C., Fleishmann, R. L., Hill, C. L., Heninger, G. R., & Charney, D. S. (1989). The Yale–Brown obsessive–compulsive scale. I. Development, use, and reliability. *Archives of General Psychiatry, 46*, 1006–1011.

Hand, I., & Tichatzky, M. (1979). Behavioral group therapy for obsessions and compulsions: First results of a pilot study. In P. O. Sjoden, D. Bates, & W. S. Dockens (eds), *Trends in behavior therapy* (pp. 269–297). New York: Academic Press.

Himle, J. A. (2000, March). Behavioral group therapy for adults and children with OCD. Paper presented at the annual meeting of the Anxiety Disorders Association of America, New Orleans.

Hope, D. A., & Heimberg, R. G. (1993). Social phobia and social anxiety. In D. H. Barlow (ed.), *Clinical handbook of psychological disorders* (2nd ed. pp. 99–136). New York: Guildford Press.

Kendall, P. C., Chu, B., Gifford, A., Hayes, C., & Nauta, M (1998). Breathing life into a manual: Flexibility and creativity with manual-based treatments. *Cognitive and Behavioral Practice, 5*, 177–198.

Krone, K. P., Himle, J. A., & Nesse, R. M. (1991). A standardized behavioral group treatment program for obsessive–compulsive disorder: Preliminary outcomes. *Behavior Research and Therapy, 29*, 627–632.

Ladouceur, R., Rhéaume, J., & Leger, E. (1996, November). *Cognitive change during cognitive treatment and behavioral treatment of checking behaviors*. Poster presented at the annual meeting of the Association of Advancement of Behavior Therapy. New York.

McLean, P. D., Whittal, M. L., Thordarson, D. S., Taylor, S., Sochting, I., Koch, W. J., Paterson, R., & Anderson, K. W. (2001). Cognitive versus behavior therapy in the group treatment of obsessive–compulsive disorder. *Journal of Consulting and Clinical Psychology, 69*, 205–214.

Obsessive–Compulsive Cognitions Working Group (2001). Development and validation of the Obsessive–Beliefs Questionnaire and the Interpretation of Intrusions Inventory. *Behaviour Research and Therapy, 39*, 986–1006.

Rachman, S., & de Silva, P. (1978). Abnormal and normal obsessions. *Behaviour Research and Therapy, 16*, 233–248.

Salkovskis, P. M. (1999). Understanding and treating obsessive–compulsive disorder. *Behaviour Research and Therapy, 37*, S29–S54.

Salkovskis, P. M., & Harrison, J. (1984). Abnormal and normal obsessions: A replication. *Behaviour Research and Therapy, 22*, 549–552.

Steketee, G. S., & van Noppen B. L. (1998). Group and family treatment for obsessive–compulsive disorder. In. M. A. Jenike, L. Baer, & W. E. Minichiello (eds), *Obsessive–compulsive disorders: Practical management* (pp. 443–468). St. Louis: Mosby.

Taylor, C. J., & Sholomskas, D. E. (1993, March). *Group exposure and response prevention for OCD*. Presented at the annual meeting of the Anxiety Disorders Association of America, Santa Monica, CA.

Telch, M. J., Lucas, J. A., Schmidt, N. B., Hanna, H. H., Jaimez, T. L., & Lucas, R. A. (1993). Group cognitive–behavioral treatment of panic disorder. *Behaviour Research and Therapy, 31*, 279–288.

van Oppen, B., Pato, M. T., Marsland, R., & Rasmussen, S. (1998). A time-limited behavioral group for treatment of obsessive–compulsive disorder. *Journal of Psychotherapy Practice and Research, 7*, 272–280.

van Oppen, B., Steketee, G., McCorkle, B. H., & Pato, M. (1997). Group and multifamily behavioral treatment for obsessive–compulsive disorder: A pilot study. *Journal of Anxiety Disorders, 11*, 431–446.

van Oppen, P., de Haan, E., van Balkom, A. J. L. M., Spinhoven, P., Hoogduin, K., & van Dyck, R. (1995). Cognitive therapy and exposure in vivo in the treatment of obsessive–compulsive disorder. *Behaviour Research and Therapy, 33*, 379–390.

Whittal, M. L., & McLean, P. D. (1999). CBT for OCD: The rationale, protocol, and challenges. *Cognitive and Behavioral Practice, 6*, 383–396.

Whittal, M. L., Rachman, S., & McLean, P. D. (in press). Psychosocial treatment for OCD: Combining cognitive and behavioral treatments. In G. Simos (ed.), *Cognitive–behavior therapy: A guide for the practicing clinician.* Hove, East Sussex: Pacific Press.

Chapter 24

Medication Effects on Obsessions and Compulsions

Gregoris Simos

Introduction

Recent advances in pharmacotherapy have led to a significant reduction in suffering and a return to productive living for many patients with obsessive compulsive disorder (OCD; Tollefson, Rampey *et al.*, 1994). However, OCD can be a chronic disorder that significantly detracts from an individual's well being. Potent inhibitors of 5-hydroxytryptamine (5 HT) re-uptake have emerged as the first-line choice in the pharmacotherapy of OCD (de Boer & Westenberg, 1997; Feighner & Boyer, 1996; Koran, 1999; Jenike, Baer, & Minichiello, 1986; Steketee, 1993). Early trials of anti-depressant drugs in OCD were apparently guided by the rationale that obsessive compulsive symptoms represent a variant of depression. Because clomipramine was a potent anti-depressant drug, and depressed mood is frequently present in patients suffering from OCD (Foa & Foa, 1982), this drug was expected to, and in fact did have, substantial beneficial effects in reducing obsessions and compulsions (van Renynghe, 1968). Findings for clomipramine and for subsequently identified serotonergic medications for OCD are reviewed below. Unfortunately, these research and clinical trials have not examined the effects of medication on cognitive aspects of OCD, such as beliefs. Thus, this chapter cannot address the role of medications in changing beliefs or interpretations associated with OCD symptoms. Some investigations have examined the separate effects of medications on obsessions, the closest available analog to cognitions for OCD. Whenever such findings are available, they are reviewed below.

Clomipramine

Two early large and lengthy studies of the effects of clomipramine came from the Maudsley Hospital (Marks, Stern, Mawson, Cobb, & McDonald, 1980; Mawson, Marks, & Ramm, 1982; Stern, Marks, Mawson, & Luscombe, 1980). In the first study, although clomipramine improved rituals, depression, anxiety and social adjustment, it helped only those patients with initial depressed or anxious mood. In the second study, where patients began with normal mood, clomipramine was less effective in reducing OCD symptomatology.

Several studies that examined the efficacy of clomipramine, as well as other anti-depressant medications, followed. Regarding obsessions, the most interesting studies are those by Thoren, Asberg, Gronholm, Jornestedt, and Traskman (1980), Volavka, Neziroglu, and Yaryura-Tobias (1985), Montgomery (1980), Yaryura-Tobias, Neziroglu, and Bergman (1976), and Insel *et al.* (1983). In the Thoren *et al.* study (1980), obsessions improved three times more in the clomipramine patients who had been the most depressed before treatment than in the remaining non-depressed patients. In the Volavka *et al.* study (1985), although initial depression did not relate to outcome, clomipramine was more potent in reducing obsessions than imipramine, another tricyclic anti-depressant. In the Montgomery study (1980), although daily dose of clomipramine was exceptionally low, clomipramine proved superior to placebo for improving obsessions and depression but not rituals. Likewise, in the Yaryura-Tobias *et al.* study (1976), clomipramine did better in reducing ruminations and depression than placebo. In the Insel *et al.* study (1983), patients suffering from obsessions without overt compulsions were also included, and assessment of progress was made with the use of the National Institute of Mental Health scales. Clomipramine was superior in reducing obsessions in comparison with clorgyline or placebo.

Taken together, the above results, as well as those reviewed by Marks (1987), indicated that clomipramine was more effective in reducing compulsions, and in some instances more effective in reducing obsessions, than placebo, and than other anti-depressant medications (imipramine, nortriptyline, amitriptiline, desipramine, clorgyline and zimelidine). Despite the evidence obtained from the Maudsley studies, the relationship between obsessive compulsive symptomatology and depression, and the differential effect medication has on these comorbid conditions still remained obscure.

The differential response of OCD and depression to clomipramine and to other anti-depressants, may give us some hints as to the underlying psychological mechanisms. The parallel decline in depression and obsessive compulsive symptoms evidenced in initially depressed OCD patients in the first few weeks of medication treatment may be due to the effect anti-depressants have on discouraged, hopeless, demoralized and easily frustrated attitudes that depressed OCD patients hold, both about themselves and their condition. Severely or moderately depressed OCD patients experience their obsessions as overwhelming and their compulsions as inescapable. Consequently, they surrender totally to them. Typical depressive biases concerning estimated severity and frequency of obsessions and time occupied by obsessions, as well as estimated ability to resist compulsions or the catastrophic consequences that obsessions and compulsions have on a patient's functioning may actually exacerbate OCD psychopathology. This, in turn, enhances depressive attitudes and cognitions. In contrast, less depressed or non-depressed OCD patients are in a better position to accurately estimate the total severity of their condition, as well as their abilities, and probably have different expectations from anti-depressant anti-obsessive medications.

The efficacy of clomipramine and the failure of other classes of anti-depressants in OCD have made researchers speculate that the principal anti-obsessive action of clomipramine is through its potent inhibitory effect on serotonin reuptake. Therefore, alterations in serotonin function are considered critical to the treatment of OCD and perhaps involved in its pathogenesis (Yaryura-Tobias *et al.*, 1976; Zohar & Insel, 1985). Although the serotonin hypothesis for the pathophysiology of OCD explains several of the above phenomena and research findings, this hypothesis is not sufficient to explain either the disorder itself or its response to potent serotonin re-uptake inhibitors (Rauch & Jenike, 1993).

Selective Serotonergic Reuptake Inhibitors

The efficacy of clomipramine in OCD and the resulting serotonin hypothesis gave birth to research with a newer category of antidepressant drugs, the selective serotonin re-uptake inhibitors (SSRI). These newer drugs, including fluvoxamine, fluoxetine, sertraline, paroxetine and citalopram, have a more selective and potent action on serotonin neurotransmission and cause minimal inhibition of other neurotransmitter re-uptake. What effect did these drugs have on obsessive thinking and, by extrapolation, on beliefs?

Fluvoxamine

Fluvoxamine, unlike clomipramine, has no known clinical metabolites; its potency for blocking serotonin re-uptake is equivalent to that of clomipramine, and it causes minimal inhibition of dopamine or norepinephrine re-uptake. Fluvoxamine was found to be equally effective to clomipramine or imipramine for depression and superior to placebo (Coleman & Block, 1982; Guelfi, Dreyfus, & Pichot, 1983; Guy *et al.*, 1984; Insel, Shrivastava, Mukheriee, Coleman, & Michael, 1983). Several placebo-controlled trials in OCD have been conducted using the Yale–Brown Obsessive Compulsive Scale (Y-BOCS) as the primary outcome measure. Patients with a principal diagnosis of OCD, with or without a secondary concurrent depression, were treated with fluvoxamine for six to eight weeks in a double-blind placebo controlled trial (Goodman *et al.*, 1989). Fluvoxamine was found to be significantly better than placebo in reducing Y-BOCS scores. There were significant but modest decreases in total Y-BOCS scores from baseline beginning at week-two of treatment. By week-three, the reduction in total Y-BOCS ratings was highly significant and was maintained at this level of significance or greater for the duration of the study. Total Y-BOCS scores at six weeks of fluvoxamine treatment were 19.4 ± 7 compared with 25.0 ± 6 at baseline (20 percent reduction), and decreased further by 25 percent of baseline values at eight weeks. Fluvoxamine was effective for both obsessions and compulsions, but a reduction in obsessional symptoms seemed to precede improvement in compulsive symptoms. In a comparison of the selective effects of fluvoxamine and placebo on obsessions and compulsions, fluvoxamine treatment resulted in a significant reduction in the obsession subtotal score of the Y-BOCS beginning at week-two and continuing through week-eight. In contrast, the compulsion subtotal did not demonstrate a significant change from baseline until week-five, after which the reduction was maintained until week-eight.

There were significantly more responders (as defined by a score of much improved or very much improved on the Y-BOCS Clinical Global Impression Scale item) among patients treated with fluvoxamine (nine out of 21 or 43 percent) than among those who received placebo (none out of 21). The percentage decrease in total Y-BOCS scores from baseline among responders to fluvoxamine was 42 percent and their mean total Y-BOCS score at the conclusion of the double blind trial was 14.3 ± 7, corresponding to a global severity rating in the mild to moderate range.

In Goodman *et al.*'s trial, although fluvoxamine exerted a significantly better antidepressant action than placebo starting with week-four and continuing through week-eight, changes in total Y-BOCS scores from baseline were significantly correlated with changes in HAM-D ratings from baseline to the end of trial. However, the response of obsessive compulsive symptoms to fluvoxamine was not related to the initial severity of depressive symptoms. In the fluvoxamine-treated group, the change in total Y-BOCS scores from baseline was not significantly different for the depressed and the non-depressed patients with OCD at any week of treatment. There were more OCD responders to fluvoxamine among the non-depressed (6 of 11) than among the depressed group (three of ten), but these differences were not statistically significant.

According to Goodman *et al.* despite clear-cut differences in the response of OCD patients to fluvoxamine and placebo, the overall magnitude of the effect as measured by the Y-BOCS was modest (25 percent decrease in eight weeks). Responders, on the other hand, had a mean decrease in Y-BOCS of 42 percent, a decrease that corresponds to substantial symptom relief, but no elimination of all obsessive compulsive symptoms. Patients who demonstrated marked improvement with fluvoxamine still reported occasional obsessive intrusions, but found themselves less distressed and having more control over obsessions. A typical comment was, "the thoughts still come, but they don't bother me as much, and I am able to shake them off better". This response appears to be within a normal range, as evident in the occasional intrusions with minimal emotional response and easy dismissal for most non-OCD individuals (see Rachman & de Silva, 1978; Salkovskis & Harrison, 1984).

At the conclusion of the double-blind phase, non-responders originally assigned to receive placebo were then openly treated with fluvoxamine for six to eight weeks. During this open phase, most patients were also treated with behavior modification techniques, including exposure and response prevention, as their clinical condition and willingness to participate permitted. Although it seems that this group of patients did not get formal structured behavior therapy, the percentage of responders increased from 25 percent to 60 percent.

Fluvoxamine was also tested in a double-blind, placebo-controlled trial in a group of OCD patients (Goodman, Kozak, Liebowitz, & White, 1996). The percentage of patients classified as responders (much or very much improved) was significantly higher in the fluvoxamine group from week six onwards, with 33 percent of fluvoxamine-treated patients and nine percent of those given placebo classified as responders at endpoint. Patients classified as responders to fluvoxamine experienced a substantial clinical benefit with marked improvements from baseline to endpoint in their Y-BOCS (47 percent). Analysis of both the obsession and compulsion sub-totals of the Y-BOCS revealed a significant treatment difference in favor of fluvoxamine at the end of the trial.

The significant treatment effect first appeared at week four for the obsession sub-total and at week ten for the compulsion sub-total. The authors give two explanations that may account for this difference. First, the optimal effect of fluvoxamine in reducing compulsions may not be achieved in some patients until they attempt to confront the situations that trigger their symptoms. Learning that it is safe to expose themselves to such situations may be a gradual process that occurs synergistically with continued medication. Second, these clinical differences in the course of response may be accounted for by the brain region specifically affected by chronic SSRI treatment.

Two studies have compared fluvoxamine to clomipramine. In a ten-week double-blind study, no significant differences with respect to the mean reduction on total Y-BOCS score were found (Freeman, Trimble, Deakin, Stokes, & Ashford, 1994). A mean Y-BOCS reduction of 33 percent was seen in the fluvoxamine group and 31 percent in the clomipramine group. Interestingly, the obsession-free interval, but not the compulsion-free interval, was significantly longer for the fluvoxamine group, suggesting that fluvoxamine may have more influence on frequency of intrusions. Whether this translates into an effect on attitudes toward intrusions is unclear.

The efficacies of fluvoxamine (100–300 mg/day) and clomipramine (100–250 mg/day) were also compared in a randomized, double-blind, parallel-group study of OCD patients without coexisting major depression (Koran *et al.*, 1996). Patients were randomized to fluvoxamine or clomipramine for ten weeks. As in the Freeman *et al.* trial, both drugs had equivalent effects. At the end of treatment, 56 percent of fluvoxamine patients were classified as responders (>25 percent decrease in Y-BOCS score), compared with 54 percent of clomipramine patients. With a >35 percent reduction in the total Y-BOCS score as the criterion for response, fluvoxamine produced 44 percent responders and clomipramine produced 38 percent responders at week ten. Mean Y-BOCS scores in the fluvoxamine group decreased by 30 percent at the end of week ten (from 25.5 ± 6 to 17.8 ± 7.7), and in the clomipramine group mean Y-BOCS scores decreased by 30 percent (from 24.3 ± 6 to 17.0 ± 8.6). Unfortunately, researchers did not evaluate differences across obsessions and compulsions separately. Both groups showed steady improvement throughout the study and no statistically significant differences were observed between the groups for any efficacy variable at any time.

Fluoxetine

The first trial of fluoxetine in OCD appeared as early as 1985 (Turner, Jacob, Beidel, & Himmelhoch, 1985). Ten out-patients meeting DSM-III criteria for OCD were selected as subjects for this study. Patients with OCD who were judged to be primarily depressed were excluded. After discontinuation of previous medication, fluoxetine was administered in a ten-week single-blind fashion in dosages beginning at 20 mg. During the first two weeks of the study, patients received one capsule of placebo each day in the morning. This period was designed to help eliminate placebo responders, but no one showed a placebo response. Fluoxetine was administered in dosages beginning with 20 mg to a high of 80 mg.

An extensive battery of self-report inventories and clinical rating scales was employed to assess OCD symptoms, depression, anxiety and social adjustment. Self-monitoring data were obtained through the use of a specially designed record form that the patient used to rate the symptoms on a daily basis. Overall degree of distress was rated on an eight-point scale. In addition, patients were required to estimate the frequency of obsessional thoughts occurring during each day by checking appropriate blocks ranging from 0 to 25+. The frequency of rituals, approximate time spent ritualizing, and the approximate time preoccupied with obsessional thoughts were assessed in a similar fashion. The effects of treatment were also assessed by global improvement rated by therapist and patient.

During the ten-week treatment period, a slow downward trend was observed in self-reported daily distress, frequency of obsessive thoughts, frequency of ritual performance, thought time, and time spent in performing rituals. Medication effects were significant for self-reported distress level, time spent obsessing, and time spent ritualizing. Frequency of thoughts and frequency of rituals improved but not significantly. Four patients indicated that they were "very much better", two were a "little better", one was "much better", one could perceive no change, and two patients dropped out of treatment. Subjects experiencing initial high levels of depression and anxiety tended to improve most on overall distress and had the greatest reduction in obsessions and compulsions, a finding suggesting that the patients with a strong affective component (depression and anxiety) benefited most from the drug.

The second trial of fluoxetine on OCD was also an open pilot study with only nine patients; in nine weeks fluoxetine produced a significant improvement in obsessional symptoms (Fontaine & Chouinard, 1986). The first large study of fluoxetine on OCD was published by Jenike *et al.* in 1989. Sixty-one outpatients completed this 12-week open trial. Fluoxetine was administered as tolerated. Fifty patients reached a dose of 80 mg/day. Mean Y-BOCS total score decreased from 22.2 (SD = 6.2) at baseline to 20.2 (SD = 6.9) at week-4, to 15.9 (SD = 6.9) at week-8, and to 13.9 (SD = 7) at week-12. The overall 37 percent decrease in mean total Y-BOCS score was statistically significant. Depressed and nondepressed subjects improved equally in OCD symptomatology as measured by the Y-BOCS and the Maudsley Obsessional-Compulsive Inventory, and change in Y-BOCS scores correlated with change in MOCI and depression scores. Unfortunately, the authors did not present separate results for the obsessions and compulsions subscales.

Levine, Hofinan, Knipple, and Kenin (1989) also evaluated the efficacy of fluoxetine in a group of 75 outpatients suffering from OCD. Patients were treated in an open clinical setting and the daily dose of fluoxetine was 80 mg in almost all cases. Assessment of obsessive compulsive symptoms was through a global scale of severity of obsessive compulsive symptoms (GOCD) similar to the NIMH Global Obsessive Compulsive Scale. Unlike the former trials, this trial was extended up to a period of five months. Patients were seen two weeks after beginning the medication and at monthly intervals thereafter. The significant reductions in GOCD achieved between the first and second visits were maintained through subsequent visits. Although a marked reduction in symptoms occurred in four weeks, this improvement represented only a partial response to treatment. By the end of the investigation period, the scores on the test instruments (GOCD, HAMD, and HAMA) had fallen by an additional 62–65 percent. Mean severity of obsessive compulsive symptoms before treatment was "severe" (an approximate value of six according to GOCD) and decreased to "normal" (an approximate value of one according to GOCD). However, according to their results, it is impossible to discriminate any differential effect of fluoxetine on obsessions and compulsions.

Fixed-dose fluoxetine (20, 40, 60 mg/d) was compared with placebo in two randomized, double-blind, parallel, 13-week trials of identical design in 355 outpatients with OCD aged 15–70 years (Tollefson, Birkett, Koran, & Genduso, 1994; Tollefson, Rampey *et al.*, 1994). To include patients in the trial, OCD symptoms had to be at least of moderate severity, as defined by a Y-BOCS score of at least 16 if both obsessions and compulsions were present or at least ten if only obsessions or only compulsions were present. Comorbid non-bipolar depression was permitted if it began after the onset of the OCD and was judged clinically to be secondary to OCD. All doses of fluoxetine were significantly superior to placebo on the Y-BOCS total score (mean baseline-to-end-point decreases of 4.6, 5.5, and 6.5 vs 0.9 respectively). More than half of all fluoxetine-treated patients achieved an end-point Y-BOCS total score of 20 or less, compared to about one third of placebo-treated patients who achieved such a score. Scores of 15 or less were twice as common with fluoxetine as placebo at end-point. Mean end-point Y-BOCS scores for the 20, 40, 60 mg/day fluoxetine treatment groups and the placebo group were 18.9 (range 0–37), 18.1 (range 0–35), 16.8 (range 0–31), and 23.6 (range 3–40) respectively. A statistically significant decreasing pattern in change in Y-BOCS total score (i.e., increasing improvement) was observed with increasing dosages of fluoxetine.

Response rates (at least 35 percent improvement in Y-BOCS total score) with fluoxetine doses of 20, 40, 60 mg/day versus placebo were 32 percent, 32 percent, 35 percent and nine percent respectively. With regard to obsession and compulsion scores, all of the fluoxetine treatment groups experienced significant improvement in baseline-to-end-point change in Y-BOCS. A significantly greater proportion of patients in the fluoxetine treatment groups than in the placebo group experienced improvement in time spent on obsessions (54 percent, 54 percent, and 48 percent vs. 19 percent respectively) and time spent on compulsions (42 percent, 50 percent, and 56 percent vs. 24 percent respectively). These effects were independent of the patients' anti-depressant response. As in some of the above studies, symptoms of OCD demonstrated a response latency; none of the fluoxetine treatment groups achieved statistically significantly greater improvement of symptoms than the placebo group until week-five. Although the 20 mg/day fluoxetine group did significantly better than placebo both in obsessions and compulsions, the effect on Y-BOCS obsession sub-score was somewhat more pronounced ($p<0.001$) than the effect on compulsions ($p<.01$), suggesting that even at low doses, fluoxetine reduced intrusions.

Data from the 355 USA patients of the Tollefson, Rampey *et al.* (1994) study were pooled together with data from 217 Europe and South Africa patients of the Montgomery *et al.* (1993) study, and were re-analyzed by Wood, Tollefson, and Birkett (1993). The Montgomery *et al.* study was identical in design to the Tollefson, Rampey *et al.* study, except that the duration of treatment in the former study was eight instead of 13 weeks. In order to ensure the closest possible comparability of data between these two protocols, the data from the USA cohort was truncated to include only the first nine weeks of treatment.

In this study, pairwise comparison of fluoxetine against placebo showed a marginally greater improvement in Y-BOCS total score for patients receiving 20 mg of fluoxetine daily, and a significantly higher response rate in those receiving 40 mg or 60 mg daily. Overall, treatment groups differed significantly in the change from baseline to end-point for Y-BOCS total score ($p = 0.002$), obsessions score ($p = 0.002$) and compulsions score ($p=0.012$). Pairwise analyses confirmed a greater effect of all three fixed doses of fluoxetine on the Y-BOCS total and obsessions score, and an effect of fluoxetine at 60 mg/day on the compulsion score in this pooled analysis. Mean baseline-to-end-point change in the Y-BOCS obsession scores for the 20, 40, 60 mg/day fluoxetine treatment groups and placebo group were 2.3, 2.7, and 3.2 versus 1.2 for placebo. These changes correspond to a mean decrease in Y-BOCS obsession scores of 20 percent, 23 percent, 27 percent, versus ten percent for placebo.

A separate responder rate analysis was undertaken to define those patients who showed a clinically useful response to treatment during the studies. The definition of response was based on both a decrease in the Y-BOCS total score of 25 percent and the more stringent threshold of 35 percent. There was clear evidence of response in fluoxetine treated patients in contrast to placebo. Using the 25 percent criterion, 40 percent to 52 percent responded in the fluoxetine groups and 29 percent in the placebo group. Using the 35 percent criterion, 29 percent to 39 percent responded in the fluoxetine groups and 17 percent in the placebo group.

Fluoxetine was also found effective in two extension studies where continuation treatment was associated with a maintained/improved symptomatic profile in most cases. In the Montgomery *et al.* (1993) study, 161 patients continued in a 16-week extension evaluation, while a group of patients from the Tollefson, Rampey *et al.* study (1994) were further followed up for an additional 24-week period (Tollefson, Birkett *et al.*, 1994). In this study, treatment responders continued blinded treatment, whereas acute fixed-dose non-responders began an open-label trial on their maximally tolerated dose (up to 80 mg daily) for 24 weeks. As in the Montgomery *et al.* study, responders maintained their acute treatment gains. In addition, all three doses of fluoxetine (20, 40, and 60 mg) were associated with further Y-BOCS improvement over the 24-week extension, and fluoxetine 60 mg achieved a statistically significantly greater reduction in Y-BOCS than placebo during the continuation. Open-label study subjects benefited from dose titration, with two-thirds achieving a clinical response during the subsequent 24 weeks.

The efficacy of fixed daily doses of fluoxetine (20, 40, or 60 mg/day) was tested again in an eight-week double-blind placebo-controlled trial in a group of 53 Austrian OCD patients where response was prospectively defined as at least a 25 percent reduction on the Y-BOCS (Eglseer & Zapotoczky, 1999). Patients treated with at least 40 mg fluoxetine per day showed significantly higher response rates than did those receiving either placebo or fluoxetine 20 mg/day. Interestingly, and contrary to previous studies, compulsions were more reduced than obsessions. This finding may be explained by the fact that the authors also observed a strong placebo effect, which, according to them, was largely reflected in the improvement in the Y-BOCS compulsion score.

Fluoxetine was also tested in children and adolescents with OCD (Riddle *et al.*, 1992). In this double-blind, placebo-controlled study, 14 children and adolescents with OCD, aged eight to 15 years old, were treated with a 20 mg/day fixed dose of fluoxetine. Assessment of symptom severity at baseline and after four and eight weeks was done through the Children Y-BOCS (CY-BOCS). After eight weeks of treatment, obsessive compulsive symptom severity for the subjects receiving fluoxetine decreased significantly. Mean total CY-BOCS decreased from 24.3 ± 4.2 to 13.6 ± 5.7 (mean decrease = 44 percent). Scores decreased substantially and significantly for both obsessions (54 percent) and compulsions (33 percent), though somewhat more for obsessions. The mean obsession score decreased from 12.3 ± 2.1 to 5.6 ± 3.3, and the mean compulsion score decreased from 12.0 ± 2.4 to 8.0 ± 4.2.

Fluoxetine was also tested against clomipramine in the treatment of OCD (Lopez-lbor Jr. *et al.*, 1996). In this eight-week, double-blind controlled study, 55 OCD patients were allocated to either 40 mg/day of fluoxetine or 150 mg/day of clomipramine. Like other comparisons with clomipramine, efficacy for both drugs was comparable. The primary efficacy criterion, the Y-BOCS total score, did not show any significant differences between treatments. Response rate was higher with clomipramine, using a 25 percent decrease in Y-BOCS total score as response threshold, but there were no significant differences between treatment groups using a 35 percent threshold.

Sertraline

Sertraline is also a selective serotonin reuptake inhibitor (SSRI) and inhibits serotonin uptake even more selectively than clomipramine, fluoxetine or fluvoxamine. This serotonergic effect made researchers suppose that sertraline would be effective in treating OCD. The first double-blind, placebo controlled trial of sertraline in OCD was published by Jenike *et al.* in 1990. In this ten-week study, ten patients received sertraline, up to 200 mg/day, and nine received placebo. Total Y-BOCS scores decreased from 22.8 (SD = 6.0) to 20.6 (SD = 9.2) in the sertraline group and from 22.8 (SD = 4.8) to 22.3 (SD = 7.8) in the placebo group. Sertraline was thus not found effective in the treatment of OCD in this small group of patients. However, subsequent larger studies have shown sertraline to be a potent medication for the treatment of OCD (Bisserbe, Lane, & Flament, 1997; Chouinard *et al.*, 1990; Greist *et al.*, 1995, and Kronig *et al.*, 1999).

In a study by Greist *et al.* (1995), 324 non-depressed out-patients with OCD were randomly assigned to 12 weeks of treatment with one of three fixed dosages of sertraline (50, 100 or 200 mg/day) or placebo. Clinical improvement according to the Y-BOCS was significantly greater in both the 50 mg/day and the 200 mg/day sertraline dosage groups compared to placebo, whereas 100 mg/day of sertraline did not show significantly greater improvement than placebo. All three sertraline treatment groups exhibited greater improvement from baseline than the placebo group, beginning at one week of double-blind treatment and continuing to the end of the study. The largest mean treatment effect was observed in the 200 mg/day group, although differences among sertraline groups were neither statistically significant nor large. In the pooled sertraline groups (*n* = 240), the Y-BOCS score decreased a mean of 23 percent from baseline to week-12, compared with 15 percent in placebo-treated patients. Treatment responders had a significantly lower baseline Y-BOCS total score (22.4 ± 4.9) than treatment nonresponders (24.4 ± 5.2). Unfortunately, the authors did not report separate results on the Y-BOCS obsession and compulsion scores; so no information is available on possible differential effects of sertraline on obsessions and compulsions.

As with the other SSRIs, sertraline was compared to clomipramine as the standard. In the 16-week, double-blind Bisserbe *et al.* (1997) study, 168 randomized patients received at least one dose of medication; 86 received sertraline and 82 clomipramine. Initial daily doses of sertraline and clomipramine were 50 mg. After a minimum of four weeks, these doses could be increased by 50 mg increments every two weeks to a maximum of 200 mg daily if the response was thought inadequate. Mean final daily doses were modest: clomipramine, 90 mg and sertraline, 129 mg. Mean baseline Y-BOCS totals were 27.7 for sertraline and 27.4 for clomipramine, placing most patients within the severe OCD range

(Y-BOCS>26). Treatment with either medication produced statistically significant decreases in Y-BOCS scores from week-one onwards, and the response profile of the two drugs was similar. Nevertheless, sertraline demonstrated greater efficacy than clomipramine in the intent-to-treat patient group: mean baseline to final visit reductions in YBOCS were 51 percent for sertraline and 43 percent for clomipramine. Seventy-two percent of sertraline-treated patients had at least a 35-point decrease in total Y-BOCS score from baseline to final visit, compared to 65 percent of clomipramine-treated patients. According to the authors, the difference in efficacy between the treatments was almost wholly accounted for by a greater number of withdrawals due to the poor patient tolerance for clomipramine.

The magnitude of improvement in obsessive and compulsive symptoms at the final visit was also greater with sertraline than with clomipramine. Further, the treatment difference was statistically significant for obsessions and approached significance for compulsions. The mean change from baseline to final visit in the amount of time occupied by obsessive thoughts (YBOCS item-1) and the amount of time spent performing compulsive behaviors (Y-BOCS item-6) also significantly favored sertraline over clomipramine. The authors did not report on the other Y-BOCS items. Treatment response was exceptionally good in this study, since approximately two thirds of patients had a greater than 35 percent reduction in total Y-BOCS. Strict entry criteria and the absence of placebo may have resulted in the selection of a more severely ill patient population in whom it was possible to detect greater therapeutic effects.

Sertraline was again compared to placebo in a double-blind multi-center study of 12 weeks duration in 167 non-depressed outpatients with moderate to severe OCD (Kronig *et al.*, 1999). Sertraline was administered at a starting dose of 50 mg/day, with flexible titration up to 200 mg/day. Patients were randomly assigned and received at least one dose of double-blind medication: 86 received sertraline and 81 received placebo. Significantly greater improvement in the sertraline group first became apparent by the end of week-three on the Y-BOCS, and all efficacy measures showed significantly greater improvement in the sertraline group from the end of week-eight until the end of week-12. Unfortunately, sertraline's effect on obsessions, relative to compulsions was not evaluated.

The sustained efficacy of sertraline in patients with OCD has also been evaluated. Rasmussen *et al.* (1997) investigated the efficacy of sertraline during long-term treatment of 59 patients with OCD. Treatment responders who completed a one-year double-blind, fixed dose-study, comparing sertraline and placebo, subsequently entered a one year open extension. Placebo responders ($n = 8$) differed from sertraline responders ($n = 51$) in that they were less impaired at baseline (Y-BOCS of 18.5 versus 23.4), and they exhibited less improvement during double-blind treatment (−6.1 versus −11.4). In the open label phase, all patients received sertraline, starting at 50 mg per day, titrated in 50 mg increments to a maximum dose of 200 mg according to clinical response. At end-point, the mean Y-BOCS score for all patients decreased by a further 3.6 points. Patients previously treated with placebo showed greater improvement after being switched to sertraline than those who received continued sertraline treatment. Patients who completed the study and received two full years of sertraline treatment ($n = 38$) exhibited a mean improvement of 15.6 points on the Y-BOCS. Again, no information about the effects of sertraline on obsessions versus compulsions was provided.

Paroxetine

Paroxetine is a potent selective inhibitor of serotonin with established effectiveness as an anti-depressant. Fewer studies have examined this newer medication. The effect of a flexible dose of paroxetine, compared with clomipramine and placebo, was assessed in a double-blind 12-week study of a large sample of 399 OCD patients (Zohar & Judge, 1996). Among other inclusion criteria, patients were included in the study if they had a base-line score of 16 or more on the Y-BOCS. Dose ranges were 20–60 mg daily for paroxetine, and 50–250 mg daily for clomipramine. In the paroxetine group, the majority of patients (53 percent) received a maximum dose of 60 mg/day. The most common maximum doses in the clomipramine group were 250 mg (30 percent) and 150 mg (21 percent). Mean daily doses across the study period were 37.5 mg for paroxetine and 113.1 mg for clomipramine. Both paroxetine and clomipramine were significantly superior to placebo in all primary efficacy variables. Reductions in Y-BOCS for both medications were apparent from week-two and continued progressively throughout the 12-week treatment period. Paroxetine and clomipramine were significantly superior to placebo at week-six, and this effect was maintained at weeks-eight and 12. Baseline depression did not appear to affect the change from baseline in the Y-BOCS total score.

Zohar and Judge defined response to treatment at week-12 as a reduction in Y-BOCS total score of 25 percent or greater. Response rates in the paroxetine and clomipramine groups were comparable (55.1 percent and 55.3 respectively) and significantly greater than the placebo response (35.4 percent) which was more substantial than in some other studies. Mean baseline-to-end-point Y-BOCS total score changes in the paroxetine and clomipramine groups were comparable (8.0 ± 8 and 8.0 ± 8.2 respectively) and significantly greater than in the placebo group (5.0 ± 7.9). These investigators also examined outcomes separately for obsessions and compulsions. Mean baseline-to-end-point Y-BOCS obsession score changes in the paroxetine and clomipramine groups were comparable (4.2 ± 4.5 and 4.1 ± 4.3 respectively) and significantly greater than in the placebo group (2.4 ± 4.4). Mean changes in compulsion scores were slightly lower and also comparable for both medications (3.8 ± 4.1 and 3.9 ± 4.5 respectively) and significantly greater than in the placebo group (2.6 ± 4.2).

Citalopram

Like other SSRIs, citalopram has been found to be effective in the treatment of OCD (Koponen *et al.*, 1997, cited in Koran, 1999; Montgomery, 1998; Mundo, Bianchi, & Bellosi, 1997). Citalopram has also been found to be effective with children and adolescents suffering from OCD (Thomsen, 1997). The potential clinical value of citalopram was examined in 11 boys and 12 girls aged nine–18 in an open-label trial of citalopram 10–40 mg (modal 40 mg) daily. After ten weeks of citalopram treatment, statistically significant improvements were reflected in CY-BOCS scores. Over 75 percent of these youth showed a marked improvement (four patients had more than 50 percent reduction in CY-BOCS scores) or moderate improvement (14 patients had 20 percent-50 percent reduction) in OCD symptoms.

Effects of Augmentation Strategies on OCD Symptoms

Although SSRIs are the mainstream of pharmacologic treatment for OCD, SSRI refractory patients seem to benefit by adding other classes of medication to the SSRI. A number of studies have examined the effect of adding various medications. In particular, risperidone, a novel anti-psychotic, was found to be effective in augmenting SSRI treatment of OCD (Jacobsen, 1995; Ravizza, Barzega, Bellino, Bogetto, & Mama, 1996; Saxena, Wang, Bystritsky, & Baxter, 1996). In the Jacobson (1995) study, nine OCD patients who had already failed to respond to one or more trials of SSRIs and/or clomipramine, participated in open add-on trials of risperidone. Before the addition of risperidone, all patients were taking sertraline 150 to 250 mg/day, and two patients were also taking clomipramine (50 and 200 mg/day). After the addition of a mean 3.6 mg dose of risperidone, the patients reported dramatic improvements in OCD symptoms and evidenced a significant decrease in mean Y-BOCS scores from 28.0 ± 8.7 to 15.6 ± 7.3.

In the Saxena *et al.* study (1996), 21 OCD patients who had failed to respond to at least one adequate trial of an anti-depressant and had a variety of comorbid disorders were treated openly with the combination of an anti-depressant (clomipramine, fluoxetine, fluvoxamine, paroxetine or sertraline) and risperidone (mean daily dose 2.75 mg). Of the 16 patients who were able to tolerate combined treatment, 14 (87 percent) had substantial reductions in obsessive compulsive symptoms, as measured by the Y-BOCS, within three weeks of initiating risperidone, and often within the first few days. Five of those patients had horrific mental imagery associated with their obsessions; all had dramatic responses to the addition of risperidone within three days. The case of a 59-year-old female patient is very interesting. She suffered from severe obsessive thoughts and horrific mental images of being violent to family members, as well as mild checking compulsions. Her obsessions had left her homebound and totally disabled. Her score on the obsession subscale of the Y-BOCS was 20. Risperidone was added to her regimen (clomipramine 150 mg/day and fluphenazine 5mg/day), and within two days her obsessions completely remitted. She remained asymptomatic for six months before experiencing a mild relapse (YBOCS obsession scale = ten).

In the Ravizza *et al.* (1996) study, 14 OCD patients who failed to respond to successive manipulations of their drug treatment were allocated to a risperidone augmentation eight week trial. Risperidone was added to 250 mg/day of clomipramine (seven patients) or to sertraline (50 mg/day) combined with 150 mg/day of clomipramine (seven patients). Both groups experienced statistically significant within-group reductions at end-point: Y-BOCS total scores decreased from 18.6 (SD = 3.2) to 14.8 (SD = 5.1) in the first group, and from 18.0 (SD = 3.2) to 13.0 (SD = 2.8) in the second group.

Since olanzapine, another novel anti-psychotic medication, has a serotonergic and dopaminergic receptor binding profile similar to that of risperidone, researchers tested the hypothesis that olanzapine augmentation would be beneficial in treatment-unresponsive OCD. Weiss *et al.* (Weiss, Potenza, McDougle, & Epperson, 1999) described a series of 10 patients with SSRI-refractory OCD who were treated with open-label olanzapine augmentation for 8 weeks. Of the nine patients who completed the trial, four demonstrated a complete remission or major improvement in OC symptoms, three had a partial remission, and two experienced no benefit. Koran, Ringold, & Elliot (2000) conducted an add-on 8-week study to a group of 10 treatment refractory OCD patients. Patients had already failed to respond to a mean of 3.3 SSRI trials, they were currently unresponsive to fluoxetine for at least ten weeks, and their mean baseline Y-BOCS was 29.0 (SD = 4.9). The addition of 10 mg/day of olanzapine had as a result a mean 16% decrease on Y-BOCS, and from the nine patients who completed the study, three were considered responders. Bogetto, Bellino, Vaschetto, & Ziero (2000) presented more favorable results from their 12-week open trial on olanzapine augmentation of fluvoxamine-refractory OCD. Twenty-three OCD non-responders to a six-month, open label trial with fluvoxamine (300 mg/day) entered a 3-month open-label trial of augmentation with olanzapine (5 mg/day). A significant decrease of mean Y-BOCS score between pre- and post-treatment (26.8 ± 3.0 vs. 18.9 ± 5.9) was found at endpoint, and ten patients (43.5 percent) were rated as responders (a decrease of 35 percent or more on Y-BOCS score and a rating of 'much improved' or 'very much improved' on the Clinical Global Impression). Interestingly, concomitant schizotypal personality disorder—a rather poor prognostic factor in SSRI studies—was a factor significantly associated with good response. Finally, the anti-obsessive effect of olanzapine was tested in a group of three schizophrenic patients with OC symptoms who were unsuccessfully treated with various conventional neuroleptics in combination with anti-obsessive agents (clomipramine or SSRIs). Within 5–8 weeks of initiation of olanzapine (10–20 mg/day) the Y-BOCS scores of the three patients decreased by 68–85 percent (Poyurovsky, Dorfman-Etrog, Hermest, Munitz, Tollefson, & Weizman, 2000).

The substantial reduction in OCD symptoms with this anti-psychotic medication is particularly interesting in view of its potent effect on psychotic mental phenomenon, delusions and hallucinations. These symptoms may be related to obsessional phenomena in the intrusive quality of the imagery and thought processes associated with both (see Chapter 14 in this volume).

Predictors of Outcome

Although a large body of evidence indicates the efficacy of pharmacotherapy in the treatment of OCD, a considerable percentage of these patients do not respond. As was evidenced in all studies, medication effects on OCD are not powerful and a large number of patients still suffer from residual symptoms, even in cases where patients were considered treatment responsive. Researchers have thus undertaken efforts to establish predictors of outcome. Unfortunately, so far, these have not included either beliefs or change in beliefs or other cognitive processing measures.

Ravizza, Barzega, Bellino, Bogetto, and Mama (1995) conducted a study to investigate clinical factors related to drug treatment response in OCD. Fifty-three OCD patients treated with either clomipramine or fluoxetine for six months, were divided into responders and non-responders to treatment. At admission, patients were evaluated using the Y-BOCS and Hamilton Rating Scales for depression and anxiety. The authors compared acute-phase patient characteristics and response to drug treatment. Response was defined as a decrease of at least 40 percent in the Y-BOCS total score and a rating of "improved" or "very improved" on the Clinical Global Impressions scale within 16 weeks of treatment and maintained over three consecutive evaluations. By the sixth month of treatment, 31 patients (58.5 percent) responded to either clomipramine or fluoxetine. Non-responders had earlier onset and longer duration of the disorder. In addition, they showed higher frequency of compulsions, washing rituals, chronic course, concomitant schizotypal personality disorder, and previous hospitalizations. A worse response to drug treatment was predicted in a stepwise multiple regression by concomitant schizotypal personality disorder, presence of compulsions, and longer illness length. These findings suggest that there are distinct types of OCD with respect to drug treatment response, and they provide indirect evidence of treatment specificity by identifying characteristics responsive to different modalities, which may be of value in the selection of patients for alternative treatments. Other personality characteristics, like avoidant, borderline, paranoid, and obsessive compulsive personality disorder, seem not to respond to an adequate trial of clomipramine (Baer *et al.*, 1992).

Pharmacotherapy research in OCD has established some tentative predictors of favorable response to drugs. The longer the duration of symptoms, the less likely they are to respond. A history of precipitating events in the development of OCD has been positively correlated with a more favorable outcome. Further, compared to all other types of symptoms, checking rituals are more likely to respond to pharmacotherapy with an SSRI, whereas patients with washing and cleaning compulsions may be more likely to improve on clomipramine.

Although there is a clinical assumption that patients who fail to respond to one SSRI trial are less likely than treatment naive patients to respond to the next SSRI trial, most patients who have failed to respond to one drug do respond to another or to an augmenting strategy. However, it may take several trials to identify the SSRI or augmenting drug that is effective for the patient (Koran, 1999). Overall, then, relatively few factors distinguish responders from non-responders to serotonergic medications. No studies have examined predictors of changes in obsessions compared to compulsions, and as noted earlier, few have attempted to determine the effect of changes in obsessions on compulsive behavior. Since beliefs and attitudes have not been routinely assessed in medication trials, their role as predictors, as well as with their role as possible mediators of outcome, is unknown.

Comparisons of Medication Treatment with Cognitive–Behavior Therapy

At the present time, behavior therapy (BT) and cognitive–behavior therapy (CBT) are the only established alternative treatments to pharmacotherapy. A meta-analysis of 16 studies of BT conducted between 1974 and 1992 reported that an average of 76 percent of patients (range 50–100 percent) were responders at behavior therapy at a mean treatment follow-up of 29 months (range 6–72 months) (Foa & Kozak, 1996). Most responders were much or very much improved, and some experienced complete freedom from symptoms. Although few of these studies included a comparison group, this meta-analysis gives a very clear picture of the effectiveness of BT in OCD.

The efficacy of combined BT and pharmacotherapy for OCD is controversial. In a review of relevant studies, Steketee (1993) concluded that this combination has shown little advantage over behavior therapy alone. Preliminary findings from a trial by Kozak, Liebowitz, and Foa (2000) also support this conclusion. However, a more recent but small sample study comparing cognitive–behavior therapy and medication in the treatment of obsessive compulsive disorder provides evidence in favor of the combination (O'Connor, Todorov, Robillard, Borgeat, & Brault, 1999). OCD patients received one of four treatments: medication and CBT simultaneously ($n = 9$), CBT only ($n = 6$), medication while on a wait-list for CBT ($n = 6$), or no treatment while on a wait-list for CBT ($n = 5$). Multi-variate analyses revealed that Y-BOCS scores and clinical ratings significantly improved after treatment in all groups except the non-treatment wait-list control group. Subjects in the two treatment groups receiving CBT showed reduced strength in their obsessional beliefs. The subsequent administration of CBT to those groups on the wait-list also decreased the strength of their primary obsessional beliefs and beliefs about the consequences of not performing the rituals. Results of this small sample study suggest that either CBT or medication alone is more effective than no treatment. The combination seems to potentiate treatment efficacy, and, according to the authors, it is more clinically beneficial to introduce CBT after a period of medication rather than to start both therapies simultaneously.

Conclusions

Certain antidepressants have proven effective in the treatment of OCD. Those anti-depressants that have a selective or more prevalent inhibition in the serotonin re-uptake are significantly potent in the reduction of OC symptomatology, whereas anti-depressants that do not affect serotonin regulation are ineffective. For those drugs that are effective in the treatment of OCD, the reduction in obsessions is almost parallel to the reduction of compulsions. Nevertheless, it seems that reduction in obsessions generally precedes reduction in compulsions. Several of these drugs seem to exhibit a trend toward a more powerful anti-obsessive than anti-compulsive efficacy. Whether this reflects a trend that would be apparent with obsessional beliefs is unclear.

Since the development of the Yale–Brown Obsessive Compulsive Scale in 1989, most studies have used reductions in Y-BOCS as their primary efficacy measure, thereby allowing comparisons among studies. Nevertheless, study-specific patient characteristics make that kind of effort difficult. Some studies, for example, used a greater than 16 score on Y-BOCS as an inclusion criterion, whereas others used a greater than 20 score. Therefore, patients in some studies were more severely ill than those in other studies. Another difficulty in comparing trials is the length of the study period; it is impossible to compare the results of an eight week trial to those from a 13 week trial, especially when the full effect of a drug may take 12 weeks to appear.

Concerning Y-BOCS as a primary efficacy measure, some studies calculated and presented only a total Y-BOCS score, whereas others also presented separate results for the obsession and compulsion scores. In the latter case, it is possible to determine the medication effect on cognitions related to obsessional thinking, but only by indirect inference. The actual effect of medications on beliefs and attitudes associated with obsessive intrusions is unknown. In fact, the only studies that have assessed cognitive factors in medicated patients have done so in the context of combined CBT or CT and medications so that the separate effect of drugs alone is unknown (e.g. van Oppen *et al.*, 1995; Emmelkamp & Beens, 1991).

In general, medications can reduce severity of obsessive and compulsive symptoms, as measured by the Y-BOCS total score, from approximately 25 percent to 50 percent, while reducing the severity of obsessions by approximately 20 percent to 30 percent. When response was defined as reduction in Y-BOCS total score of 25 percent, response rates ranged from 33 percent to 55 percent. When response was defined as reduction in Y-BOCS total score of 35 percent, response rates ranged from 30 percent to 45 percent. Response rates were higher in patients with an initial severe condition, or those naive to medication, like children and adolescents.

In summary, although it seems likely that medications do change OCD cognitions and consequently, obsessions and compulsions, their effect usually results in a partial response, and seldom in a complete remission. Nevertheless, OCD is a difficult condition to treat and even partial reduction in obsessive and compulsive problems is welcome on the part of both patient and treatment provider.

References

Baer, L., Lenike, M. A., Black, D. W., Treece, C., Rosenfeld R., & Greist J. (1992). Effects of Axis I diagnoses on treatment outcome with clomipramine in 55 patients with obsessive–compulsive disorder. *Archives of General Psychiatry, 49*, 862–866.

Bisserbe, I. C., Lane R. M., & Flament M. F. (1997). A double-blind comparison of sertraline and clomipramine in out-patients with obsessive–compulsive disorder. *European Journal of Psychiatry, 12*, 82–93.

Bogetto, F., Bellino, S., Vaschetto, P., & Ziero, S. (2000). Olanzapine augmentation of fluvoxamine-refractory obsessive–compulsive disorder (OCD): A 12-week open trial. *Psychiatry Research, 96*, 91–98.

Chouinard, G., Goodman, W., Greist, J., Jenike, M., Rasmussen, S., White, K., Hackett, E., Gaffney, M., & Bick, P. (1990). Results of a double-blind placebo controlled trial of a new serotonin n uptake inhibitor, sertraline, in the treatment of obsessive–compulsive disorder. *Psychopharmocology Bulletin, 26*, 279–284.

Coleman, B. S., & Block B. A. (1982). Fluvoxamine maleate, a serotonergic anti-depressant: A comparison with clomipramine. *Progress in Neuropsychopharmacology and Biological Psychiatry, 6*, 475–478.

den Boer, J. A., & Westenberg, H. G. M. (1997). *Focus on obsessive–compulsive spectrum disorders.* Amsterdam: Syn Thesis Publishers.

Eglseer, K., & Zapotoczky, H. G. (1999). Efficacy of fluoxetine in Austrian patients with obsessive–compulsive disorder. *Wiener Klinische Wochenschrift, 111*, 439–442.

Emmelkamp, P. M. G., & Beens, H. (1991). Cognitive therapy with obsessive–compulsive disorder: A comparative evaluation. *Behaviour Research and Therapy, 29*, 293–300.

Feighner, J. P., & Boyer, W. F. (1996). *Selective serotonin re-uptake inhibitors.* Chichester: Wiley.

Foa, E. B., & Foa, U. G. (1982). Differentiating depression and anxiety: Is it possible? Is it useful? *Psychophamocology Bulletin, 18*, 62–68.

Foa, E. B., & Kozak, M. I. (1996). Psychological treatment of obsessive–compulsive disorder. In M. R. Mavissakalian & R. F. Prien (eds) *Long-term treatments of anxiety disorders*. Washington, DC: American Psychiatric Press.

Fontaine, R., & Chouinard, G. (1986). An open clinical trial of fluoxetine in the treatment of obsessive–compulsive disorder. *Journal of Clinical Psychopharmacology, 6*, 98–100.

Freeman, G. P. L., Trimble, M. R., Deakin, W. J. F., Stokes, T. M., & Ashford, J. J. (1994). Fluvoxamine versus clomipramine in the treatment of obsessive–compulsive disorder: A multi-center, randomized, double-blind, parallel group comparison. *Journal of Clinical Psychiatry, 55*, 301–305.

Goodman, W. K., Kozak, M. I., Liebowitz, M., & White, K. L. (1996). Treatment of obsessive–compulsive disorder with fluvoxamine: a multi-centre, double-blind, placebo-controlled trial. *Journal of Clinical Psychopharmacology, 11*, 21–29.

Goodman, W. K., Price, L. H., Rasmussen, S. A., Delgado, P. L., Heninger, G. R., & Charney, D. S. (1989). Efficacy of fluvoxamine in obsessive–compulsive disorder. *Archives of General Psychiatry, 46*, 36–44.

Greist, J., Chouinard, G., DuBoff, E., Halaris, A., Kim, S. W., Koran, L., Liebowitz, M., Lydiard, B., Rasmussen, S., White, K., & Sikes, C. (1995). Double-blind parallel comparison of three dosages of sertraline and placebo in outpatients with obsessive–compulsive disorder. *Archives of General Psychiatry, 52*, 289–295.

Guelfi, I. D., Dreyfus, I. F., & Pichot, P. (1983). A double-blind controlled clinical trial comparing fluvoxamine with imipramine. *British Journal of Clinical Pharmacology, 15*, 411S–417S.

Guy, W., Wilson, W. H., Ban, T. A., King, D. L., Manov, G., & Fjetland, O. K. (1984). A double-blind clinical trial of fluvoxamine and imipramine in out-patients with primary depression. *Drug Development Research, 4*, 143–153.

Insel, T. M., Shrivastava, R. K., Mukheriee, S., Coleman, R. S., & Michael, S. T. (1983). A double-blind placebo-controlled study of fluvoxanime and imipramine in out-patients with primary depression. *British Journal of Clinical Pharmacology, 15*, 433S–438S.

Insel, T. R., Murphy, D. L., Cohen, R. M., Alterman, I., Kilts, C., & Linnoila, M. (1983). Clomipramine and clorgyline in OCD. *Archives of General Psychiatry, 40*, 605–612

Jacobsen, F. M. (1995). Risperidone in the treatment of affective illness and obsessive–compulsive disorder. *Journal of Clinical Psychiatry, 56*, 423–429.

Jenike, M. A., Baer, L., & Minichiello, W. E. (1986). *Obsessive–compulsive disorder: theory and management*. Chicago: Year Book Medical.

Jenike, M. A., Baer, L., Summergrad, P., Minichiello, W. E., Holland, A., & Seymour, R. (1990). Sertraline in obsessive–compulsive disorder: a double-blind comparison with placebo. *American Journal of Psychiatry, 147*, 923–928.

Jenike, M. A., Buttolph, L., Baer, L., Ricciardi, J., & Holland, A. (1989) Open trial of fluoxetine in obsessive–compulsive disorder. *American Journal of Psychiatry, 7*, 909–911.

Koponen, H., Lepola, U., Leinonen, E., Lakinen, R., Penttinen, J., & Turtonen, J.(1997). Citalopram in the treatment of obsessive–compulsive disorder: an open pilot study. *Acta Psychiatrica Scandinavica, 96*, 343–346.

Koran, L. M., McElroy, S. L., Davidson, J. R. T., Rasmussen, S. A., Hollander, E., & Jenike, M. A. (1996). Fluvoxamine versus clomipramine for obsessive–compulsive disorder: A double-blind comparison. *Journal of Clinical Psychopharmacology, 16*, 121–129.

Koran, L. M. (1999). *Obsessive–compulsive and related disorders in adults: A comprehensive clinical guide*. Cambridge University Press, Cambridge.

Koran, L. M., Ringold, A. L., & Elliot, M. A. (2000). Olanzapine augmentation for treatment-resistant obsessive-compulsive disorder. *Journal of Clinical Psychiatry, 61*, 514–517.

Kozak, M. J., Liebowitz, M. R., & Foa, E. B. (2000). Cogniotive behavior therapy and pharmacotherapy for obsessive–compulsive disorder: The NIMH-sponsored collaborative study. In W. K. Goodman, M. V. Rudorfer, & J. D. Maser (2000). *Obsessive–compulsive disorder: Contemporary issues in treatment.* London: Erlbaum Associates.

Kronig, M. I. J., Apter, I., Asnis, G., Bystritsky, A., Curtis, G., Ferguson, I., Landbloom, R., Munjack, D., Riesenberg, R., Robinson, D., Roy-Byrne, P., Phillips, K., & Du Pont, I. J. (1999). Placebo-controlled, multi-center study of sertraline treatment for obsessive–compulsive disorder. *Journal of Clinical Psychopharmacology, 19,* 172–176.

Levine, R., Hofinan, I. S., Knipple, E. D., & Kenin, M. (1989). Long-term fluoxetine treatment of a large number of obsessive–compulsive patients. *Journal of Clinical Psychopharmacology, 9,* 281–283.

Lopez-lbor, Jr., I. L., Saiz, I., Gottraux, I., Note, I., Villas, R., Bourgeois, M., Hernandez, M., & Gomez Perez, I. C. (1996). Double-blind comparison of fluoxetine versus clomipramine in the treatment of obsessive–compulsive disorder. *European Neuropsychopharmacology, 6,* 111–118.

Marks, I. M. (1987). *Fears, phobias, and rituals: Panic, anxiety, and their disorders.* New York: Oxford University Press.

Marks, I. M., Stern, R. S., Mawson, D., Cobb, I., & McDonald, R. (1980). Clomipramine and exposure for OCD-compulsive rituals. *British Journal of Psychiatry, 136,* 1–25.

Mawson, D., Marks, I. M., & Ramm, E. (1982). Clomipramine and exposure for chronic OC rituals: III. Two-year follow-up. *British Journal of Psychiatry, 140,* 11–18.

Montgomery, S. A. (1980). Clomipramine in obsessional neurosis: A placebo-controlled trial. *Pharmacological Medicine, 1,* 189–195.

Montgomery, S. A. (1998, December). *Citalopram treatment in OCD: Results from a double-blind, placebo-controlled trial.* Paper presented at the 37th American College of Neuropsychopharmacology Annual Meeting, Puerto Rico.

Montgomery, S. A., Mcintyre, A., Osterheider, M., Sarteschi, P., Zitterl, W., Zohar, I., Birkett, M., Wood, A. J., Beckmann, H., Gassachia, M., Freeman, C. P. L., Giberti, F., Hand, I., Kemali, D., & Lauwers, C. (1993). A double-blind, placebo-controlled study of fluoxetine in patients with DSM-III-R obsessive–compulsive disorder. *European Neuropsychopharmacology, 3,* 143–152.

Mundo, E., Bianchi, L., & Bellosi, L. (1997). Efficacy of fluvoxamine, paroxetine, and citalopram in the treatment of obsessive–compulsive disorder: a single-blind study. *Journal of Clinical Psychopharmacology, 17,* 267–271.

O'Connor, K., Todorov, C., Robillard, S., Borgeat, F., & Brault, M. (1999). Cognitive–behavior therapy and medication in the treatment of obsessive–compulsive disorder: A controlled study. *Canadian Journal of Psychiatry, 44,* 64–71.

Poyurovsky, M., Dorfman-Etrog, P., Hermesh, H., Munitz, H., Tollefson, G. D., & Weizman, A. (2000). Beneficial effect of olanzapine in schizophrenic patients with obsessive-compulsive symptoms. *International Clinical Psychopharmacology, 15,* 169–173.

Rachman, S., & de Silva, P. (1978). Abnormal and normal obsessions. *Behavior Research and Therapy, 16,* 233–248.

Rasmussen, S., Hackett, E., DuBoff, E., Greist, J., Halaris, A., Koran, L. M., Liebowitz, M., Lydiard, R. E., McElroy, S., Mendels, J., & O'Connor, K. (1997). A 2-year study of sertraline in the treatment of obsessive–compulsive disorder. *Journal of Clinical Psychopharmacology, 12,* 309–316.

Rauch, S. L., & Jenike, M. A. (1993). Neurobiogical models of obsessive–compulsive disorder. *Psychosomatics, 34,* 20–32.

Ravizza, L., Barzega, G., Bellino, S., Bogetto, F., & Mama, G. (1995). Predictors of drug treatment response in obsessive–compulsive disorder. *Journal of Clinical Psychiatry, 56,* 368–373.

Ravizza, L., Barzega, G., Bellino, S., Bogetto, F., & Mama, G. (1996). Therapeutic effects and safety of adjunctive risperidone in refractory obsessive–compulsive disorder. *Psychopharmacology Bulletin, 32*, 677–682.

Riddle, M. A., Scahill, L., King, R. A., Hardin, M. T., Anderson, G. M. Ort, S. I., Smith, J. C., Leckman, J. F., & Cohen, D. J. (1992). Double-blind crossover trial of fluoxetine and placebo in children and adolescents with obsessive–compulsive disorder. *Journal of the American Academy of Child and Adolescent Psychiatry, 31*, 1062–1069.

Salkovskis, P. M., & Harrison, J. (1984) Abnormal and normal obsessions: A replication. *Behaviour Research and Therapy, 22*, 549–552.

Saxena, S., Wang, D., Bystritsky, A., & Baxter, L. R. (1996). Risperidone augmentation of SRI treatment for refractory obsessive–compulsive disorder. *Journal of Clinical Psychiatry, 57*, 303–306.

Steketee, G. S. (1993). *Treatment of obsessive–compulsive disorder*. New York: Guilford.

Stern, R. S., Marks, I. M., Mawson, D., & Luscombe, D. K. (1980). Clomipramine and exposure for compulsive rituals: II. Plasma levels, side effects and outcome. *British Journal of Psychiatry, 136*, 161–166.

Thomsen, P. H. (1997). Child and adolescent obsessive–compulsive disorder treated with citalopram: findings from an open trial of 23 cases. *Journal of Child Adolescent Psychopharmacology, 7*, 157–166.

Thoren, P., Asberg, M., Gronholm, B., Jornestedt, L., & Traskman, L.(1980). Clomipramine treatment of obsessive–compulsive disorder. *Archives of General Psychiatry, 37*, 1281–1285.

Tollefson, G. D., Birkett, M., Koran, L., & Genduso, L.(1994). Continuation treatment of OGD: Double-blind and open-label experience with fluoxetine. *Journal of Clinical Psychiatry, 55*(10/Suppl), 69–78.

Tollefson, G. D., Rampey, A. H., Potvin, J. H., Jenike, M. A., Rush, I. A., Dominguez, R. A., Koran, L. M., Shear, K. M., Goodman, W., & Genduso, L. A. (1994). A multi-center investigation of fixed dose fluoxetine in the treatment of obsessive–compulsive disorder. *Archives of General Psychiatry, 51*, 559–567.

Turner, S. M., Jacob, R. G., Beidel, D. C., & Himmelhoch, J. (1985). Fluoxetine treatment of obsessive–compulsive disorder. *Journal of Psychopharmacology, 5*, 207–212.

van Oppen, P., de Haan, E., van Balkom, A. J. L. M., Spinhoven, P., Hoogduin, K., & van Dyck, R. (1995). Cognitive therapy and exposure in vivo in the treatment of obsessive–compulsive disorder. *Behaviour Research and Therapy, 33*, 379–390.

van Renynghe de Voxvrie (1968). Use of anafranil (G34586) in obsessive neurosis. *Acta Neurologica Belgique 68*, 787–792.

Volavka, L., Neziroglu, F., & Yaryura-Tobias, J. A. (1985). Clomipramine and imipramine in obsessive–compulsive disorder. *Psychiatric Research, 14*, 83–91.

Weiss, E. L., Potenza, M. N., McDougle, C. J., & Epperson, C. N. (1999). Olanzapine addition in obsessive-compulsive disorder refractory to selective serotonin reuptake inhibitors: An open-label case series. *Journal of Clinical Psychiatry, 60*, 524–527.

Wood, A., Tollefson, G. D., & Birkett, M. (1993). Pharmacotherapy of obsessive–compulsive disorder: Experience with fluoxetine. *International Clinical Psychopharmacology, 8*, 301–306.

Yaryura-Tobias, J. A., Neziroglu, F., & Bergman, L. (1976). Clomipramine for obsessive–compulsive neurosis: An organic approach. *Current Therapeutic Research, 20*, 541–547.

Zohar, I., & Insel, T. R. (1985). Obsessive–compulsive disorder: psychological approaches to diagnosis, treatment and pathophysiology. *Biological Psychiatry, 22*, 667–687.

Zohar, I., & Judge, R. (1996). Paroxetine versus clomipramine line in the treatment of obsessive–compulsive disorder. *British Journal of Psychiatry, 169*, 468–474.

Commentary on Therapy Effects on Cognition

Jose A. Yaryura-Tobias

As Emmelkamp, van Oppen, and van Balkom (2002) clearly state ". . . until the early 1970s, obsessive compulsive disorder (OCD) was considered a treatment refractory condition. . . ." Currently, therapy has advanced very much indeed, including the administration of specific anti-obsessive compulsive agents. Nonetheless, the negative response to treatment oscillates between 50 and 60 percent. This lack of response still requires an answer for those dedicated to the study of the treatment of OCD.

Emmelkamp and colleagues accept that the therapist's presence and the participation of a spouse during exposure exercises are unnecessary. However, the size of the samples and the small number of studies described here suggest caution in reaching definite conclusions. Another aspect to take into account is an absence of combined cognitive–behavior therapy (CBT) and pharmacotherapy. Some research indicates that the addition of medication does not enhance exposure and response prevention (ERP) efficacy.

Accepting that thought pathology may trigger obsessive compulsive behavior, the role of cognitive factors must be examined. Cognitive dominions may influence therapeutic outcome; for instance, inflated responsibility attached to checking, perfectionism, and thought–action fusion (TAF). This latter cognitive distortion is defined as an intrusive thought that can directly influence an external or internal event. In the context of this chapter, an intrusive thought is a synonym for an obsession. Historically, the description of an obsession includes the quality of intrusiveness. That is to say, an obsession is intrusive because it does not require a permit "to walk into the brain." Furthermore, it seems important to clarify for those who are not acquainted with cognitive semantics, that TAF has the same connotation as magical thinking. TAF *per se* may be a type of thought process closely related to a delusion. If so, TAF may influence the therapeutic outcome with CBT and/or pharmacotherapy in a different manner from the treatment of an intrusive thought. Consequently, patients suffering from TAF should be differently grouped for research and statistical purposes.

Emmelkamp *et al.* note that washing and cleaning may have a moral or purifying action (TAF). It is also possible that the symptom of a motor washing compulsion may occur without a cleaning or contamination cause. This behavior may have an ethological component, perhaps basal ganglia related, and may not respond to exposure and response prevention (ERP) intervention.

The authors examined three studies focused on the advantage or disadvantage of CT over ERP. Nine patients treated with rational emotional therapy were compared to nine patients treated with ERP. Results indicated that both forms of treatment were equally effective, and both lead to a reduction of social anxiety. For patients with depressed mood CT led to more significant improvement. In a second study a crossover design was carried out to compare ERP ($n = 11$) and CT ($n = 10$). Both treatment procedures were equally effective, but the small number of patients may have masked any significant differences between groups. Finally, a third study with a larger sample ($n = 71$) randomly assigned showed a better yet minimal improvement with CT over ERP. However, currently there is no evidence to justify one form of therapy over the other. One step forward is to investigate if there is a subset of OCD patients that responds more favorably to a specific type of therapy.

Emmelkamp *et al.* also examined the modifications of irrational beliefs as a result of treatment. Here, the term irrational belief is used in the context of cognitive therapy rather than as the irrational belief of a delusion. Some researchers use the word "unreasonableness" as part of the behavior therapy glossary with the same connotation as "irrational belief." We may assume that CT, by challenging the false belief structure, will better modify irrational beliefs. Findings from the study comparing CT and ERP confirm this. Once again, caution is advised when stating that CT leads to changes in irrational beliefs.

It seems important that therapy protocols analyze the factors influencing outcome. Research must search not only for the best therapeutic model, but also for successful clinical applications. Several outcome modifiers come to mind. The normal aspects of family participation, and the pathology of the patient's family are two equations to consider when assessing prognostic indicators. As we know, over 50 percent of the families of patients with OCD suffer from major psychiatric disorders. This psychopathology will undoubtedly affect the progression of OCD.

The presence of overvalued ideas and delusional components in OCD subtypes may require assessment and evaluation before starting therapy. Obsessiveness, delusions, and overvalued ideas, may replace each other, confounding the therapist and distorting the diagnostic assessment scales. One important factor is readiness for change. Many patients come for therapy to appease family members' concerns and demands. Another important yet neglected factor is the evaluation of personality disorders that can be strong determinants in therapeutic outcome. When we are faced with comorbid or parallel conditions, the treatment scenario becomes rather complex. For example, the presence of organicity (e.g., cerebral structural damage) will certainly demand a very different treatment approach and may suggest a guarded prognosis. Finally, is the patient being supported morally? One suggestion to improve treatment choice is to improve diagnostic procedures and the screening of factors mentioned above.

It is important to consider that behavior therapy modifies serotonin availability without the presence of medication (Neziroglu *et al.*, 1990) and that behavior therapy, without medication, changes the levels of cerebral glucose metabolic rate measured by positron emission tomography (Schwartz, Stoessel, Baxter, Martin, & Phelps, 1996). These two pieces of pilot and original research assist in integrating CT, BT, and pharmacotherapy and may eventually lead to a better understanding of the pathophysiology of OCD. However, this evidence is limited and further research is required.

Emmelkamp *et al.*'s chapter offers not only original results, but opens an avenue of ideas to advance the complex territory of OCD and its partially putative treatments.

Whittal and McLean's chapter (2002) presents the possibility of treating patients in groups when trained cognitive–behavior therapists are in short supply. This possibility is also an enticing way of reducing the cost of therapy. At the onset these authors state that medication and behavioral treatments are not the perfect solution to the problem of OCD. Currently, therapists choose between neurobiological or psychological models. Severe obsessionality may respond better to pharmacotherapy, as may OCD symptoms with a delusional flavor. In addition, patients demanding rapid solutions to their affliction may want to follow this model. CBT is indicated when medication is ineffective, a patient is a child, there is pregnancy, or the patient has other conditions that prevent the use of medication. The ideal situation is for psychologists and psychiatrists to work on a team basis.

Group treatment for OCD has been studied in eight uncontrolled studies that focused on exposure and response prevention. In total, 424 patients participated in these studies. The number of sessions varied from a total of seven to 24. In general, the outcome was of moderate efficacy, with an average degree of severity of 22 percent by YBOCS standards. Thus, moderately ill patients may be more suitable for participating in a group treatment model. This is encouraging because patients suffering from OCD not only are secretive but very self-centered, and will often choose individual therapy and attention.

Among the several group treatment trials presented, Himle's (2000) large uncontrolled study with 113 patients compared patients in a seven- or a 12-week behavioral treatment. Results were favorable, in spite of the short duration of the study, but the high attrition rate requires a cautious interpretation of the data. Further, good results were achieved after the exclusion of patients with comorbid depression or axis II pathology, two important factors that play a negative role in treatment outcome. Even combining CBT with medication may not remedy this situation. McLean, Whittal and colleagues report on an interesting study comparing contemporary group CBT with standard ERP. However, in this study medication was given to a substantial number of patients in the ERP group (62.5 percent) and in CBT group (35.5 percent). Although this combination may indirectly contaminate the design, this innovation of a combined approach speaks once again in favor of the need to blend treatment as much as possible. In this way the idea of treatment competition gives place to a better use of every therapeutic tool available.

As Whittal and McLean's chapter suggests, several principles may help to improve therapeutic outcome. These include: (1) a working alliance, (2) interpretation of the meaning of their thoughts, (3) appraisal of intrusive thoughts, (4) the power of thoughts, (5) the overimportance of thoughts, (6) the challenge to TAF, (7) the challenge to control over thoughts, (8) to challenge responsibility, (9) overestimation of danger, (10) challenge tolerance of uncertainty, and (11) challenging perfectionism. The therapeutic alliance is a pivotal factor to establish a working relationship between therapist and patient and vice versa. Some elements of suspiciousness are not alien in patients with OCD. Therefore, the alliance will reinforce trust, much needed for a better outcome.

The task of thought interpretation as an endeavor devoid of unwanted judgement seems important, and constitutes a phase of cognitive treatment that may not be put aside. Whittal *et al.* emphasize the need to modify the power of thoughts to foreshadow negative events. How effective is this challenge remains to be seen. An intrusive or obsessional thought is certainly characterized by the inability of the patient to reject it and to modify it. The modification process to weaken the belief will eventually take place, but this stage is closely related to the depth of the belief.

Can the patient reduce the overimportance of his/her thoughts? If not, the thought may remain because it is important. Gradual appraisal of the thought may help to change the attitude of the patient towards the importance of the thought. Not every thought that emerges from our brain is important. Most thoughts are inconsequential, and fall rather quickly into oblivion. However, an intrusive thought or obsession as per its own description remains present, and hence it is important, and difficult to displace, even if the patient agrees that it is useless, a common belief.

Perhaps it is not always possible or useful to challenge TAF beliefs. TAF seems to be constructed in a rather delusional system, or, with children, in neurodevelopmental elements of fantasy or grandiose thinking. TAF has been a common element in religion and magic as well. Unfortunately, except for schizophrenia and schizotypic disorders, TAF has not drawn the interest of those investigating OCD.

The greatest need of the patient with OCD is to be in control, although actually, it is the OCD process that controls the patient 100 percent. Are there alternate options to make the life of the patient less constricted, and how can this be added to the therapeutic plan?

Overwhelming responsibility accompanies moral issues, perfectionism, and over-importance of thoughts and the need to control thoughts (Salkovskis, 1985, 1989). The right and wrong posture, scrupulosity, the perfect moral response and attitude all interface in this challenging feature of cognitive treatment. Overestimation of danger is coupled with anxiety, a symptom quite frequent in OCD, and primary in any type of phobia. In this case objective and subjective probabilities are measured, and the general context is usually projected into the future. Intolerance of uncertainty or doubting creates two major problems: the need to check to be sure that nothing will occur, and the inability to make decisions. The latter affects the social and emotional growth of the affected person. In this case exposure over time (e.g., nothing will happen tomorrow) may play an important role. Perfectionism may be related to the rigidity of the thought process. Perfectionism is coupled to symmetry, and symmetry to the geometric desire of the brain for visual equilibrium. Therefore, OCD patients experience not only the need to be best, but also the need to be surrounded by the best as well.

In conclusion, this important chapter explores the need to supply skillful therapists for the growing number of untreated patients, and a recognition of the lack of money required to treat this population. In the USA the presence of HMO insurers plays an unacceptable function to hamper the treatment of the mentally ill.

References

Emmelkamp, P. M. G., van Oppen, P., & van Balkom, A. J. M. L. (2002). Cognitive changes during exposure and response prevention for OCD. In R. O. Frost & G. Steketee (eds), *Cognitive approaches to obsessions and compulsions: Theory, assessment and treatment*, (pp. 391–401). Oxford: Elsevier.

Himle, J. A. (2000). Behavioral group theapy for adults and children with OCD. Paper presented at the meeting of the Anxiety Disorders Association of America.

Neziroglu, F., Steelye, J., Yaryura-Tobias, J. A., *et al.* (1990). Effect of behavior therapy on serotonin level in obsessive–compulsive disorder. In C. N. Stefanis, A. D. Rabavilas, & C. R. Soldatos (eds), *Psychiatry: A world perspective* (Vol. 1). Amsterdam: Elsevier.

Salkovskis, P. M. (1985). Obsessional–compulsive problems: A cognitive–behavioral analysis. *Behaviour Research and Therapy, 25,* 571–583.

Salkovskis, P. M. (1989). Cognitive–behavioral factors and the persistence of intrusive thoughts in obsessional thoughts. *Behaviour Research and Therapy, 27,* 677–682.

Schwartz, J. M., Stoessel, P. W., Baxter, L. R., Martin, K. M., & Phelps, M. E. (1996). Systematic changes in cerebral glucose metabolic rate after successful behavior modification treatment of obsessive–compulsive disorder. *Archives of General Psychiatry, 53,* 109–113.

Whittal, M. L., & McLean, P. D. (2002). Group cognitive–behavioral treatment for OCD. In R. O. Frost & G. Steketee (eds), *Cognitive approaches to obsessions and compulsions: Theory, assessment and treatment,* (pp. 417–433). Oxford: Elsevier.

Commentary on Treatment

Paul M.G. Emmelkamp

The effects of behavior therapy, i.e. exposure in vivo and response prevention, with obsessive compulsive patients have been well established. Little evidence is yet available with respect to changes in cognitions as a result of behavioral treatment and even less so as a result of pharmacotherapy. The controlled studies discussed by Emmelkamp, van Oppen, & van Balkom (Chapter 21 in this volume) and Bouvard and Freeston (chapter 22 in this volume) found only limited changes in beliefs of obsessive compulsive disorder (OCD) patients, but only global measures were used, not specifically devised to assess specific beliefs associated with OCD.

Recently, McLean *et al.* (2001) reported the results of a controlled study in which the results of cognitive–behavior therapy were compared with the results of exposure and response prevention on specific measures for OCD beliefs: Thought–Action Fusion (TAF), Inventory of Beliefs Related to Obsessions (IBRO), and the Responsibility Attitude Scale. Unfortunately, results on these specific measures were rather meager. Neither at post-test, nor at follow-up was there differential improvement in OCD-related beliefs between cognitive–behavior therapy and exposure and response prevention. Perhaps even more disappointing, of the seven subscales used to assess cognitive changes (TAF-Moral; TAF-Likelihood for Others, TAF-Likelihood for Self; IBRO-Inflated Responsibility, IBRO-Overestimation of Threat, IBRO-Intolerance for Uncertainty, and the Responsibility Scale), only the Responsibility Scale was found to improve more in both treatment conditions than in the no-treatment control condition. Further, none of the cognitive measures predicted improvement.

As far as the Obsessional Beliefs Questionnaire (OBQ) and the Interpretation of Intrusions Inventory (III) are concerned, Emmelkamp and colleagues (Chapter 21 in this volume) found significant changes on these measures in OCD patients treated with exposure and response prevention. Thus, behavioral intervention without any cognitive therapy led to changes in OCD-related beliefs. Several recent studies (see Chapter 22 in this volume) indicate that cognitive–behavior therapy for OCD also results in significant reduction in certain beliefs or appraisals as measured by the OBQ and III. However, it has yet to be demonstrated that cognitive therapy for OCD will lead to significant larger changes in OCD-related beliefs than pure exposure and response prevention, though Whittal, Thordarson, and McLean (2001) reported some preliminary data suggesting this possibility. Unfortunately, studies have not yet investigated whether pharmacotherapy will also lead to changes in OCD-related belief domains as reviewed by Simos (this volume).

Cognitive Approaches to Obsessions and Compulsions – Theory, Assessment, and Treatment
Copyright © 2002 by Elsevier Science Ltd.
All rights of reproduction in any form reserved.
ISBN: 0-08-043410-X

This would not be that surprising, given the fact that behavior therapy, cognitive therapy and pharmacotherapy resulted in comparable changes in cognitions in social phobia (e.g. Mersch, Emmelkamp, & Lipa, 1991; Oosterbaan, van Balkom, Spinhoven, van Oppen, & van Dyck, in press; Scholing & Emmelkamp, 1993), hypochondriasis (Visser & Bouman, 2001), and depression (Emmelkamp, in press). Thus, while changes in OCD-related beliefs might be an important outcome measure and perhaps prophylactic in terms of relapse prevention, it is far from clear yet whether cognitive therapy is the only way to achieve those changes in beliefs.

An important question is whether the OBQ and the III are able to differentiate between responders and non-responders. Unfortunately, in the study of Emmelkamp and colleagues (see Chapter 21 in this volume) the pre-post changes on the OBQ did not discriminate responders from non-responders. However, on the intrusion measure responders could be clearly differentiated from non-responders. Both on the III-total score, as well on the subscales Importance of Thoughts and Responsibility, responders improved more than non-responders. Although more studies are needed before we may be in a position to evaluate the validity and utility of the OBQ and III as outcome measures, at present there is reason for some concern with respect to the OBQ.

Another question is whether these measures really tap the most important belief domains of OCD patients. In the study of Emmelkamp and colleagues (Chapter 21 in this volume) Tolerance for Uncertainty proved to be the main obsessional belief domain of the OBQ. The other belief domains of the OBQ were of much less importance for these patients. For example, responsibility was the most important belief domain for only four out of 28 patients. There was also some evidence that other belief domains not included in the OBQ may also be of importance in OCD. For example, in a study by Emmelkamp and Aardema (1999), Responsibility hardly accounted for any variance in obsessive compulsive behavior as assessed with the Padua-R (van Oppen, Hoekstra, & Emmelkamp, 1995). In contrast, Inverse Inference which is not included in the OBQ and III was found to be related to three of the five scales (checking, rumination and impulses) of the Padua-R. Inverse Inference is a confusion between what might be there (a probability), what is actually there (a certainty), and what is purely imaginary (fictitious identity) (O'Connor & Robillard, 1995) and is highly prevalent among OCD patients. Therefore, a scale to assess Inverse Inference would be a good candidate to assess additional belief changes in OCD patients beyond those assessed with the OBQ. Further, the study of Emmelkamp and Aardema (1999) clearly demonstrated that specific domains of obsessional beliefs accounted for specific obsessive compulsive behaviors. This latter finding suggests that perhaps we should use more idiosyncratic measures to assess belief changes in OCD patients.

Further, it is questionable whether scores on the III and the OBQ reflect irrational beliefs, or alternatively reflect mood states. The relative primacy of cognition and affect is an important issue in contemporary cognitive theories on emotional disorders. Changes on irrational belief questionnaires may represent epiphenomena of changes in mood states rather than changes in deeper cognitive structures. It is still an unresolved issue whether it is possible to measure deeper cognitive structures by means of self-report.

In sum, the validity of self-report measures of irrational beliefs to assess treatment outcome is still questionable: changes in scores on such questionnaires may not accurately reflect the timing and degree of changes in beliefs and may be confounded by changes in mood states.

References

Emmelkamp, P. M. G. (in press). Behavior therapy with adults In M. Lamberts (ed.), *Bergin and Garfields' Handbook of Psychotherapy and Behavior Change*. New York : Wiley.

Emmelkamp, P. M. G., & Aardema, A. (1999). Metacognition, specific obsessive–compulsive beliefs and obsessive–compulsive behavior. *Clinical Psychology and Psychotherapy, 6,* 139–145.

McLean, P. D., Whittal, M. L., Thordarson, D. S., Taylor, S., Sochting, I., Koch, W. J., Paterson, R., & Anderson, K. W. (2001). Cognitive versus behavior therapy in the group treatment of obsessive–compulsive disorder. *Journal of Consulting and Clinical Psychology, 69,* 205–214.

Mersch, P. P., Emmelkamp, P. M. G., & Lips, C. (1991). Social phobia; individual response patterns and the long term effects of behavioral and cognitive interventions. A follow-up study. *Behaviour Research and Therapy, 29,* 357–362.

O'Connor, K., & Robillard, S. (1995). Inference processes in obsessive–compulsive disorder: Some clinical observations. *Behaviour Research and Therapy, 33,* 887–896.

Scholing, A., & Emmelkamp, P. M. G. (1993). Exposure with and without cognitive therapy for generalized social phobia: Effects of individual and group treatment. *Behaviour Research and Therapy, 31,* 667–681

Oosterbaan, D. B., van Balkom, A. J. L. M., Spinhoven, Ph., van Oppen, P., & van Dyck, R. (in press). Cognitive therapy versus moclobemide in social phobia: A controlled study. *Clinical Psychology and Psychotherapy.*

van Oppen, P., Hoekstra, R. J., & Emmelkamp, P. M. G. (1995). The structure of obsessive–compulsive symptoms. *Behaviour Research and Therapy, 33,* 15–23.

Visser, S., & Bouman, T. K. (2001). The treatment of hypochondriasis: Exposure in vivo plus response prevention versus cognitive therapy. *Behaviour Research and Therapy, 39,* 423–442

Whittal, M. L., Thordarson, D. S., & McLean, P. M. (2001, July). *Cognitive change in cognitive and behavioral treatments for OCD.* Paper presented at the World Congress of Behavioral and Cognitive Therapies, Vancouver, BC.

Chapter 25

Studying Cognition in Obsessive Compulsive Disorder: Where to From Here?

Gail Steketee, Randy Frost and Kimberly Wilson

In his opening address to the World Congress of Behavioral and Cognitive Therapies in Vancouver, British Columbia, in 2001, Jack Rachman posed a conundrum for cognitive therapists. Notwithstanding the growing evidence for the efficacy of cognitive therapy (CT) in treating anxiety disorders, there is still little or no evidence that cognitive components of treatment add to the effectiveness of traditional behavior therapy. This is certainly the case with obsessive compulsive disorder (OCD) where CT or cognitive–behavior therapy (CBT) has compared favorably with exposure and response prevention (ERP), but has not added to its efficacy. Initial enthusiasm for CBT for OCD has been tempered by these findings. One interpretation of them is that we do not yet understand enough about cognition in OCD, especially how to measure and change it. This challenge brought the Obsessive Compulsive Cognitions Working Group (OCCWG) together in 1995 and served as the impetus for this book. In this chapter we draw on the work reviewed in this volume to pose questions we hope will lead to a clearer understanding of the role of cognition in OCD.

As Chapter one indicates, one of the first objectives of the OCCWG was to address the problem of too many measures of beliefs in OCD. By 1995 more than a dozen self-report measures were under development (OCCWG, 1997). With so many definitions and measures of similar constructs, research on cognitive aspects of OCD could be seriously delayed because results could not be compared across studies. We therefore identified as many researchers as possible who were involved in developing measures of beliefs to see if a group could be assembled to develop and test measures of OCD-related beliefs. This required a series of steps that Steve Taylor has outlined in Chapter one. The first phase of this goal has been accomplished. As reported in Chapter seven and discussed in several of the chapters on belief domains, two self-report measures, the Obsessive–Beliefs Questionnaire (OBQ) and Interpretation of Intrusions Inventory (III) were developed and tested in two waves of data collection (OCCWG, 2001, in preparation). The total sample of participants with OCD in these studies exceeded 350, certainly a very large group of patients. The instruments appear to be very promising with regard to reliability and validity. The existence of these measures opens the door for researchers studying cognition in OCD to speak the same language. The chapters in this volume suggest numerous directions for research on OCD-related beliefs. Here, we focus on some of the most important questions to answer with regard to these new measures.

Cognitive Approaches to Obsessions and Compulsions – Theory, Assessment, and Treatment
Copyright © 2002 by Elsevier Science Ltd.
ISBN: 0-08-043410-X

To What Extent are the Belief Domains Found in the OBQ and III Trait-like or State-like?

Cognitive theory regarding OCD holds that certain general belief domains (i.e., perfectionism, intolerance of uncertainty, overestimation of threat, responsibility, overimportance of thoughts, need to control thoughts as assessed by the OBQ) are trait-like and form a general predisposition for OCD and probably for other disorders. Some of these (e.g., responsibility, need to control thoughts, overimportance of thoughts) are also thought to occur in the context of immediate appraisals of ongoing processes and are thereby more state-like (OCCWG, 1997, 2001). However, findings from the first two stages of data collection and analysis did not reveal more stability in the OBQ, the measure of beliefs thought to be trait-like, than the III, the measure of appraisals thought to be state-like. One reason why a discussion of state versus trait may be useful beyond the stability of measurement issue is that trait-like beliefs resemble schemas or core beliefs as described by Beck, Rush, Shaw, and Emery (1979). These are long-standing, pervasive beliefs about the self that have obvious implications for development of disorders, treatment and relapse prevention. More research is needed to fully understand the way these play out in OCD, how to measure them, and what types of schemas dominate the clinical picture.

To What Extent are Belief/Appraisal Domains Independent?

As is evident from OCCWG research on importance and control of thoughts, threat estimation, tolerance for uncertainty, responsibility and perfectionism, there is considerable overlap among these cognitive domains. The most recent factor analyses of these domains from the OBQ suggest that only three themes are distinct for those with OCD: significance attached to thoughts, responsibility and perfectionism (OCCWG, in preparation; see also Chapter seven in this volume). Further examination of these domains may help to clarify the distinctive features of cognitive domains in OCD.

Which Domains are OCD-relevant and Which are OCD-specific?

One of the issues raised by Salkovskis (see Chapter four) and others is the need to distinguish beliefs and cognitive processes that are OCD-specific from beliefs and processes that are OCD-relevant. Certain of the dimensions of the OBQ, in particular, the tendency to overestimate the probability or severity of threat and intolerance of uncertainty, have been found in other disorders characterized by anxious and depressed mood (see also Chapters five and 11–13 in this volume). High levels of perfectionism have also been found in a number of other disorders as well (see Chapter six in this volume). Findings from the OBQ also suggest that these three domains are as prevalent among those with anxiety disorders as those with OCD (see Chapter seven). These cognitive domains may still be important for understanding the phenomenology, severity, development and even successful treatment of OCD, but it seems likely that they are not specific to OCD.

On the other hand, a full understanding of the etiology of OCD requires identification of OCD-specific phenomena as well. The recent study examining the OBQ and III provides some evidence that certain dimensions (i.e., responsibility, importance and control of thoughts) characterized OCD patients more than other anxiety disorder patients (OCCWG, in preparation). OCD-specific phenomena are important for understanding why OCD develops in some individuals but not others. To date almost no research is devoted to prevention of OCD, probably precisely because the factors that cause it are not yet clear. Although many investigators concur that OCD is most likely provoked by multiple factors (biological, genetic, environmental), we have no reliable formulae to predict who will develop OCD and who will not. It is difficult to conduct the longitudinal studies necessary to identify causal factors, and it is unlikely that researchers will receive funding to do so without defining markers for this disorder in children who can then be followed over time. Some cognitive features may prove to be markers, and therefore identification of cognitive aspects of children with clinical and subclinical OCD seems especially important. For this type of research, it is important to identify OCD-relevant features that are precursors to OCD (and to other disorders, especially anxiety and affective disorders), and OCD-specific ones that lead only to this condition.

Notwithstanding the importance of etiology and prevention, most research activity has focused on understanding the psychopathology of OCD (what is wrong rather than why) and on effective interventions (how to fix it), both biological and psychological. Especially in the latter case, understanding OCD-relevant features may be as important as understanding OCD-specific ones. If CT methods such as examining the evidence, downward arrow to identify core beliefs, and behavioral experiments help modify automatic thoughts and beliefs that maintain symptoms (whether depression, panic, worry or obsessions), it is of little import how OCD-specific these elements are. What is important is their relevance to the correction of maladaptive aspects of the condition. How clinicians correct these faulty appraisals and beliefs (e.g., by using a pie chart technique to reduce assumptions about responsibility) may be more peculiar to OCD than other conditions, but is probably not exclusive to this disorder.

So, when is it important to identify OCD-specific beliefs, appraisals, or other cognitive processes and when is OCD-relevance sufficient? We suggest that although specificity is important for understanding etiology and to some extent for prevention, it may be less critical to correcting the problem. With regard to assessment, then, cognitive measures must at least be relevant to OCD so pertinent pathology and outcomes can be measured. Measures that include pathology specific to OCD will be very useful in helping patients develop an understanding of their symptoms so they can participate fully in treatment procedures.

How are the Belief/Appraisal Domains Related to other Cognitive Phenomena like Insight and Motivation?

Insight into the problematic nature of OCD symptoms is discussed in Chapter ten. It is not yet clear how this cognitive feature relates to appraisals, beliefs and cognitive processes involved in OCD. Perhaps insight should be considered a representation of the strength of belief about probability and severity of danger pertinent to obsessive symptoms. Low insight may simply reflect strong beliefs that threat is likely and that harm will be serious. An extreme form may occur in those with psychotic thinking processes. Future research might address these questions.

We suspect most clinicians would agree that insight directly influences motivation for treatment, but that motivation is also affected by beliefs about what is to be gained and lost by engaging in therapy and by reducing symptoms and improving mood. Thus, insightful clients who believe that their behavior does not reflect reality are more likely to engage fully in treatment, as indicated by prompt attendance at sessions, completion of homework assignments, and expressions of interest in the treatment method and their learning. Consequently, their beliefs may be more malleable. Other factors affecting motivation may be beliefs about capacity to function successfully in other areas (e.g., employment, social situations) if symptoms are alleviated or beliefs about loss and/or gain of resources (e.g., disability payments, sympathy from others, special privileges). Again, we are not aware of research that has focused on linking types and strength of beliefs to motivation and insight in OCD. It seems important to identify impediments to engaging fully in therapies (whether CT, ERP or medications) and corrective strategies that will ultimately improve outcomes.

Are Some Belief/Appraisal Domains Identifiable in Children and Related to the Etiology of OCD?

A number of investigators have become interested in determining whether certain types of OCD symptoms are driven by certain beliefs or appraisals. As mentioned earlier, beliefs and cognitive appraisals in childhood may be important for the development of OCD. Thus, expanding the measurement of beliefs/appraisals to children may provide markers for later development of OCD. It is not clear yet whether the OBQ or III can be adapted for use with children and adolescents, and research on this topic is currently underway. In light of cognitive theories of OCD, it is of considerable interest to determine whether early onset of OCD is in fact associated with childhood interpretations of teachings, observations or experiences that subsequently can be identified, assessed and modified. For example, John March's therapy for children with OCD (e.g., "How I ran OCD off my land") contains a cognitive component that focuses on increasing understanding of OCD symptoms and altering attitudes toward them by externalizing the OCD as an oppressive illness (March & Mulle, 1998).

Another area that seems useful for future research is identifying cognitive buffers in children who have some predisposing factors (e.g., family history of OCD) who then do *not* go on to develop the disorder. Are there certain patterns of thinking that these children endorse beyond the *absence* of distorted thinking (e.g., a balanced view of responsibility, general cognitive flexibility, an attitude of acceptance)? Thus, working on cognitive assessment and intervention in children seems a promising avenue.

How Broadly Applicable is Cognitive Theory of OCD?

The theoretical models described in several chapters of this volume indicate a sequence of experiences thought to give rise to obsessions and compulsions. Intrusive internal experiences in the form of thoughts, images, impulses and even physical sensations are followed by interpretations or appraisals of these experiences. When these interpretations are negative, they are accompanied by unpleasant emotions such as guilt, anxiety, frustration and sadness. The individual seeks to reduce these emotions and gain control over the original intrusions by avoidance and also by mental or behavioral acts that become compulsive habits as they are repeated. A number of factors contribute to the negative interpretations, including pre-existing negative mood (e.g., depression) and beliefs based on parental teachings and modeling and prior experiences. This basic model of intrusions → beliefs → emotions → behaviors has been supported by various research studies too numerous to detail here, although further study is clearly needed.

This model applies not only to OCD, but also to other problems, a number of which are identified as OC-spectrum conditions (see Chapters 11–14). Differences among these disorders lie in which type (domain) of cognitive interpretations and beliefs are applied and what behaviors are used to cope with discomfort. For example, individuals with body dysmorphic disorder experience intrusive thoughts about their appearance, accompanied by appraisals and beliefs about the probability of social rejection that engender anxiety and depression and efforts to hide or alter the presumed defect. The model also appears to apply well to other anxiety disorders. For instance, in panic and generalized anxiety disorder intrusions occur in the form of body sensations or worrisome thoughts, accompanied by negative appraisals about threat and coping, anxiety and sometimes depression, and behavioral or mental efforts to reduce the presumed threat. Similar models can also be applied to hypochondriasis, eating disorders and perhaps depression (see Chapters 12 and 13). Elements of this cognitive model also pertain to schizophrenia (see Chapter 14) in which intrusions take the form of delusional thoughts, hallucinated images, or impulsive ideas accompanied by interpretations of these as real and often threatening and by negative emotions that drive corrective behaviors. Of course, other features such as biological substrates may also play important roles in many of these conditions, but the general model in which cognitive features (appraisals, beliefs and core beliefs) are central appears to be robust in its explanatory capacity for a wide variety of behavioral disorders. Thus, efforts to assess and modify various types of cognitions have become of paramount importance in moving research and intervention ahead.

How do Belief/Appraisal Domains Relate to OCD Relevant Cognitive Processes?

Although cognitive processes such as attention, perception, and memory are not specifically detailed in this cognitive model, it seems likely that they play important roles at least in the ease with which appraisals and beliefs (and accompanying emotions and behaviors) can be modified. For example, Savage and colleagues are presently examining whether a certain cognitive process, visuospatial organization, which has been identified as problematic for those with hoarding and OCD problems can be improved with skills training (Savage *et al.*,

2000). Improvement in this cognitive process may lead to improved memory and confidence in memory and to reductions in symptoms. We (Frost & Steketee) are also experimenting with deliberate attempts to modify organization and decision-making in hoarders to determine whether this will improve their ability to discard and store possessions. Do processes like organization, decision-making, and memory influence OCD symptoms or beliefs that mediate these symptoms? More research on this issue is warranted.

Do Certain Types of Beliefs and Appraisals Predict Outcome?

Research in other areas has suggested that certain cognitive domains (i.e., perfectionism) interfere with the treatment process (Blatt, 1995). It is not hard to imagine that strong beliefs about responsibility, importance of thoughts, and the necessity of controlling thoughts would interfere with attempts to get patients to expose themselves to feared situations and therefore interfere with ERP outcomes if unaddressed. This seems an area of fruitful research.

Does Cognitive Therapy Improve OCD Symptoms?

Once we confirm that treatment produces improvement in OCD symptoms, we can begin to determine whether changes in cognition play a role in this process. It is obvious from much foregoing research that ERP methods are highly successful in reducing obsessions and compulsions. Recent research detailed by Bouvard in Chapter 22 of this volume also suggests that CT based on a Beckian model produces good effects for OCD symptoms. In fact, it appears that symptoms improve approximately as much with CT as with ERP, and the overall effectiveness of combined CBT was verified by a reduction of OCD symptoms, and of related pathology, in all of the relevant studies.

Although combined CT and ERP seems clinically most likely to provide the best treatment package, it is not yet clear whether the combination affords any advantage for OCD symptoms over either therapy alone. Studies by Neil Rector and colleagues and by Maureen Whittal and colleagues (and no doubt others) are now underway to examine this question. But, as in the case of combinations of medications and ERP, demonstration of differences will be difficult because the potent effects of ERP tend to obscure any additional benefit conferred by other therapies. It will be of some interest to determine whether CT or CT combined with other methods works best for certain individuals, and this will require further study of large and diverse samples. Questions to be addressed include whether the addition of CT decreases the dropout rate of approximately 25 percent seen in many studies of ERP? Will it work for those who do not improve with ERP? Further, will the addition of CT improve outcome for those with certain types of OCD symptoms (e.g., hoarding or obsessions without overt compulsions) or those with comorbid conditions that may otherwise interfere with gains (e.g., major depression, generalized anxiety disorder)? Will CT be easier to disseminate given the reluctance of many community therapists and patients to engage in exposure?

Do OCD Beliefs and Appraisals Change with Treatment?

As Bouvard suggests in Chapter 22 in this volume, a number of researchers have demonstrated that CBT produces change on measures of beliefs considered relevant and/or specific to OCD. These studies are still preliminary at this point, but nonetheless promising. Several groups of researchers have demonstrated significant reductions in measures of beliefs associated with OCD following CBT. Further, changes in beliefs following CT or CBT have correlated with improvement of OCD symptoms. The majority of reported studies have combined CT with ERP so that it is difficult to differentiate which changes derive from behavior therapy and which from CT. As some researchers and theoreticians have noted, ERP may influence cognition indirectly by providing ideal conditions for the disconfirmation of beliefs associated with obsessive illness. As van Oppen and colleagues note in Chapter 21 in this volume, there is some evidence that successful treatment with ERP is related to significant changes in obsessional beliefs and interpretations, but results are far from conclusive. It is important to note that treatment that is successful in producing symptom improvement may not alter relevant beliefs. For example, elevated perfectionism persisted with successful weight restoration in patients with anorexia nervosa (Bastiani, Rao, Weltzin, & Kaye, 1995).

Further, it is unclear whether changes in obsessional beliefs precede or follow changes in OCD behavior, or whether they are merely epiphenomena of changes in mood state. Thus, causal inferences cannot yet be drawn and it is not yet clear whether changes in cognition for ERP are more limited than those noted with CBT when specific measures of OCD cognitions are used. Much work remains to be done in order to clarify the results obtained by either method alone or in combination.

What are the Best Ways of Assessing Cognition in OCD?

Several researchers have reported on the use of idiographic assessment methods for OCD relevant cognitions. For example, Mark Freeston and Debbie Sookman and their colleagues have developed daily ratings of the intensity of idiosyncratic beliefs that can be tracked across treatment sessions and weeks. Using this method, patients recorded the strength/ intensity of several identified beliefs throughout the day on small cards they carried with them and charted these graphically. This permitted the therapist and patient to determine the immediate effect of specific intervention methods on the problematic beliefs. Other studies have also used idiographic methods to good effect in studying beliefs and interpretations (e.g., Jones & Menzies, 1997; Rhéaume & Ladouceur, 2000).

The internal material of interest to researchers of OCD is represented by both cognitive content and cognitive processes. Self-report and idiographic measures of cognition have typically focused on the cognitive content of interpretations and beliefs. Although cognitive content can also be assessed via laboratory tasks, traditionally such tasks have focused on determining cognitive processes as participants engage in a task designed to identify the type and intensity of cognitive deficits or skills. Of particular interest to researchers of OCD are attentional focus, perception (e.g., of threat, usually using linguistic or visual cues), memory (e.g., verbal, visual), and other information processing tasks (e.g., categorization, decision-making). Recently, Rector and colleagues reported preliminary findings from a study of CT in OCD in which results were assessed by traditional outcome measures and also by a laboratory task (Rector, Richter, Gemar, Denisoff, & Cassin, 2001). Such methods are underused in intervention research and a concerted effort is needed to identify laboratory assessments that are reliable and valid and can be used across treatment centers. Whether cognitive processes may also be linked to cognitive belief and appraisal domains is not yet clear.

Where to From Here?

Overall, we are impressed by the amount of research on cognitive features of OCD that has emerged in recent years, sparked by theoretical models that have strong bases in research findings for other disorders (e.g., depression, panic disorder). There is obviously a great deal more research and thinking to be done in this area. An important field of study will be the development of reliable and valid assessment strategies that move beyond self-report of beliefs. Idiographic and laboratory measures seem promising avenues for measuring beliefs and cognitive processes that are instrumental in maintaining OCD symptoms. Obviously, it will be most useful to the field if these methods can be systematized somewhat so that they are replicable across clinical settings. Another area for future study is certainly cognitive intervention. Several immediate questions come to mind: Can we detect any additional immediate or long-term benefit if CT is added to other effective treatments (ERP, serotonergic medications)? What are the most effective methods for modifying immediate interpretations and long-standing beliefs, and are changes in these cognitive aspects the mediators of symptomatic outcome? Can therapy modify cognitive processes like attention, organization of information and memory and will these improve outcomes?

References

Bastiani, A. M., Rao, R., Weltzin, T., & Kaye, W. H. (1995). Perfectionism in anorexia nervosa. *International Journal of Eating Disorders, 17*, 147–152.

Beck, A. T., Rush, A. J., Shaw, B. F., & Emery, G. (1979). *Cognitive therapy of depression*. New York: Guilford.

Blatt, S. J. (1995). The destructiveness of perfectionism: Implications for the treatment of depression. *American Psychologist, 50*, 1003–1020.

Jones, M. K., & Menzies, R. G. (1997). The cognitive mediation of obsessive–compulsive handwashing. *Behaviour Research and Therapy, 35*, 843–850.

March, J. S., & Mulle, K. (1998). *OCD in children and adolescents: A cognitive–behavioral treatment manual*. New York: Guilford.

Obsessive–Compulsive Cognitions Working Group (1997). Cognitive assessment of obsessive–compulsive disorder. *Behaviour Research and Therapy, 35*, 667–681.

Obsessive–Compulsive Cognitions Working Group. (2001). Development and initial validation of the Obsessive–Beliefs Questionnaire and the Interpretation of Intrusions Inventory. *Behaviour Research and Therapy, 39*, 987–1006.

Obsessive–Compulsive Cognitions Working Group (in preparation). *Reliability and validity of the*

Obsessive–Beliefs Questionnaire and the Interpretation of Intrusions Inventory. Part I.

Rector, N. A., Richter, M. A., Gemar, M., Denisoff, E., & Cassin, S. (2001). *Cognitive and behavioral treatment of obsessive–compulsive disorder: The role of cognitive factors in treatment response and relapse prevention.* Paper presented at the World Congress of Behavioral and Cognitive Therapies, Vancouver, British Columbia.

Rhéaume, J., & Ladouceur, R. (2000). Cognitive and behavioral treatments for checking behaviors: An examination of individual cognitive change. *Clinical Psychology and Psychotherapy, 7,* 118–127.

Savage, C. R., Deckersbach, T., Wilhelm, S., Buhlmann, U., Reid, T., Nelissen, I., Hoffman, E., & Jenike, M. (2000). Cognitive retraining in obsessive–compulsive disorder. Paper presented at the annual meeting of the Association for Advancement of Behavior Therapy, New Orleans, LA.

Appendices

Appendix A

Obsessional–Beliefs Questionnaire (OBQ-87)

This inventory lists different attitudes or beliefs that people sometimes hold. Read each statement carefully and decide how much you agree or disagree with it.

For each of the statements, choose the number matching the answer that *best describes how you think*. Because people are different, there are no right or wrong answers.

To decide whether a given statement is typical of your way of looking at things, simply keep in mind what you are like *most of the time*.

Use the following scale:

1	2	3	4	5	6	7
disagree very much	disagree moderately	disagree a little	neither agree nor disagree	agree a little	agree moderately	agree very much

In making your ratings, try to avoid using the middle point of the scale (4), but rather indicate whether you usually disagree or agree with the statements about your own beliefs and attitudes.

1. Having bad thoughts or urges means I'm likely to act on them.　　　　　1 2 3 4 5 6 7

2. Having control over my thoughts is a sign of good character.　　　　　1 2 3 4 5 6 7

3. If I am uncertain, there is something wrong with me.　　　　　1 2 3 4 5 6 7

4. If I imagine something bad happening, then I am responsible for making sure that it doesn't happen.　　　　　1 2 3 4 5 6 7

5. If I don't control my unwanted thoughts, something bad is bound to happen.　　　　　1 2 3 4 5 6 7

6. I often think things around me are unsafe.　　　　　1 2 3 4 5 6 7

7. When I hear about a tragedy, I can't stop wondering if I am responsible in some way.　　　　　1 2 3 4 5 6 7

1	2	3	4	5	6	7
disagree very much	disagree moderately	disagree a little	neither agree nor disagree	agree a little	agree moderately	agree very much

8. Whenever I lose control of my thoughts, I must struggle to regain control.   1 2 3 4 5 6 7

9. I am much more likely to be punished than others are.   1 2 3 4 5 6 7

10. If I'm not absolutely sure of something, I'm bound to make a mistake.   1 2 3 4 5 6 7

11. There is only one right way to do things.   1 2 3 4 5 6 7

12. I would be a better person if I gained more control over my thoughts.   1 2 3 4 5 6 7

13. Things should be perfect according to my own standards.   1 2 3 4 5 6 7

14. The more distressing my thoughts are, the greater the risk that they will come true.   1 2 3 4 5 6 7

15. I can have no peace of mind as long as I have intrusive thoughts.   1 2 3 4 5 6 7

16. Things that are minor annoyances for most people seem like disasters for me.   1 2 3 4 5 6 7

17. I must know what is going on in my mind at all times so I can control my thoughts.   1 2 3 4 5 6 7

18. The more I think of something horrible, the greater the risk it will come true.   1 2 3 4 5 6 7

19. In order to be a worthwhile person, I must be perfect at everything I do.   1 2 3 4 5 6 7

20. When I see any opportunity to do so, I must act to prevent bad things from happening.   1 2 3 4 5 6 7

21. It is ultimately my responsibility to ensure that everything is in order.   1 2 3 4 5 6 7

22. If I fail at something, I am a failure as a person.   1 2 3 4 5 6 7

23. Even if harm is very unlikely, I should try to prevent it at any cost.   1 2 3 4 5 6 7

24. For me, having bad urges is as bad as actually carrying

1	2	3	4	5	6	7
disagree very much	disagree moderately	disagree a little	neither agree nor disagree	agree a little	agree moderately	agree very much

them out.	1 2 3 4 5 6 7
25. I must think through the consequences of even my smallest actions.	1 2 3 4 5 6 7
26. If an unexpected change occurs in my daily life, something bad will happen.	1 2 3 4 5 6 7
27. If I don't act when I foresee danger, then I am to blame for any consequences.	1 2 3 4 5 6 7
28. If I can't do something perfectly, I shouldn't do it at all.	1 2 3 4 5 6 7
29. I must be ready to regain control of my thinking whenever an intrusive thought or image occurs.	1 2 3 4 5 6 7
30. Bad things are more likely to happen to me than to other people.	1 2 3 4 5 6 7
31. I must work to my full potential at all times.	1 2 3 4 5 6 7
32. It is essential for me to consider all possible outcomes of a situation.	1 2 3 4 5 6 7
33. Even minor mistakes mean a job is not complete.	1 2 3 4 5 6 7
34. If I have aggressive thoughts or impulses about my loved ones, this means I may secretly want to hurt them.	1 2 3 4 5 6 7
35. I must be certain of my decisions.	1 2 3 4 5 6 7
36. If someone does a task better than I do, that means I failed the whole task.	1 2 3 4 5 6 7
37. If I have an intrusive thought while I'm doing something, what I'm doing will be ruined.	1 2 3 4 5 6 7
38. In all kinds of daily situations, failing to prevent harm is just as bad as deliberately causing harm.	1 2 3 4 5 6 7
39. Avoiding serious problems (for example, illness or accidents) requires constant effort on my part.	1 2 3 4 5 6 7
40. Small problems always seem to turn into big ones in my life.	1 2 3 4 5 6 7

1	2	3	4	5	6	7
disagree very much	disagree moderately	disagree a little	neither agree nor disagree	agree a little	agree moderately	agree very much

41. For me, not preventing harm is as bad as causing harm. 1 2 3 4 5 6 7

42. I should be upset if I make a mistake. 1 2 3 4 5 6 7

43. I should make sure others are protected from any negative consequences of my decisions or actions. 1 2 3 4 5 6 7

44. If I exercise enough will-power, I should be able to gain complete control over my mind. 1 2 3 4 5 6 7

45. For me, things are not right if they are not perfect. 1 2 3 4 5 6 7

46. Having nasty thoughts means I am a terrible person. 1 2 3 4 5 6 7

47. I often believe I am responsible for things that other people don't think are my fault. 1 2 3 4 5 6 7

48. If an intrusive thought pops into my mind, it must be important. 1 2 3 4 5 6 7

49. Thinking about a good thing happening can prevent it from happening.1 2 3 4 5 6 7

50. If I do not take extra precautions, I am more likely than others to have or cause a serious disaster. 1 2 3 4 5 6 7

51. If I don't do as well as other people, that means I am an inferior person. 1 2 3 4 5 6 7

52. I believe that the world is a dangerous place. 1 2 3 4 5 6 7

53. In order to feel safe, I have to be as prepared as possible for anything that could go wrong. 1 2 3 4 5 6 7

54. To avoid disasters, I need to control all the thoughts or images that pop into my mind. 1 2 3 4 5 6 7

55. I should not have bizarre or disgusting thoughts. 1 2 3 4 5 6 7

56. For me, making a mistake is as bad as failing completely. 1 2 3 4 5 6 7

57. It is essential for everything to be clear cut, even in minor matters. 1 2 3 4 5 6 7

58. Having a blasphemous thought is as sinful as committing a sacrilegious act. 1 2 3 4 5 6 7

1	2	3	4	5	6	7
disagree very much	disagree moderately	disagree a little	neither agree nor disagree	agree a little	agree moderately	agree very much

59. I should be able to rid my mind of unwanted thoughts.   1 2 3 4 5 6 7

60. I should be 100 percent certain that everything around me is safe.   1 2 3 4 5 6 7

61. I am more likely than other people to accidentally cause harm to myself or to others.   1 2 3 4 5 6 7

62. For me, even slight carelessness is inexcusable when it might affect other people.   1 2 3 4 5 6 7

63. If something unexpected happens, I will not be able to cope with it.   1 2 3 4 5 6 7

64. Having bad thoughts means I am weird or abnormal.   1 2 3 4 5 6 7

65. I must be the best at things that are important to me.   1 2 3 4 5 6 7

66. Having an unwanted sexual thought or image means I really want to do it.   1 2 3 4 5 6 7

67. If my actions could have even a small effect on a potential misfortune, I am responsible for the outcome.   1 2 3 4 5 6 7

68. Even when I am careful, I often think that bad things will happen.   1 2 3 4 5 6 7

69. Having intrusive thoughts means I'm out of control.   1 2 3 4 5 6 7

70. It is terrible to be surprised.   1 2 3 4 5 6 7

71. Even if I think harm is very unlikely, I should still try to prevent it.   1 2 3 4 5 6 7

72. Harmful events will happen unless I am very careful.   1 2 3 4 5 6 7

73. I should go to great lengths to get all the relevant information before I make a decision.   1 2 3 4 5 6 7

74. I must keep working at something until it's done exactly right.   1 2 3 4 5 6 7

75. Being unable to control unwanted thoughts will make me physically ill.   1 2 3 4 5 6 7

76. Having violent thoughts means I will lose control and

1	2	3	4	5	6	7
disagree very much	disagree moderately	disagree a little	neither agree nor disagree	agree a little	agree moderately	agree very much

become violent.   1 2 3 4 5 6 7

77. To me, failing to prevent a disaster is as bad as causing it.   1 2 3 4 5 6 7

78. If I don't do a job perfectly, people won't respect me.   1 2 3 4 5 6 7

79. Even ordinary experiences in my life are full of risk.   1 2 3 4 5 6 7

80. When things go too well for me, something bad will follow. 1 2 3 4 5 6 7

81. If I take sufficient care, I can prevent any harmful accident from occurring.   1 2 3 4 5 6 7

82. When anything goes wrong in my life, it is likely to have terrible effects.   1 2 3 4 5 6 7

83. Having a bad thought is morally no different than doing a bad deed.   1 2 3 4 5 6 7

84. No matter what I do, it won't be good enough.   1 2 3 4 5 6 7

85. I often think that I will be overwhelmed by unforeseen events.   1 2 3 4 5 6 7

86. If I don't control my thoughts, I'll be punished.   1 2 3 4 5 6 7

87. I need the people around me to behave in a predictable way.   1 2 3 4 5 6 7

Score Key

U = Tolerance for Uncertainty
T = Threat Estimation
C = Control of Thoughts
I = Importance of Thoughts
R = Responsibility
P = Perfectionism

Use the following scale:

1	2	3	4	5	6	7
disagree very much	disagree moderately	disagree a little	neither agree nor disagree	agree a little	agree moderately	agree very much

I   1   Having bad thoughts or urges means I'm likely to act on them.   1 2 3 4 5 6 7

C   2.   Having control over my thoughts is a sign of good character.   1 2 3 4 5 6 7

U   3.   If I am uncertain, there is something wrong with me.   1 2 3 4 5 6 7

R   4.   If I imagine something bad happening, then I am responsible for making sure that it doesn't happen.   1 2 3 4 5 6 7

C   5.   If I don't control my unwanted thoughts, something bad is bound to happen.   1 2 3 4 5 6 7

T   6.   I often think things around me are unsafe.   1 2 3 4 5 6 7

R   7.   When I hear about a tragedy, I can't stop wondering if I am responsible in some way.   1 2 3 4 5 6 7

C   8.   Whenever I lose control of my thoughts, I must struggle to regain control.   1 2 3 4 5 6 7

T   9.   I am much more likely to be punished than are others.   1 2 3 4 5 6 7

U   10.   If I'm not absolutely sure of something, I'm bound to make a mistake.   1 2 3 4 5 6 7

P   11.   There is only one right way to do things.   1 2 3 4 5 6 7

1	2	3	4	5	6	7
disagree very much	disagree moderately	disagree a little	neither agree nor disagree	agree a little	agree moderately	agree very much

U = Tolerance for Uncertainty; T = Threat Estimation; C = Control of Thoughts; I = Importance of Thoughts; R = Responsibility; P = Perfectionism.

C 12. I would be a better person if I gained more control over
my thoughts. 1 2 3 4 5 6 7

P 13. Things should be perfect according to my own
standards. 1 2 3 4 5 6 7

I 14. The more distressing my thoughts are, the greater the
risk that they will come true. 1 2 3 4 5 6 7

C 15. I can have no peace of mind as long as I have intrusive
thoughts. 1 2 3 4 5 6 7

T 16. Things that are minor annoyances for most people seem
like disasters for me. 1 2 3 4 5 6 7

C 17. I must know what is going on in my mind at all times so
I can control my thoughts. 1 2 3 4 5 6 7

I 18. The more I think of something horrible, the greater the
risk it will come true. 1 2 3 4 5 6 7

P 19. In order to be a worthwhile person, I must be perfect at
everything I do. 1 2 3 4 5 6 7

R 20. When I see any opportunity to do so, I must act to
prevent bad things from happening. 1 2 3 4 5 6 7

R 21. It is ultimately my responsibility to ensure that
everything is in order. 1 2 3 4 5 6 7

P 22. If I fail at something, I am a failure as a person. 1 2 3 4 5 6 7

R 23. Even if harm is very unlikely, I should try to prevent it
at any cost. 1 2 3 4 5 6 7

I 24. For me, having bad urges is as bad as actually carrying
them out. 1 2 3 4 5 6 7

R 25. I must think through the consequences of even my
smallest actions. 1 2 3 4 5 6 7

1	2	3	4	5	6	7
disagree very much	disagree moderately	disagree a little	neither agree nor disagree	agree a little	agree moderately	agree very much

U = Tolerance for Uncertainty; T = Threat Estimation; C = Control of Thoughts;
I = Importance of Thoughts; R = Responsibility; P = Perfectionism.

U 26. If an unexpected change occurs in my daily life, something bad will happen.   1 2 3 4 5 6 7

R 27. If I don't act when I foresee danger, then I am to blame for any consequences.   1 2 3 4 5 6 7

P 28. If I can't do something perfectly, I shouldn't do it at all.   1 2 3 4 5 6 7

C 29. I must be ready to regain control of my thinking whenever an intrusive thought or image occurs.   1 2 3 4 5 6 7

T 30. Bad things are more likely to happen to me than to other people   1 2 3 4 5 6 7

P 31. I must work to my full potential at all times.   1 2 3 4 5 6 7

U 32. It is essential for me to consider all possible outcomes of a situation.   1 2 3 4 5 6 7

P 33. Even minor mistakes mean a job is not complete.   1 2 3 4 5 6 7

I 34. If I have aggressive thoughts or impulses about my loved ones, this means I may secretly want to hurt them.   1 2 3 4 5 6 7

U 35. I must be certain of my decisions.   1 2 3 4 5 6 7

P 36. If someone does a task better than I do, that means I failed the whole task.   1 2 3 4 5 6 7

C 37. If I have an intrusive thought while I'm doing something, what I'm doing will be ruined.   1 2 3 4 5 6 7

R 38. In all kinds of daily situations, failing to prevent harm is just as bad as deliberately causing harm.   1 2 3 4 5 6 7

T 39. Avoiding serious problems (for example, illness or accidents) requires constant effort on my part.   1 2 3 4 5 6 7

T 40. Small problems always seem to turn into big ones in my life.   1 2 3 4 5 6 7

1	2	3	4	5	6	7
disagree very much	disagree moderately	disagree a little	neither agree nor disagree	agree a little	agree moderately	agree very much

U = Tolerance for Uncertainty; T = Threat Estimation; C = Control of Thoughts; I = Importance of Thoughts; R = Responsibility; P = Perfectionism.

R 41. For me, not preventing harm is as bad as causing harm. 1 2 3 4 5 6 7

P 42. I should be upset if I make a mistake. 1 2 3 4 5 6 7

R 43. I should make sure others are protected from any
negative consequences of my decisions or actions. 1 2 3 4 5 6 7

C 44. If I exercise enough will-power, I should be able to
gain complete control over my mind. 1 2 3 4 5 6 7

P 45. For me, things are not right if they are not perfect. 1 2 3 4 5 6 7

I 46. Having nasty thoughts means I am a terrible person. 1 2 3 4 5 6 7

R 47. I often believe I am responsible for things that other
people don't think are my fault. 1 2 3 4 5 6 7

I 48. If an intrusive thought pops into my mind, it must be
important. 1 2 3 4 5 6 7

I 49. Thinking about a good thing happening can prevent it
from happening. 1 2 3 4 5 6 7

T 50. If I do not take extra precautions, I am more likely than
others to have or cause a serious disaster. 1 2 3 4 5 6 7

P 51. If I don't do as well as other people, that means I am
an inferior person. 1 2 3 4 5 6 7

T 52. I believe that the world is a dangerous place. 1 2 3 4 5 6 7

U 53. In order to feel safe, I have to be as prepared as possible
for anything that could go wrong. 1 2 3 4 5 6 7

C 54. To avoid disasters, I need to control all the thoughts or
images that pop into my mind. 1 2 3 4 5 6 7

I 55. I should not have bizarre or disgusting thoughts. 1 2 3 4 5 6 7

P 56. For me, making a mistake is as bad as failing
completely. 1 2 3 4 5 6 7

1	2	3	4	5	6	7
disagree very much	disagree moderately	disagree a little	neither agree nor disagree	agree a little	agree moderately	agree very much

U = Tolerance for Uncertainty; T = Threat Estimation; C = Control of Thoughts; I = Importance of Thoughts; R = Responsibility; P = Perfectionism.

U 57. It is essential for everything to be clear cut, even in minor matters.   1 2 3 4 5 6 7

I 58. Having a blasphemous thought is as sinful as committing a sacrilegious act.   1 2 3 4 5 6 7

C 59. I should be able to rid my mind of unwanted thoughts. 1 2 3 4 5 6 7

U 60. I should be 100 percent certain that everything around me is safe.   1 2 3 4 5 6 7

T 61. I am more likely than other people to accidentally cause harm to myself or to others.   1 2 3 4 5 6 7

R 62. For me, even slight carelessness is inexcusable when it might affect other people.   1 2 3 4 5 6 7

U 63. If something unexpected happens, I will not be able to cope with it.   1 2 3 4 5 6 7

I 64. Having bad thoughts means I am weird or abnormal.   1 2 3 4 5 6 7

P 65. I must be the best at things that are important to me.   1 2 3 4 5 6 7

I 66. Having an unwanted sexual thought or image means I really want to do it.   1 2 3 4 5 6 7

R 67. If my actions could have even a small effect on a potential misfortune, I am responsible for the outcome. 1 2 3 4 5 6 7

T 68. Even when I am careful, I often think that bad things will happen.   1 2 3 4 5 6 7

C 69. Having intrusive thoughts means I'm out of control.   1 2 3 4 5 6 7

U 70. It is terrible to be surprised.   1 2 3 4 5 6 7

R 71. Even if I think harm is very unlikely, I should still try to prevent it.   1 2 3 4 5 6 7

T 72. Harmful events will happen unless I am very careful.   1 2 3 4 5 6 7

1	2	3	4	5	6	7
disagree very much	disagree moderately	disagree a little	neither agree nor disagree	agree a little	agree moderately	agree very much

U = Tolerance for Uncertainty; T = Threat Estimation; C = Control of Thoughts; I = Importance of Thoughts; R = Responsibility; P = Perfectionism.

U 73. I should go to great lengths to get all the relevant
information before I make a decision.   1 2 3 4 5 6 7

P 74. I must keep working at something until it's done exactly
right.   1 2 3 4 5 6 7

C 75. Being unable to control unwanted thoughts will make
me physically ill.   1 2 3 4 5 6 7

I 76. Having violent thoughts means I will lose control and
become violent.   1 2 3 4 5 6 7

R 77. To me, failing to prevent a disaster is as bad as
causing it.   1 2 3 4 5 6 7

P 78. If I don't do a job perfectly, people won't respect me.   1 2 3 4 5 6 7

T 79. Even ordinary experiences in my life are full of risk.   1 2 3 4 5 6 7

T 80. When things go too well for me, something bad will
follow.   1 2 3 4 5 6 7

R 81. If I take sufficient care, I can prevent any harmful
accident from occurring.   1 2 3 4 5 6 7

T 82. When anything goes wrong in my life, it is likely to
have terrible effects.   1 2 3 4 5 6 7

I 83. Having a bad thought is morally no different than doing
a bad deed.   1 2 3 4 5 6 7

P 84. No matter what I do, it won't be good enough.   1 2 3 4 5 6 7

U 85. I often think that I will be overwhelmed by unforeseen
events.   1 2 3 4 5 6 7

C 86. If I don't control my thoughts, I'll be punished.   1 2 3 4 5 6 7

Appendix B

Interpretation of Intrusions Inventory (III-31)

We are interested in your experiences with unpleasant and unwanted thoughts or images or impulses that pop into your mind unexpectedly. Nearly everyone has such experiences, but people vary in how frequently these occur and how distressing they are. Some examples of the many possible negative intrusions are given below:

X   an impulse to do something shameful or terrible
X   the idea or image of harming someone you don't want to hurt
X   the idea that something terrible will occur because you were not careful enough
X   an unwanted sexual urge or image
X   the thought that you or someone else will become dirty or contaminated by a substance that may cause harm
X   the thought that you left an appliance on that might cause a fire
X   an image of a loved one having an accident
X   the thought that objects are not arranged perfectly
X   a thought or image that is contrary to your religious or moral beliefs
X   an impulse to say something rude or embarassing
X   the thought of running the car off the road or into oncoming traffic
X   the thought that you didn't lock the door and someone may break in

Please note that we are NOT talking about daydreams or pleasant fantasies. Nor are we interested in general worries about health or finances or other family matters. Also, we are NOT talking about the sort of thoughts that accompany depression or low self-confidence. Rather, we ARE interested in thoughts, mental images or impulses that pop into your mind and that you experience as intrusive and inappropriate.

In the spaces below please write down two unwanted mental intrusions that you have experienced:

(1)

(2)

Using the rating scales provided below, please answer the following questions *about these and other similar intrusions*. Please circle the appropriate number for the following questions:

A. When did you last experience an intrusion of this kind?

Within the last year	Within last 6 months	Within last 4 weeks	Within last 2 weeks	Within last week	Within last 24 hours
1	2	3	4	5	6

B. In the last six months, how frequently did you experience an intrusion of this kind?

less than once a month	about once a month	about once a week	a few times per week	about once a day	several times per day
1	2	3	4	5	6

C. On average, how much distress do you usually experience when you have an intrusion of this kind?

none	minimal	a little	moderate	great	extreme
0	1	2	3	4	5

When you were bothered by intrusive thoughts like the ones you described above, rate how much you believed each of the ideas listed below. Circle the number that best represents your belief when an intrusion is occurring.

Use the following scale:

0	10	20	30	40	50	60	70	80	90	100

| I did not believe this idea at all | | | | I was moderately convinced this idea was true | | | | | I was completely convinced this idea was true | |

1. I must regain control of this thought.

0	10	20	30	40	50	60	70	80	90	100

2. Having this unwanted thought means I will act on it.

0	10	20	30	40	50	60	70	80	90	100

3. Because I've thought of bad things that might happen, I must act to prevent them.

0	10	20	30	40	50	60	70	80	90	100

4. Because I have this thought, it must be important.

0	10	20	30	40	50	60	70	80	90	100

5. I should be able to rid my mind of this thought.

0	10	20	30	40	50	60	70	80	90	100

6. Thinking this thought could make it happen.

0	10	20	30	40	50	60	70	80	90	100

| I did not believe this idea at all | | | | I was moderately convinced this idea was true | | | | I was completely convinced this idea was true | | |

7. This intrusive thought could be an omen.

0   10   20   30   40   50   60   70   80   90   100

8. Because I've had this intrusive thought, what I'm doing will be ruined.

0   10   20   30   40   50   60   70   80   90   100

9. If I don't do something about this intrusive thought, it will be my fault if something terrible happens.

0   10   20   30   40   50   60   70   80   90   100

10. I am irresponsible if I don't resist this unwanted thought.

0   10   20   30   40   50   60   70   80   90   100

11. Because this thought comes from my mind, I must want to have it.

0   10   20   30   40   50   60   70   80   90   100

12. It's wrong to ignore this unwanted thought.

0   10   20   30   40   50   60   70   80   90   100

13. Because I can't control this thought, I am a weak person.

0   10   20   30   40   50   60   70   80   90   100

14. I cannot take the risk that this thought will come true.

0   10   20   30   40   50   60   70   80   90   100

15. Now that I've thought of something bad that could go wrong, I have a responsibility to make sure it doesn't happen.

0   10   20   30   40   50   60   70   80   90   100

16. Because I've had this thought, I must want it to happen.

0   10   20   30   40   50   60   70   80   90   100

17. Having this intrusive thought means that I could lose control of my mind.

0   10   20   30   40   50   60   70   80   90   100

18. I would be a better person if I gained more control over this thought.

0   10   20   30   40   50   60   70   80   90   100

19. I need to be certain something awful won't happen as a result of this thought.

0   10   20   30   40   50   60   70   80   90   100

20. This thought could harm people.

0   10   20   30   40   50   60   70   80   90   100

I did not believe this idea at all				I was moderately convinced this idea was true				I was completely convinced this idea was true		

21. Having this intrusive thought means I'm out of control.

| 0 | 10 | 20 | 30 | 40 | 50 | 60 | 70 | 80 | 90 | 100 |

22. Having this thought means I am weird or abnormal.

| 0 | 10 | 20 | 30 | 40 | 50 | 60 | 70 | 80 | 90 | 100 |

23. I would be irresponsible if I ignored this intrusive thought.

| 0 | 10 | 20 | 30 | 40 | 50 | 60 | 70 | 80 | 90 | 100 |

24. Having this intrusive thought means I am a terrible person.

| 0 | 10 | 20 | 30 | 40 | 50 | 60 | 70 | 80 | 90 | 100 |

25. If I don't control this unwanted thought, something bad is bound to happen.

| 0 | 10 | 20 | 30 | 40 | 50 | 60 | 70 | 80 | 90 | 100 |

26. I must have control over this thought.

| 0 | 10 | 20 | 30 | 40 | 50 | 60 | 70 | 80 | 90 | 100 |

27. The more I think about these things, the greater the risk they will come true.

| 0 | 10 | 20 | 30 | 40 | 50 | 60 | 70 | 80 | 90 | 100 |

28. I'll feel guilty unless I do something about this thought.

| 0 | 10 | 20 | 30 | 40 | 50 | 60 | 70 | 80 | 90 | 100 |

29. I should not be thinking this kind of thing.

| 0 | 10 | 20 | 30 | 40 | 50 | 60 | 70 | 80 | 90 | 100 |

30. If I don't control this thought, I'll be punished.

| 0 | 10 | 20 | 30 | 40 | 50 | 60 | 70 | 80 | 90 | 100 |

31. If I ignore this thought, I could be responsible for serious harm.

| 0 | 10 | 20 | 30 | 40 | 50 | 60 | 70 | 80 | 90 | 100 |

Score Key

A. When did you last experience an intrusion of this kind?

Within the last year	Within last 6 months	Within last 4 weeks	Within last 2 weeks	Within last week	Within last 24 hours
1	2	3	4	5	6

B. In the last six months, how frequently did you experience an intrusion of this kind?

less than once a month	about once a month	about once a week	a few times per week	about once a day	several times per day
1	2	3	4	5	6

C. On average, how much distress do you usually experience when you have an intrusion of this kind?

none	minimal	a little	moderate	great	extreme
0	1	2	3	4	5

C = Control, I = Importance of Thoughts, R = Responsibility

0	10	20	30	40	50	60	70	80	90	100

I did not believe this idea at all	I was moderately convinced this idea was true	I was completely convinced this idea was true

C 1. I must regain control of this thought

0	10	20	30	40	50	60	70	80	90	100

I 2. Having this unwanted thought means I will act on it

0	10	20	30	40	50	60	70	80	90	100

R 3. Because I've thought of bad things that might happen, I must act to prevent them

0	10	20	30	40	50	60	70	80	90	100

I 4. Because I have this thought, it must be important

0	10	20	30	40	50	60	70	80	90	100

C 5. I should be able to rid my mind of this thought

0	10	20	30	40	50	60	70	80	90	100

I did not believe this idea at all				I was moderately convinced this idea was true				I was completely convinced this idea was true		

I   6. Thinking this thought could make it happen

0	10	20	30	40	50	60	70	80	90	100

I   7. This intrusive thought could be an omen

0	10	20	30	40	50	60	70	80	90	100

C   8. Because I've had this intrusive thought, what I'm doing will be ruined

0	10	20	30	40	50	60	70	80	90	100

R   9. If I don't do something about this intrusive thought, it will be my fault if something terrible happens

0	10	20	30	40	50	60	70	80	90	100

R   10. I am irresponsible if I don't resist this unwanted thought

0	10	20	30	40	50	60	70	80	90	100

I   11. Because this thought comes from my mind, I must want to have it

0	10	20	30	40	50	60	70	80	90	100

R   12. It's wrong to ignore this unwanted thought

0	10	20	30	40	50	60	70	80	90	100

C   13. Because I can't control this thought, I am a weak person

0	10	20	30	40	50	60	70	80	90	100

R   14. I cannot take the risk that this thought will come true

0	10	20	30	40	50	60	70	80	90	100

R   15. Now that I've thought of something bad that could go wrong, I have a responsibility to make sure it doesn't happen

0	10	20	30	40	50	60	70	80	90	100

I   16. Because I've had this thought, I must want it to happen

0	10	20	30	40	50	60	70	80	90	100

C   17. Having this intrusive thought means that I could lose control of my mind

0	10	20	30	40	50	60	70	80	90	100

C   18. I would be a better person if I gained more control over this thought

0	10	20	30	40	50	60	70	80	90	100

R   19. I need to be certain something awful won't happen as a result of this thought

0	10	20	30	40	50	60	70	80	90	100

I did not believe this idea at all		I was moderately convinced this idea was true		I was completely convinced this idea was true	

I 20. This thought could harm people
0   10   20   30   40   50   60   70   80   90   100

C 21. Having this intrusive thought means I'm out of control
0   10   20   30   40   50   60   70   80   90   100

I 22. Having this thought means I am weird or abnormal
0   10   20   30   40   50   60   70   80   90   100

R 23. I would be irresponsible if I ignored this intrusive thought
0   10   20   30   40   50   60   70   80   90   100

I 24. Having this intrusive thought means I am a terrible person
0   10   20   30   40   50   60   70   80   90   100

C 25. If I don't control this unwanted thought, something bad is bound to happen
0   10   20   30   40   50   60   70   80   90   100

C 26. I must have control over this thought
0   10   20   30   40   50   60   70   80   90   100

I 27. The more I think about these things, the greater the risk they will come true
0   10   20   30   40   50   60   70   80   90   100

Author Index

Subject Index